HEALTHY OPTIONS

&

Vegetarian Guide to Eat -

1997

ESSENTIAL INFORMATION FOR A HEALTHY LIFESTYLE

*Nutrion * Vitamins * Organics * Herbal Remedies*

*Aromatherapy * Whole Body Healing * Gluten Free & Allergy Diets*

*Health & Beauty * Vegetarian Living * Vegan Issues * Organic Wines*

Recipes

Product Analysis

&

VEGETARIAN & VEGAN VENUES TO EAT OR STAY.

PLACES TO VISIT

HEALTH FOOD SHOPS.

" The quintessential good health book "   The Times.

" A must for every health conscious family " The Telegraph.

" Written with integrity by experts " The Daily Express.

AN INVALUABLE GUIDE TO BETTER HEALTH & ENVIRONMENT PROTECTION

£12.50

The Editor wishes to thank the team of writers, also Stephen Terrass, Peter Phillips, Freda Dawydowskjy, Richard Mistlin, Mr.Tophill, Ian Pethers, Angella Dowden and Arthur Ling for their enthusiasm and support, without whom this book would not have been possible.

Thanks are also given to Shirley Hembrow, Sue Dymock, Nikki Miles and Paul Bugge for their invaluable assistance in bringing this book to you. I hope you will have as much enjoyment reading and using the book as we have in preparing it.

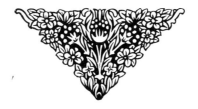

ISBN ..09526555 0 0..

Healthy Options & Vegetarian Guide to Eat - Stay & Visit.

Published by
Kingsley Media Ltd. - Plymouth.

Copyright :- Kingsley Media Ltd.
Copyright (Travel Guide Section) Joy David.

The purpose of Healthy Options is both to educate and entertain. Our objective is to provide accurate and useful information to the consumer. Whilst every care is taken the publisher accepts no responsibility for any errors or misinformation contained in the articles or claims made by advertisers. The information included is not intended as advice for self diagnosis, readers are advised to consult a medical practitioner prior to adopting dietary guidelines or any form of nutritional or medical treatments. The views expressed are those of the authors and not necessarily those of the publisher or advertisers.

Origination and typesetting by Typestyle, Ivybridge, Devon.
Printed and bound in the United Kingdom by BPC Wheatons - Exeter, Devon.

Concept by M.Willcocks. Phd.Dom.Sc.

Edited by JOY DAVID.

CHAPTER CONTENTS

Preface
by Stephen Terrass

𝕎elcome to the *Healthy Options Guide - your guide to discovering the most practical way to a healthy and happy life for you and your family!*

In today's world you have been bestowed with one of the greatest gifts in the history of humankind - the freedom to choose how you live your life. One area where this freedom is especially vital is through the expression of your lifestyle. Lifestyle means more than merely whether or not you choose to smoke or how frequently you exercise. It encompasses a vast range of expressions of your daily life which also includes your personal ethics and your views about nature and the rest of humanity. Lifestyle is not just your way of expressing your daily activities; it is the avenue to ensure enjoyment and happiness. Another area, which is often under-rated, is your right to take control of your own health. Health, of course, is more than just a physical state, it also includes mental and emotional wellness. Lifestyle and health intermingle with one another perhaps more than any other areas of your life. What you choose as your lifestyle expression invariably affects your physical, emotional and mental health. The state of your physical, emotional and mental health dictate the type of lifestyle you are able to maintain. As a result, in order to get the most out of your life - the key would be to create a *healthy lifestyle.*

Creating a healthy lifestyle may be among the most important goals in order to gain personal happiness, but it can only be achieved with knowledge. This is where difficulties can occur, especially as there are so many issues to consider such as:

How do I know what to eat to remain healthy? How can I play a part in reducing the use of damaging pesticides? I am interested in treating myself with herbal medicine, but I don't know where to begin! I want to be a vegetarian/vegan, but can I get everything I need *without meat?..... and how can I make it taste good? I want to help the environment in any way I can. but where do I start? If I eat a good diet would I still benefit from taking vitamins? How can aromatherapy work on the outside to help me on the inside? I want to eat healthily, but I seem to be allergic even to healthy foods! I've always wanted to explore alternative therapies, but which one is best for me? I now know what I want to do for myself, my family and the world, but where can I go for guidance? I have created an environment at home which meets my needs and makes me healthy and happy -.but what can I do when I am away from home?*

As it happens, there are so many sources of information on these issues that it can be quite confusing, and it is not unusual for the information from one source to contradict another. Unfortunately the challenge of accumulating enough knowledge to create a healthy lifestyle is often so daunting that many people give up on the idea altogether. This is a tragic waste and completely unnecessary.

What is needed to remedy this situation is a manual which discusses the most important facets of a healthy lifestyle all in one place. The optimal manual should be in a format that is easy to understand and use, and written from the standpoint of recognised experts in *each field - not one person who takes a 'crash course' in an attempt to do every subject justice.*

The *Healthy Options Guide is just such a manual!*

In this up-to-date guide book to healthy living, the following chapters are presented by recognised experts in each field in a comprehensive and fascinating manner:

Travel Section

As you may have already experienced, creating a healthy and nurturing environment can be very satisfying. As you may also know, at first it can also be a challenge, especially for those with special dietary requirements, such as vegetarians or vegans, and those who wish to take advantage of alternative therapies. Fortunately, the number of opportunities for such people is certainly on the rise, and almost anywhere you go you can find some, or perhaps many healthy options. It is a wonderful feeling when you have discovered an ample selection of health-promoting activities close to home to keep your life enjoyable and rewarding, such as some creative and affordable vegetarian restaurants, a friendly gym or perhaps a great place to get a relaxing massage. But what if you are travelling on business or are away visiting relatives? A person with a healthy lifestyle certainly does not want to have to settle for a lower standard of health when travelling, and yet trying to re-create your optimal environment somewhere new can be very time consuming. The secret is, of course, knowing where to look. Even if you do not have to be away, discovering new and exciting ideas on places to visit which cater to your health-promoting interests can even further enrich your life. Whatever your situation, this chapter takes the guess work and the excessive time investment out of finding healthy options no matter where you happen to be. This section is divided into ten different regions, with each region packed full of choices of where to eat and stay (with a special emphasis on vegetarian and vegan interests), and what to see and do - all with an emphasis on a healthy lifestyle.

Nutrition

The subject of nutrition is, without doubt, one of the most important to understand in order to achieve vibrant health. Here you will learn the role that your diet plays in health, and how best to obtain the optimum benefits from the food you eat. This chapter also discusses the function of vitamins, minerals, protein, carbohydrates and fats as well as other classes of food compounds which have been found to be vital in health maintenance and disease prevention. In the chapter you will learn the best types of food to eat to help provide a rich source of these nutrients from your diet. Here you will experience some of the best reasons why a natural, 'wholefood' meal is one of the keys to vibrant health.

Vegetarian Nutrition

Very useful information is included in this chapter, both for current vegetarians and vegans as well as those who are considering eliminating meat and other animal products from their diet in the future. There are many scientifically supported benefits to vegetarianism and the main areas are clearly explained here. There is a special emphasis on the proven association between vegetarians and a lower risk of the most common and serious diseases afflicting western society today. Also discussed are the special focus areas for both vegetarians and vegans in order to help them achieve adequate levels of essential nutrients within the context of their dietary restrictions.

A Vegetarian Swing to Vegan

The number of people choosing to avoid animal products is clearly on the rise. The majority of these people choose a diet avoiding products of animal slaughter and become vegetarians. Others go a step further and eliminate all products of animal origin and become vegans. The major arguments for becoming vegan are well covered in this chapter - the unfortunate fate of commercial dairy cattle gaining well-deserved focus. Potential health benefits and environmental implications are also looked into. In addition, you will learn how to find your way around ambiguous product labelling to obtain vegan-friendly products. The addition of the interesting results of a vegan questionnaire adds to the usefulness of this chapter.

Revolution is the Solution

Many are familiar with at least some of the negative publicity of how commercial livestock and fowl are treated during their lives. However, it is doubtful that most have come across such a compelling and thorough justification for the banning of such practices as you will find in this chapter. As it happens, the animals and birds are not the only ones to suffer from such practices - the environment is also ravaged due to commercial rearing, which, in turn, harms us all. Always thought-provoking, this section is a must-read for anyone concerned with the future of the planet and all who live on it.

Could it be a Food Allergy?

People are increasingly taking advantage of the benefits afforded by eating a healthier diet, which often involves changes such as eating more whole grains and reducing meat intake. However, there are those who face the problem of not being able to tolerate even some of the most healthy and nutritious foods due to allergies. For instance, many people are allergic to wheat and some are even intolerant to most other cereal grains such as oats, rye and barley. Even more common is the sensitivity to dairy products, which is particularly problematic to vegetarians who rely heavily on dairy foods as a replacement for meat in their diet. Fortunately, even for those with the most wide-ranging allergies to food, there are alternatives available, and this chapter provides very useful guidance and meal-planning tips to help such people enhance their quality of life.

Herbal Remedies

Herbal medicine has been used throughout the world for both health maintenance and the treatment of disease for thousands of years. Unfortunately, in many western countries the advent of the orthodox drug culture has caused an unjustified de-emphasis of the healing power of nature. Over the last decade, the huge volume of medical and scientific research proving the benefits and high level of safety to herbal remedies has led to a renaissance in herbal medicine. Also instrumental in this process of re-discovery has been the increasingly obvious limitations of orthodox drugs, such as the high risk of side effects and toxicity, not to mention the high cost. Here you will find an interesting explanation of the evolution of herbal medicine, which provides strong justification for it once again becoming a primary form of health maintenance, rather than merely the last resort for those who become 'fed up' with orthodox medicine. There is also a useful discussion of some of the more common herbs used medicinally, which makes a handy reference guide for any family. Also, should you choose to seek the advice of a qualified herbalist, this will be made much easier with the information found in this chapter.

Organic Foods

A very compelling argument for the move to an organic diet and lifestyle, not only for the health of you and your family, but also for the environment. This chapter leaves no doubt that the implications of commercial agriculture, as well as commercial rearing of livestock, poultry, etc., represents one of the greatest threats to society and the planet as a whole. Additionally, while many proponents of the 'commercial' approach may encourage the belief that organic approaches are a step backward, the information in this chapter clearly shows that organic living is actually the most desirable way forward in the future.

Organic Wines

Winemaking is clearly an art, and considering what is involved in the process many regard it as a science as well. As winemaking is so heavily influenced by agricultural factors, this has led most large-scale producers to improve the end result through the use of potentially damaging pesticides. In addition, the use of preservatives and other chemical treatments is commonplace. Like all other forms of food production there is strong justification for applying organic principles in winemaking, a subject discussed in depth in this chapter. What drinkers the world over universally care about is taste. The myth that such chemicals are needed to produce high quality wine is effectively put to rest here. Included is a wonderful guide to the best organic wines throughout the world.

Aromatherapy

The interest in aromatherapy is very much on the rise. How aromatherapy works, and the potential benefits of this gentle practice to the body and mind are looked at in depth. You will become aquainted with the use of aromatherapy in your own home to fight the effects of stress or aid in recovery from various health complaints, and you will discover how a qualified aromatherapist can be especially useful to the wellbeing of you and your family. The proper use of aromatherapy is both beneficial and safe, and is well deserving of the positive emphasis it receives in this section.

Beauty and Health for Men and Women

Many of the principles focused on improving your health on the inside also are of great value to your appearance on the outside. The adage "when you look good you feel good, and when you feel good you look good" certainly applies here. This chapter outlines some of the most effective tips to achieve this aim. As you will see, slowing the effect ageing has on the way you look, enhancing the quality and lustre of your hair, correcting different kind of skin problems and many other goals can all become a reality through a natural approach to health and beauty.

It is no secret that there is more to you than just your body, and equally there is more to your state of well-being than merely enhancing your physical state of health. An increasing number of people are choosing to adopt an approach to health and happiness which is holistic, or that which addresses the 'whole person' - body, mind and spirit. As it happens, there are many forms of complementary therapy which aid in achieving holistic health. Some of the most interesting and widely used are discussed here, including, among others, reflexology, massage, Reiki and rebirthing. This chapter outlines the importance of a balanced perspective on healing, and as such, is a brilliant tool to helping you achieve *total health*.

The world has changed so much, with people becoming increasingly aware of the need to take responsibility for their health, and well directed guidance always makes this much easier and rewarding. The fact that the most effective ways to accomplish personal well-being typically benefit the health of the entire planet is particularly satisfying. The *Healthy Options Guide is a guide which can be referred to over and over again, and represents a vital step on the path towards vibrant health and happiness!*

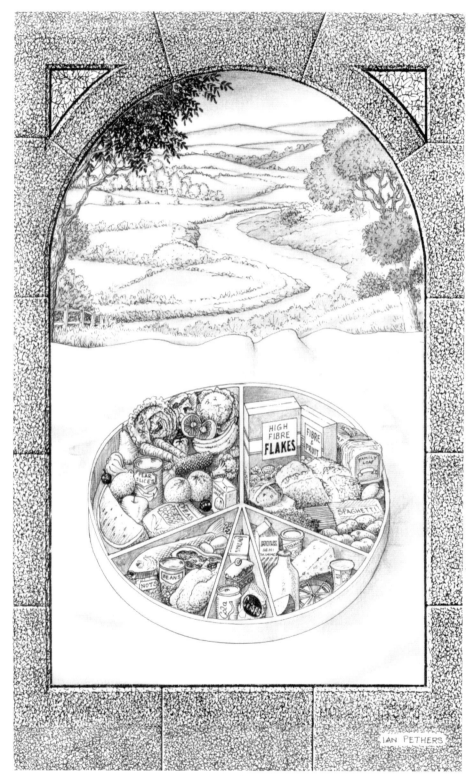

NUTRITION FOR ALL
by Stephen Terrass

utrition refers to the essential relationship of the food you eat to the health of your body. Such a simple definition, but clearly it is the most important issue of human health over which you have control.

Your initiation into the subject of nutrition probably began in childhood when your parents said that you must eat your broccoli because 'it is good for you', or that you couldn't have this piece of chocolate because 'it was bad for you'. Such basic reasoning is appropriate for a young child who will not otherwise understand the more specific reasons why they should eat one way or another. However the problem in western society today is that relatively few adults are much more aware of the reason for addressing proper nutrition than they were taught in their youth.

Considering the noticeable benefits of improving nutritional status and considering that poor nutrition is strongly linked to most diseases, learning how best to nourish yourself deserves to be one of the biggest priorities in life. As nutrition is the relationship between your food and your health, the first step to a new approach toward health is to understand how different types of food impact on your nutritional status and why.

Nutrients in food
A nutrient is a substance found in food which plays a part in the process of nourishing the body. By nourishing, this refers to providing the components your body needs to maintain essential biological functioning, such as energy production; growth, repair and maintenance of organs and tissues; production of blood, hormones, etc.; resistance from disease, and so on - basically everything accounted for in your physical body.

The nutrients in your diet encompass primarily five different categories:

proteins, carbohydrates, fats
protein, carbohydrates and fats are sometimes referred to as macronutrients
vitamins, minerals
vitamins and minerals are classed as micronutrients

These five categories represent essential nutrients. They are referred to as essential because they are needed in order for your life to be sustained, but they cannot be manufactured in your body, either at all, or at least not in adequate quantities; thus they must be supplied through your diet.

Aside from the essential nutrients, foods also contain many other classes of compounds which can beneficially influence your health. They are sometimes referred to as accessory nutrients or anutrients. This category consists of:

Fibre, carotenoids, flavonoids, chlorophyll and many others

The role of essential nutrients
As mentioned, essential nutrients are needed for life to exist. A lack of even one essential nutrient will lead to defects in biological functioning. If the deficiency is persistent and substantial

enough, disease, and possibly even death, will occur as a result. (You will be familiar with the implications of essential nutrient deficiencies through diseases such as scurvy, rickets, beriberi and so on.) The function of essential nutrients in manufacturing every one of the trillions of cells in your body and their role in countless chemical reactions which keep you alive make the expression 'you are what you eat' not so far fetched. Each category and sub-category of essential nutrients has its own list of functions in the process of maintaining human life.

Protein
Proteins are components which the body uses to manufacture hormones, blood, enzymes, genes, muscles, skin, hair and nails, tendons and ligaments, etc. In fact, protein is a constituent of every cell in the body. The fact that they are needed to make the vast quantity of both structural and non-structural compounds is what accounts for the fact that protein is the second most abundant component in your body (after water).

As it happens, the body does not use the proteins as they are found in foods, but rather breaks the food proteins down into their component parts and restructures them into new proteins as required. The component parts of proteins are known as amino acids. There are 20 amino acids found in human tissue, and 8 (and sometimes 10) are considered as essential. As essential amino acids are, in fact, essential nutrients, they must all be supplied through diet in order to sustain life. The eight essential amino acids are; isoleucine, leucine, lysine, methionine, phenylalanine, threonine, tryptophan and valine. (Histidine and arginine are considered to be essential under certain circumstances.)

Natural sources of dietary proteins can be found both in animal and non-animal foods. The richest natural sources of animal proteins include:
      Meat, poultry, fish, eggs, dairy products

The best non-animal sources of proteins are:
      Beans/legumes, grains (e.g. wheat, rye, oats, barley, rice, corn, millet)
      (Vegetables and fruits also contain protein but in comparatively small amounts.)

As your supply of at least eight of the amino acids is dependant on your diet, ensuring that these amino acids are in your food in adequate quantities is clearly a priority. It is a common assumption that if a food has protein, that it will have all the essential amino acids in ample amounts. This is not always the case. Animal proteins do contain all eight essential amino acids, and thus are referred to as 'complete' proteins. However many non-animal protein sources lack one or more of the essential amino acids and thus are incomplete. (Remember that a lack of even one essential nutrient leads to deterioration of health.)

As you might expect, maintaining this balance is especially an issue for those on diets which restrict the intake of animal foods. Vegetarians often consume ample dairy products to supply sufficient complete protein. However for vegans, who consume no animal products whatsoever, achieving ample amounts of the eight essential amino acids is more of a challenge, although not impossible. Most beans/legumes and whole grains, the richest vegetable sources of protein, are lacking in one or two essential amino acids. However, the amino acids which are lacking in a particular legume will typically be supplied in a member of the grain family and vice versa. So the rule of thumb for those subsisting on non-animal diets is to ensure that you diet is rich in both the legume family as well as the grain family. Combining them together assures that you will avoid essential amino acid deficiencies. Soybeans are one of the few vegetable sources which supply complete protein, thus giving you more flexibility with your dietary combining.

In spite of the advantage meat eaters have in getting complete protein, the excessive consumption of meat is clearly associated with some of the most common and severe diseases which afflict western society, such as cancer, heart disease and osteoporosis. Much of this correlation is due to the fact that meat lacks many important nutritional compounds which prevent these diseases in the first place. In addition, certain contents of meat, in and of themselves, increase the risk of such diseases. For instance, the high saturated fat and cholesterol content in meat is particularly linked to heart disease. In addition, meat lacks dietary fibre which is known to lower heart disease risk, in part by reducing the absorption of dietary fat and cholesterol in the intestines. The slow elimination of meat from the intestines allows for potentially cancer causing toxins to be produced.

Fibre and the protective antioxidant nutrients such as vitamins C and E, selenium and carotenoids would provide protection from these concerns, but as mentioned, meat contains no fibre and also lacks antioxidants. On the other hand, vegetable sources of protein such as legumes and whole grains are very rich in fibre and protective nutrients and anutrients, and liberal consumption is associated with a reduced risk of many diseases. It should be noted that certain types of fish such as the cold-water varieties (e.g. mackerel, salmon, herring) are associated with a reduced risk of heart disease due to certain protective fats that they contain.

From a health standpoint, one needn't be obsessive about the avoidance of meat. It is advisable, however, to reduce red meat intake to no more than once or twice per week and substitute with fish (not fried), white meat of poultry and liberal intake of vegetable protein sources. As dairy products also lack fibre and often contain high levels of saturated fat and cholesterol, it is best to moderate their intake and/or consume low-fat varieties whenever possible.

Carbohydrates
Carbohydrates are the dietary sources of sugars, the primary function of which is to provide your body with a source of energy to keep all of your cells running and able to carry out bodily functions. The carbohydrates you eat are broken down into two categories: simple and complex. Simple carbohydrates are sugars which are already in a form which can be readily absorbed and used by the body as an energy source. They include:

> White table sugar (sucrose), brown sugar, glucose, honey, fructose/levulose (fruit sugar) dextrose, lactose (milk sugar), fruits and fruit juices, molasses, corn syrup

Complex carbohydrates, or starches, are composed of many sugars which are molecularly linked together. They cannot be used as a source of energy until the links holding the sugars together are separated. The following are among the best natural sources of complex carbohydrates:

> Whole grains (e.g. whole wheat, brown rice, oats, barley, rye, corn, millet), beans/legumes, potatoes

When sugar is absorbed into your bloodstream it provides a primary energy source to your body. On the surface this elevation in blood sugar levels would seem most appealing, as you would think, 'the more sugar in the blood, the more energy'. This accounts for many people's decision to eat a chocolate bar or some sugary food when they want energy. This approach to diet, while logical on the surface, is actually built on an erroneous assumption and will have the opposite effect in the long term.

Simple vs. complex
Sugar can only carry out its function as an energy nutrient when it has been carried into your body's cells by the action of the hormone insulin. When you eat sugar, the body releases insulin to compensate for the high blood sugar, temporarily raising available energy. Unfortunately, insulin release can be quite excessive and erratic in response to the consumption of concentrated amounts of sugar. As a result, the high insulin release causes the blood sugar to 'crash' soon after, leading to a loss of energy which is experienced both physically and mentally.

This crash from low blood sugar (hypoglycaemia) causes you to crave sugar again to elevate blood sugar levels and the cycle is repeated again and again. This roller-coaster ride of blood sugar can have destructive influences on health and can increase the risk of permanent malfunction of blood sugar control such as chronic hypoglycaemia or even diabetes (high blood sugar).

Since complex carbohydrates are broken down gradually, they are absorbed gradually. As a result they succeed in elevating blood sugar, but in a slow, consistent and most importantly, a controllable manner. This accomplishes the goal of raising energy levels, but without the peaks and crashes associated with concentrated sugars. In addition, complex carbohydrates are not associated with health disorders - as a matter of fact, the consumption of starchy foods such as legumes and whole grains is associated with a decreased risk of many diseases.

'Whole' foods vs. processed foods
While all starches break down slower than simple carbohydrates, there are certain forms of starches that are better than others. Starches in 'whole' foods (foods that have not been processed) are found inter-linked with substances such as fibre, vitamins and minerals. As it happens, fibre further slows the release of the sugars in the food and many of the vitamins and minerals help in the proper utilisation of the carbohydrates.

Food processing methods, especially in the case of grains and flour, often remove the fibre, vitamins and minerals, leaving the starch in a form which is converted to simpler sugars more quickly, and which is metabolised less efficiently. Examples of this are the conversion of whole wheat into white four and the creation of white rice from brown rice.

Beans and other legumes are not generally processed in this manner. Potatoes represent an excellent whole food starch and are surprisingly low in calories (that is, of course, provided that they are not fried or slathered in butter and sour cream). If you eat the skins, potatoes are especially rich in vitamins, minerals and fibre.

Although the sugar found in fruit is in its simple form, eating fruit has many advantages over other simple carbohydrate sources. The high fibre content in fruit slows the release of the contained sugar and slows the emptying of the sugar from the stomach into the intestines. Fruit is also generally very high in carbohydrate-metabolising vitamins and minerals. In addition, fruit has a high natural water content which helps dilute the sugar concentration.

Hidden sugars

It should be noted that sugar (especially sucrose) may be hidden in many prepared foods. Sometimes the sugar will be veiled on a label by the use of technical terminology. For example, many people are unaware that dextrose is a form of sugar. Other times the sugar will be made to seem more 'natural' or healthier, with terms such as 'pure cane sugar' or 'natural sugar'.

Recent research has highlighted many reasons to make a conscious effort to reduce refined and concentrated sugars in your diet. For instance, the excessive intake of concentrated or refined sugar is associated with heart disease, cancer and obesity. One would therefore logically assume that dietary trends would steadily improve in response to these findings. Unfortunately, in the western diet, the opposite is true; while the percentage of dietary calories from carbohydrates has dropped since the turn of the century from about 60% to 45%, the percentage of sweeteners and other refined sugars has risen dramatically in proportion to carbohydrates found in legumes, grains and vegetables (from 30% to over 50% of total carbohydrate intake).

The implications of this trend are, of course, disastrous. The increase in obesity is a case in point. The research shows children to be the most susceptible sugar-related obesity. As it happens, obese children statistically have a very high likelihood of becoming an obese adult. Children of obese adults are statistically more likely to become obese themselves - a truly vicious cycle. On the other hand, if a more balanced approach to intake of carbohydrates occurs in the future, we will undoubtedly see a commensurate drop in such risks. The best way to accomplish this balance would be to revert back to the dietary trends of the turn of the century, with total carbohydrates making up 60-65% total calories, with at least 70% of that being of the complex form.

Fats

As with carbohydrates, fats also function to supply a source of energy for your body, but this is far from their only function. There are many properties of fats which can not be accomplished by any other food component, and since certain substances found in fat are classed as essential, they too must be supplied through your diet.

Fat is not as simple a subject as many think - as a matter of fact, its properties are among the most detailed and fascinating of all the nutrients. As with both proteins and carbohydrates, dietary fats are not used by the body in their 'whole' form, but rather are broken down in the body to other compounds which carry out fat's important functions. These compounds are known as fatty acids. There are two essential fatty acids found in the diet, linoleic acid and linolenic acid. They are used by the body to produce hormone-like substances called prostaglandins. The prostaglandins carry out numerous functions such as regulating blood clotting, inflammatory mechanisms, hormone balance, immune function and so on. Fatty acids are also major components of all of the membranes found in every cell of your body, and are especially prominent in nerve cells.

The best natural sources of dietary fats include:

Vegetable oils (e.g. safflower, sunflower, corn, etc.), dairy products, meats, fish, poultry eggs, nuts and seeds, avocados, olives, soybeans

Dietary fats come in different forms, each having its own implication on health and nutrition. The best sources of the essential fatty acids (linoleic and linolenic) are those that are rich in

WE BELIEVE IN

universal wellness

WHERE ALL LOVES HAVE

liberty

ALL BODIES ARE

nourished

AND ALL MINDS ARE

open

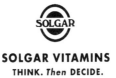

SOLGAR VITAMINS
THINK. *Then* DECIDE.

polyunsaturated fats. These are found in high concentration in the vegetable oils, nuts and seeds and soybeans. Oils such as olive and rapeseed (canola) are rich in the monounsaturated fats. Saturated fats are prominent in animal foods such as meat, dairy products, eggs and poultry, although can also be found in large quantities in tropical nuts (e.g. coconut). Dietary cholesterol is only found in foods containing animal fat such as meat, poultry, eggs and dairy products.

At the beginning of this century the typical fat intake in the western diet was around 30% of total calories. Now it is hovering nearer to 50%! Recent public awareness campaigns regarding the dangers of too much fat have been effective in influencing many to restrict their intake, but unfortunately they have also been effective in misleading many. It is clear that the western diet contains far too much fat, but people are often unaware of the distinction between the different forms of fat. As a result, many people excessively restrict the necessary forms of fat, compromising health due to a deficiency in essential fatty acids.

What is clear is that total fat intake must be reduced to alleviate the alarming rise in cardiovascular disease, obesity and cancer over the last few decades. Many experts recommend that fat comprise no more than 20-30% of total calories. The key is to strike the correct balance between the types of fats - in other words, eating more of the 'good' and less of the 'bad'. As it is primarily the vegetable fats which provide you with the essential polyunsaturated fats, these should make up the vast majority of your total fat intake. Experts also recommend that saturated fats, such as those found in animal foods, be reduced to less than 10% of total calories.

Calories in food
Aside from the amino acids, sugars and fatty acids macronutrients also provide your dietary source of calories. Calories are a unit of measure for energy from foods. The protein, carbohydrates and fats each possess a maximum energy potential.

> protein - provides 4 calories per gram
> carbohydrates - provide 4 calories per gram
> fats - provide 9 calories per gram

Calories in excess of what can be used immediately to meet your body's demand for energy can then be stored for use at a later time. Unfortunately, excess calories normally store as fat. This is why obesity is so often linked with over-eating. The speed in which your body burns calories depends on many factors such as exercise, stress levels, age and your over-all metabolic rate.

The metabolic rate is controlled by what is known as a 'set point', which acts as a sort of thermostat. In other words, when you take in more food than usual, in theory your metabolic rate should speed up in order to compensate for the additional calories.

Conversely, if you reduce your food intake, your metabolic rate should slow down. This appears to be why short term dieting does not generally aid fat loss, and short term overeating does not usually cause a gain in body fat. This adjustment may be more efficient in some people than others, and it is only a temporary compensation. The longer you increase or decrease your typical calorie intake, your set point begins to change its 'setting'. As a result, any consistent decrease or increase in calories will eventually begin to influence body-fat percentage one way or another.

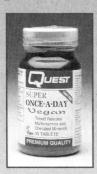
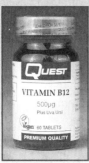 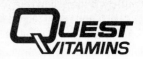

Vitamins

There are currently thirteen vitamins classed as essential to life, which are divided into two sub-classes - fat soluble and water soluble. Each vitamin has its individual roles and many of them work inter-dependently in facilitating hundreds of necessary processes. Many vitamins are used to make enzymes, and/or work along with enzymes to carry out their beneficial effects. Enzymes are the compounds in your body which initiate all chemical processes.

The following represents some of the basic properties of each vitamin and its best natural sources:

Fat soluble:

> * vitamin A
> essential for proper respiratory function, skin health, vision, immune and reproductive function (liver, yellow and green vegetables, yellow fruits, dairy products)

> * vitamin D
> - necessary for calcium absorption and proper skeletal growth and maintenance (fish, eggs, butter)

> * vitamin E
> powerful antioxidant; protects all fats and fatty components in the body from oxidation and is vital to circulation and a healthy cardiovascular system in general (vegetable oils, leafy green vegetables)

> * vitamin K
> - needed for proper blood clotting and bone health (leafy green vegetables, dairy products, liver)

The water-soluble vitamins are:
the B-vitamins

> * B1 (thiamine)
> - releases energy from carbohydrates and helps maintain healthy nerves (brewer's yeast, liver, legumes, whole grains)

> * B2 (riboflavin)
> - releases energy from foods and is essential for growth and development (brewer's yeast, liver, milk, whole grains)

> * B3 (niacin)
> - releases energy from foods and is needed for proper brain and nerve functioning (brewer's yeast, whole grains, meat, fish, milk)

> * B5 (pantothenic acid)
> needed for health of adrenal glands and stress tolerance and is a major factor in energy production (brewer's yeast, legumes, whole grains, liver)

HEALTHCRAFTS - KEEPING YOU IN PEAK CONDITION, WHATEVER THE WEATHER!

Maintaining our good health is essential if we are to live life to the full. Experts agree that it is essential that we take care of our bodies by adopting the right diet and lifestyle yet the modern and hectic world we live in does not always provide us with the nutritional requirements our bodies need. Stress and overworking, exercise and environmental conditions can all reduce our energy levels, and the amount of nutrients in our bloodstreams can also be reduced.

To keep fit and healthy, it is important to maintain levels of nutrients in the bloodstream. They act in conjunction with enzymes to control biochemical reactions within the cells and tissues of the body, and are vital to growth and healthy maintaineance of the body's organs, structure and tissues. In addition, they are essential for metabolic processes and for maintinaing the healthy function of the body's nervous, immune and digestive systems.

Despite occurring naturally in foodstuffs, many vitamins and minerals are destroyed by food processing and cooking methods. Our vitamin and mineral requirements can also change during our lives, so safeguarding optimum health by taking vitamin or mineral supplements is particularly important.

Healthcrafts, the vitamins and minerals experts, recommend taking the following steps to ensure optimum health is maintained, whatever the weather:

* Take regular and gentle exercise
* Stop smoking
* Learn to relax and enjoy life - this will help to reduce stress levels
* Keep to a healthy diet and lifestyle

Many of us will find that we need a vitamin and mineral supplement to help keep our nutritional intake at its peak:

Vitamin A is essential for sound growth and healthy skin, tissue and eyes. Vitamin D is important for maintaining healthy bones and teeth and is necessary for absorption of calcium and vitamin E is an antioxidant which helps to maintain healthy circulation. Healthcrafts High Strength Cod Liver Oil (£2.99 for 30 capsules) provides the EC recommended daily allowance of all three vitamins ensuring sufficient levels are provided. It is also rich in Omega - 3 fatty acids which help to maintain mobility and health of the joints, as well as keeping the heart and circulation healthy, as part of a healthy diet and lifestyle.

You may find that a multivitamin and mineral supplement is most appropriate, to fulfil all your nutritional needs. Healthcrafts Chewable Multivitamins, in a one-a-day formulation, contain 12 key nutrients - Vitamins A, D, E, C, Thiamin, Riboflavin, Niacin, Vitamin B6, Folacin, Vitamin B12, Biotin and Pantothenic acid - each giving 100 per cent EC RDA.

Ginseng helps the body to adapt to changing circumstances and helps to maintain optimal physical and mental performance. Vitamin B complex helps to ensure general good health, while vitamin C helps to maintain the health of every cell and tissue of the body. Meanwhile, Healthcrafts Acidophilus Extra is a unique dietary supplement which provides more than four billion "friendly" bacteria to maintain our digestive systems in peak condition, a fact confirmed by independent research.

The full Healthcrafts vitamins and minerals range is available from leading chemists and healthfood stores nationwide. So, whether you're facing winter frosts or summer sunshine, your health can be in peak condition, the whole year round.

* B6 (pyridoxine)
- essential for energy production, protein metabolism and nervous system health
(brewer's yeast, whole grains, poultry, fish)

* B12 (cobalamin)
- essential for cellular development, nervous system health and red blood cell formation
(liver, eggs, dairy products, fish)

* biotin
- releases energy from foods and is needed to make proteins and fatty acids in the body
(brewer's yeast, nuts, whole grains, eggs)

* folic acid
- needed for red blood cell formation and the metabolism of amino acids and fats
(brewer's yeast, legumes, whole grains, greens, liver, mushrooms)

* vitamin C
needed for collagen production, immune function and red blood cell formation, and is a
powerful free radical scavenger (antioxidant)
(citrus fruits, peppers, tomatoes, potatoes)

Minerals

At present there are over twenty minerals which are known to be of utmost value to human health - and the list keeps growing as more research accumulates. Many of them are officially classed as essential, with others being obviously beneficial but still on the periphery of being considered essential. Minerals, like vitamins, often play a role in the production or activity of the body's chemical catalysts, the enzymes. Additionally they are often found as major components of the actual structure or composition of the skeletal system as well as other tissues.

There are two main classes of essential minerals: macro-minerals and trace minerals. Sometimes they are called major and minor minerals, but these terms can give the wrong impression about the importance of one over the other. In truth, the minor minerals are just as important to health as the major minerals, but the major ones are found in the body in much larger quantities.

The following is a list of minerals, their functions and best food sources:

macro-minerals:

* calcium
essential for building bones and teeth, and needed for proper nerve and muscle function
and blood clotting (dairy products, dark green vegetables, seeds)

* phosphorus
needed for skeletal structure and calcium utilisation, as well as being involved in
metabolism of energy (meat, dairy products, eggs, legumes and whole grains)

Shape up to another busy day

Like many people constantly on the go today, you would like your diet to include all the vitamins and minerals you need. But in practice it's never easy to be sure of your intake, which is why FSC Liquid Gel Multi-Vits can be a good safeguard.

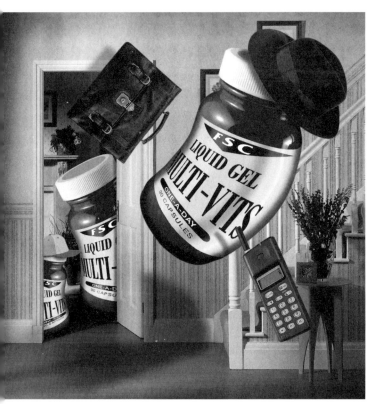

Each capsule contains a comprehensive variety of nutrients including vitamins, minerals and anti-oxidants in a carefully selected formulation which, as part of a healthy diet, helps to ensure that your body is getting everything it needs.

Being in Liquid Gel form they're more easily digestible, without the risk of reflux of the B vitamin content which can bring back an unpleasant aftertaste.

So start each busy day fresh, with FSC Multi-Vits.

A healthier approach to life that you can build on with the full range of FSC vitamin and mineral daily supplements, available from leading health stores.

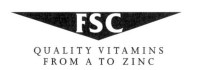

FSC

QUALITY VITAMINS
FROM A TO ZINC

FSC Quality Vitamins, Europa Park, Radcliffe, Manchester M26 1GG. Telephone 01204 707420.
Available from General Nutrition Centres (GNC), Health & Diet Centres and all good health food stores.

* magnesium
needed for skeletal structure and calcium utilisation and distribution; it is also involved
in proper nerve and muscle function, energy utilisation and over-all cardiovascular health
(nuts, legumes, whole grains)

* electrolytes (e.g. potassium, sodium and chloride)
- regulate water balance, and nerve and muscle activity, cardiovascular function, etc.
(potassium - fruits, vegetables, whole grains / sodium - table salt and salty foods / chloride
- table salt)

* sulphur
needed for proper structure and integrity of the hair, skin, nails, joints and other body
tissues and acts as a powerful detoxifier (garlic, legumes, eggs, broccoli, cabbage)

trace minerals:

* boron
aids in calcium utilisation and appears to be needed to activate vitamin D and the hormone
oestrogen (vegetables, legumes, whole grains)

* chromium
needed to make GTF (glucose tolerance factor) which works with insulin to regulate
blood sugar and facilitate carbohydrate metabolism
(brewer's yeast, whole grains, liver, potatoes)

* copper
- a major component of certain protective enzymes and essential for red blood cell
formation (nuts, liver, whole grains)

* iodine
- required for the production of active thyroid hormone
(kelp and other seaweed, iodised salt, seafood)

* iron
essential for haemoglobin production, thereby facilitating transport of oxygen throughout
the body
(brewer's yeast, liver, eggs, meat, beets, blackstrap molasses, dark green vegetables)

* manganese
required for the production of various enzymes involved in protein and energy metabolism
and important for bone integrity (nuts, whole grains)

* molybdenum
- involved in producing various enzymes and is needed for proper growth and development
(legumes, whole grains, brewer's yeast)

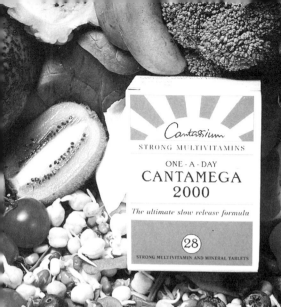

Cantamega 2000

Unbeatabl[e]

After 15 years i[t]
is still the most
comprehensive
and best value
multi-nutrient
supplement on
the market.

Vitamins:	per tablet	%RDA
Vitamin A (7500iu)	1250µg	156.3
Vitamin B1	80mg	5710
Vitamin B2	100mg	6250
Vitamin B6	83.8mg	4190
Vitamin B12	100µg	10000
Biotin	0.1mg	66.7
Folacin (folic acid)	400µg	200
Niacin	100mg	556
Pantothenic Acid	100mg	1667
Vitamin C	300mg	500
Vitamin D (400iu)	10µg	200
Vitamin E (200iu)	136mg	1360
Vitamin K	10µg	-
PABA	50mg	-
Choline Bitartrate	100mg	-
Inositol	100mg	-

Minerals:	per tablet	%RDA
Boron	100µg	-
Calcium	108.4mg	13.5
Chromium	40µg	-
Copper	0.3mg	-
Iodine	232µg	154.7
Iron	3.9mg	28.2
Magnesium	39.5mg	13.2
Manganese	1mg	-
Molybdenum	100µg	-
Potassium	2.3mg	-
Selenium	10µg	-
Silica	1mg	-
Zinc	7.5mg	50

	per tablet
Energy	1.1kJ/0.3kcal
Protein	21.1mg
Fat	6.2mg
Carbohydrate	29.6mg

Herbs	
Alfalfa	10mg
Kelp	10mg
Horsetail Grass	3mg
Golden Seal Root	5mg

Enzymes/Assimilators	
Bromelain	5mg
Papain	5mg
Betaine Hydrochloride	25mg
Glutamic Acid Hydrochloride	25mg
Lecithin	10mg

Bioflavonoid Group	
Citrus Bioflavonoids	50mg
Hesperidin	10mg
Rutin	25mg

Fibre Sources	
Acacia	20mg
Guar Gum	10mg
Apple Pectin	5mg

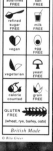

artificial additives FREE · salt FREE · refined sugar FREE · milk FREE · vegan · egg FREE · vegetarian · yeast FREE · calorie counted · grain FREE · GLUTEN FREE (wheat, rye, barley, oats)

British Made
© Rita Greer

Cantamega 2000 provides an exceptiona[l]
range of vitamins, minerals and enzymes
in a timed release, one-a-day tablet. Man[y]
years of research have provided the
experience needed to produce this spec[ial]
state-of-the-art formula, which provides
essential nutrients and their important co[-]
factors in the most easily utilised form,
continuously over 6-8 hours. For those
who find larger tablets hard to swallow, w[e]
also offer the formula in a divided dose o[f]
four small tablets.

The Cantamega 2000 Challenge

*We are so confident that Cantamega 2000 is
unbeatable that we offer a challenge to anyone
who has bought this supplement. Just compare
the formula (as printed on the carton) with that [of]
any other manufacturer. If their product is bette[r]
value than ours, then we will give you your
money back
– and you can keep your Cantamega 2000!*

Cantamega 2000 is available from healt[h]
stores and selected chemists nationwide.

For further information & free nutritional
advice please contact one of our nutritionists [at]
Larkhall Green Farm
225 Putney Bridge Road, London SW15 2PY

Tel: 0181-874 1130

* selenium
component of powerful antioxidant (free radical scavenging) and detoxification enzymes, and works synergistically with vitamin E (whole grains, brazil nuts, garlic, vegetables)

* silicon
needed for proper integrity of connective tissue, such as that found in the skin, blood vessels, etc. and is required for strong bones   (whole grains)

* zinc
component of vast array of enzymes, and is essential for properly functioning immune system, tissue healing; in men zinc is vital for prostate function
(oysters, seeds, nuts, whole grains, legumes)

Fibre
Although strictly speaking dietary fibre is not essential to life, it is one of the most vital components of a healthy diet. Fibre is the primarily indigestible portion of non-animal foods. The richest sources of fibre include:

Vegetable, fruit, beans/legumes, whole grains ('whole' should be emphasised as fibre is eliminated from processed grains such as white flour and white rice), seeds, nuts

There are many different forms of fibre which fall under two main classes; insoluble fibre and soluble fibre. Each type has its own functions and attributes. The main function of fibre, regardless of the type, is to facilitate the elimination of food from your body. This fact is what gives fibre the label of an 'intestinal cleanser'.

Insoluble fibre is particularly prevalent in whole grains (especially wheat bran), fruit and vegetables. Its form and texture do not alter much after you have eaten it, and it is primarily insoluble in water, although it does bind moisture. Some of the health benefits attributed to insoluble fibre are as follows:

* increases the bulk and weight of the stool, thereby aiding in elimination and relieving constipation
* aids in the production of short chain fatty acids which help reduce the number of disease-causing bacteria in the intestinal tract

Rich sources of soluble fibre include fruit (e.g. apple and citrus pectin), legumes (e.g. guar gum), seeds (especially psyllium and flax) and oats. Soluble fibre is especially diverse in its promotion of health. Among its attributes are the following:

* facilitates elimination, thereby relieving constipation
* absorbs moisture, thereby helping to relieve diarrhoea
* absorbs disease-causing toxins in the gut and helps eliminate heavy metals
* reduces the absorption of dietary fat and cholesterol
* stimulates short chain fatty acid production, thus producing a more favourable intestinal bacterial balance
* aids in blood sugar control by delaying release of carbohydrates from the stomach

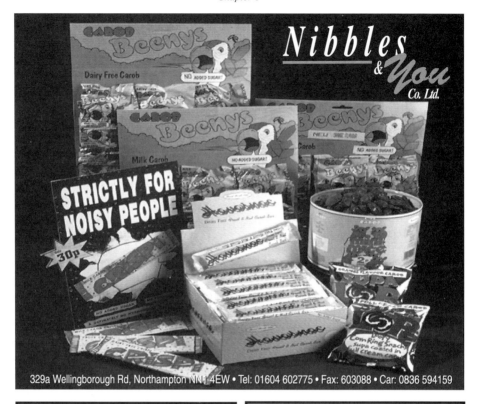

* softens when exposed to moisture, thereby soothing the intestinal wall
* swells in volume when exposed to water, thus aiding in appetite control when taken
with water prior to meals

The benefits of fibre reach far beyond the environment of the gut. After all, much of what is harmful to our entire body is eliminated through the digestive tract and all of what is essential for life is absorbed through it. It is clear that increasing the amount of fibre in the diet is one of the greatest priorities in improving your health.

A major focus of scientific and medical research of late has been in the area of plant pigments, such as carotenoids, flavonoids and chlorophyll. Although plant pigments are not classed as essential to life, this research has uncovered a very impressive track record of various pigments in terms of preventing disease and benefiting health in general.

Carotenoids
The fat-soluble pigments in fruits, vegetables and herbs are carotenoids. There are several hundred which have been discovered to date. Among the most important of these include:
Alpha carotene, beta carotene, gamma carotene, lycopene, lutein, zeaxanthin capsanthin

Although more research is needed to uncover the potential of carotenoids in disease prevention, it is known that those who consume the highest amount of carotenoids typically have a lower risk of diseases such as cancer and cardiovascular disease. Carotenoids are known to be powerful antioxidants and free radical scavengers (free radicals are a causative factor in many diseases such as cancer, cardiovascular disease, arthritis and in the ageing process in general).

Flavonoids
Flavonoids are the water-soluble pigments in fruits, vegetables and herbs. There are several thousand which have been discovered, each of which falls into one of many classes. Among the most heavily studied classes are proanthocyanidins, anthocyanidins and flavonols. Flavonoids have many different health benefits, which vary depending on the type. Among the most common include:

* augmenting the formation of collagen
(collagen is the main protein in connective tissue)
* free radical scavenging/antioxidant activity
* anti-inflammatory effects
* anti-allergic effects

Many of the properties of common flavonoids would have far-reaching benefits in terms of disease prevention, especially due to their free radical scavenging and connective tissue-stabilising attributes.

The different classes of flavonoids account for different colour ranges in the plants they are found in. As a result, it is recommended to eat a diet containing fruits and vegetables which encompasses as wide a variety of colours as possible. Of course, these foods will typically be rich sources of vitamins, minerals and fibre as well.

Chlorophyll

This pigment, which is responsible for the green colour of plants, is familiar to most in terms of the process of photosynthesis. As it happens, chlorophyll also possesses significant health benefits, such as:

> * free radical scavenging/antioxidant effects
> * aiding in wound healing
> * augmenting haemoglobin production

Eating chlorophyll-rich foods is especially useful in that the chlorophyll is found as part of a complex containing other beneficial substances such as the antioxidant beta carotene and vitamin K, which is necessary for proper blood clotting and bone health
.

Water

Although it often gets overlooked, water is one of the most important dietary compounds. It is your most abundant constituent, comprising over 60% of your body. Water is involved one way or another in every bodily process, and is especially needed to carry all essential compounds to your cells and to remove all toxins from them. As a result, every effort must be made to maintain an intake of water which is adequate to meet your needs.

How much is necessary to drink each day varies from person to person and from time to time in the same person. Certain factors such as exercise, sodium and potassium intake, stress levels and so on will cause your needs to fluctuate. Many experts suggest a general recommendation of six to eight glasses per day. Due to their caffeine content, beverages such as tea, coffee or cola drinks act as diuretics (remove water from the body) so it is not recommended to rely on these exclusively for you daily water intake.

There are many other classes of compounds found in foods which are known to be beneficial to health, but the above represent some of the most prominent. In order to ensure the widest range of nutrients and anutrients, it is advisable to eat a wide variety of whole foods, while limiting the intake of animal foods and processed foods. Unless you have exceptional circumstances, there is generally no need to be compulsively restrictive. As a result, any changes you make can be gradually phased in so that you and your family can begin to develop a way of eating which promotes health and vitality, while still allowing you to enjoy your food.

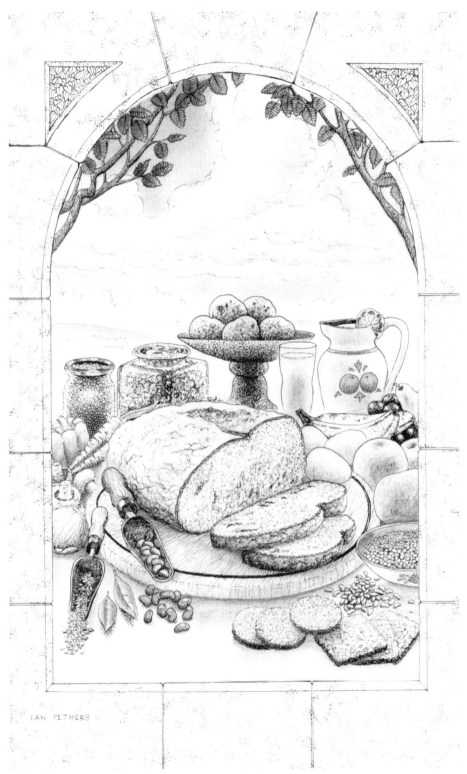

IAN PETHERS

VEGETARIAN NUTRITION
by Angella Dowden

very week, the three million-strong band of British vegetarians is joined by a further two thousand people pledging to give up meat. No longer is vegetarianism the preserve of sandal-wearing hippy types or radical animal liberationists: moderate, down-to-earth people of all ages and walks of life are making an educated decision to embrace the vegetarian way of life. Meanwhile, such a broad change in the dietary landscape has stimulated detailed scientific research into the vegetarian diet, and has forced traditional nutritionists and health professionals to rethink their commonly prejudiced view that meat is a vital part of a healthy diet.

So what exactly is a vegetarian? It may seem like an obvious question, but there are many subtle gradings of "meat avoidance", ranging from the exclusion of red meat only, to the elimination of animal-derived products and ingredients in their entirety. A small minority follow highly restrictive - and potentially dangerous - practices, for example macrobiotic diets, which at the extreme allow for the consumption of brown rice only.

The Vegetarian Society defines a vegetarian as: "one who eats no fish, flesh or fowl and avoids all by-products of slaughter". It is generally accepted that vegetarians consume dairy products and eggs, but the term "lacto-ovo" vegetarian is sometimes used to clarify this. This term also distinguishes vegetarians from vegans; the latter choose to exclude all animal-derived products - including eggs and dairy products - from their diets.

Vegetarianism is nothing new, and diets containing very little or no animal products have been practised by various populations for many centuries - either on cultural grounds, or for reasons of poverty or non-availability of animal foods. Today, in Western society, ethical considerations are a common motivating factor in changing to a vegetarian diet - ranging from an outright objection to the killing of animals, to more subtle concerns about modern animal production and welfare methods. Environmental awareness is another commonly cited reason for becoming vegetarian, with the vegetarian diet recognised as a more efficient provider of energy and nutrients against the backdrop of finite world resources, and world hunger issues. A further major reason for making the switch to vegetarianism is the health benefits perceived to accompany such a lifestyle.

In practice, there are a plethora of personal reasons for an individual becoming a vegetarian. However, large-scale surveys of UK vegetarians indicate that the principal factors provoking the switch to vegetarianism are usually moral or ethical; belief in the health benefits of a vegetarian diet are usually of secondary importance. Whether this emphasis will change now we are living with the reality of BSE remains to be seen.

Food is undoubtedly an intensely emotional subject, and many myths about the vegetarian diet still abound. However, old-fashioned warnings of dire consequences for those who give up meat are completely unfounded, and based on ignorance. The fact is that both vegetarian and meat-containing diets can be healthy or unhealthy; it is the particular balance of foods eaten by the individual that determines nutritional worth.

Nevertheless, vegetarians as a population group generally suffer less from many of the diseases of modern Western society. These include obesity, coronary heart disease, diet-related cancers, gall stones, bowel disease and certain types of diabetes.

Coronary Heart Disease

Coronary heart disease is the biggest cause of death in Britain, but on average, vegetarians display less risk factors for the disease than the population as a whole. For example, vegetarian groups generally have lower levels of LDL cholesterol - the cholesterol fraction associated with clogged arteries and increased risk of heart attack. There is also evidence that vegetarians have lower blood pressure than their meat-eating counterparts.

Some of the classical studies investigating heart disease risk in vegetarians have been carried out amongst religious groups advocating life-long vegetarianism. For example, amongst a group of Seventh-Day Adventists, death rate from coronary heart disease was found to be 40 per cent lower in those who ate meat less than once a week, than in those who ate it every day. However, Seventh-Day Adventists have other lifestyle traits which could also be affecting their risk - for example they avoid alcohol, tobacco and caffeine.

One large UK study which eliminated possible bias from such factors, still found a benefit of the vegetarian diet in heart disease. The study looked at two groups of people with broadly similar lifestyles and attitudes to health; both groups - one vegetarian and the other not - were recruited via health food shops. After five years, the data showed a below average mortality rate from coronary heart disease for both groups; however the vegetarians were at a significantly lower risk than the meat-eaters.

The Oxford Vegetarian Study, published in the British Medical Journal in 1994 also found lower rates of heart disease in vegetarians. In this study, after adjustment for the possible effects of smoking, socioeconomic status and body weight, mortality rate from the disease was 28 per cent lower than in meat-eating subjects.

Not all vegetarian population groups appear to be safeguarded against heart disease however. For example, British Asians, following a Hindu vegetarian diet, actually have a higher incidence of heart disease than the general population, including meat-eaters.

Cancers

It is estimated that at least one third of cancers are diet-related, and several studies have examined the cancer mortality patterns of vegetarians in relation to omnivores.

In the Oxford Vegetarian Study, non-meat eaters had a 39 per cent reduction in risk for all cancers compared with omnivores, after taking into account the effect of other common risk factors for the disease. Other studies have not found such substantial differences between cancer rates in meat-eaters and vegetarians.

One cancer that may be particularly influenced by the vegetarian diet is colon cancer. In a study amongst nearly 90,000 American nurses, the relative risk of colon cancer in those who ate beef, pork or lamb as a main dish every day was two and a half times greater than in those consuming these meats less than once a month.

There is also particular interest in cancer of the breast in relation to vegetarianism. Studies investigating breast cancer differences between vegetarians and non-vegetarians have mostly been inconsistent in their conclusions, indicating that any dietary association is likely to be weak. However, a developing line of research suggests that a diet rich in soya, rather than a more generalised vegetarian diet, could be the key to a lower breast cancer risk in specific population groups, for example the Japanese. Soya beans provide naturally high levels of substances called phyto-oestrogens which to some degree may mimic the action of oestrogen. It is thought that phyto-oestrogens may block the oestrogen receptor sites in tissues such as the breast, thus reducing the risk of tumours which are dependent on hormones for their development.

In men, prostate cancer has been associated with a high meat intake, and vegetarianism may consequently act as a safeguard. More specifically, lycopene, a substance found richly in tomatoes, appears to be the protective agent. In an assessment of the diet of nearly 48,000 male doctors, dentists and other health professionals, Boston researchers found that the risk of prostate cancer was reduced by 45 per cent amongst those who ate at least ten servings of tomatoes a week compared with those who ate none. Men with an intake of four to seven servings of tomatoes weekly had a 20 per cent reduction in risk.

A vegetarian diet also appears to be linked with a lower incidence of lung cancer, although smoking is obviously by far the biggest risk factor for this disease.

Osteoporosis
Osteoporosis (sometimes known as brittle bone disease) is not exclusively a disease of women, but does affect many more women than men, as a result of reducing levels of the hormone oestrogen at the menopause. Because vegetarian women tend to have lower oestrogen levels throughout life (and incidentally a higher rate of menstrual irregularity), it would seem probable that they are more prone to osteoporosis than meat-eaters. However, scientific studies do not bear this out; in fact high animal protein intake is associated with leaching of calcium from the body, and some studies have shown vegetarians to have better bone strength than their meat-eating counterparts.

Other Diseases
Vegetarians are less likely to be overweight than meat-eaters, and this could be one of the reasons that they are lower risk of developing non-insulin dependent diabetes (the type which responds through dietary modification). Vegetarians are also only around half as likely to develop gall stones and, probably as a result of their high fibre intake, have less incidence of bowel disorders such as diverticular disease, irritable bowel syndrome and constipation.

What scientists don't yet know, is exactly which aspects of the vegetarian diet confer its health-giving benefits: is it the exclusion of meat per se which makes people healthier, or is it the inclusion of greater amounts of other dietary components, e.g. vegetables, wholemeal bread, pulses?

It seems increasingly likely that the increased consumption of fruit and vegetables could be a major key. A wealth of research now shows that fruit and vegetables collectively provide a complete cocktail of disease-protective constituents. The most well known of these are the antioxidant vitamins C, E and beta carotene which help neutralise the effects of excess free radicals in the body. Free radicals are unstable molecules which can damage our tissues, play havoc with the genetic material of our cells, and possibly lead to mutations and cancerous changes. They arise as a natural part of metabolism, but also come from environmental sources such as smoking, exposure to the sun and x-rays. Whilst a certain number of free radicals are required for the normal functioning of our immune system, an excess is associated with the development of many diseases, including cancer, heart disease and even arthritis. Antioxidants are our natural defence mechanism to ensure that free radicals don't get out of hand.

Other important components of fruit and vegetables are the flavonoids and the carotenoids. Carotenoids - of which beta carotene is only one - are found most concentrated in richly coloured fruit and vegetables such as peppers, mangoes, apricots and carrots. Flavonoids are found concentrated in the pith of citrus fruits, but apples, onions and tea are also important sources in our diets. Both groups of compounds are also thought to help protect against cancer and other major diseases such as heart disease.

Nutrient Intakes of Vegetarians
In the diets of omnivorous adults, meat and fish provide on average 18 per cent of energy intake, more than 50 per cent of vitamin A intake, and around a third of the intake of protein and certain minerals. When meat and fish products are not consumed, other foods replace them which have slightly different nutritional profiles: these profiles explain the higher or lower intakes of some nutrients in the vegetarian diet.

Energy and Protein
Energy (calorie) intakes are almost always adequate in vegetarians, usually being on a par with or perhaps slightly lower than those of meat eaters. However the protein content of the vegetarian diet has historically been considered its major shortcoming. Animal foods are superior sources of protein, as they provide all the essential amino acids in a balance which closely matches the body's own needs. By comparison, vegetable sources of protein are usually inadequate in one or more amino acids, and a diet based purely on plant protein can theoretically lead to protein deficiency. However, in practice, a balanced vegetarian diet provides proteins from a number of different sources, with the result that they complement each other to provide a perfectly adequate amino acid profile overall. Furthermore, dairy products provide an excellent amino acid profile, so only vegans, or those with particularly restrictive dietary practices need to take particular care to complement proteins. However, as a guide, complementary protein mixes include grains and pulses (e.g. beans on toast), and seeds or nuts with pulses (e.g. chickpea dahl sprinkled with sesame).

Fat
The total intake of fat, and the percentage of energy provided by fat, is about similar in both vegetarians and meat-eaters. In vegetarians, the lack of fat from meat is made up for by an increased consumption of fat from other sources; including dairy products and possibly convenience dishes. Whilst fat intake may not differ significantly between vegetarians and meat-eaters, vegetarians consistently have a higher ratio of polyunsaturates to saturates in their diet. This may help to account for their lower risk of coronary heart disease. Vegetarian diets also provide less cholesterol than the diets of meat-eaters; and vegan diets contain none.

Two polyunsaturated fatty acids must be present in the diet because they cannot be made by the body. These fatty acids are called linoleic acid and alpha linolenic acid: linoleic acid is particularly abundant in the vegetarian diet, whilst alpha linolenic acid is much more scarce. The long-chain fatty acids - EPA and DHA - which are derived from alpha linolenic acid, are particularly important for foetal development, and are also helpful in maintaining cardiovascular health. EPA and DHA are only found preformed in fish, so it is very important for vegetarians to obtain a good intake of alpha linolenic acid to act as the starter material for these derivatives. Good supplies of alpha linolenic acid can be found in linseed, soya bean and rapeseed oils, whilst pulses, walnuts, and green leafy vegetables supply smaller amounts.

Carbohydrate and Fibre
Many studies confirm that there are minimal differences between vegetarians and meat-eaters in respect of their total carbohydrate intake, although strict vegans usually obtain a higher proportion of their energy intake from starches. When it comes to fibre, vegetarians generally have substantially higher intakes than omnivores - often eating amounts in excess of the recommended intake of 18g per day.

Vitamins
Most vitamins can be adequately supplied by a mixed vegetarian diet, but intake of those which only occur naturally in animal foods - such as vitamins D and B12 - may be borderline. Vitamin D, which is needed for maintaining bone strength, can be formed in the skin by the action of sunlight, and is also found in small amounts in dairy products or margarines.

However vegetarians who do not spend much time out of doors, or who have a low intake of dairy products, should ideally take a vitamin D supplement. Alternatively, they can eat foods such as breakfast cereals which are fortified with the nutrient.

Vitamin B12 can usually be obtained in sufficient amounts from dairy products, but vegans almost invariably have low intakes. If dairy products are not a feature in the diet, vitamin B12 - which is needed for healthy red blood cells and a properly functioning nervous system - needs to be taken as a supplement. It may also be obtained from certain fortified foods such as breakfast cereals, yeast extract and soya milk. Seaweed and fermented soya products may not be the useful source of the vitamin once thought, as up to 90 per cent of vitamin B12 measured from these sources may actually be inactive analogues.

Other members of the B complex group may also be consumed at lower levels by vegetarians, as meat is the primary source of these vitamins. However most vegetarians still eat adequate amounts from sources such as dairy products and whole grains. Intakes of folic acid - especially important in women who may become pregnant - are in fact generally higher in vegetarians, as this particular B vitamin predominates in green leafy vegetables.

Vitamin A is another nutrient that only occurs preformed in animal foods, but adequate amounts of the vitamin - important for the skin and immune system - can be synthesised in the body from beta carotene and certain other carotenoids. It is particularly important for vegetarians to maintain a high intake of carotenoids from brightly coloured fruit and vegetables, as in addition to fulfilling the body's vitamin A requirement, they play an important antioxidant role in the body.

Maintaining health and vitality with Premence.

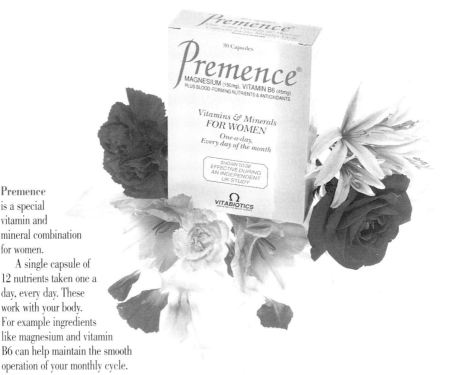

Premence is a special vitamin and mineral combination for women.

A single capsule of 12 nutrients taken one a day, every day. These work with your body. For example ingredients like magnesium and vitamin B6 can help maintain the smooth operation of your monthly cycle.

Blood forming nutrients

Research has shown that many women may not be getting all the iron they need. Premence provides iron, vitamin B12 and folic acid which help the body replace lost blood.

Antioxidants

Premence also gives you the protection of natural vitamin E, and vitamin C you've read so much about.

Reassuringly, Premence was found to be highly effective by an independent UK study. Plus, with Premence there's no need to splash out on another multivitamin as well.

So you really are getting the best of all worlds.

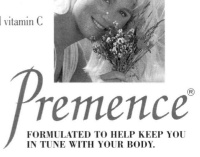

Premence®

FORMULATED TO HELP KEEP YOU IN TUNE WITH YOUR BODY.

Available from health food stores. £4.95 per months supply.
For further information, please contact: VITABIOTICS Ltd., 3 Bashley Road, London NW10 6SU. Tel: 0181 963 0999.

Vitamin C and vitamin E - two other major dietary antioxidants - are generally better supplied in the vegetarian diet than in the diet of omnivores. Both are found predominantly in plant foods, with vitamin E being particularly concentrated in the oils of vegetables, nuts and seeds.

Minerals

Contrary to popular belief, most vegetarians actually consume a higher amount of iron in their diets than meat eaters. However the absorbability of the mineral from vegetable sources is very much poorer than from meat, and in theory at least, vegetarians are at greater risk of developing iron-deficiency anaemia. In practice, vegetarians tend to adapt to their diet by an increased ability to absorb iron, and their higher intake of vitamin C is also useful as this vitamin markedly enhances the uptake of iron from non-meat sources. However, vegetarians should avoid drinking tea with meals, as the tannins in the drink can have an adverse affect on iron absorption from plant sources.

Dietary intakes of bone-strengthening calcium are generally no lower in vegetarians than in omnivores, as both groups include dairy products - which are the richest source of this mineral - as part of their diets. Magnesium is also essential for bone structure, and actually tends to be higher in the diets of vegetarians, as it features richly in green vegetables.

The intake of zinc - another mineral which is important for many aspects of health - can be marginal in vegetarians, and it's availability may be reduced by fibre, phytate and either dietary factors present in plant material. Despite this, in vegetarians eating a varied and balanced diet, zinc levels are generally within normal limits.

A further mineral of theoretical concern for vegetarians is iodine. This mineral plays an important role in regulating the metabolism, and seafood is the only consistently rich source. Vegetarians who regularly drink milk can obtain enough iodine from this source, but vegans need to include fortified foods or seaweeds in their diet in order to ensure an adequate supply.

Sodium (salt) intakes are usually about equal in vegetarians and omnivores. However, potassium levels are generally higher in vegetarians, creating a favourable potassium to sodium ratio which may help explain the lower blood pressure levels often noted in vegetarian subjects.

Groups With Special Dietary Needs

Some population groups have higher needs of certain nutrients, and are more likely than the general population to have a poor nutritional status. In these groups, vegetarian diets may require more careful planning to ensure no deficiencies develop.

Pregnant or Breastfeeding Women

During pregnancy, women have increased calorie requirements, as well as extra needs for vitamins A, B2 (riboflavin), B12 and D. Increased energy needs are relatively easy for vegetarian women to meet through increasing their food intake, and likewise the extra vitamin B2 and B12 requirements may be covered by regularly drinking milk. Similarly, vitamin A needs can be met by eating more carrots or other carotenoid-rich vegetables. However, a supplement of vitamin D may be advisable as it is virtually impossible to achieve the levels of intake required in pregnancy through a vegetarian diet. In addition, all women, including vegetarians, should take a 400

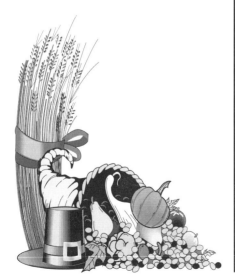

microgramme folic acid from prior to conception until at least the twelfth week of pregnancy. This important vitamin has been shown to reduce the risk of spina bifida in the developing child. During breastfeeding, the requirements for energy plus vitamins A, B2 and B12 increase still further and there are also additional demands for zinc and calcium. Nature does all it can to keep up the nutritive content of breast milk, so the woman's body reserves of nutrients will be plundered if her dietary intake is inadequate. Whilst a carefully chosen vegetarian diet can provide enough nutrition to support a mother whilst she is breastfeeding, many women, whether vegetarian or not, can benefit from the safeguard of a multivitamin and mineral at this time. Most formulations are suitable, but pregnant women are advised not to take tablets or capsules providing more than 800 microgrammes (the Recommended Daily Allowance) of vitamin A per day.

Infants and Children
Studies have shown that vegetarian children given a balanced diet show similar patterns of growth and development to non-vegetarian children. In fact youngsters brought up in a vegetarian household, may often be healthier because they have learned a nutritious eating pattern with less reliance on "junk" food from an early age. The only danger that vegetarianism may hold for children, is amongst those who relinquish meat without any knowledge of how to balance their diet with nutritious alternatives. And extreme practices, such as macrobiotic diets, may have more severe consequences for a child's development.

Recently, the poor iron status of infants below school age has been highlighted. All infants, but especially vegetarian infants, should ideally consume foods fortified with iron (e.g. breakfast cereals and formula milks). A good intake of vitamin C from fruit and fruit juices will also enhance iron status by enhancing its uptake from vegetable sources.
What Should Vegetarians Eat?

As a basic guide, the Vegetarian Society recommends that a healthy vegetarian diet should include the following each day:

> 3 or 4 servings of cereals or grains
> - to provide energy, fibre, B vitamins, calcium and iron.
>
> 2 or 3 servings of pulses, nuts or seeds
> - to provide protein, energy, fibre, calcium, iron and zinc.
>
> 4 or 5 servings of fruit and vegetables, including:
> >   Dark green leafy vegetables - for folic acid, calcium and iron;
> >   Red, orange and yellow vegetables - for beta carotene;
> >   Fresh fruit - for vitamin C;
> >   Dried fruit - for fibre and iron.
>
> 2 servings of dairy or soya products
> - to provide protein, energy, calcium and other minerals; vitamin B12, vitamin D.
>
> A small amount of plant oils, margarine or butter
> - to provide energy, essential fatty acids, vitamin E (plant oil)
> and vitamins A and D (margarine and butter).

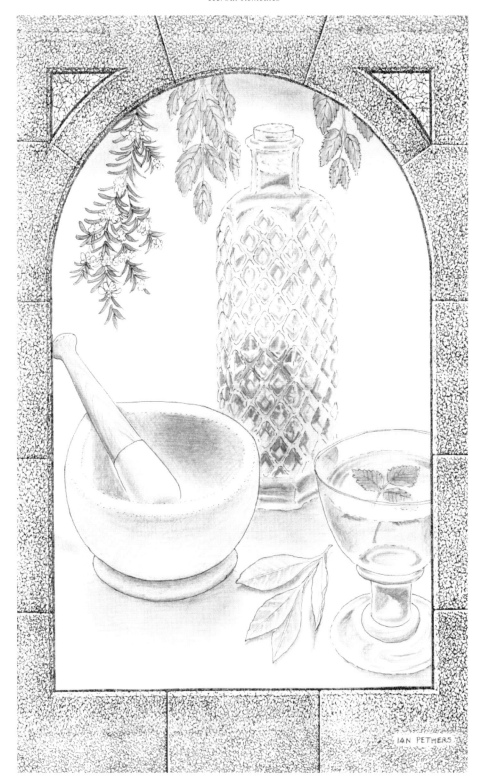

IAN PETHERS

Herbal Remedies
by Penelope Ody

Herbs have been used medicinally for at least 5,000 years that we know of, probably longer. Babylonian records going back to around 3,000BC talk of taking garlic for coughs and colds while the Chinese credit a mythical figure, known as the Divine Husbandman, with discovering such remedies as angelica root Angelica sinensis or known as Dang Gui in Chinese is used for menstrual irregularities.

Both herbs are used in much the same way today and can be found in neat shrink-wrapped packs in high street chemists and health food chains. They have not always been so readily available: while doctors depended on herbs for thousands of years the growth of modern synthetic drugs has wiped many from the pharmacistis shelves in recent decades. Even in the 1930s many of the prescriptions written by GPs were still for herbal products and pharmacists would regularly dispense tinctures of apothecaryis rose for sore throats or ipecacuanha for coughs. Successive Medicines Acts during and after the Second World War severely restricted the use of herbs by both professionals and lay people and it is only in the past few years that popular demand has resulted in the current revival and boom in ready-made herbal products.

It's quite different elsewhere in Europe. In France herbalists (known as phytotherapists) are qualified GPs who have studied herbs at post-graduate level and tend to use aromatic oils both internally and externally while in Germany around two-thirds of all doctor's prescriptions still recommend herbal extracts. There, the most widely used anti-depressant is not a man-made drug like amitriptyline or clomipramine, but the common hedgerow plant St John's wort (Hypericum perforatum), which is now known to have a potent and restorative effect on the nervous symptom. Although the product is licensed as a medicine in Germany, in the UK it can only be sold at present as a food supplement so tends to be described simply as a sunshine herb or one for grey days.

Over the counter

Regulations on what can and cannot be sold as a medicine are understandably tight, but the rules mean that many unlicensed herbal remedies can only be sold over-the-counter as food products in packs which do not give any indication of their therapeutic uses.

This can be confusing for those new to herbs as the names, especially if given in formal botanical versions, are complicated and unfamiliar. Licensed products which have been approved by the Medicines Control Agency as safe and efficacious, can give details of recommended use and dosage but herbal remedies tend only to be awarded licences for minor, self-limiting disorders. So devils claw (Harpagophytum procumbens) which is a strong anti-inflammatory widely used in many parts of the world to treat arthritis, would only be licensed as a remedy for muscular aches and pains or mild rheumatic pain rather than a chronic condition like arthritis. Similarly, the purple cone flower or echinacea (Echinacea angustifolia, E. purpurea, or E. pallida) is a very effective antibacterial, antiviral and antifungal herb that can be useful for treating a very wide range of infections including common colds, influenza and some kidney disorders. It is also sometimes used for skin problems like acne where bacteria can cause some of the familiar pustules and inflammation. As a licensed remedy it is often sold for treating minor skin conditions so if you are looking in the health food shop for something to help your coughs and sneezes, you'd probably miss this valuable herb.

In recent years there has been a great upsurge of interest in over-the-counter herbal remedies and the market which is now reputedly worth around £35-40 million a year. Products on offer range from traditional remedies such as garlic to more recently discovered exotic herbs. Peruvian catis claw (Uncaria tomentosa), for example, was first discovered in the Amazon forests in the 1970s and has recently been identified as having anti-tumour and immune stimulant properties. In trials it has been used to treat AIDS and certain cancers. In many ways it is still a very experimental product and one with which few professional herbalists would claim familiarity, but it can now be found powdered in capsules on numerous herbal suppliers' lists generally offered as a vaguely tonic herb.

Among the more familiar herbs likely to be found on the chemist's shelves are:

Arnica (Arnica montana) - used externally in creams to encourage wound healing and tissue repair. It should only be taken internally in homoeopathc doses (e.g. Arnica 6X)

Bearberry (Arctostaphylos uva-ursi) - a urinary antiseptic often included in over-the counter remedies for cystitis.

Bladderwrack or kelp (Fucus vesiculosis) - nutritious and a good source of iodine used in treating thyroid problems; this herb can be helpful in debility and arthritic problems. Because it tends to stimulate the thyroid and thus increase metabolism it is sometimes promoted as a slimming aid, although long-term use of the plant in this way is inadvisable.

Borage (Borago officinalis) - borage leaves have a stimulating effect on the adrenal glands, but it is the seed oil extract that is most likely to be found in proprietary products today. Like evening primrose (see below), borage seeds are rich in essential fatty acids which may be lacking in those suffering from certain skin and rheumatic disorders. The same acids can be helpful in menstrual irregularities as well . Borage oil is often marketed as starflower oil.

Buchu (Agathosma betulina) - a South African herb which has a pleasant blackcurrant taste and is a diuretic and kidney stimulant used mainly in over-the-counter products for cystitis and water retention problems.

Cascara sagrada (Rhamnus purshianus) - a strong laxative very widely used in constipation remedies. The herb is generally combined with carminatives like fennel seed or ginger to counter the griping pains that such purgatives can produce. It should be avoided in pregnancy.

Chaste tree (Vitex agnus-castus) - chaste tree, also known as monkis pepper, stimulates the production of female sex hormones and is useful for menopausal and menstrual irregularities. Although it acts as an aphrodisiac for women it has the opposite effect on men and was reputedly taken by mediaeval monks to encourage celibacy, hence its name.

Comfrey (Symphytum officinalis) - like arnica this herb encourages tissue repair and is used in creams for bruises and sprains. It contains potentially toxic alkaloids and its internal use is restricted in many countries.

Evening primrose (Oenetheris biennis) - although the leaves of this North American plant were once used for digestive upsets, like borage it is the seed oil that is most highly prized. During the 1970s gamma-linolenic acid (GLA) was found in the oil and this is one of the essential fatty acids vital for much body chemistry, including the production of prostaglandins. it is now an important commercial crop for farmers in many parts of the world and a very wide assortment of products based on the oil is available over-the-counter. Supplements of GLA can be helpful for chronic skin and joint disorders such as psoriasis and rheumatoid arthritis and it can also be beneficial for menopausal and menstrual irregularities.

Feverfew (Tanacetum parthenium) - research in the 1970s identified various chemicals in this herb which can help counter the symptoms of migraine and many sufferers find that simply eating a couple of fresh leaves daily will prevent attacks. The leaves have a very unpleasant bitter taste so many people prefer to take the herb dried in capsules. The active constituent is parthenolide and many OTC products will specify the content of this chemical. Feverfew can cause mouth ulcers so should be avoided by sensitive individuals; it also effects the blood's clotting mechanism so should not be taken by those on blood-thinning drugs such as warfarin. It should be avoided in pregnancy.

Garlic (Allium sativa) - a useful antibacterial and antifungal herb for treating chest infections, colds and 'flu, and also a herb that can help reduce blood cholesterol levels so is popularly used as a heart tonic especially by those at risk of heart attacks.

Ginkgo (Ginkgo biloba) - another recent addition to the herbal repertoire, ginkgo leaves are now known to improve circulation and strengthen blood vessels notably in the brain. This can be especially helpful in the elderly, for stroke victims or for those suffering from ear disorders such as MeniÅreis disease.

Ginseng (Panax ginseng) - used in China as a tonic herb for more than 5,000 years, ginseng products have long been widely available in the West. The herb makes a good general stimulant for the elderly and is useful to take before winter sets in to strengthen the system ready to combat winter chills. A similar herb is Siberian ginseng (Eleutherococcus senticosus) which also improves the body's ability to cope with stress so is ideal to take before exams, long-distance travel or peaks in workload. Both should only be used with caution in pregnancy.

Isphaghula (Plantago psyllium) - also known as flea seeds, isphaghula acts as a bulking laxative. Soak a teaspoonful of seeds in a cup of boiling water and they will swell to form a gelatinous mass which then needs to be swallowed to lubricate the gut. Many people find this mix rather unpleasant so it is not surprising that isphaghula is more commonly processed and flavoured in numerous OTC formats.

Liquorice (Glycyrrhiza glabra) - familiar from confectionery and as a flavouring, liquorice is also anti-inflammatory, antispasmodic, expectorant and will also help heal stomach ulcers. It is soothing for the digestive system and mildly laxative so is generally used in OTC digestive products.

Passion flower (Passiflora incarnata) - a sedative herb, often combined with hops or valerian, which is recommended for nervous tension and insomnia.

Senna (Cassia alexandrina) - like cascara sagrada, senna is a strong purgative with a long history of use in treating constipation. Both plants contain irritant compounds (anthraquinone glycosides) which spur the digestive tract into action. However in long-term use these can weaken the system and should be avoided in pregnancy.

Slippery elm (Ulmus rubra) - a mucilaginous herb which is very soothing for the digestive system and is sold either as powder which needs to be mixed with water to make a paste before swallowing or tablets.

Tea tree (Melaleuca alternifolia) - a highly antiseptic oil used by Aborigines in Australia as a cure-all and now well-established in Europe as a healing remedy for grazes, fungal infections, or head lice.

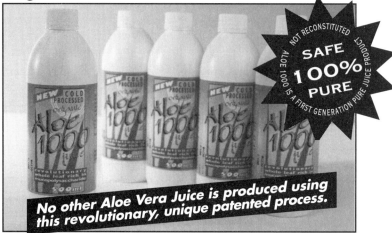
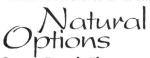

Valerian (Valeriana officinalis) - a natural tranquilliser useful for nervous tension, anxiety and insomnia.

Making your own

Although there is now a good choice of ready-made herbal remedies, growing, gathering and making your own remains a highly satisfying and cost-effective alternative.

The easiest way to take home made products is as infusions using either the dried or fresh plant to make a tea. In general one needs 25 gm (1 oz) of dried herb to 500 ml (1 pt) of boiling water. and the tea should be left to infuse for about 10 minutes before straining and taking in wine glass doses, three times a day. Roots and berries need more cooking so are made into decoctions. This involves heating 25 gm (1 oz) of herb in about 750 ml (1.5 pts) of water and allowing the brew to simmer for about 20 minutes or until the total volume has been reduced by about a third. Because fresh plant material contains so much more water one needs three times as much herb (75 gm to 500 ml for an infusion) to compensate. Teas like this can either be made from a single herb often known as simples or combined in various mixtures. The total amount of herb used should not exceed the standard quantities given above.

Although easy to make, herbal teas can be something of an acquired taste and are often rather bitter. Many people find that adding a squeeze of lemon juice or a teaspoonful of honey will improve the flavour, but if the first sip is off-putting, persevere the flavours do grow on you!

When gathering herbs in the wild it is important to ensure that you have the right plant: comfrey leaves, for example, are easily confused with foxglove, which is toxic while the flowers of valerian are very similar to both cow parsley and hemlock another poison. One also needs to avoid herbs growing close to roads as they are likely to be polluted by traffic fumes, while those on farmland may have been accidentally sprayed with pesticides or other agricultural chemicals. Growing herbs organically at home is safest: many are easy to grow and a single well-established plant can often provide enough leaves for all year round teas.

Useful herbs to keep in the garden and use in infusions include:

Chamomile (Matricaria recutita) - the flowers make a very popular relaxing tea which is good for insomnia and ideal for restless children. it is also helpful for indigestion, nausea and stomach upsets although not everyone likes the taste.

Lavender (Lavandula angustifolia) - the flowers can be used in teas for headaches and nervous tension while an infused oil (see below) can be helpful for muscular aches and pains.

Lemon balm (Melissa officinalis) - a useful carminative and anti-depressant herb and one to encourage relaxation at the end of a stressful day.

Peppermint (Mentha X piperita) - pleasant as an after dinner drink or to combat indigestion.

Rosemary (Rosmarinus officinalis) - a stimulating herb to counter tiredness and fatigue while a compress soaked in the infusion can relieve aching muscles.

Sage (Salvia officinalis) - ideal as a gargle for sore throats or to drink for menopausal problems. Large doses should be avoided in pregnancy.

PROPOLIS

For thousands of years, man has reaped the benefits of bee products for health and cosmetic purposes. With this in mind, API Natural has developed a large range of food supplements and skin care items, as well as our own tasty slimming drink.

API Natural health supplements are produced naturally, full of goodness from the hive. Our customers have reported benefits ranging from helping skin complaints and arthritis, to generally feeling better. Our best-selling product is the amazing Propolis, but also popular are Royal Jelly Capsules, Pollen Granules and Capsules, Propolis Liquid, Honey and Propolis Cream and we have just added Evening Primrose Oil, Cod Liver Oil and Aloe Vera, all in capsule form, to our range.

Cosmetics come gently fragranced with floral essential oils, and are suitable even for sensitive skins. Honey and beeswax are two of the main ingredients used, and these have been renowned for the beneficial properties in cosmetics for centuries. Our bath and skin care range treat hair and skin with the gentleness and respect they deserve, at the same time as cleansing thoroughly. These products are not tested on animals, and are free from lanolin and artificial colourings.

For an information sheet and order form, please write to:-

API Natural

Health Supplements, Bee Products And Natural Cosmetics
FREEPOST NEA 1447, Sheffield S18 6LZ
NO STAMP REQUIRED!

Thyme (Thymus vulgaris) - is a very potent antiseptic and expectorant that is often included in cough remedies to counter chest infections. It can be made into an ideal cough syrup by adding 500 gm of honey to 500 ml of the infusion and the juice of two lemons, and heating to form a thick syrup which can be taken n teaspoon doses up to 6 times a day,

Vervain (Verbena officinalis) - very popular in France, vervain helps to stimulate the liver to improve digestion as well as having a relaxing effect on the nervous system. It should be avoided in pregnancy.

Wood betony (Stachys betonica) - one of the most popular herbs in Anglo-Saxon times, betony is now mainly used to counter headaches, nervous stress and digestive upsets. It also has a tonic effect on the blood circulation and it makes a very pleasant tasting tea. It should be avoided in pregnancy.

Many of our most useful medicinal herbs are the sorts of plants that gardeners tend to dismiss as weeds. Dandelion leaves (Taraxacum officinale), for example, are strongly diuretic and can be helpful where fluid retention is part of the problem while the root can be made into a decoction and used as a stimulant for sluggish digestions and liver tonic. Shepherd's purse (Capsella bursa-pastoris) another invasive perennial weed is very effective at stopping bleeding both externally as a first aid remedy, or taken internally for severest cystitis or menstrual irregularities (but avoid in pregnancy) while goosegrass (Galium aparine), that persistent climber that winds around shrubs, is an excellent cleanser for the lymphatic system and can also be helpful with swollen glands and in glandular fever.

Useful combinations for herbal teas include elderflowers (Sambucus nigra) with equal amounts of peppermint and yarrow (Achillea millefolium avoid in pregnancy) which is an anti-inflammatory, anti-catarrhal and cooling mixture for colds and influenza or one can mix equal amounts of lavender flowers, St John's wort (Hypericum perforatum) and Californian poppies (Eschscholzia californica) for insomnia. Mild cases of high blood pressure can often be helped by teas containing yarrow, hawthorn flowers (Crataegus oxycantha) and lime flowers (Tilia europaea) while raspberry leaf (Rubus idaeus) mixed with St John's wort can ease period pains. Raspberry leaf tea is also helpful in preparing the womb for childbirth and a daily cup can be safely drunk in the last six weeks of pregnancy although is best avoided before then.

While creams and ointments are more complicated to make at home, infused oils are quite simple and can be ideal for external use. Infused flower oils are easily made by filling a large screw-top jar with the blooms and then covering with a good quality sunflower oil and leaving on a sunny windowsill for two or three weeks. The oil absorbs various chemicals from the flowers and will change colour. St John's wort oil is a bright red colour and is ideal for using on minor burns and inflammations, while marigold (Calendula officinalis) oil is deep orange and is useful for cuts and grazes as well as dry eczema.

Leaves need rather more rigorous treatment, they have to be heated in the sunflower oil for about three hours using a double saucepan. Simply cover the dried leaves with sunflower oil and heat over water for at least three hours or until the oil has changed colour.

Useful for infused oils to make at home include:

Rosemary which is useful as a massage for aching joints, stinging nettle (Urtica dioica) which

If you don't see this seal on the outside...

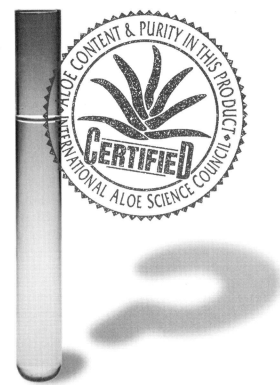

It may not be Aloe Vera on the inside!

ESI introduce Europe's first certified Aloe Vera range. Purity and activity guaranteed.

What does IASC certification mean to you?

The IASC is the International Aloe Science Council, an independent organisation that works to provide information and establish standards for Aloe Vera.

In an industry where the adulteration of Aloe Vera products is increasingly common, now there is independent verification guaranteeing unrivalled quality and purity.

Do I really care if my Aloe Vera is pure?

Yes, you do. The implications of using impure Aloe Vera are staggering. Is the product labelled correctly? How much Aloe Vera does the product really contain? Have all the properties of Aloe Vera been destroyed in production? And therefore, are you getting the results you want?

Aloe Vera from ESI Laboratories is certified—and purity is guaranteed. In turn, our products deliver the maximum benefits of pure Aloe Vera to you.

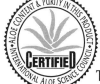

ESI Laboratories
38/39 St Mary Street, Cardiff CF1 2AD
Tel (01222) 388422 Fax (01222) 233010

There are just two kinds of Aloe Vera, certified, and everything else.

can be soothing for irritant skin rashes and psoriasis, and chickweed (Stellaria media) which is also useful for skin rashes and makes an alternative to St John's wort for burns. Chickweed oil can also help to draw stubborn splinters.

Many people prefer taking regular doses of herbal teas to more orthodox drugs but caution is needed in chronic conditions or if you are taking regular medication as occasionally there can be conflicts in therapeutic approach. It is generally simplest for newcomers to herbal medicine to regard these sorts of teas as alternatives to the sort of self-medication one would generally buy from the chemist, simple remedies for self-limiting complaints like common colds, mild stomach upsets, indigestion or minor sprains rather than trying to treat serious or chronic conditions. For these problems it is best to seek professional help from a qualified herbal practitioner.

Consulting a specialist

At one time every village boasted its local 'herb wife' well skilled in the traditions of folk medicine who could be relied upon to treat most ills. These days herbal medicine is a rather more orderly affair. The National Institute of Medical Herbalists was founded in 1864 and its members who use the initials MNIMH or FNIMH after their names can be found in most large towns and cities. Members undergo a four-year training period in medicine, diagnosis and clinical skills, and are well-qualified to treat a wide variety of ailments. A second professional herbal body is the General Council and Register of Consultant Herbalists.

In general NIMH members regard herbs as working with the body to overcome health problems and will generally prescribe in quite large quantities and will offer dietary advice as well. The General Council members usually prefer smaller amounts of herbs and many adopt homoeopathic techniques. Individual approach does, however, vary with some herbalists adding oriental herbs, massage skills or counselling to their repertoire while others may focus on food allergies or use esoteric techniques like iris diagnosis, radionics or kinesiology.

In general the first consultation with a medical herbalist will include a lengthy session taking full details of the case history, a clinical examination or simple tests such as blood pressure or urine analysis. It can last for an hour or more and is usually followed at three to four week intervals by shorter consultations checking on progress.

In the UK herbalists are allowed to dispense their own medicines so after each consultation and review of the therapeutic approach, the patient will be sent home with a collection of herbal potions. These might include dried herbs to be made into teas but are more likely to be herbal tinctures which are alcoholic extracts that simply need diluting with water rather than brewing into an infusion. The herbalist might also prescribe creams, ointments, herbal capsules or pessaries. Many of these will be made by the practitioner and all will be matched to the individual patient's set of symptoms. Western herbalists very rarely use standard formulations to treat patients preferring to see each as an individual with unique health problems rather than simply as a standard disease label.

As well as practitioners following Western herbal traditions, there is growing interest in Eastern use of herbs with Ayurvedic medicine, which originates in India and Traditional Chinese Medicine (TCM). A recently formed organisation is the Register of Chinese Herbal Medicine which reflects

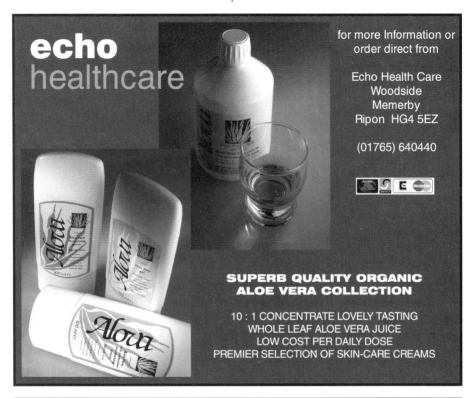
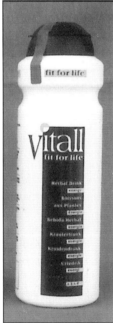

this growing popularity. Oriental herbs have long been used in the West: the 11th century herbalist Hildegard of Bingen, mentions such Eastern exotics as long pepper (Piper longum) - a digestive stimulant, also used for colds and chest problems and galangal (Alpinia galanga) which she recommended for various heart conditions. More recently we have seen herbs like Dang Gui (also labelled as Tang Kwai thanks to an older system of transliterating Chinese names) and reishi mushroom (Ganoderma lucidem) a tonic and immune stimulant fungus joining the ranks of over-the-counter products. Interest has come, too, from orthodox medicine with well publicised clinical trials such as the programme for using Chinese herbs at Great Ormond Street Hospital to treat children suffering from eczema.

Chinese herbalists often use classic combinations of herbs, many dating back thousands of years, in their prescriptions and a number of these standard formulae are available as over-the-counter pills and powders.

Remember ....

However you choose to take your herbs, as simple teas brewed at home or in complex factory-made pills and potions, always remember that they are potent medicines. Never assume that taking twice as much will be twice as good for you or increase recommended dosages without professional advice. Remember, too, that herbs can have side effects or may cause an allergic reaction in sensitive individuals, and that particular caution is needed even with quite commonplace plants in pregnancy and with small children.

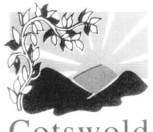
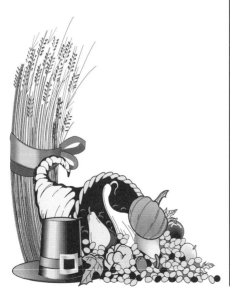

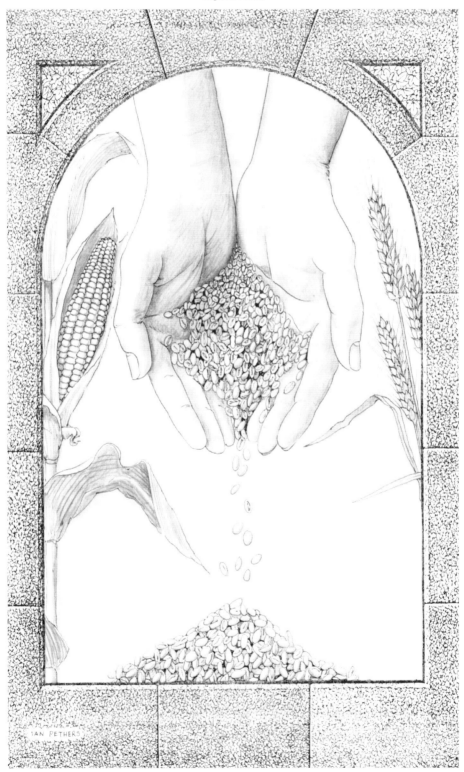

ORGANIC FOODS
by Judy Steele

Organic food from farm to table - better for you and better for the environment Every week there is new evidence that our food is not always safe - animal diseases threaten humans, pesticides are linked to low sperm counts that may threaten our very existence. More and more people are concerned about the conditions that farm animals are forced to live in, and many are turning away from meat as a result. It is not surprising that in this climate of fear consumers are looking for a source of healthy food that they can trust - and organic food, whether it is vegetable or animal, is the answer.

Organic produce is far more than food grown without chemicals - it is pure, safe, responsibly and independently regulated and is good for human health, animal health and the environment. Organic farmers are farming for the future. Their system is designed to be sustainable - to meet the needs of our generation without compromising the ability of future generations to meet their own needs. The idea is not to fight to dominate nature, but to work with it. One organic farmer says he is aiming for a system that will be around for thousands of years.

How can you be sure your organic food is genuine? After all, it would be easy enough for an unscrupulous trader to put up a sign saying "organic produce for sale", and very hard for a consumer to tell the difference.

In fact the organic food chain is very carefully regulated, and anyone falsely claiming food is organic can be prosecuted. Farms and food processing premises are regularly inspected, and operators must keep careful records of everything that comes into and leaves the business. Processed foods should have an easily accessible "audit trail" for every ingredient, so that it can be traced back to its place of origin. There are European regulations covering most aspects of organic production, and if you have any suspicions about the food you are buying you should contact your local trading standards officer.

While conventionally produced food only has to follow general guide-lines on health and safety, every aspect of organic production has been thought out, and the standards are always being re-assessed in the light of new research.

All organic standards in this country are approved by the government's United Kingdom Register of Organic Food Standards (UKROFS). It administers its own standards, and also oversees several bodies which set and police their own standards: the Scottish Organic Producers Association, Organic Farmers and Growers Ltd, the Soil Association, Irish Organic Farmers and Growers and the Biodynamic Agricultural Association. Biodynamic farming is an organic farming system based on the principles of Rudolf Steiner.

The Soil Association certifies 90% of all organic food and farming in the UK, as well as operating overseas. Not surprisingly, its symbol is the one that most consumers recognise as an assurance that food is organic, and all the information contained in this chapter is based on its standards. Other standards may vary somewhat, and if you are concerned about something it would pay to contact the relevant body for more information.

A healthy, fertile soil is the key to the success of any organic farm, and it is carefully managed as a precious resource. We tend to take soil for granted, but a good soil is full of beneficial microbes - one teaspoonful can contain millions of bacteria and more than a kilometre of vital fungal material. The standards followed by organic farmers oblige them to keep soils healthy, with high levels of humus, earthworms, plant foods and microbes.

Crops are not grown in the same place in successive years - they are carefully rotated. This practice is a major weapon in the fight against pests and diseases. It helps to stop them building up. Different crops take different nutrients out of the soil, too, so moving them around makes the most of the plant food that is available.

Compost and manure are the obvious tools used for building fertility. Green manures - short-lived crops like rye or clover - are used to cover bare soil and prevent nutrient loss caused by rain. They are dug straight into the soil to provide instant food. Where arable crops like wheat are grown, a farmer will grow a mixture of grass and clover for several years beforehand. When this "ley" is ploughed up, the soil will have built up its fertility naturally. Many conventional farmers may grow three or four crops of cereals in a row, relying on chemical fertiliser to feed what is often a very lifeless soil. Soil erosion is carefully guarded against in organic systems. Soil is kept covered whenever possible with crops or vegetation. Care has to be taken when soil is cultivated, or the structure may be damaged. Organic farmers don't use tram-lines - regular tracks used for tractor sprayers on conventional farms. These can become very compacted, and act like a mini-stream in heavy rain allowing soil to wash down them.

Herbicides and pesticides are not allowed. We know that they can be present in the innocent-looking carrot and lettuce, and it is impossible to tell what effect a life-time's exposure to the cocktail of chemicals in our food will have. The recent evidence of the ability of certain commonly used chemicals to disrupt hormones in both humans and animals adds weight to the argument against their use. Chemicals can creep in in places the consumer might not suspect, and the regulations deal with this - most chemical seed dressings are not permitted, nor are chemical soil sterilants. Organophosphorus and other chemicals are often used when conventional cereals and potatoes are stored, or may coat citrus fruits. They are also prohibited.

Biological control - using natural predators to kill pests - is used when necessary. A minute wasp called Encarsia is introduce to control whitefly in greenhouses, for example. This was first used in the 1920s, but after the war DDT became the wonder chemical, and encarsia was forgotten for years. Organic farmers aim to build up natural predators on their land anyway. Because they don't spray pesticides into the bottoms of hedges, the plants there encourage insects that attack pests. A few nettles around a farm are not regarded as a sign of slack weeding - they can support predators too, as can other "weeds".

There are a few products that an organic farmer can use against pests, but prevention by good management is always preferred. Soft soap can be used against aphid, a sulphur compound against fungus diseases and a copper compound against blight. Natural insecticides like derris and pyrethrum are allowed, but not encouraged.

Because manure is an important fertiliser, many organic farms are mixed - they keep animals and grow arable crops as well. This means that they don't have to buy manure, a practice which is also restricted. There is usually more grassland on their farms, so the soil is not over-exploited. One or two farmers are starting to compost green and vegetable waste brought from nearby towns by their local councils, and are returning urban waste back to the land.

One charge levelled by the sceptical is that organic farming is a step back to our grandfather's day. This is far from the truth. Although it does not command the research budget devoted to agrochemicals and fertilisers, organic farmers make the most of modern research techniques, and are accumulating a wealth of knowledge based on modern information and machinery. But they always adopt the attitude that any technology has to be proved safe before it is used. DDT seemed like a wonder chemical, but it devastated wildlife. Now there are problems with organophosphorus sheep dips, found to harm the people that use them by damaging their nervous systems. In the light of experiences like these, genetically engineered crops and products have been banned from organic food for the time being.

Animal welfare is important to organic farmers, and is incorporated into their regulations. Animals must be kept in a way which meets their physiological, behavioural and health needs, say the Soil Association standards. All animals must have access to natural daylight, and although they may be allowed to be kept indoors in the winter, they can't be kept permanently indoors. Battery cages and farrowing crates are not allowed. Nor is the routine debeaking of poultry, or the clipping of piglets' teeth and trimming of tails. These practices are often necessary in intensive farming: animals kept in crowded conditions, where they can't follow their natural behaviour patterns, get bored and disturbed, and will start to hurt themselves and others. Chickens will peck out their own feathers or those of their neighbours, pigs will bite at each others' tails.
Every aspect of the animal's welfare has been considered by the Soil Association standards, including transport. Electric goads are not used, vehicles must not be overcrowded, and animals are only allowed to travel for eight hours before they are rested and watered. And organic animals cannot be exported for slaughter.

In the early 1980's the Soil Association banned animal protein from food intended for ruminants - the accepted source of the BSE outbreak. No animal born and reared on an organic farm has ever contracted BSE, so no animal eligible for sale as organic beef could have been contaminated. But although meat and bonemeal was removed early from the diet of organic cows, this does not mean that there is no BSE at all on organic farms. Livestock sometimes has to be bought in, and conventional herds are sometimes converted to become organic, and the disease may come in with them. But wherever it occurs, that animal and its sons and daughters are removed from the herd immediately. Farmers are usually very willing to talk to consumers about these matters, and the Soil Association can give advice.

Some uninformed people assume that because the routine use of drugs like growth promoters, hormones and antibiotics is not allowed, sick organic animals are not treated. This is not true. A sick animal will not be allowed to suffer, and will always be treated by a vet if need be. It will be isolated from the rest of the herd, and its organic status may be affected. Organic farmers need to be very good stockmen - they must spot a problem early, because they want to avoid emergency treatment or the spread of a disease. They often use homoeopathic and herbal remedies as both preventatives and treatments. Homoeopathic remedies have been found to be very effective, especially against intractable problems like skin diseases. Some specific conventional medicines cam be used for cases of anaemia or magnesium deficiency, and wormers are allowed if there is

WESTMILL FOODS LTD

Customer Services,
Vanwall Road,
Maidenhead,
Berks SL6 4UF

Tel: 01279 658473
Fax: 01279 657723/657952

Dr Tom Allinson established his first mill in 1895 and, even today, Allinson wholemeal flours are still stoneground in the traditional way so that none of the wheat grain is lost during milling. This gives the flour a unique texture and flavour. All made from the finest wheats, the full range of Allinson Wholemeal and Bread Flours consists of:

Allinson 100% Wholemeal Plain Flour
Allinson 100% Wholemeal Self-Raising Flour
Allinson Strong White Bread Flour
Allinson Softgrain Strong White Bread Flour
Allinson Strong 100% Wholemeal Bread Flour
Allinson Organic 100% Wholemeal Flour - this carries the Soil Association Symbol of Organic Quality and is produced from wheat grown totally naturally, without the use of artificial fertilisers or chemical sprays.
Allinson Harvester Strong Brown Bread Flour - this has added malted wheatflakes which give a delicious, nutty flavour to your baking.

Each bag has the attraction of an original recipe and a handy table detailing the uses of each kind of flour. If you need more information, then call the **Allinson Baking Club Hotline** on **0990 200 623** where you can obtain expert hints, tips and recipe ideas. There is also a chance to enter the monthly free prize draw; or else call the Hotline, leave your name and address and receive the latest **Allinson Baking Club Recipe Cards** absolutely free. New cards are issued each month, enabling you to build up a comprehensive collection of delicious and exciting recipes for your family.

Allinson Yeast is a vital addition to any baker's cupboard. Traditional **Dried Active Yeast** is a long-standing favourite, while with **Allinson Easybake Yeast** great bread-making becomes even easier; there is no need to reconstitute it as you simply stir the yeast into the dry flour and it requires only one kneading and proving, saving you time and energy.

Last , but by no means least, are **Allinson Wheat Germ, Broad Bran** and **Bran Plus** (a unique blend of bran and wheat germ). These can be used in all sorts of nourishing recipes from bread to thick sauces and soups.

The complete range of Allinson's products is widely available in all major supermarkets and good health food shops. It is comforting to know that when you use the wholesome, unbleached goodness of the Allinson range you are giving your family and yourself the very best in healthy eating.

a specific problem, but their use must be recorded. Organic farmers don't dip their sheep unless they are required to by law when there is an outbreak of sheep scab, but use alternative methods.

Conservation is so important that again it is incorporated into the standards farmers are expected to meet. They must consider enhancing the landscape and the habitat for wild plants and animals. The ministry of agriculture has acknowledged the environmental value of organic farming in a very positive report based on research it has commissioned.

The British Trust for Ornithology has discovered that there are more birds on organic farms. Skylarks, for example, under most threat at the moment with 58% of the population lost between 1969 and 1994, may do better on organic farms. The way the land is managed, especially the lack of pesticides, means there is more insect and plant food, and more nest sites for birds. Another survey found more butterflies on organic farms. It is not possible to say whether there are more mammals and amphibians, but it seems likely.

One of the main reasons why wildlife is more abundant on organic farms is the way that hedgerows and trees are looked after. Hedges are wildlife corridors and larders. Hedges must be trimmed between January and March, when birds are not nesting. Ditches are cleared in rotation, so some uncleared ditches, valuable for wildlife, are left undisturbed each year. Wetlands must not be drained where they have conservation value.

Woodlands, too, should be managed in the traditional way. They are allowed to regrow naturally, or they may be coppiced - that is they are cut down once every eight to twelve years. This practice is valuable for wildlife, with the different phases encouraging different types of wildflowers. If woodlands are replanted, native trees and shrubs should be used. There are even guide-lines about buildings, aimed at protecting traditional buildings, and conserving bats and barn owls which use farm buildings as a roosting place.

But as well as conserving what is already on the farm, Soil Association farmers are encouraged to start new conservation projects. It is also recommended that they maintain rights of way.

Farming can cause water pollution - whether it is effluent from manure or silage killing fish or nitrates from fertilisers in drinking water. Although every farm is different, a well managed organic farm produces less pollution than a conventional one. Manure is regarded as a resource, rather than the problem it is on some conventional farms, and it is carefully spread at times when nitrate leaching is least likely to occur. A greater proportion of organic livestock is bedded on straw, so there is less of the liquid slurry that is so devastating to fish if it leaks into a stream. Heavy metals are often used as growth promoters in conventional systems, and can cause pollution, but they are not allowed on organic farms. There is also less risk of phosphate pollution.

How about your fruits and vegetables? They are grown along the guide-lines we have already looked at. Demand for them is so strong that quite a lot of fresh organic produce has to be brought in from abroad. Britain does not seem to put a lot of effort in to growing even conventional vegetables, and they don't attract any subsidies. Efforts are being made to get more people to grow vegetables organically, but not much progress has been made yet.

At one time, most produce was sent to wholesale markets or supermarkets. That made organic

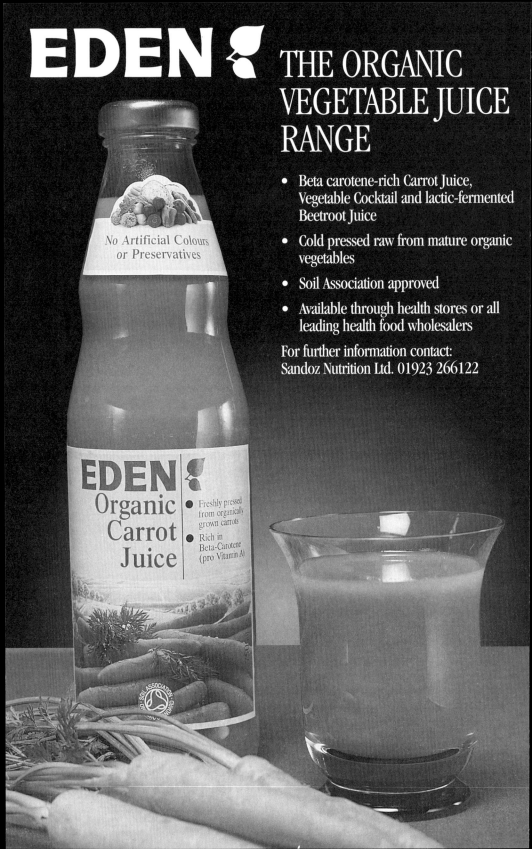

EDEN JUICES FOR HEALTH

Germany's leading range of fresh vegetable juices is now available in the UK. Eden Organic Vegetable Juices are produced using an organic gardening method developed by a group of vegetarian German farmers who started the company in the 1890s.

There are three pure juices to choose from, each free from artificial colours and preservatives and rich in nutrients – Eden Organic Carrot Juice, Vegetable Cocktail and Beetroot Juice.

Eden Organic Vegetable Juices are cold pressed raw from freshly grown organic vegetables, picked when they are mature, ensuring that the nutrient levels are at their peak. The juice is flash pasteurised once bottled to maintain shelf life for maximum freshness, without loss of vitamins and minerals.

Approved by the Soil Association in meeting it's organic standard, Eden Organic Vegetable Juices are packaged in 750ml bottles and available in health food stores or through all leading health food wholesalers.

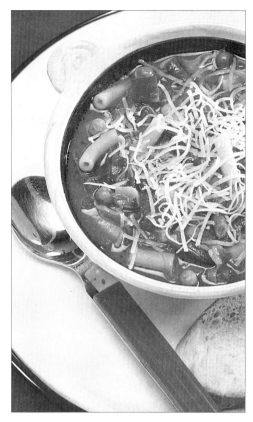

Above: *Eden Mr Stroni's Supper Soup.*

JUICE UP YOUR COOKING WITH EDEN

Eden Juices are excellent when used as ingredients in cookery. JUICE UP FAMILY MEALTIME is Eden's latest recipe booklet featuring eight vegetarian dishes created by leading home economist Roz Denny with both adults and children in mind.

Copies are available free from CBPR, PO Box 1089, Pulborough, West Sussex. RH20 2YX.

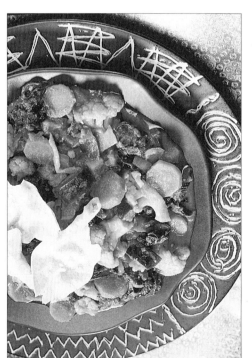

Left: *Eden Indian Vegetable Curry.*

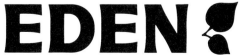

food more widely available, but it also led to some problems. Wholesalers did not always honour their bills, and often kept farmers waiting for their money. Some did not survive. Supermarkets demand a high standard of packaging, and their transport system is centralised. All the organic vegetables for supermarkets all over the country are packed by two companies. The produce travels many miles to reach them, and is then re-distributed on the supermarkets' lorries. To survive the rigours of this process, growers must grade so severely that they throw a good deal of food away. Size is very closely restricted too, and the length of runner beans and the diameter of tomatoes has to fit the packaging.

You will be able to buy good quality organic food from a supermarket, and that's fine. But the range will not be enormous and the system doesn't always suit the small family horticulturist. In a few areas they have grouped together to form co-operatives, but many of them have decided to sell directly to their customers. Customers get food which is really fresh. They can buy a lettuce or bag of spinach cut on the day and eat it shortly afterwards. Some crops will be harvested more than once a day to ensure peak freshness. Farm shops and stalls do a steady trade with customers who trust their grower, with whom they often have a personal relationship.

Then there is the Vegetable Box Scheme. These have taken off all over the country, and are successful with growers and customers alike. What happens is that the grower packs a box with a certain value of vegetables - often in small, medium and large sizes - that are in season at the time. The customer does not know what will be in the box, except that the basics - carrots onions and potatoes will be included most weeks. They may be allowed a couple of "dislikes" that they never, ever, want. The box is delivered once a week, and payment is either a week in advance or a week in arrears. Groups of boxes are usually dropped off at a collection point.

The beauty of the scheme is that growers know that they can sell what they grow, and that they won't have to wait long to be paid for it. It is not too much of an exaggeration to say that some organic growers would not have been able to survive without the box scheme. The crop is picked on the day it is delivered and it's food value is all the higher. Really fresh food tastes better, and some claim that organic food is more nutritious.

Supermarket growers have to specialise, and may grow about 10 crops. Box scheme and shop growers usually have 50 types of vegetables and fruit - maybe even more. Customers at box schemes and farm shops don't mind if their beans are a little bit too long, or their tomatoes are a mixed size, as long as the quality is good. And if there is a crop failure, there are plenty of other crops around to eat. They will probably come across things that you can never find in local supermarkets like organic aubergines, peppers and spinach. Vegetables they never dreamt of buying could appear at any time - often with recipes supplied - and children are likely to become curious and interested, and regard vegetables as friends not foes.

The main advantage of buying directly from an organic farmer is that "Food Miles" are reduced. The cost of processing, transporting and packaging food takes up an enormous amount of resources, and the environmental cost is not being taken into account. In some cases we can hardly consider this necessary. Why do you want to eat strawberries in January? Why not enjoy them when they are in season, and eat a crisp stored apple or a mellow pear in the winter? Why eat green beans, imported from Kenya and grown on land that could be feeding the local population. If you waited till summer you could eat green beans for several months, and in winter enjoy root crops, crisp cabbages, or summer vegetables you have frozen yourself. One of the first studies on Food Miles in Germany discovered that over 6000 miles of travel had gone into producing a pot of yogurt. This can hardly be called sustainable. The SAFE Alliance, with colleagues in other countries, is trying to devise a sustainable menu for each area, substituting food we can grow in our own countries for things we import.

Another advantage of supporting local food growing is that the money stays local. Your producers will probably be spending what they earn locally, and if the business is successful it will probably be providing employment. This all adds up to a more sustainable economy in your area. And perhaps to a more vibrant small town or village.

It is amazing how much food can be grown on a small area. A market garden of only a few acres could feed 60 families for a good proportion of the year. Many growers take a break during the "hungry gap" - when the winter crops have finished and the summer crops have not started - but gradually the season is being extended with the use of polythene tunnels, glass houses, cloches and crop covers.

Many of those wedded to the old way of doing things will tell you that we couldn't feed the world if we went organic. But a recent study showed that even Norway, much farther north than Britain and with less fertile soils, could feed itself organically without too drastic a change of diet. In fact, the diet would be healthier, with less emphasis on meat.

At the moment the demand for organic food is greater than the supply available. It takes two years to convert a farm to organic, and at least five years before it achieves full fertility and a natural balance. The government provides very limited help to organic farmers through the Organic Aid Scheme. This is to help them convert to organic production, but although it can be used together with other subsidies it is a very small amount. If an arable farmer wants to convert, he can lose thousands of pounds worth of subsidy, because he won't get it on the fertility building phase of his rotation - the grass-clover ley. This state of affairs is not likely to encourage newcomers, given that it takes a good deal of courage for a farmer who has been relying on fertiliser out of a bag and instant remedies for insect pests to go organic.

Organic food deserves our whole-hearted consideration. We should be growing some of our own, however small our gardens, and remembering the seasons and their meaning. Children appreciate food all the more when they know where it has come from. Although everyone is so busy these days, it can be well worthwhile making an effort to sit down together a few times each week to a meal made with food that has been grown nearby with care and consideration for the environment. If everyone can help prepare it, without too much bother about mess, so much the better. That's an easy way to passing on an appreciation of good healthy eating to our children which will last them for life.

The Soil Association, 86 Colston St, Bristol BS1 5BB

Note on Judy Steele: Freelance journalist, specialising in organic food and farming and environmental issues attached to agriculture, writes for Soil Association and British Organic Farmers magazines. Author of Local Foodlinks: new ways of getting organic food from farm to table. Published by and available from the Soil Association.

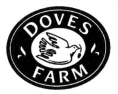
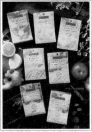

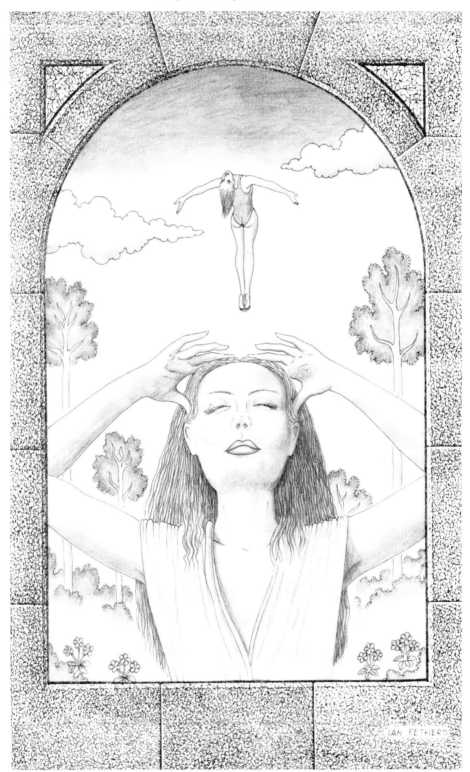

Beauty and Health for Men and Women
by Frances Nicholls

𝕴 t is my firm and proven belief that we can all achieve an ideal state of beauty, but not necessarily from what we put onto ourselves - it is more from what we put into ourselves!

This may seem a strange opening statement but over my many years in practice I have seen men, women and children increase their levels of vitality, optimism and hope for the future, through simple and sensible nutrition, adjusting life-styles and utilising one or more forms of back-up complementary therapy.

Aromatherapy has become very important to people in recent years, however it could easily be denigrated for commercial gain. Thankfully there are a number of organisations who maintain the standards of therapists, check insurance and work for the publics' better gain. Other 'well-being' therapists might include osteopathy which works well with massage therapies, freeing muscles and therefore circulation, martial arts, meditation practice, yoga etc. The key element in any of this is time. Do you, the reader, have time for yourself? If not, why not, and anyway 'why bother?', might be your reply.

My answer is that our bodies, and therefore our minds and spirits too can only suffer so much stress, albeit environmental, personal etc. When we get to 'snap-point' the body rebels, with perhaps early warning signs such as headaches, changed digestive patterns, skin eruptions, insomnia, joint pains etc. Obviously it is wise to consult your GP if your symptoms persist, but just taking a little time for yourself could be all you need to do.

I hope that this article might inspire you with some ideas to do just that. It is amazing how much you can do for yourself at home. Think in terms of a 'home-spa' and a regular pattern of visits to a really good hairdresser and beauty salon where you can be severely pampered. Many now do 'special treat days' with refreshments included, and it can be a real unwind. They make superb gifts, and are an excellent method of introducing you to the treatments now available.

Before embarking on outlining these sybaritic concepts of well-being let me remind you of the value of exercise. It gives some people a tremendous 'buzz' and it is easy to join gyms and clubs for a work-out.

Water

Water is one of the four elements, and because it is so fundamental, its importance to us as human beings can be forgotten. Use water to clean and balance yourself. It can be used in so many ways - baths, showers, jacuzzis, steam rooms, saunas etc.

Our bathrooms are generally used functionally, but in fact the healing potential in that one room is enormous. Rituals and healing using water were employed by ancient civilisations emanating from Egypt, Italy, Greece and India. Spas were the focal points of many cities all over Europe in the 18th and 19th centuries, but as allopathic health care emerged hydrotherapy was less and less utilised.

However there is a come back now with a wealth of natural products available so that your bathroom can serve a positive health purpose. Balneology and Thalassotherapy are two increasingly popular treatments with many benefits. Balneology is the use of substances such as clays, peats, and muds of a particular region added to the bath. Thalassotherapy is the use of sea products into the bath, (seaweed, brine, and sea water.) The French are particularly good at the latter.

Baths can be beneficial through the effect of temperature, the effect and feel of the water itself, and the results of any additional products added to the water.

Let us briefly look at temperature and the effect on the skin. In this context we should remember our skin absorbs and excretes as well as regulating most of our body temperature, therefore it is sometimes known as the third kidney. Heat on the skin dilates the blood vessels in it, demonstrated by flushing followed by extra perspiration. The opposite happens when cool temperatures are used, resulting in shivering. When the skin temperature rises there is a metabolic exchange between the skin tissues and blood, resulting in ultimately a faster removal of waste products. The extra blood used in this process has been diverted from the internal organs therefore slowing down their functions. However the heart rate increases to move blood to the skin.

The body loses heat through perspiration, so if it is encased or wrapped the heating effect is intensified, and the third kidney moves into action once you have left the water. The 'encasing' principle is now fashionable in salons, and provides another aspect of hydrotherapy. Bath temperature should generally be similar to body temperature thus creating a comfortable environment for a relaxing soak.

Hotter baths will stimulate the excretory function of the skin, and give a sedative effect. Stay in one for up to fifteen minutes, and then go to bed! Cold baths up to 85oF and 29oC are not for the faint hearted. They stimulate metabolic function, tone the skin, strengthen one, but should only be used by people who do not have cardiac problems. If you want to be accurate get a bath thermometer.

Treatment baths can involve a variety of ingredients, one of the most simple using Epsom Salts. Take about 500 grams and put into a tepid bath. Get in and gradually increase the temperature to hot. Rest there for around ten minutes. Shower off with tepid water and then wrap up for bed as the perspiration action will take place all night. Use two to three times a week to keep the skin healthy, and ease niggly muscle and joint pains. Oatmeal has an ancient history long associated with exfoliation and skin softening. To about 500 grams add dried herbs of your choice, tie in a cloth under the hot tap, so that the water runs fragrant and soft. Rest in the tepid bath for up to 30 minutes.

Muds, clays and peats are also used in bath products. In general there is a two fold action - absorption of some of the natural components through the skin and the induction of a detoxification process.

Thalossotherapy is freely available in different forms, and has the advantage that as the brine increases the water buoyancy, so is the body partially supported, becoming more weightless. Use common salt, as for an Epsom bath. A fine paste can be made with water and rubbed over the body towards the heart, avoiding the genital area and face. Seaweed products can be added or used on their own as can also a variety of essential oils.

Here are a few words of caution for home/spa users.

1.   Get up slowly after a hot bath or wrap up in case you have a drop in blood pressure which may cause dizziness or fainting.
2.   Allow at least three hours to pass after a heavy meal if you want a hot bath.
3.   Do not have hot baths if you are feeling low.
4.   Close the pores down with a tepid shower after a hot bath.
5.   Do not use seaweed in a bath if there is a known allergy to iodine.
6.   Always drink extra water after a hot bath.

A selection of the wide array of products available may be found at the end, but whatever else you do, think about how you could transform your bathroom into a home spa - dimmer switches, candles, fragrant oils, music and thick warm towels. It will form a base for all your in-house self-care programmes.

Waxing

A leg wax makes you feel good about yourself and may inspire you to have some foot beauty too! Hot wax is an older method and not generally used today because it can be too hot, and certainly for most of us, quite painful. Sensitive skin can be inflamed for a few hours afterwards. Cool wax is much more tolerable and hygenic as strips are used and then discarded.

The latest technique is of ancient origin, going back to the Egyptians, and is called sugaring. It was brought back to the UK in 1986, and has many advantages over traditional methods in that it can be used on all skins, and for all types of hair, it is less painful, dead cells are removed, and there is a slowing down of the hair growth. There is also a very cooling and antiseptic soothing lotion that can be applied after your home or professional treatment. The products are not tested on animals. As with all forms of epilation the paste should not be used over moles, septic or broken skin or enlarged varicose veins.

Honey products are also available for leg waxes. Honey is a real product of nature and very healing and restorative to the skin. (It is well known for its healing of minor burns and scalds.) Your local beauty salon will be able to advise you which waxing method is best for you.

Fingers and Toes

Women are usually very conscious of their hands and take time to have them looking their best. Men are now finding it acceptable to have basic manicures and it adds enormously to the overall image. Think of the number of times we use our hands -just on a social/professional basis: in restaurants, in relationships, in body language generally for emphasis, even using the ubiquitous mobile! Our hands will also age quickly and be even more of a give-away in the age-stakes unless we protect them from excessive sun, harsh detergents, and extreme weather conditions. The most obvious thing to do is to use plenty of hand cream, rich in natural products like vitamin E, and get into the habit of putting some on after hand-washing, or before you go out.

Have some by every set of taps! Work it well into the nails, as the cuticles are often the first to dehydrate. Keep some in the car too. Barrier creams have been around for a long time; many are formulated and in conjunction with household gloves will protect your hands from harsh detergents and rough work.

Keep appropriate gloves at your work stations and use them before touching anything. This may seem excessive but people with allergies triggered by various products know the importance of stage one protection.

Home care for hands and feet is easy and fun but do invest in good quality emery board nail files, steel clippers and scissors, orange sticks etc. Nail files are notorious for splitting nails especially if a see-saw action is used. Work alternately in one direction from the side to the middle of the nail, using emery, not metal boards.

To hydrate and soften rough nails and cuticles, soak in a small bowl of warmed almond oil, to which a little sugar has been added. Massage the finger tips with this oily sugar and it will really help to soften and feed the cuticles. Have tissues nearby to wipe fingers. This treatment can of course be adapted to your toes. With newly softened cuticles ready, use an orange stick to push them back gently to follow the natural shape of your nail. A healthy way to finish your home manicure is a brisk buffing with a leather buffer, which will increase the blood circulation and thus feed the nail bed.

Artificial nails have reached a new peak of excellence using gels, resins and acrylics. They need to be applied by a salon nail technician who will give you all the advice needed to maintain them. Once on they must not be pulled off, because the nail will be damaged and show this for around six months. There is no risk of fungal or other infections unless the tip is damaged. Henna extract, an ancient plant for use in beauty is incorporated to help strengthen weak nails, so obviously an already strong nail will grow faster. As they grow you will need to go back to the salon for a resin infill, and your technician will also give a general consultation.

Endless fun can now be had with traditional nail polishes and jewellery. There is so much to choose from, and when you go for a professional manicure you will no doubt see a wide selection to choose from.

Feet are disdained by most of us, but in fact if they are not maintained problems can set in - fungal infections being the most common.

Also, diabetics need regular foot checks by practice nurses and chiropodists. Home and professional pedicures always look better if the chiropodist has been visited first. Corns and calluses will be checked amongst a myriad of things that can make our feet uncomfortable. Our whole body weight goes through our knees into the feet.

They are composed of many tiny bones and ligaments which can get cramped with ill-fitting shoes, or distorted if you are walking unevenly. It is easier to have a salon pedicure to maintain the nails, and there are ranges of aromatic plant-based products available for foot health generally in use by salons. They really nurture all of the foot, and the best bit is the massage!

Cellulite

This is a perennial problem for many women, that has been much exploited by a variety of markets. Miracle cures are advertised constantly, but in my experience an understanding of self and an analysis of life-style are very helpful.

With my aromatherapist's hat on I can honestly say that essential oils have given the best overall results but it involves a great deal of work and thought by the woman and support by her therapist. Attention to food is paramount and certain aspects of life-style would need in all probability, to be adjusted.

However, if aromatherapy is not for you try some of the clay body wraps which will absorb the toxins that we all accumulate, or robot lymphatic massagers which move lymph very efficiently and improve circulation. Lymph movement circulation and toxins are three physical aspects of cellulite that can also be treated variably by G5 massagers and vacuum cup suction, especially when pre-blended essential oils are used too.

I have also known food allergies contribute to the problem so, seeking help via perhaps vega-testing would be a useful starting point.

Cellulite can be triggered amongst other things by puberty, pregnancy, severe stress, altered life-style, debilitating illness and drug treatments. In my opinion the mind, body, soul aspect is an important part of the care programme for cellulite sufferers, as it can take a few weeks before any radical change is noticed.

There is hope but you will need a dedicated and experienced practitioner to take you through, and you will need to give yourself time each day for your home care routine, be it body brushing, exercise, massage or making delicious food.

The fine detail of cellulite is a topic all of its own, covered well in a book out in April 1997, 'The Complete Anti-Cellulite Plan' - Liz Hodgkinson. £5.99 by Thorsons Harper Collins.

This should inspire you all!

Massage

We all benefit from having a massage, even if it is only shoulders and neck in the office lunch hour. Why?

Someone else is taking charge and care of you. The well-being factor is good because, post massage, the blood is circulating more freely through the tissue, sweeping away build-ups of lactic acid and bringing a fresh burst of oxygen to the tissue as well.

Before aromatherapy became as acceptable as it is now, massage used to be done with, generally, an unfragranced oil in the 'Swedish' style. This is not an intuitive approach - it is strictly physical and can be quite painful, but it is the 'right sort of pain'! The feel good factor emerges usually after 24 hours, but it depends really on how often you have a massage.

Our skin is a very large and busy organ. It not only regulates temperature and protects us from bacteria, but it is also part of the excretory system. Massage will greatly enhance its performance and therefore maintain your health levels. The quality of the skin will change becoming more supple, hydrated and smooth and also a better colour. It is very easy to purchase massage oil for use at home, but try avoiding a cheap mass market product, or a product that is over-packaged. You need the contents of the bottle - not the box! Oils are absorbed into our tissue, and further dissolved by the lipids in the blood, so you will see now that you should choose carefully.

Face

The face is permanently targeted for the latest in creams and colour cosmetics. Some of the product ranges are quite complicated, so it is advisable to read all the literature, talk with the sales girls, and try out some samples before you finally commit yourself. No amount of money can give you beauty - that comes from within. The most radiant women that I have met are those that are at peace with themselves and the world -they have sorted LIFE out! Any make-up they use enhances an already lovely skin and face, but to be fair, genetics are also a major contributory factor.

Skin problems like acne can be the result of a stress problem, but they are aggravated by junk food, drugs, etc. Sun and sand holidays help many acne sufferers, and Dead Sea salts help psoriasis, but it is difficult to deal with these problems alone. Professionally selected essential oils can also have excellent results. Whatever you do, remember that your skin is sensitive and should be treated with great care. Alcohol based solutions dry up the skin, and to compensate, the sebaceous glands go into overdrive, and the problem continues.

As a society, we drink everything that we shouldn't and not very much of what we should - namely water. Water cleans the blood, body tissue and organs, and ideally at least a litre a day should be consumed along with other drinks. The greatest percentage of our body make-up is water. Bottled water can be very hard - Evian seems to be one of the best, but what is wrong with drinking boiled water at any temperature? It is cheaper! You can always add a slice of lime or lemon.

Some people like to go on fruit or juice fasts to clear the mind and the skin, which is excellent, but do this at a time when not under pressure so that you can rest. The result of this may be some spots, a general feeling of lassitude, and maybe a headache. Take these as positive signs and plan your next 'health day'.

Colour cosmetics and many other products may have been tested on animals, particularly in France, but new European legislation is coming into force in 1997 banning this. This is a serious issue for many of us, and once again, I direct you to aromatherapy because it is excellent for skin care and our consciences. New ways of testing are being used, and also human volunteers, but if in doubt, ask the sales team for your intended products.

To complete the immediate impact we make in society our hair is the next stage for consideration.

Hair and Scalp

Hair reflects our health, its shine, swing and style can make heads turn. Hair is in fact an extension of the skin, and can be affected by the same problems. The scalp is of major importance as the hair bulb is to be found in the subcutaneous tissue. It is nourished by a supply of blood and sebaceous glands to keep the hair soft and pliable through the secretion of sebum. Sebum also waterproofs the skin and helps to protect it from microbes. Hair growth is affected by the condition of the scalp. If it is tight the blood flow will be restricted, so new hair growth will be stunted.

The old fashioned way to keep a scalp healthy is to bend from the waist and brush downwards a hundred times. There is a multiple benefit from doing this - loose hairs (we lose at least 40 a day!) and dust are brushed out. Sebum is distributed along the length of the hair and the scalp is exercised by the brush bristles (invest in a really good bristle brush). By bending down you also increase blood supply to the hair bulb. Follow the brushing by a minute of head massage - just your finger pads working into the scalp and moving it about - then come up slowly. Hair growth can also be affected by long and severe illness, debilitation and pregnancy. Stress is a major growth inhibitor as the body molecules tense and reduce a healthy circulation. Permanent hair loss is the unfortunate lot of many men, and some women. Normally it is inherited or is part of the ageing process, but some illnesses can be responsible - typhoid and hyper thyroidism being two. Other causes may include drugs, some type of dermatitis, frequent x-rays and hormonal factors.

Excessive hair drying can cause mechanical root damage which may result in temporary hair loss, and patchy baldness can occur resulting from shingles dermatitis, fungal infection, syphilis or other scalp diseases.

It behoves us therefore to treat our scalps and hair as well as we treat the rest of our bodies. The choice of shampoos, conditioners and other hair care products. Some brands have genuine essential oils added giving a good effect, and others have herbal, seaweed extracts or sea salts and even mud! They are more costly because of the natural ingredients included in the formula, but they are less aggressive for the hair and scalp.

A really natural way to end your hair wash is to pour a water-based rinse through and leave it to dry on your scalp if you can. Make your own infusions of rosemary, sage or chamomile flowers (for blond hair) or rub about 20mls of organic flower water through the scalp. No alcohol is involved so the sebum secretion will remain at a normal level.

Very dry and brittle hair can be much improved by a hot oil treatment. Jojoba oil is odourless and very stable. Heat about 25mls in a cup standing in a pan of hot water , then work it through with your fingers and a comb. Cover up with a hot towel, and leave as long as possible, to allow the jojoba oil to penetrate.

If you have serious problems with your hair and scalp see your doctor and/or a trichologist. There may be a hidden reason which needs professional understanding - after all, your hair is an immediate barometer of your overall health.

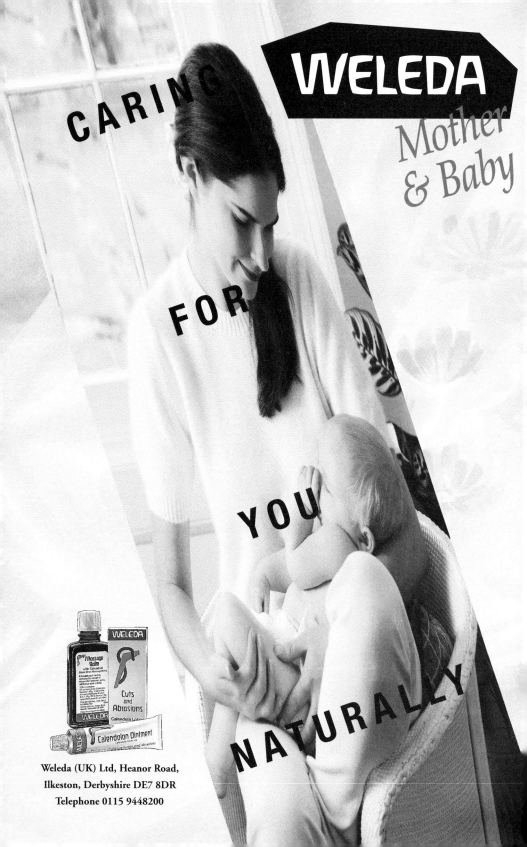

Black Beauty

World society is multi-ethnic and this section of the book would be incomplete if I did not acknowledge black skins. White skins have a fragility that does not occur in the more exotic and sultry skins of black people. The heightened level of melanin in black skins means that light is absorbed, but white skins reflect light. Melanin protects skins from ultraviolet light, and can also protect it from skin cancer. Black skins are also endowed with more sweat glands, and therefore pores, which are also larger than those in white skins. The water and salts that exude from the pores gives black skin a sheen, which is a miracle deterrent against ageing, so if you are black, you can hide the passing of the years for longer.

The normal care routines should be observed as for white skins, and make sure you have enough oils in your diet so that the skin does not dehydrate, especially if you are living in a less exotic climate. I have found that black people coming to live in Europe have had problems with skin dehydration, partly due to central heating and pollution which they do not have at home, and partly due to the change of food, especially the easy availability of fast food.

Exfoliation techniques are especially good to use, not only on your face, but the whole body. Cheloid (scar) tissue shows up on black skin and there is a greater tendency to acne, blackheads and other annoying skin conditions. However, certain essential oils used under professional advice can work wonders without aggravating any skin function. Bath and shower times are occasions when you can indulge yourself with thalasso and balneotherapy, and if you can get to a steam room, sauna or jacuzzi, so much the better for your skin.

Black hair can lend itself to the most exotic and colourful hairstyles, but trying to tame it to become 'European' can cause much damage to the hair itself. Keep an eye on its condition especially if you've had it relaxed, or frequently wear it corn-rowed or plaited (this means that the scalp can't move!) Use a warm oil conditioner as for European hair, but if possible leave it on the hair for a day or two so that it can really penetrate, and have a very simple hair style. Spend a little extra money on good quality shampoos with natural ingredients, especially essential oils or herbal extracts, and use a conditioner too!

Your hair reflects your health so look at your whole self as often as you can!

Black skinned women are recorded as having used make up from 3500BC. Egyptian tombs and hieroglyphics have revealed evidence of eye make up and aromatic ointments. We know that they and many later civilisations used bathing as part of mainstream beauty rituals, so, with history behind you, and professional advice from colour cosmetic companies you can bring colour and exotism to society that white skins can never achieve.

Pregnancy

This topic is included under Health and Beauty because I have seen so many different attitudes by women to themselves when pregnant. It is a time when a woman can be at her most naturally beautiful especially as the pregnancy progresses. After the first trimester, the skin and hair settle down, and the most important thing for many women is to keep their skins supple to prevent

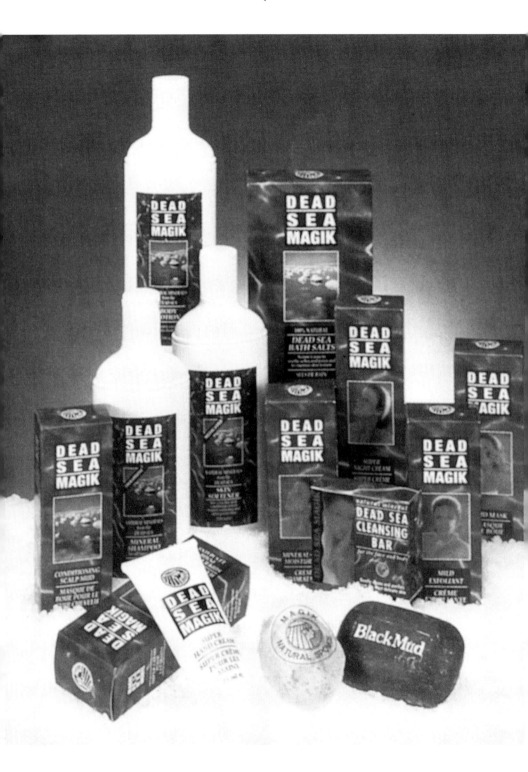

stretch marks. It is always better to prevent them as there is no real cure once they are there. Creams and lotions are available, but they do not really have the long term hydrating power of vegetable carrier oils - something as simple as almond, wheatgerm or jojoba oil can be used as often as required. Some women like to have aromatherapy treatments to nurture the skin, and help to ease the muscular aches as the pregnancy progresses. Osteopathy is also extremely beneficial and can help 100% if the tail-bone becomes misaligned during labour and delivery. Reflexology also induces a feeling of well-being and can help with the minor problems of pregnancy. Most women work for as long as they can before delivery and should make time for themselves and take advantage of their salaries, because it can be quite tiring working and being pregnant.

As the pregnancy advances some women have leg oedema and fatigue which is much eased by massage, and a regular routine of resting with the legs up. It has been my experience that mothers make a positive effort with food and life style and they also look to complementary medicine to see what options are available.

Once delivered, the new mother will mostly only think of her baby, but there is usually a father around and he needs to recover from it all too! It may seem idealistic, but with a bit of team work mothers can take a long bath, get their hair done etc. and begin to feel themselves again. However it will not happen overnight, so aim at a little self-care every day. Try and find a slot in the day that is for you!

Conclusion

We are each one of us, quite unique, and it is up to us to recognise and develop our inner and outer potentials. At our conception we are given 'chi' - inherited energies, which will help to make us who we really are. As we grow older, so we grow in wisdom, which we draw on, and maybe call it 'life experience' Look for the positive and beautiful things in life, and learn to give and receive, however simply. It will bring you joy, and joy to others, and, more wonderfully can have a chain effect, which helps to make our world a better place. Philosophy this may be - but it is not unrelated to the overall topic of Health and Beauty.

The companies listed below are known to me in many different ways. They will provide you with products and information to inspire you to a higher level of well being. Needless to say they have been vetted with reference to animal testing and they make every effort to package in recyclable materials. The R.S.P.C.A. publish a handbook with further names and addresses. Send an A5 S.A.E. to their Horsham office.

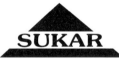

THALGO -   Thalassotherapy and skin care products.   0171- 512 0872
AHAVA -   Thalassotherapy. Dead Sea Salts and skin care products.
                                                                                  01452 - 864574
FINDERS INT. LTD. - Thalassotherapy. Dead Sea Salts and skin care products.
                                                                                  01580 - 211055
ELEMIS -   An excellent range of skin care, bath products, shampoos etc.
                                                                                  0181- 954 8033
TISSERAND -   Aromatherapy - interesting shampoos and bath products.
                                                                                  01273 - 325666
BODYTREATS INT. LTD. -   Specialists in organic essential oils, flower waters
                             (Mail Order) and other aromatherapy products.
                                                                                  0181- 543 7633
AVEDA -   Plant based products from the bath to colour cosmetics. (Mail Order)
                                                                                  0171- 636 7911
GENWOL -   Foot care products with aromatic extracts. (At MEDIFORCE)
                                                                                  01274 -844220

SIXTUS -   Foot care products with balsamic extracts.
                                                                                  0181 - 979 7261
E'SPA -   Plant based products for complete body care.
                                                                                  01483 -454444
SUKAR ORIGINAL SUGARING - Home care kits available. (Mail Order)
                                                                                  01937 - 572711
NAILS TODAY -   Artificial nails advice line.   01625 - 510343
HARBOURNE PRODUCTS LTD. - 'Salon Beauty' range of skin care and massage oils.
                             (Mail Order)   01372 - 729629
WELEDA (UK) LTD. - Aromatic product range for skin and hair care and baths.
                             (Mail Order)   0115 - 944820
NOMA -   Enquiry line for vega testing.   01703 - 770513
BEAUTY WITHOUT CRUELTY COSMETICS. -   01732-365291
BEAUTY WITHOUT CRUELTY CHARITY. -   01983-731491
NATURE WATCH (Campaigning against animal cruelty) -   01242-252871

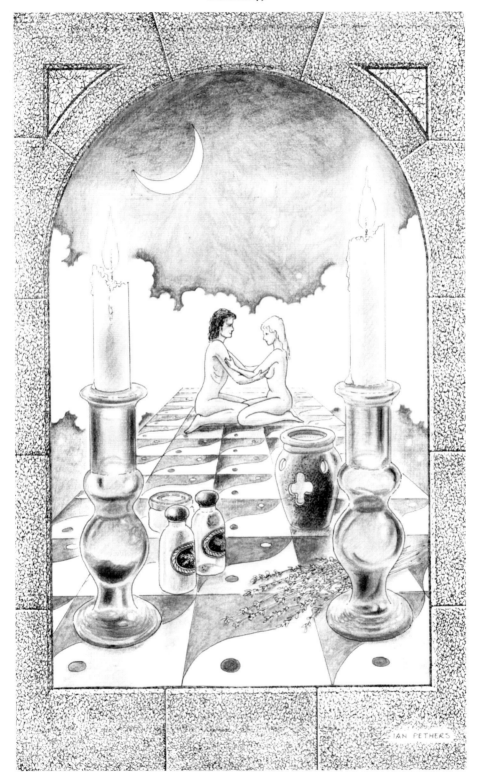

by Ms. Nicole PEREZ IFA

en years ago Aromatherapy was almost unknown but in the last few years it has attracted a great deal of attention which in turn has resulted in extensive media coverage making the public aware of its existence. One could assume from this fast development that it is just another trend, something new and interesting to do which will soon die down. This has turned out not to be the case as Aromatherapy has proven itself to offer a wonderful remedy for stress and many people have directly benefited from it already. In fact as it is much in demand from the general public, in the last two years a number of Hospital Trusts have elected to add Aromatherapy to their range of care for patients. Recently a major hospital in Liverpool made it known that Aromatherapy was available on the NHS in this Hospital, as reported in the National Press. The purpose of this chapter is to present a brief account of Aromatherapy for the guidance of those embarking on either a self-help treatment or a visit to the local Aromatherapist.

What is Aromatherapy? It is a therapeutic treatment which makes systematic use of essential oils, the wonderfully scented essences of aromatic plants, to relieve physical and psychological discomfort, stress and to promote good-health and well-being.

Aromatic plants have been known to mankind, from remote antiquity, having been utilised in the prevention of illness or the curative treatment of numerous ailments affecting the human body. Aromatherapy truly owes its roots to Aromatic Medicine whose origins have been lost in the past. Many practices have been around a long time and may easily be traced in various accounts and texts from Ancient China, Ancient Egypt and Ancient Greece. Many such classical references emphasise the inter-dependence of Health and Hygiene, showing that protecting and cleansing 'body and soul' were at the forefront of the concerns of the people of these days. Aromatic ointments, wines, vinegars, powders, medicated aromatic oils, inhalants, creams, poultices, compresses, deodorants and many healing perfumes are found comprehensively described in the writings of some of the most famous physicians of all times: Hippocrates, Gallen, Dioscorides, Avicenna, Parascelsus and the Englishman Culpepper and many others had great respect for the world of Aromatics.

Aromatherapy owes its success story to the essential oils from aromatic plants as these have the similar qualities as the plants they are extracted from but in a more concentrated form. Modern Aromatherapy has the same capacity as its ancestor and is a safe therapy when applied correctly. It can be used alone or alongside conventional medical treatment where it appears to boost efficacy of such treatment, helping in recovery and in avoiding recurrences. At this point it is appropriate to say that comprehensive research is still in its infancy and will require further investigation to assert why it seems to work in this way. The practice of Aromatherapy in the UK started some thirty years ago or so and was brought to this country by a lady called Marguerite Maury whose motto was: - 'We are not trying to add years to life, but to add life to years' (quote from her book: The Secret of Life and Youth. 1968) Marguerite Maury was a pioneer of Aromatherapy who not only investigated the properties of essential oils, particularly the effect of their scents on the Nervous System, but who also developed a unique way of working with

REAL

aromatherapy

Here's Health
NATURAL PRODUCT
AWARDS
1997
WINNER
OVER THE BEST
ESSENTIAL OIL
PRODUCTS

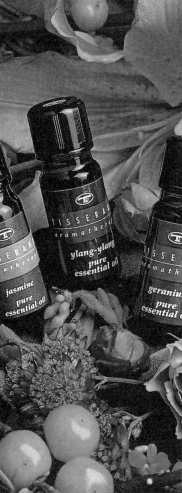

TISSERAND

PURE ESSENTIAL OILS

VAPORISERS

BODY OILS & LOTIONS

SHOWER GELS & SOAPS

BATH OILS & SOAKS

HAIRCARE

HAND & NAIL CREAM

FOOTCARE

TEA TREE RANGE

LAVENDER RANGE

MOIST TISSUES

CRUELTY FREE

Purity and Quality

CALL 01273 325666 FOR STOCKISTS DETAILS

Natural Therapies. She employed massage and Reflex zone Therapy and probably created one of the first Aromatherapy Massage treatments which is the standard form of treatment today. Who can use Aromatherapy today and what can be gained from it? - Anyone who is healthy and fit and wants to keep that way.

- Anyone who is healthy and fit but whose lifestyle is taxing and wants to avoid becoming overstressed.
- Anyone who is not so well and whose symptoms can be alleviated by Aromatherapy.
- Anyone who is physically or psychologically impaired and who needs comfort and support.

Aromatherapy's healing capacity revolves around the use of essential oils whose remarkable therapeutic properties tend to stimulate the body's own healing process. However it must be understood that the use of physical therapies such as massage is also an important factor in the therapy. Touch has its own rewards and an expert massage will clear the body of unwanted tensions as well as decrease any Nervous hyperactivity thus restoring a sense of balance. If one adds the Aromatic dimension through including essential oils to the massage it will activate another important sensory organ in the body, the Sense of smell. This will work at a very deep and unconscious level and result in a further beneficial transformation.

Essential oils are the fragrant chemical substances extracted from Aromatic plants and represent the scent of such plants. Occuring naturally in a plant, they can be found in the roots, stems, flowers, leaves, bark and other parts of any aromatic plant. They are obtained by various modes of extraction, the most suitable being distillation and expression to ensure that they retain their therapeutic properties. e.g.: prophylactic, antiseptic, anti-spasmodic, etc. They are very powerful chemicals which tend to become even concentrated after the process of extraction.

Rene M Gattefosse (1881-1950) who was a French Perfumer chemist and who had many interests in various sciences, thoroughly researched the therapeutic properties of essential oils. His amazing findings are recorded in his well-known book 'Aromatherapy' in 1937 and this remains a leading textbook on the subject. R. M. Gattefosse is responsible for inventing the term 'Aromatherapy', to designate a previously unnamed area of medicine where essential oils can be used as antiseptic and anti-bacterial agents in pharmaceutical compositions for the treatment of certain diseases. Currently, essential oils are widely used in pharmacy and complementary medicine. They have been found to be particularly efficient with ailments which are not responding to conventional drugs and they do not seem to have particular side-effects if applied correctly. * Buying & storing essential oils To get the most from essential oils, they need to be relatively fresh as different essential oils have a different lifespan , stored in dark glass container with a screw on top and a special dropper cap to facilitate easy pouring and kept away from direct sunlight and heat as these would damage them. Essential oils for Aromatherapy use should only be bought from a reliable source where the supplier has a competent knowledge of aromatherapy as well as a responsible awareness of their shelf-life.

The versatility of essential oils and their multi-uses in cosmetic preparation + houshold cleaning products has led to much confusion and concern. Their inclusion in such products should not imply any therapeutic properties. So now one can buy aromatherapy soaps, shampoos, creams, car deodorants, house deodorants and not a day passes without something coming on to the market with the glorious title 'Aromatherapy something'. Obviously, Aromatherapy business is booming. The Cosmetic Industry seem to get away with many claims such as 'rejuvenation',

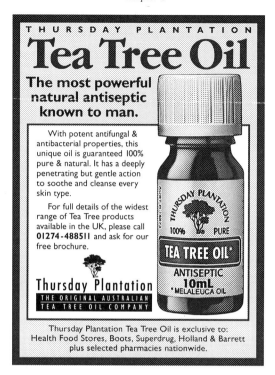
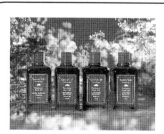

'regrowth', 'skin improvement' and many other things. This may be true for some products and not for others, there is no way to tell by the label. Although superficial benefits in some cases cannot be denied, it cannot automatically be attributed to the Aromatherapy factor within the product as many other ingredients might have been incorporated. Beauty Aromatherapy treatment, Many Beauty Therapists regularly make use of essential oils in dilution to cleanse and rejuvenate the skin of the face and this no doubt will have some benefits too. This is often presented as an Aromatherapy treatment and advertised in the Hairdresser shop. It should really be made clear that this is not a Complementary therapy. Because of these confusing claims it must be stated that the emphasis of an Aromatherapy Beauty treatment and the training of a beautician is very different from the Complementary Therapy practitioner approach as the former only addresses very superficial problems. Further to this, the outcomes of a treatment are more concerned with self-image than with Health and well-being.

'A little bit of this or a little bit of that can't do any harm'. This is what the many current books on Aromatherapy often claim, many may even contradict each other as to what is best for what. Many recipes are given for all sorts of ailments and seem to be encouraging the reader to make many assumptions about their health. This is worrying as not everyone is qualified to ascertain what the problem is to begin with. Essential oils like all chemicals have their do's and don'ts and their dangers, and it is wise to follow a reliable guide of instructions if intending to create one's own treatment. The key is, if applied correctly it is 100% safe.

The Professional approach: Having established the differences between various facets of Aromatherapy we can now take a serious look at what it really means. Clinical Aromatherapy usually refers to essential oils used in the same manner as any pharmaceutical drugs or prescriptions and within the same conditions. First, it is necessary to establish what the problem or symptoms of the sufferer are and second to prescribe the right remedy and use it only as instructed. HOLISTIC Aromatherapy includes the Clinical approach if required. This approach is concerned with the overall Healing process but will still look at physical problems and symptoms. But the analysis will go further and include an emotional and spiritual outlook before the final assessment and the specific treatment is decided. This insures that the recommended treatment (or course of treatments) addresses the state of the person as a whole. These two approaches are compatible and work very well together.

Health and fitness, lifestyles, stress and emotional responses are all important factors in our life. So what can be considered an Aromatherapy treatment? Here is a list of the various aspects of a treatment: - An essential oil used neat or in dilution applied to an area of the body - if diluted, it is likely to be in a medium such as: * Alcohol, Grapeseed oil, Sesame oil, Virgin olive oil, Peach Kernel oil, Sweet Almond oil. - essential oils to be inhaled directly or by a steam method - to be applied as local or full body massage - for use in a compress on the skin - it can be by in self-application or application by a qualified professional aromatherapist. - it can be applied for medical or psychological reasons - applied simply to enhance the quality of life and well-being - finally, it can be a 'one off' treatment or a course of treatments. The result: Aromatherapy often seems to have an undefined but noticeable overall healing effect.

Aromatherapy works in a twofold dynamic action: 1. The trigger of physiological response from the body's own repair system from the application of essential oils. e.g.: for medical, for psychological reasons or simply to enhance the quality of life and well-being. e.g.: a drop of an

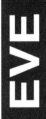
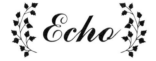
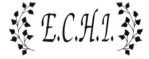

antispasmodic on an aching muscle or a compress on a skin wound or by massage treatment. 2. Aromatic scents affect the psychological state of the receiver, particularly the moods, through olfactory stimulation. Most people will say that after treatment they felt wonderful

AROMATHERAPY - A NATURAL CONNECTION?

Taking a breath is something that we do all the time and without thinking yet this simple everyday action is the most important life-sustaining process in our body. Maybe then, it is not by pure chance that Nature designed the human nose with the sense of smell sitting at its top, guarding the entrance of our inner realm.

Physio-AROMATHERAPY Physiological workings of Aromatherapy: Aromatherapy goes much further than just 'skin-deep' as it is an accepted fact that minute quantities of essential oils when applied are absorbed by the skin and taken up by the capillaries under the skin and eventually are circulated around the body in the blood stream. Although the exact explanation and implications have not as yet been properly analysed or proven, there is no doubt that it works and that benefits are derived by the receivers.

OLFACTORY THERAPY/PSYCHO-AROMATHERAPY

The psychological effect of aromatherapy: To understand aromatherapy further it is important to explain how people are likely to be affected by the interaction of essential oils with our olfactory system. The human brain is extremely elaborate in comparison to its cousins' in the animal world, it is also a lot larger. In terms of evolution, the Brainstem (which sits on top of the spinal cord) seems to be the first structure to have emerged. This is where the control for pre-programmed reflexes which ensure survival and keep the body running are located. Later, from this original structure evolved the Limbic system (Limbic derives from Latin meaning: a ring because of its shape) which itself controls our feelings, emotions and our emotional responses to situations. This area is the seat of our irrational behaviour where our instinctive nature predominates. The core factor in this part of our brain is our sense of smell which allows us to determine what is dangerous (smoke/fire), what is edible (cooking, food), what is desirable (love & sex) and finally what we should do about it according to whether it awakens fear or the promise of pleasure. Although we might not notice most of these scent sensations consciously. It is true that most living things have their own scented key signature and that the human brain is pretty good at recognising a great number of them. This of course, is even more prominent for anyone who use's their 'nose' as part of their job as is the case with a trained aromatherapist. It is in this same area of the brain that memories of our long forgotten past are hidden and will be 'recalled' by certain smells as these probably contributed to 'fixing' these events in our mind in the first place. Looking at the way it all works together : - Various scents find their way to our little olfactory receptors at top of our nose and tickle (the receptors) creating small but distinct sensations. Some of the sensations will have an instant effect such as making us take a deep breath or making us feel suddenly more alert and awake. But others sensations will be received by our 'smell brain' in the Limbic system, will be analysed, possibly recognised and may 'recall' a previous experience. Depending on the brain's perception of these sensations a response will ensue. This response might be pleasant, signal danger or stimulate repulsion although a great deal of our response will be pre-conditioned by our early experiences. Often we are not even aware of it but many of our likes and dislikes of other people are actually triggered by their own scent which our brain may interpret as a threat. So, when our olfactory sensors encounter these naturally scented substances called essential oils it is not surprising that a reaction also

occurs. The difference is that in this case the reaction is intentionally created. Essential oils from Aromatic plants have the particularity to carry the 'smells of the Earth' and 'Nature', some of which are carefully stored in our Limbic system. It often results in putting the receiver in touch with this more instinctive part of human nature. The person becomes more aware of these underlying feelings of deep tiredness, sadness, weariness or anger and these may come as a surprise as most people try their best to keep control of their emotions. It is not unusual to hear someone who has experienced aromatherapy say that a particular scent tends to make them feel calmer and that inhaling that scent at different times of the day keeps them from becoming very stressed.

Which conditions can benefit most from an aromatherapy treatment? It is important to note that one does not need to be ill to receive a treatment. INSTANT OR LONG TERM BENEFIT The effect of the therapy can be quite immediate as in the relief of symptons such as muscle spasms or sore throat or long term as when dealing with chronic ailments or illnesses. Apart from the improvement of health it can provide support for people who are undergoing major surgery or those life threatening situations. Chronic conditions such as arthritis or bronchitis can make the life of the sufferer very uncomfortable. Aromatherapy can calm down the symptoms and make the person more relaxed thus improving the quality of life and sometimes even help to improve the condition. This is also the case with 'flu' viruses, infections, muscular tensions, poor circulation etc., etc.... For people with a tendency to experience 'on & off' ailments such as aches & pains, tiredness, colds, headaches, constipation, eczema and other similar problems, natural remedies like essential oils have a well earned reputation for being efficient. An Aromatherapy treatment can give a quick boost to the nervous system, is gentle on the body's organs and keeps the receiver's outlook on life on a more positive footing. One of the greatest benefits which aromatherapy can claim over many other therapies is that it is the most efficient therapy in the release of stress. Many ailments are caused by acute stress over a prolonged period of time and stress reduction is very important today.

i. Aromatic baths: For stress or insomnia: Application of a chosen blend to the whole body followed by relaxation in a hot bath for 10 to 15mn. Do not use soap, repeat as necessary. ii. Inhalations: The easiest way is to add a few drops of essential oils to half a pint of hot boiling water for colds, chest congestion, or alternatively a few drops on a tissue to be inhaled as a 'calm- me- down' measure. iii. Compresses: 1 pint of hot boiling water in a bowl, add recommended essential oils, skim surface of water and apply warm to the area of skin needing treatment, usually used for things like: abscesses, acne, wounds, grazes.

1. Lavender: the 'first aid oil' best for its relaxing effects on adults, children and even pets.
2. Geranium: The 'stress oil', one of the most efficient oils for stress.
3. Rosemary: the 'get up & go' oil, excellent when you need to see yourself through a hard schedule, exercise, long journey.
4. Benzoin: the 'children's oil' it is very soothing for coughs and any itchy skin condition.
5. Cinnamon leaf: the 'anti-infection' oil, best used as prevention of flu viruses, etc.
6. Niaouli: the 'natural antibiotic' oil, for any viral infection e.g.: flu.
7. Mandarin: the 'gently calming oil' best oil for baby and children.

A professionally qualified aromatherapist will be someone who has trained over a period of time rather than on a short course, by a teacher who not only is a qualified teacher but also a

practitioner of the therapy, so as to impart a good standard of practice. The aromatherapist will be insured and have a qualification with a certificate indicating which professional association they belong to. These associations are important as they have a code of practice and ethics which the Aromatherapist has agreed to follow. A competent aromatherapist will work towards improving the state of mind of a person as this is strongly related to the natural healing process of the body. AROMATHERAPY IS A VOCATION AND REQUIRES DEDICATION The role of an aromatherapist is very difficult to define as it requires the therapist to be gifted with human qualities such as warmth and patience but also to possess a sound understanding of the workings of the human body, and to be accomplished in aromatic science.

THE PRACTICE OF AROMATHERAPY:

A professional practitioner is someone who will ensure that the client/patient fulfils the required prerequisites before treatment takes place. After being assured by the aromatherapist that all personal details remain strictly confidential, the client will be expected to answer some questions relevant to their current state of mind and physical health. This will allow the therapist to design the treatment best suited for the particular individual's needs. Once this is done, the client will be informed of the routine and explained what will happen next. If massage is the form of treatment, as it is in many instances the client will be asked to undress the parts of the body to be worked on and enabled to get ready in privacy. Once on the massage couch, the client's modesty will be protected at all times. It is important to understand that to obtain the most effect from a treatment it is necessary that the clients feel that they can trust the practitioner and let go. This is why all these precautions are taken in the same manner as would be expected from any other healthcare practitioner. A blend of essential oils and unrefined, organic vegetable oil (such as grapeseed oil or sweet almond oil) will be made up for the massage. The room should be kept warm at all times to meet the needs of the client. The massage, if given in full, will be from 'head to toe' and might possibly include the face and the scalp. The pressure applied will depend on the state of tension of the client's muscular system but in many cases the aromatherapist will concentrate on a gentle touch to help the client relax. After the treatment the client will be given further advice as to what to expect and what to do if any uncomfortable feelings develop later on. The whole procedure is designed to give a feeling of gentle care and relaxation. On many occasions the blend will include specific oils appropriate for particular conditions. This will depend on the specialised expertise of the aromatherapist.

The Aromatherapist's standards of training has to be acceptable to the main Professional Bodies which are currently involved in setting National Standards for the whole of the Aromatherapy Profession. One such Organisation is the International Federation of Aromatherapists whose members carry the initials MIFA after their name. Differentiation between aromatherapists is necessary as to protect the public from incompetent practice. There are many levels at which a practitioner can train in aromatherapy at the present. Aromatherapists in the UK do not automatically receive the same training, as the standards for the profession are still being discussed by government appointed organisations who are in consultation with the main Aromatherapy Associations. An aromatherapist carries a great responsibility towards the public and Schools offering tuition do not always impart this message to their trainees. One more point, not everyone is suited for the work or has the right background as Aromatherapy should never be treated as 'just' another means to earn a living. Again, one will have to turn to the Associations to obtain information about the various Schools available and choose whether the aim is to work in Complementary Therapies, as a beautician adding a nicely scented dimension

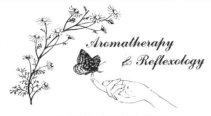
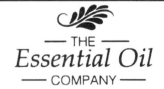

to the normal routine. Studies in Anatomy and Physiology, basic and advanced body massage, theory of aromatherapy, design of an individual treatment, counselling skills, a love of people, patience, warmth and empathy are all necessary to the practice of Aromatherapy. PROFESSIONAL ORGANISATIONS & REGULATING BODY The International Federation of Aromatherapists is an organisation founded ten years ago, by pioneers of Aromatherapy, in the UK and has some of the most experienced practitioners in its membership. It is a registered Charity, and its main aim is to play an informative role to the public and promote and maintain standards in Aromatherapy. It holds a Register of IFA Professional Aromatherapists and a list of accredited Centres for Aromatherapy training. It is worth noting that most Aromatherapists welcome the government intervention and the setting of a Regulatory Body with defined Standards for the whole profession, as this will help the public to recognise who is a genuine practitioner and who is not.

This chapter was written by Nicole PEREZ who is currently the Chairperson of the International Federation of Aromatherapist and has many years experience as an Aromatherapy Practitioner and Teacher at her own School. For further details on Courses please write including an s.a.e to:

The School of Holistic Aromatherapy, 108B Haverstock Hill LONDON NW3 2BD
Fax: 0171 284 1315

Anyone wishing to find out where there is an IFA Aromatherapist in their area or a Training Centre need to write with a self-addressed envelope to:
THE INTERNATIONAL FEDERATION OF AROMATHERAPISTS
Stamford House 2/4 Chiswick High Road, LONDON W4 1TH

AROMATHERAPY EVERYTHING?
"NO WAY!"
says Michael Van Moppes
Chairman of EOTA95, a trade association devoted to consumer protection.

Editors note: Michael has been accused of having a hobby of exposing the tricks of the trade.
His views are his, not ours.

When you visit Britains shops, take your hype detector with you.
Don't buy when it rings!

Watch for the ultimate overstated marketing buzzword; look for "aromatherapy everything" labels, and ignore them. They are the adman's dream, hatched in the get rich quick marketing dept. of large companies. By not buying their rubbish, we defend a wonderful branch of complimentary medicine from a highjack.

My family spends over £1000 per month in one of Britains top retailers. In 1994, I purchased a "Cinnamon and Myrrh aromatic bath oil, with the essential oil Neroli, 250ml for 75p." Myrrh was, at the time of Christ, one of the most valuable substances known to humanity, the first Christmas gift with frankincense and gold; it is still valuable today. Neroli is one of this planet's most precious liquids, retailing for £5000 to £12,000 per litre. I wondered how high the stopper was, when it was waved above the vat! In 1995, I purchased 3 bars of soap, beautifully boxed and costing £1.50 per 100gm. One contains (if we can believe the label) 1.2% of melissa oil, which costs about £5000 per litre (£6 for 1.2% of 100gms) from the farm that produces it: it takes 8,000 lemon balm plants to make one ounce of the oil. Another apparently contains Sandalwood oil at 0.45%. Sandalwood is a protected species and the market in its oil is greatly restricted, I would expect the retail price of 0.45gm to exceed £0.50p for the essential oil alone. All this in soaps costing £1.50: who do they think they are kidding?

How are these seemingly impossible claims made on supermarket shelves, without involving the Trades Descriptions Act? There are 2 reasons, and you can help on both. Firstly, the Trading Standards Dept rarely acts because they rarely get complaints (hint). Secondly, there is little protection for the word "natural" in English law (another hint; please write to your MP, and ask why the law does not oblige makers of synthetic and artificial products, which are packaged to fool you into believing they are natural, to be truthful about the goods they sell.

Why does this matter? Suppose you were a consumer with a medical condition that could be helped by herbal medicine. You buy a product in a supermarket which claims to contain that substance, (but does not) and you are disappointed with the result. Not knowing you have been sold a fake, you assume that herbs do not work for you, so you forsake aromatherapy. While you may lose the chance to improve your quality of life, consider who has benefited from selling you a 75p bottle containing "Myrrh" and "Neroli?" Well, the supermarket will have made a few pennies, and may actually be very happy to have evidence of malpractice by a supplier: they consider your satisfaction to be more important than the supplier's profits. So, please complain to Trading Standards, whose number you will find in the phone directory, under your local council. The shop will take Trading Standards very seriously.

Research into the testing of essential oils and other natural products is one of our prime functions. I have written a long series of articles about falsification and testing, and they are being published in Aromatherapy Quarterley and Health Food Business magazines.

EOTA95 can help with false (illegal) essential oils, which are usually sold by market traders, who retail "pure essential oils" for 99p or £1.99. Please read our advert in this book!

Why do you have to pay for wonderful complimentary medicine, when doctors have been allowed to employ practitioners within their surgeries since 1992, and would save a fortune on their synthetic drugs bill if they did? Many doctors do respect other branches of medicine, but many more don't: their reasons may have little to do with patient care. Although we are an association of essential oil suppliers, EOTA95 does not promote any particular branch of medicine against another: we believe that the only therapy that matters in each case; the one that is in the best interest of the patient. For example, we do not know of any remedy that can repair a worn and arthritic joint, so we support the surgeon who is able to replace it and the aromatherapist who can often ease the pain while waiting for the hospital lists to shorten. Write to us, and we will send you information that you can show your doctor.

In 1994, a Government Dept called the Medicines Control Agency (MCA) attacked herbal medicine. Millions of people (probably including you) rushed to defend it by writing your sincere views to your MPs: thank you. The civil servants who had said their Euro-law was irreversible, got the shock of their lives when Parliament climbed down and changed it. A great victory for our British system of Parliamentary democracy!

The MCA is very active in in consumer protection, and is your ultimate legal protection against firms making false medicinal claims for dubious products. The MCA has EOTA95's full support in this area, and we prefer to leave aromatherapy's contacts with the MCA to the other trade association, the ATC (Aromatherapy Trades Council), which we respect.

Since 1994, there has been a continuing series of media attacks against complimentary medicine, which EOTA95 monitors and answers when we know untruths have been published. You can help, by sending us such media articles; newspaper cuttings with the name of the paper, the author and the date; audio tapes or transcripts of radio programs with dates, programme names and times; and video tapes with the same proof of broadcast. Any such help may be of immeasurable value, it could even provide proof of malpractice.

Finally, EOTA95 intends to put an end to the product misrepresentations which are illustrated in this article. Dishonest businesses thrive in ignorance, so we intend to put all the knowledge of the scams in the public domain, just as we are doing now, by writing this article. We want to support a "public domain database," where matters like the price of the chemicals used to adulterate essential oils can be compared with the percentages of those same chemicals in this years crop, thus enabling you to prove how a 75p product containing neroli oil cannot possible be real.

EOTA is a non profit organisation. Our ultimate goal is to provide you, the consumer, with the knowledge to resist trade misconduct, through commonsense, education and the truth..

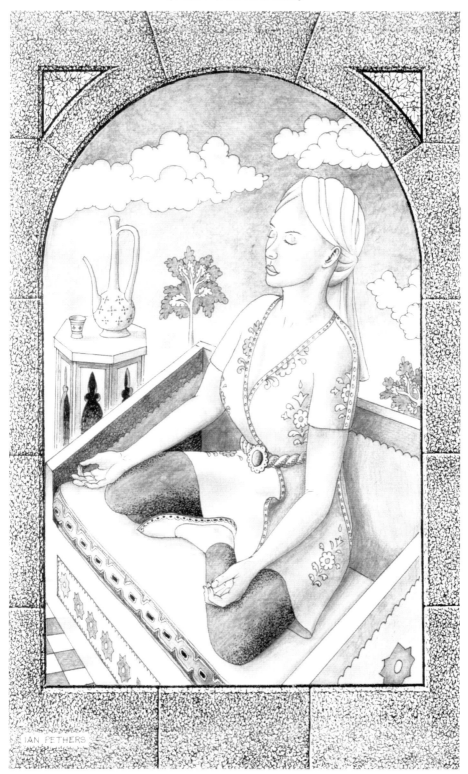

Spiritual Awarenes and Healing by Isis Nixon

A hundred years ago we would be living at a much slower pace than we do today. Communications were very much slower, transportation was not so readily available or as speedy and there was more time for contemplation and contact with nature for a great many people. When we look around our world today, we wonder what has happened. Everyone seems to be in a rush and there never seems to be enough time, particularly enough time to sit quietly and make a sense of peace and deep meditation within. The third dimensional materialistic world appears to hold sway and a deeper spiritual connection with all life is not so evident. Stress is common place and the doctors' surgeries are full of those who are invariably sent away with tranquillisers or antibiotics as a gesture of healing. What has happened to the balance and harmony of our lives? Does the pursuit of money, ambition and prestige truly take precedence over our health and well-being and indeed happiness?

In a world where we are inundated with persuasive advertising wherever we look and whatever we read, where subliminals are common-place, what can we do to find truth of ourselves and recreate the joy of the mind, the body and the soul. Fortunately, there are many who have opted out of the so called 'rat race' and the stress that can bring and are looking for alternatives. Alternatives that are truly very ancient indeed. Last year in America for the first time, alternative medicine was used more than allopathic medicine and the trend towards natural remedies and techniques to relieve pain, suffering and create ease where there was dis-ease, is on the increase. At last, the cause and not the effect of dis-ease is being looked at and the days of taking a painkiller for all ills can, with intention, be a thing of the past. Virtually all physical level dis-ease has an emotional co-ordinate. And dis-ease and painful emotions go together, so that by healing the dis-ease means also healing the emotions that go with it.

Mostly our lives are filled with emotional pain and with traumas and with shocks of some degree and most of us are taught from young children not to express our feelings, but to swallow them deep down inside. Instead of allowing ourselves to feel the pain and release it, emotions get stuck. And where pain remains within and has no other release, it manifests as physical illness. The answer as always has been in healing the emotional cause and as this happens and the love goes deep inside, then all the painful emotions and traumas come to the surface and we are able to re-connect with the pain long enough to finish it and let it go. With the emotion released, physical dis-ease usually goes also.

Anger, frustration, grief, loneliness and fear are more often the cause of human dis-ease than any bacteria, virus or organic malfunction. So the key for us all to look at is how we can become whole and healed and the various methods available to us to make this a reality. By understanding that we create our own stress and our own dis-ease and that we are responsible for our own lives, gives the understanding that because our intention and thoughts created our situation, then of course by changing the thoughts and intentions, everything can change as well.

We all tend to repeat the patterns of our parents and our habits and our beliefs about ourselves condition our responses. Luckily, there are wonderful techniques available today to overcome and alter the patterns of our lives and far more joyful, spontaneous and happy ways of living.

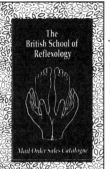

A number of techniques are available, such as relaxation, visualisation, counselling, meditation, altogenic training and healing that can create the necessary change. The key is the willingness to explore what is available and to find out what suits you best, remembering always that you yourself have the power to be your own best healer by working with energies such as Reiki.

Reiki

This most powerful 'hands-on' healing technique can be learnt in a weekend and is the way that Jesus and the Buddha were able to heal those that came to them in the past. Reiki is simply translated as Universal Love Force and is received by a series of attunements from a Master who touches the head, the heart and the hands. To receive a Reiki treatment you simply lie quietly and allow the practitioner to move their hands across your body while listening to soft music and a wonderful sense of euphoria and bliss can result. Receiving regular Reiki treatments can move the most stubborn physical, mental and emotional blocks, but to do it yourself is even more beneficial , as of course you can give yourself a treatment every day, when ever you wish. After an attunement, healing energy will pour through your hands and feet and once you have been 'switched on' by a Master, then you have it for life. Reiki brings about a cellular change, rejuvenation and a balance and harmonising and even blending of mind, body and spirit. It is the most wonderful healing method available on the planet at this time. There are no examinations and there is no long training involved, simply a willingness to help others and an open heart. It can also be used most effectively for distant healing, whether a person, a situation or the planet. Because Reiki healing affects the whole mind, body and spirit and does not always necessitate putting the hands on the body, it can be used for the more extreme cases of shock, accident, burns and of course childbirth. It is the greatest gift.

Massage

Massage is probably one of the most sought after as well as the oldest and simplest skills because it is something we all do instinctively. Not only does it improve circulation and relaxes tense muscles, but aids digestion, stimulates the lymphatic system and speeds elimination of waste products. Massage can stimulate or sedate and is very much part of a sense of nurturing and nourishment between one person and another. The value of touch cannot be over estimated, for without touch we die. Children brought up in families that touch each other and hug each other are healthier and more able to withstand pain and infection than children deprived of touch. As a result they are happier and more at peace. Ideally massage starts from childhood, providing warmth and security and soothes tension and stress.

Many businesses now have a massage therapist on hand because so much stress is alleviated by it. Deep tissue massage is probably the most effective for most as it gets to the tension that is held, that most of us don't even recognise. A lighter massage with essential oils can be delightful and therapeutic as the oils bring their properties into the blood stream and this is known as aromatherapy. Herbs and spices, woods and resins, flowers, berries, leaves, twigs and grasses give their oil to be blended by the aromatherapist to great effect. The pituatary gland of the body, situated within the brain is affected by essential oils and as the master-gland, determines the whole of the body's physical well-being and the balance of our personality. Scent is as important as touch and smells help us to recall the past and can bring much pleasure. A truly sensual experience that can release stress build up from the mind and physical tensions from the body as the oils are massaged into the skin. This most ancient art has been developed over thousands of years and we are discovering it again.

THE HEALTHY OPTIONS FOR
MIND, BODY AND SPIRIT

Shambhala is a sacred site on the slopes of the legendary Glastonbury Tor. We overlook the Vale of Avalon and you can enjoy our themed bedrooms, gardens, pond, flock of doves, wonderful vegetarian food. Come and enjoy a few days rest and relaxation; or feel loved and looked after with one of our two, three, or four day healing breaks; you'll find peace, love and laughter.

We offer therapies for your personal, spiritual and physical needs.
Reiki Healing
Powerful, 'hands on ' healing on many levels, from a Reiki Master.
Reflexology
Working on the feet to relieve stress, emotional, and physical pain.
Holistic massage
Gentle full body massage with fragrant oils.
Aromatherapy
Massage with essential oils specially mixed for each person.
Warm water Rebirthing
Conscious energy breathing clears emotional and physical blocks.
Private counselling
Get problems eased, new pictures of reality and fresh insights.
Deep tissue massage
Resistances held deep within the body are released and healed.
Learn to channel
Learn to talk with your guardian angel or guide for clarity.
Sauna and Jacuzzi
Relax, unwind and let go of stress and tension in the perfect setting.

Shambhala

The heart of the Heart
Centre for Spiritual Growth and Healing
Coursing Batch, Glastonbury, Somerset, BA6 8BH UK.
Telephone: 01458 831797 / 833081 Fax: 01458 834751
Email: shambhala@dial.pipex.com
Internet: http://www.isleofavalon.co.uk /shambala.html

Reflexology

A delightful form of massage is reflexology, which stimulates the reflex points of the feet, the hands and the head. Another ancient therapy being used for over five thousand years, it is one of the most popular today. It not only works well with all other forms of medicine, but is simple, safe and very effective and of course you have no need to undress! Particularly after surgery, reflexology comes into its own and can also be used to reduce or eliminate the side-effects of allopathic drugs. A state of relaxation is induced, tension eased, circulation improved and toxins released and eliminated from the body.

Homeopathy

Many are now turning to homeopathy rather than allopathic medicine and this natural system of medicine, using extremely low doses of remedies derived from plants, minerals and metals is available to treat all types of ailment, by stimulating the body's own healing power. Harmless in themselves, these remedies do not have the side-effects of modern medicine and can be taken safely, even by the youngest children.

Nutrition

Nutrition forms the basis of alternative medicine, because without the right raw materials, our bodies can never be truly healthy. We are literally what we eat and no one's needs are the same as anyone elses. A well balanced diet is essential and knowledge of additives, chemicals and pesticides on our food needs to be understood. Using organic, naturally produced foods will pay the greatest dividends of all and a rise in health shops and health projects is well known. Fast-food is not the way to good health, nor is a diet of chips and chocolate! By eating well, energy increases, the immune system is strengthened and degenerative disorders such as cancer, diabetes, heart disease and arthritis can be prevented. Perhaps the most basic and important part of our lifestyle, your diet is vital for a healthy body and mind.

Often in life we have a major trauma and can go into deep shock. If you have been abused sexually or emotionally as a child, the trauma is often locked deep inside the sub-conscious and it is only later on that you are able in a safe space to recall exactly what happened. Although various methods are available to bring up the past to be healed it is always the memory that haunts us. If you are seeking to let go such a memory and to bring anger, frustration, hatred or grief out of the body once and for all, then energetic rebirthing is the answer. Because it works at a cellular level, the memory fades and the 'charge' of the emotion taken out. And like all the best natural remedies, it is so simple.

All you have to do is breathe in a particular way, floating in the warm water of a jacuzzi! Although very few practitioners can do this, it is well worth seeking out those who offer it. It is such a treatment and a release of negative energies, it is profoundly life changing and is literally a 'rebirth'. It is possible to be 'in therapy' for 20 years and not achieve what can be done with three rebirthing sessions. For it is not so much the understanding of the mind that is needed, or the recreation of the past and its emotional tugs, but a total release and a complete clearing on all levels. Extreme cases, such as rape, incest, violence of all kinds, depravation and not surprisingly, lack of love, can be let go of and a true rebirth of spirit can occur.

Often in life, we simply need someone to talk to. Someone outside the situation we find ourselves in, someone who doesn't take sides or who is giving us platitudes or judgement. This is where counselling comes in and is so very valuable. It has been said that if there were professional listeners, then the mental hospitals would be empty. We all need a helping hand during a crisis, whether it is a relationship breakdown, a bereavement or a change of lifestyle or circumstances. A good counsellor will let you talk and also by bringing you into a heart space rather than a mind space, allow you to feel what is really going on. As the heart is the place where the 'knowing' is and the intuition functions, here the answers lie. Decisions made from the heart work, decisions made from the mind sometimes work! Samaritans do a wonderful job of listening. Perhaps in our lives we could do a better job for ourselves.

Although there is a pot pourri of therapies and remedies available through alternative medicine, the most important thing of all is to remember balance. Without the balance and harmonising of mind, body and spirit, we cannot function well. If our connection to the divine is not strong and acknowledged, then very little else has value. It is this spark of life, this joy, this spontaneous vivacity and aliveness that makes life worth living. Children have it, they do not worry about the mortgage or the next promotion. This is because they live in the now moment. They are not concerned about the past or the future. Contentment comes from inside, by being at peace with yourself and with your creator. Remembering that thoughts can pollute as much as actions harm and destroy. Remembering that arms are for hugging and hearts for feeling and the giving and receiving of love. And above all, we are all here for a purpose. We all have a vision of how to create a world of peace and joy and it begins right here and now. In you.

Chapter 8

Company News

I n this day and age with a vast selection of similar products to choose from it is important to have some knowledge of why a particular product could be suitable for your requirement. Therefore to assist the reader a selection of the advertisers have submitted an analysis of the products they have featured in this publication. Should you require more information please contact the relative company directly.

Tea Tree Oil is the most powerful antiseptic known to man, can help to ease many minor skin problems and is also a natural bactericide, it also has a slight anaesthetic effect.

There are many Tea Tree products available, from pure oil to shampoos, conditioners, toothpaste, antiseptic cream, soap, skin wash and hand/body lotions.

Information was supplied by;- **Thursday Plantation Tea Tree Oil . Telephone 01274488511**

Robert Tisserand - Aromatherapy Guru and an exponent on essential oil safety describes three exquisite, popular Tisserand oils and their usage.

" The three essential oils described here all have floral aromas and are safe to use in a variety of ways from bathing to general massage to vaporisation ".

GERANIUM - is suitable for all skin types with a balancing effect on the emotions.

YLANG - YLANG - is a sensual and soothing oil with a euphoric fragrance. To elevate and stabilise emotions.

JASMINE - is a delicate floral scent which is sensual and luxuriant - used widely in fragrances.

Information supplied by:- **Tisserand Aromatherapy Products Ltd., Tel:- 01273325666**

An enchanting world of Essential Oils.

Welcome to the world of Echo Essential Oils and Associated Products. Echo has earned a reputation associated only with high quality products and service. As a company EHCO do not believe in or use any animal testing whatsoever, hence our CAT A listing with the RSPCA and BUVA.

We are approved suppliers to many teaching colleges, hospitals, clinics, professional therapists and High Street stores. We are an established exporter to Europe and Japan.

Echo Essential Oils hold full membership of NORA and we are currently working under the guidelines of the BSI. We expect to gain our BSI Quality Assurance Award in the Spring of 1997.

We are stockists of :- pure essential oils, carrier oils, the Elimay range of self-help and sport aid blends. Aroma shampoo, conditioner, foam bath, beautiful wooded presentation boxes, burners and a very select range of fragrance oils.

Comprehensive mail-order, trade and professional price lists available from:-

Echo Essential Oils,44 Chestnut Drive, Congleton, Cheshire CW12 4UB.

Information supplied by :- **ECHO Essential Oils. Tel :- 011260277680.**

A new product.

New to the natural health market is **Lavender Componiom** in a unique roll-on-bottle. It is a blend of natural oils featuring the most versatile lavender. It has a diversity of uses from treating cuts, grazes, spots etc, use on temples to soothe headache pains and to induce sleep. See mail order offer in "Readers Offer" section of this book.

Information supplied by :- **RAH Ltd. Tel ; 01706229779**

Can Aromatherapy Help Me?

Everyone can benefit at some level from aromatherapy treatment. There are many conditions which can be helped directly by aromatherapy, ranging from such things as Eczema and backache to stress and depression. You do not need to be ill to consult an aromatherapist. How many of us can honestly say that the stresses of the 20th century life have no adverse effect on our lives. What better way to unwind that with a deeply relaxing massage from a skilled and sensitive person. Obviously if you are receiving treatment from a Doctor or a have a serious medical condition you should consult your Doctor first.

For more information on Aromatherpy please contact :- The London School of Aromatherapy, for complete details please see advertisement in Aromatherapy chapter of this book.

Information supplied by :- **The London School of Aromatherpy.**

Essential Balms

This popular and versatile product is Meadows version of the popular Essential type balms.

The difference is that Elephant balm is totally natural, the ingredients are:- Beeswax, Lavender Oil, Rosemary, Tee Tree, Peppermint and Cinnamon Leaf.

This balm can be used on aches, pains, muscle strains, headaches, minor burns, bites and as a chest rub.

10p from the sale of every jar is donated to Howells and Port Lympne wild animal parks, which has a charity status.

Information supplied by :- **Meadows of Canterbury Ltd. Tel:- 01227731489.**

Massage

Dog Oil to be used wherever massage is beneficial.

Information supplied by :- **Masons Products. Tel :- 01706379817.**

Natural Health Science

The School of Natural Science is a correspondence college providing 'home study' courses in most alternative therapies, E.G. Homeopathy, herbalism, reflexology, nutrition, acupuncture. There are 20 courses which are all individually tutored. Successful students are awarded a diploma which enables them to start their own business, should they wish.

Information supplied by :- **The School of Natural Health Sciences. Tel :- 01714139577.**

Summerbee Products.

Summerbee Products is a company supplying in excess of eighty health products. The products are food supplements, honeybee products, aromatherapy oils and products and cosmetics. High quality is guaranteed and prices are very competitive.

Summerbee is an advertiser in this publication.

For full details please contact :- Summerbee Products, Windsor House, Lime Avenue, Torquay. TQ2.5 JL. Tel:- 01803212965.

Information supplied by :- **Summerbee Products. Tel:- 018033212965**

Tee Tree Pure Essential Oil.

Used by the Aborigine people in the outback, tee tree is one of the few essential oils that can be used undiluted on the skin yet is potent against fungal, bacterial and viral infections. The sometimes fatal superbug (MRSA) that is becoming resistant to antibiotics has found an adversary in this ancient remedy. Research has shown that *in-vitro* tea tree can kill the bacterium responsible. Described as the medicine kit in a bottle, tea tree can help many conditions including Influenza, athletes foot, thrush, dandruff and spots.

For more information contact The Essential Oil Co.Ltd., quoting ref: HO.

Tel:- 10256332737.Fax:- 01256332119. E-mail ESSOIL@AOL.COM

Information supplied by :- **The Essential Oil Co. Ltd.**

Aromatherapy Treatments

AROMATHERAPY AND THE COMMON COLD

One pleasant and often highly effective way of fighting the common cold is by using Pure Essential Oils to help clear congestion and boost the immune system.

The Natural Life Aromatherapy laboratory produces one outstanding mixture of Essential oils for this purpose called '*Care for Sinus*`. It is a carefully balanced mixture of *Eucalyptus*, *Pine Needle, Peppermint and Tea Tree* Pure Essential Oils. '*Care for Sinus* 'can be used diluted in an essence burner, sprinkled onto a handkerchief, or just a drop on the pillow may help ease nasal congestion during the night.

An effective method if the nose is very blocked is to put just two drops of '*Care for Sinus*` oil into a bowl of hot water. Close your eyes, cover your head with a thick towel and inhale the steam vapour - though this potent inhalation method should not be used by people suffering from asthma.

'*Care for Sinus*' has become the company's top seller this winter and the oil is now available by post direct from :-
Natural Life Aromatherapy Ltd,
Lifestyle Natural Health,
4, The Centre, Hersham Green, Walton-on-Thames, Surrey, KT12 4HL
Tele/Fax; 01932 228285 Tele; 01932 269245 / 01242 252007

* *Natural Life Aromatherapy* is committed to producing only pure and natural essential oils and teaching people how to effectively and safely use such oils at home, through their *'Leisure Learning*` *Programme.*

AROMATHERAPY AND STRESS

Stress overload is a common complaint of today's lifestyle - and one which can frequently be helped by aromatherapy. In fact more and more people are using Pure Essential Oils as part of a regime to help alleviate stress and aid relaxation

There are several ways of using these incredibly useful and effective oils - such as adding a few drops into a bath, vaporising them in an essence burner, or blending them with a carrier oil and gently massaging them into the body where they are absorbed into the system.

The Natural Life Aromatherapy laboratory has introduced a special mixture of Pure Essential Oils called '*Care for Stress*` - a carefully balanced mixture of pure essential oils of French *Lavender* and *Vetiver* - a musky smelling oil that is known as the 'Oil of Tranquillity` in the East because of its deeply relaxing qualities.

Adding a few drops of **'Care for Stress** ` to your bath and relaxing in the warm water for ten minutes, or just a drop on a handkerchief under your pillow may help you relax and sleep more restfully.

'Care for Stress ` is now available by mail order from
Natural Life Aromatherapy Ltd, Lifestyle Natural Health, 4 The Centre, Hersham Green, Walton-on-Thames, Surrey. KT12 4HU.
Tele/Fax: 01932 228385   Tele 01932 269245 / 01242 252007

* *Natural Life Aromatherapy Ltd*, is committed to producing only Pure and Natural Essential oils and teaching people how to effectively and safely use such oils at home, through their *'Leisure Learning Programme* `

AROMATHERAPY AND INSECT CONTROL

The longed for Summer and holidays in the sun can so often be spoilt by those irritating insects and painful insect bites that accompany these delightful times - especially in the evening when many insects are most likely to bite and particularly near water!

Natural Life Aromatherapy **Insect Repellent** ` is a carefully balanced mixture of the Pure Essential Oils of *Lavender, Lemongrass* and *Citronella* and is the perfect answer to averting the little pests from spoiling your enjoyment..

There are several ways of using this useful and effective product - such as sprinkling a few drops onto rugs and cushions; or diluted in an essence burner. If you do not have a burner, try adding just two drops to a candle wick before lighting or a few drops to a bowl of hot water.

Another method of use is by blending *Natural Life Aromatherapy* premier grade **Aloe Vera Gel** with **Insect Repellent** and massaging this into the skin before going our. Blend just *10 drops* of Insect Repellent with *100ml* of **Aloe Vera Gel** and massage into the skin. *Natural Life Aromatherapy* **Aloe Vera Gel** is also an excellent 'after sun` skin treatment, being soothing, cooling, healing and moisturising.

Insect Repellent and **Aloe Vera Gel** are now available by mail order from
Natural Life Aromatherapy Ltd, Lifestyle Natural Health, 4 The Centre
Hersham Green, Walton on Thames, Surrey. KT12 4HL.
Tele/Fax: 01932 228285   Tele: 01932 269245 / 01242 252007

* *Natural Life Aromatherapy* is committed to producing only Pure and Natural Essential Oils and teaching people how to use them effectively and safely at home, through their *'Leisure Learning Programme* `.

'REVITALISING` AROMATHERAPY

Lethargy, exhaustion and fatigue are all far too familiar occurrences for many people in all walks of life - these are conditions which can very often be helped by *Aromatherapy*
In fact *Aromatherapy* includes a vast range of Pure Essential Oils which can help relieve   many ailments.

There are several ways of using these incredibly useful and effective Essential Oils - such as adding a few drops to the bath water...vaporising them when they are diluted in water in an essence burner...or blending them with a carrier oil and gently massaging them into the body, where they are absorbed into the system.

The *Natural Life Aromatherapy* laboratory has introduced several special mixes of Pure Essential Oils which best combine to help a number of conditions.

Revitalising is one such blend of Pure, Natural Essential Oils. It contains a carefully balanced mixture of *Basil,* an oil reputed to help clear the head and aid concentration and *Grapefruit* to uplift and refresh - also useful for helping to relieve headaches. **Revitalising** is particularly helpful to relieve lethargy, exhaustion and fatigue.
(If symptoms persist always consult a medical practitioner.)
Basil should be avoided during pregnancy.

Suggested uses: Ideal for the business traveller and useful for 'jet lag` Sprinkle a few drops of **Revitalising** mixed Essential Oils in your car or onto a handkerchief to help you through your day of hurry and bustle. An essence burner is another good way of experiencing the benefits of these **Revitalising** Essential Oils; or just four drops in your early morning bath can invigorate you for the day ahead

Revitalising is now available by mail order form *Natural Life Aromatherapy Ltd,*
Lifestyle Natural Heath, 4 The Centre, Hersham Green, Walton on Thames, Surrey KT12 4HL
Tele/Fax: 01932 228285 Tele; 01932 269245 / 01242 252007

* *Natural Life Aromatherapy Ltd*, is committed to producing only Pure and Natural Essential oils and teaching people how to effectively and safely use such oils at home, through their *'Leisure Learning Programme`*

Information supplied by:- Natural Life Aromatherapy

Arbonne Pure Skin Care.

Arbonne uses concentrated herbal and botanical extracts. These products have never contained any petrolatum, mineral oil, wax, paraffin, artificial perfumes or harmful levels of preservatives. The company philosophy is to help protect the earth's natural resources and they are an active proponent of recyclable packaging, no animal testing and no use of animal or human by-products is in their skin care products.
Information supplied by :- **Arbonne (UK) Ltd., Tel :- 01280824599.**

Health & Beauty from the Dead Sea.

Finders International Ltd., the pioneers and market leaders in Dead Sea Mineral skin care, first introduced the therapeutic and healing properties of Dead Sea minerals to the United Kingdom fifteen years ago.

The beneficial effects of the Dead Sea minerals on the skin have been known for centuries. The Legendary Queen Cleopatra knew well the extraordinary properties of the minerals found in the waters of the Dead Sea- the lowest place on earth. These minerals have the remarkable ability to attract and retain moisture, and moisture retention is the most important factor in maintaining a healthy skin. Since the launch of the Dead Sea Magik, the thousands of users have reported to us the wonderful effect these products had on their skin.

By adopting the Finders Dead Sea Magik therapeutic skin and scalp routine, which is affordable, practical and easy to follow, your mind and body will feel revitalised. Finders Dead Sea Magik health and beauty natural skin care range helps to reduce scars or blemishes, brighten dull complexions and revitalise dehydrated skin. It is also beneficial for skin disorders, such as eczema, psoriasis and other skin complaints.

The Dead Sea Magik products are a naturally based range, which are ideal for all skin types. The range consists of products for the face, body and hair, and a soothing, relaxing additive for the bath.

The Dead Sea Magik facial routine consists of cleansing morning and evening with the Magik Cleansing Bar and pat dry. In he morning follow with Magik Moisturiser and in the evening follow with Magik Super Night Cream. For a deep cleansing routine once a week, apply the Magik Mud Mask, leave on for 1- 5 minutes, then rinse thoroughly. Follow with Magik Super Night Cream.

The Dead Sea Magik body routine, which will help normalise and rebalance the skin, consists of adding 1-4 handfuls of Magik Bath Salts to a warm bath and soak for twenty minutes. Rinse with clear water and pat dry. Apply Magik Body Lotion after your bath. Apply the Magik Body Lotion twice daily for dry skin.

Finders International also operates a free Helpline facility on 01580211055, for personal advice on your skin care regime.

Finders Dead Sea Magik range can be obtained nationwide via health food stores, including Holland & Barret and General Nutrition Centres (GNC), independent chemists and department stores, or by mail order on 01580211055.

Infromation supplied by :- **Finders International.**

Vegan Beauty.

An exclusive range of high quality perfumes, toiletries and skin care products, all carefully blended from safe, long established animal free ingredients are marketed by Dolma.

For more information on Vegan cosmetics please contact:- Lesley Peters, CICAW, P.O.Box 5, Manchester M26 1PE. Tel. 01204578119.

The Animal Free Shoppers can be purchased from:- The Vegan Society, 7 Battle Road, St. Leonard's - on- Sea. East Sussex. TN37. 7AA.

Information supplied by :- **Dolma Tel :- 01159634237.**

Gluten free bread

Latest technology in specialised baking has made it possible to produce well raised gluten-free loaves without the need to use de-glutenized wheatstarch. This means that wheat allergy sufferers in particular now have proper well-raised, tasty loaves to enjoy. Normal wheat-starch-based gluten-free breads can not be used in a wheat-free diet.
Information supplied by :- **General Dietary Ltd., Tel :- 01813362323.**

Organic Cheddar Cheese

Mature cheddar cheese made by Alvis Bros Ltd., uses organic milk from Soil Association approved farms, it is suitable for vegetarians and the health conscious consumer.
Information supplied by :- **Alvis Bros Ltd. Tel :- 01934862320.**

Soya Cheese

Scheese is a soya based 100% free alternative to cows milk cheese. It is available in nine varieties and suitable for any animal free product diet.
Information supplied by :- **Bute Island Foods. Tel :- 011700505117.**

Meat Free Haggis.

Macsween produce Vegetarian haggis, it is approved by the Vegetarian Society and is vegan friendly. The ingredients are kidney beans, lentils, mixed vegetables, nuts, seasonings and spices.
Information supplied by :- **Macsween of Edinburgh. Tel :- 01314402555.**

Preserves.

Thursday Cottage Ltd., marmalades, jams, curds and diabetic preserves are traditionally made in small open pans. The best quality whole fruit is used with raw sugar (fructose in the case of diabetic preserves) to make preserves which are wholesome and delicious.
Information supplied by :- **Thursday Cottage Ltd., Tel :- 01297445555.**

Fruit Spreads & Vegesauces.

100% all fruit spreads are not like ordinary jams, they are made entirely with fruit and fruit juice and sugars derived from the fruit and the juices. The high fruit and low sugar content allows a full fresh flavour of the natural fruit, the low calorie content is approximately half that of ordinary jams, this is helpful for slimming and diabetics.

Vegesauces are made with vegemince, a blended vegetable protein that contains no meat but has a satisfying hearty taste and texture. There are many varieties, the most popular being Bolognese, Chilli and Curry.

Both the Preserves and Vegesauces are suitable for Vegetarians.

Information supplied by :- **Meridian Foods Ltd., Tel :- 01490413151.**

Organic fruit juices

Eden is Germany's leading range of fresh vegetable juices. The range comprises of three pure juices, each free from artificial colour and preservatives and rich in nutrients- Carrot Juice, Vegetable Cocktail and Beetroot Juice. The juices are produced using an organic gardening method developed by a group of vegetarian farmers in the 1890's.

Eden vegetable juices are cold pressed raw from freshly grown organic vegetables which are picked when mature to ensure that nutrient levels are at their peak.

To help demonstrate the suitability of its three juice products in cookery as well as for drinking neat, Eden has produced a recipe booklet "Juice Up Family Mealtime". This spotlights eight vegetarian recipes which combine beta carotene rich organic vegetables with Eden juices. Copies are available by calling 01798875527.

Approved by the Soil Association in meeting its organic standard, 750 ml bottles of Eden Organic Vegetable Juices are available from health food retailers or by contacting Sandoz Nutrition on 01923266122.

Information supplied by :- **Christine Ball PR . Tel :- 01798875527.**

Pure fruit juice

La Verja 100% pure fruit juices are available in most health foods stores.

Produced in Spain the juices are made from locally grown crops of Grade A fruits, picked and processed when ripe. They are additive and preservative free, with no added sugars or artificial sweeteners.

Vitalia organic pressed juices are made in France by a leading manufacturer, the range consists of red and white grape, prune, vegetable, carrot, and beetroot. All of the varieties are suitable for Vegetarians.

Information supplied by :- **SDF. Trade & Promotion Limited. Tel :- 01713800906.**

Wheat free Oatcakes

Traditional oatcakes are baked in Scotland by Nairns, the No.1 Oatcake producer, these traditional oatcakes are baked solely with oatmeal and without wheat flour.

They can be topped with cheese, pate, marmalade, jams or almost anything, even eaten with soups.

Outside of Scotland most larger branches of the supermarket chains are stockists.

Nairns Rough Oatcakes, a rougher blend of oatmeal has been used to bake these traditional Scottish oatcakes, the recipe is free from sugar and wheat flour. These can also be topped with virtually anything.

Outside of Scotland they are available from Holland & Barret, Waitrose and Wm Morrison.
Information supplied by :- **Simmers of Edinburgh., Tel :- 01313340853.**

Food Hampers.

Healthy Hampers™ offer a vegetarian and vegan hamper gift service with foods (many organic) that contain no artificial colours, additives or preservatives. The hampers provide a fast, reliable and courteoius service all year round. Coupled with excellent value for money at a national and international level. For more information call **01252878698.**
Information supplied by :- **Healthy Hampers. Tel :- 01252878698.**

Oil of peppermint.

Oil of peppermint has many diverse uses from relieving the symptoms of irritable bowel syndrome to helping clear a blocked nose. This traditional herbal remedy is a useful and versatile addition to the family first aid kit, it is available in capsules or tablets, there is also pure Japanese oil of peppermint.
Information supplied by :- **Bennet Natural Products.**

Pure Honey

Manuka honey is a high purity mono-floral honey. This honey is prized by the Maoris in its native New Zealand for its curative properties, it is known to have a very high anti-bacterial action and is also believed to help with stomach ulcer discomfort, as well as having an excellent flavour.
Information supplied by :- **Anmark Ltd. Tel :- 01718334187.**

Herbal Drink

Vitall the herbal *"Health & Fitness"* drink, taken like a tonic, 53 mls twice a day, is a unique blend of 16 herbs ands has been used professionally over many years by leading international herbalists before now being available commercially. Whatever age, level of activity, or state of health, most people soon acquire more energy, better sleep and clearer thought. This increased energy and the detoxifying and strengthening effect of the herbs can give a better chance of avoiding or dealing with the many illnesses of this stressful age.

Being overweight is becoming a national problem, not just a personal one and **Vitall** *natural weight loss* products provide a natural, well researched and safe solution. *Citrimax* changes the way the body processes fat and *Cookies*, which are oat and herb based and high in fibre, provide a delicious, healthy alternative snack.

Vitall *Botanics* have been designed to give the skin the care it deserves. It is the largest organ of the body, and has to cope with increasing stress and pollution. The skin treatment products nourish the skin to help it retain a natural radiance. They are high in natural active ingredients but free of substances considered to be skin irritants.

Overall the Vitall range is the ideal choice for people who want to radiate well-being.
Information supplied by :- **Vitall Ltd. Tel :- 01203351356.**

Aloe Vera.

Aloe vera has been used for thousands of years. Among the many benefits sited by users, aloe vera has become best known for its soothing and cleansing properties and is often taken to promote digestive well being. ESI is a leading manufacturer of organic, certified aloe vera which uses the whole leaf and inner gel. The products are cold pressed, non pasteurised and high in mucopolysaccharides.

ESI are the first European company to have been awarded the IASC independent seal of approval for their aloe vera products. This certification guarantees purity and quality of the complete range from ESI. Aloe Vera comes in several forms so read on to find out which one best suits your needs.

Aloe Vera plus colon cleanse juice uses double strength organic aloe vera and aloe pulp to provide natural fibre; FOS which promotes friendly intestinal bacteria and milk thistle; dandelion and liquorice are added for their cleansing properties. The resultant formula maintains digestive regularity and helps promote intestinal well being.

Aloe Vera double strength juice has a unique formation where the water content naturally present in the leaf is halved providing twice the enzyme and nutrient level to maximise beneficial activity.

Aloe Vera plus digestive aid juice is a unique blend of double strength organic aloe vera with peppermint oil, papaya, camomile and slippery elm combined to soothe the digestive system.

Aloe Vera Capsules are a convenient "one a day" method of taking aloe vera. Equivalent to 123ml of 12,000 mg juice the formulation is a unique blend of organic whole leaf and inner gel available in 30 and 90 capsule packs.

Aloe Vera Skin Care System is 100% pure aloe gel from the inner leaf. The bio active treatment moisturise, softens and helps restore dry and damaged skin. The gel is useful in treating minor burns, sun burn, scars and general skin irritations.

Information supplied by :- **ESI Ltd. Tel :- 01222388422.**

Aloe Vera Juice.

Natural Options Aloe 1000.
Setting a higher standard for Aloe Vera Juice. Aloe 1000 is the finest aloe vera juice in the world. It is produced using a revolutionary, patented, whole leaf cold pressing process, making Aloe 1000 up to five times stronger than filleted products. Aloe 1000 exceeds the International Aloe Council standard.

Information supplied by :- **R&B Marketing . Tel :- 01482870962.**

Aloe Vera a Natural Herb.

Aloe Vera, a natural Herb given to us by God has been known for centuries for its healing properties. In the 6000 years or more since its qualities were first recognised, aloe vera has been called the " fountain of youth" and the " first aid plant" because it has been known to act as a palliative for medical problems from food allergies to sore throats, from digestive problems to rheumatism and arthritis, colitis, ulcers and inflammatory problems of all kinds. For more information on organic supplies please contact Echo Healthcare, Woodside, Melmerby, Ripon, N.Yorks.

Information supplied by :-   **Echo Healthcare. Tel :- 01765640440.**

Iron + Oxygen = Energy.

Spatone Iron Plus is clinically proven, easily absorbed and guarantees no constipation. This natural Spa Water contains iron and helps to relieve lethargy, sluggishness and improves your general health.

Information supplied by:- **Trefriw Wells Spa Ltd. Tel:- 01492640057.**

OxCgen TM

OxCgen ™ capsules are a truly unique product releasing activated oxygen-, a unique and powerful mixture of oxygen and ozone initially into the digestive tract (where it will eliminate anaerobic pathogens, bacteria and fungi such as candida) and then throughout the body where oxygen deficient diseases such as Aids, cancer, colds, flu, arthritis and other anaerobic invasions can be addressed.

Information supplied by :-   **Resonance Tel:- 01519205306**

Research shows Calcium supplements should also contain Magnesium.

It is well known that you need plenty of calcium to maintain strong bones, but new research is showing that an optimum intake of another material, magnesium, is also essential.

Daily intakes of calcium and magnesium together have been shown to help maintain the calcium content of weight bearing bone. In one study the Medical Tribune reported almost 75% of women taking a magnesium supplement experienced bone density increases.

Dairy produce is rich in calcium, but lower in the magnesium required to utilise calcium properly. Magnesium when taken with calcium may also provide other benefits, such as the prevention of kidney stone formation.

Information supplied by :- **Vatabiotics Ltd., Tel:- 01819631880.**

Solgar gold label range of vitamins

Established in 1947, Solgar Vitamins is well respected for its leading-edge product development and quality of manufacture.

The Solgar gold label range of vitamins, minerals, herbs and amino acids is available from health foods stores nation-wide and in more than 30 countries internationally. For details of your local stockist and a *free Desk Reference* write to Solgar Vitamins, Aldbury, Tring, Herts HP23 5PT.

Information supplied by :-   **Solgar Vitamins.**

Hypoallergenic supplements from Quest.

Quest provide a range of hypoallergenic supplements all manufactured to the highest pharmaceutical standards. Within the range are comprehensive multivitamin formulations, chelated mineral supplements, vitamin C, B complex, evening primrose oils, Kyolic aged garlic and amino acids. The vast majority of products are free from all the following ingredients: yeast, wheat, gluten, artificial preservatives, colours and flavours; added starch sucrose, lactose and salt. The range is also free from hydrogenated fats.

Information supplied by :- **Quest Vitamins.**

An essential potent daily supplement.

Cantassium Cantamega 2000, from Larkhall Green Farm, is a potent, synergistically combined formulation developed to provide over 45 'active' key nutrients and co-factors essential for optimum health, including vitamins, minerals, trace elements, herbs and digestive enzymes.

Available in health food stores and chemists nation-wide, Cantamega 2000 is probably the most comprehensive multi health food supplement available in the United Kingdom.
It retails at £8.25 for 28 one-a-day tablets or £6.25 for 60, easy to swallow, quarter size tablets, which should be taken four times daily. For further information please contact Garys Thomas, Jo Orchard or Sue Ash, at Ash Associates, 122 St. Martins Lane. London WC2N4AZ. Tel:- 01712406005. Fax:- 01712408005. E-mail 1006634,3446 @compuserve.com.
For details of stockists or free nutritional advice, telephone 01818741130.

Information supplied by :- **Larkhall Green Farm Ltd.**

Superfood with 28 nutrients.

Greens Plus is an alkaline, whole food, containing 28 nutrients, derived from all food classifications be they vitamins, minerals, herbs or anti-oxidants that have been concentrated as a powder. A Superfood such as Greens Plus R can help to supply the body's nutritional requirements in the optimal manner as it receives those essential substances which may be in short supply in its everyday nutrition. Each daily three teaspoon serving is equal to six full servings of raw vegetables. Greens Plus contains no yeast, sugar, sweeteners of any type, salt, egg, colouring, flavours, preservatives, fats, oils, irradiation, MSG, gluten or dairy products. Some of the benefits of Greens Plus R are :-

1:-Gently sweeps the intestine clean with its 17.2% soluble and insoluble fibres.

2:- Expels toxins and poisons from the body. As an alkaline food it neutralises acidity.

3:- Sets the right pH in the intestines.

4:- Supports the "immune", adrenal and lymphatic systems.

5:- Assists with menopause and PMS.

6:- allows extended energy throughout the day without any stimulants.

7:- Increases mental acuity and supports brain functioning.

Ingredients:- Soy Lecithin, Hawaiian Spirulina Pacifica, Barley, Alfala, Wheat Grass, Red Beet Juice, High Pectin Apple Fibre, Chlorella, Wheat Sprout Complex, Brown Rice Germ, Barley Malt, Vitamin E, Dairy Free Probiotic Cultures, Royal Jelly, Montana Region Bee pollen, Acerola Berry Juice Powder, Natural Licorice Root, Dunaliella Salina, Nova-Scotia Dulse.

Available from Greens Plus Ltd.,Parallel House, 32 London Road, Guildford, Surrey GU1 2AB. Tel :- 01483454225.
Information supplied by :- Greens Plus Limited.

Tempeh.

The ingredients of the above product are Organic soya beans, Rhizopus oligosporus culture and Organic cider vinegar. The nutritional analysis is:- Energy 664Kjoules. 150 Kcalories. Protein 10.9grams. Carbohydrate 9.9.grams. Fat 7.5grams. Vitamin B1 0.28 mg. Vitamin B2 0.65 mg. Calcium 142mg. Iron.5mg.
Information supplied by :- Impulse Foods.

Keeping you in peak condition,whatever the weather.

Maintaining our good health is essential if we are to live life to the full. Experts agree that it is essential that we take care of our bodies by adopting the right diet and lifestyle, yet the modern and hectic world we live in does not always provide us with the nutritional requirements our bodies need. Stress and overworking, exercise and the amount of nutrients in our bloodstream can also be reduced.
To keep fit and healthy, it is important to maintain levels of nutrients in the bloodstream.
They act in conjunction with enzymes to control biochemical reactions within the cells and tissues of the body, and are vital to growth and healthy maintenance of the body's organs, structure and tissues. In addition, they are essential for metabolic processes and for maintaining the healthy function of the body's nervous, immune and digestive systems.

Despite occurring naturally in foodstuffs, many vitamins and minerals are destroyed by food processing and cooking methods. Our vitamin and mineral requirements can also change during our lives, so safeguarding optimum health by taking vitamin or mineral supplements is particularly important.

Healthcrafts, the vitamins and minerals experts, recommend taking the following steps to ensure optimum health is maintained, whatever the weather.

* Take regular and gentle exercise.

* Stop smoking.

* Learn to relax and enjoy life - this will help to reduce stress.

* Keep to a healthy diet and lifestyle.

Many of us will find that we need a vitamin and mineral supplement to keep our nutrition intake at its peak.

Vitamin A is essential for sound growth and healthy skin tissue and eyes. Vitamin D is important for maintaining healthy bones and teeth, and is also necessary for the absorption of calcium . Vitamin E is an intoxicant which helps to maintain healthy circulation.

Healthcraft's High Strength Cod Liver Oil (£2.99 for 30 capsules) provided the EC recommended daily allowance of all three vitamins ensuring sufficient levels are provided. It is also rich in Omega- 3 fatty acids which help to maintain mobility and health of the joints, as well as keeping the heart circulation healthy, as part of a healthy diet and lifestyle.

You may find that a multivitamin and mineral supplement is most appropriate to fulfil all your nutritional needs. **Healthcraft's** Chewable Multivitamins, in a one-a-day formulation, contain 12 key nutrients - Vitamins A,D,E & C, Thiamine, Riboflavin, Niacin, Vitamin B6, Folacin, Vitamin B12, Biotin and Pantothenic acid - each giving 100 % EC RDA.

Ginseng helps the body to adapt to changing circumstances and helps maintain optimal physical and mental performance. Vitamin B complex helps to ensure general good health, whilst Vitamin C helps to maintain the health of every cell and tissue of the body. Meanwhile, **Healthcrafts Acidopphilus Extra** is a unique dietary supplement which provides more than four billion "friendly" bacteria to maintain our digestive systems in peak condition, a fact confirmed by independent research.

The full Healthcrafts vitamins and minerals range is available from leading chemist and healthfood stores nation-wide. So, whether you are facing winter frosts or summer sunshine, your health can be in peak condition for the whole year.

Information supplied by :- Healthcrafts.

Healing Gifts of the Plant Kingdom

Each plant has its own unique essence, its "life-force", as its individual beauty. Each person has their own energy pattern as unique as their fingerprint or DNA profile. Energy medicine contains the vibrations of flowering plants which act upon our own personal energy pattern bringing balance and harmony and releiving disease.

Information supplied by:- Ebergos Ltd Tel:- 01958 338742

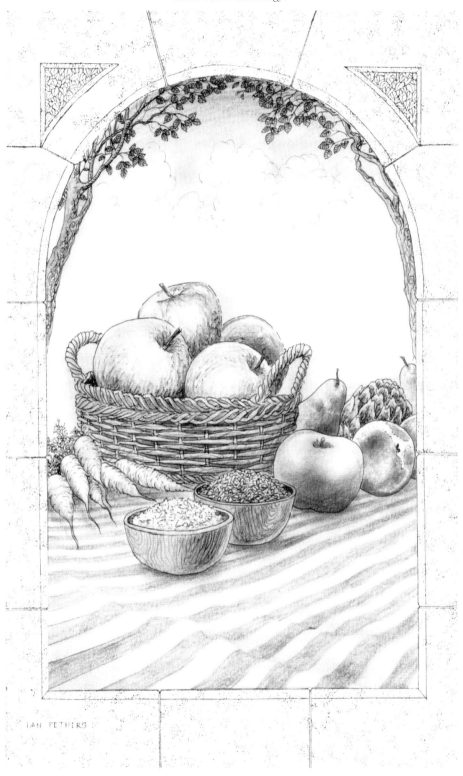

IAN PETHERS

llergy and intolerance to certain foods present considerable difficulties to a fast growing number of people. Unfortunately, only a few individuals find the help they need to sort out their problems, be they complex ones, or just simple ones.

The very word "Allergy" has already become overworked and is used to describe all manner of symptoms including not just those caused by food but household chemical sensitivity, stress, environmental and domestic sensitivities, plus allergy to clothing, nickel, moulds, house dust mite, agricultural chemicals and so on. The common word to describe it all is ALLERGY.

Is it a Food Allergy or Not?

Following recent research, there is a body of opinion which says that, whilst the incidence of allergy is increasing every year, in fact only an extremely small percentage of the population is actually 'truly' allergic to food, i.e., the body produces an anti-body reaction, via the immune system, to a particular food. This is the official, medical view because true allergy is scientifically proven and can be replicated in tests.

But if this is so, why then has the word 'allergy' become so increasingly used to describe all the irritating and ghastly symptoms, aches, pains and ailments we all suffer, from time to time or in some cases endlessly but which are not necessarily provable as a true allergy with an anti-body reaction? Unfortunately, the word 'allergy' is greatly misused, and it is used to describe all types of food allergy, intolerance, sensitivity, irritation, hostility, craving or even indigestion.

Evolutionary Description

Whilst this evolutionary description is understandable, the fact remains that by far and away the largest percentage of people who at first suspect they have an 'allergy' to a food, don't in fact have one, at least not as far as the official medical definition says so. But they may well have an intolerance, a sensitivity, or an irritation, hostility, craving or indigestion. And those can be equally nasty.

These other 'allergic' responses to certain foods can also be triggered by all manner of things, even exercise, emotion, temperature changes, the menstrual cycle, a hot bath, psychological problems ... Smoking often provokes a migraine, never mind chocolate, red wine, yeast, cheese, broad beans, canned fish or bananas. Take your pick! Wheat, grains, rye, garlic, eggs etc. can create misery for IBS sufferers.

Then there's all those chemicals, additives, flavourings, colourings, emulsifiers, fungicides and insecticides. All of these, or even just one of them are quite capable of triggering or producing an 'allergic' response in the wider definition of the word.

True Allergy

True allergy then, is triggered by the body's own immune system, whereby the antibodies attack the food molecules, and the symptoms are usually immediate. They would include asthma, eczema, hay fever, urticaria, nausea, vomiting, diarrhoea, gut spasm, oedema and similar type reactions. If you have a 'true' allergy, you know about it and will usually avoid the food which triggers it. The common foods implicated in true allergy are cows milk, eggs, wheat, yeast, citrus, nuts, beans and pulses.

Food Intolerance, Sensitivity, Hostility

Food intolerance on the other hand is an umbrella term covering all the other adverse reaction to foods. The main symptoms here are:

Headache, Migraine, Fatigue, Hyperactivity in children, Mouth ulcers, Aching joints, Arthritis, Nausea, Stomach ulcers, Irritable bowel syndrome, Candidiasis, Wind, bloating, Itchy skin, Earache, Depression and mood swings, Pins and needles, Catarrh and runny nose, Heartburn

Difficult to Identify

This type of reaction can often take longer to appear and is so hard to identify. People feel they are just not getting any help from anyone. Usually, their symptoms are mild at first but then they get steadily worse and inevitably they feel generally unwell, often tired and exhausted, lacking in any sense of enthusiasm, never mind the discomfort.

Elimination

Despite all the claims that this or that method of detection is the best (and probably the most expensive), the only way to find out if food or drink is affecting an individual is to ELIMINATE the potentially difficult foods for a period of one month and then to re-introduce each item, one at a time to monitor any symptoms.

If the symptoms re-appear then it is probably best to avoid the food responsible for at least 6 months to a year then try again. If the symptoms do not re-appear, then you can usually eat the food again, but in moderation lest all the old symptoms come flooding back! "IF IN DOUBT, LEAVE IT OUT" is the most sensible attitude. If you know that a certain food gives you gyp then why bother to eat it in the first place?

Why the Growth in Allergic Responses?

Today, in the advanced countries of the world, food has never been more plentiful, varied and available but yet, despite these fantastic advances in the food supply chain, as much as one in ten people suffer from digestive disorders of some sort and one in five of all patients going through a Doctor's surgery have a problem in their gut somewhere.

The Increase in Allergic and Digestive Disorders

In recent years, the reported incidence of food allergy and disorder has grown dramatically and many reasons are put forward to explain this increase. Apart from a few exceptions, it is no small coincidence that in countries where there is little industrial power and fresh food is eaten straight from the land where no sprays have been used there appears to be a low allergy situation.

So, is allergy therefore, in all its different types, a possible side effect of the more affluent, industrialised societies, in addition to the usual statements about pollution, food colourings, additives, fast and convenient foods etc? Yes it is!

We can't change it now

The problem here, is that we can't all go off and change our lifestyles that easily - like going back to nature - cutting out the stress - living off the land - making sure the food is organic and fresh every day, living in non-allergic houses/offices - wearing non-allergic clothes - using non-allergic detergents, cosmetics, cleaners, polishes, paints etc.

We have to put up with, reluctantly, the side effects of the modern world and thus the increasing incidence of allergy, be it through family genetics, environmental positions, the very air we breathe, our work places, our houses and yes, the FOOD WE EAT. Consider the evidence.

Reliance on Drugs

As we approach the end of this century, we are already being promised all sorts of new drugs to cure cancer, aids, arthritis, asthma, heart disease and so on...

Not a week goes by without reports being carried in the media about a scientific breakthrough or a vaccine for this disease or that. This is great news and everyone welcomes it - science must indeed break new barriers of discovery just as it always has done - but we must also hope that any new and even more powerful drugs produced for these cures will have much less side effects than their predecessors, and certainly reduce the total number of drugs in use at this time. Currently, there are some 6,000 licensed antibiotics!

Reduction in Drug Culture

Conventional medicine relies heavily on drugs, all of which are essentially toxic substances and, if we really are looking to the year 2,000 where this past century's diseases can all be cured and our life span lengthened, then let's hope that these fantastic advances will also see a drastic reduction in the drug culture of the 1990's.

50 Million Prescriptions per year

In the UK alone there are some 50 million medical prescriptions written each year or just under 1 million a week, and this figure carries on rising. Even worse, between 30% and 50% of all outpatients given a drug prescription, then fail to finish the course or listen to the advice they have been given. The very laws of nature surely tell us that we can't keep putting unnatural things into the human body without there being side effects or a build-up of undesirable toxins or bacteria. No-one here is condemning antibiotics for that would be absolutely foolish and irresponsible, bearing in mind the millions of lives they have saved and the illnesses and infection they relieve.

But in the Process

It is the misuse, overuse, and ever growing potencies of antibiotics administered to us medically, plus those found in low level residues in our foodstuffs and in intensively reared livestock, plus other drugs, steroids, the contraceptive pill, chemicals, additives, flavourings in our food, stress and all the other wonderful advances of the last 30 years which have helped to create allergies to our food and the environment.

In the most simplistic terms, the advances of the last 30 years have also helped to weaken the body's own immune system to the point where it has difficulty in continuing to fight its own battles, and then it needs further and more powerful drugs to help it do so.

New and even more powerful Immune Suppressant drugs are designed to 'switch off' the immune system, and one does begin to wonder why on earth we should actually allow ourselves to switch off the most precious thing we've got going for us.

A Typical case of the Graduation into the Allergy Syndrome
If we look at a quite typical case, we might look at a young girl who has been on antibiotics from an early age for things like ear infections, tonsillitis and the usual collection of minor illnesses.

As she gets older she may have been give a broad-spectrum antibiotic for cystitis. She may have used steroid creams for eczema, acne and then possibly developed asthma leading on from that with the use of steroids.

Typical Lifestyle
Next, as she gets into her late teens she goes on the contraceptive pill. Chances are she may also smoke, drink too much alcohol socially, and live on a diet of sugar, burgers and chips!

Childbirth arrives and the new arrival stands a wonderful chance of inheriting a weakened immune system and allergies aplenty. Moving on to middle age, the menopause and all the years in between when vaginal thrush, cystitis and PMT were problems our lady in question may also have arthritis as she gets older. She may also feel tired all the time.

Classic Symptoms
Is all this being negative or sceptical? NO! It happens, and a weakened immune system is created. Inadequate nutrition through lack of nutrient absorption, multiple allergies, unexplained fatigue and many other problems - there you have it - classic symptoms of total mismanagement.

This may sound dramatic or, perhaps a classical piece of sensational journalism, but it is not. It simply describes, quite typically, how a middle-aged woman can have what she believes is an allergy to perhaps everything. In this case, careful management, with inner cleansing and detoxification and then a more balanced diet to suit the individual's nutritional needs, will often go a long way to recovery for this allergic person.

Our Children
It is quite possible that many allergic problems can be traced to the diets our mothers had in the latter stages of pregnancy, or what a baby eats and drinks in the all important weaning period. Certainly, cow's milk comes in for a lot of criticism with the suggestion that 20% of the population has a problem with it. It is known to be associated with conditions related to psoriasis, eczema, colitis, diverticulitis, asthma and angina. There are other, equally nutritionally acceptable milks which can replace cow's milk.

White Flour Products
White flour was used in the 1940's to make glue when wallpaper needed to be stuck on a wall, and quite frankly that just about sums up its use to allergy sufferers.

A loaf of white, sliced, 'supermarket' bread, must be the most tampered with, unnatural food of all time. It has masses of additives. When the wheat grain is milled, it is then processed so much that the millers have to add-back important vitamins and minerals.

50 Additives can be Involved

There are bleaches, oxidising agents, anti-fungals, mould inhibitors, stabilisers, maturing agents, carriers, free-flowing agents, extra yeast to aid smooth fermentation, and so it goes on. One would need to be an industrial chemist to understand them all and there are some 50-odd additives which are available and can be involved. And they call it the staff of life!

White flour also glues up the walls of the small intestine which then develops bacteria and yeasts. It is an easy job to dispense with white flour. There are so many far better quality substitutes available. Some examples are:

Wholemeal, Spelt, Brown Rice, Amaranth, Quinoa, Buckwheat, Millet, Tapioca, Chickpea, Red, Lentil, Sago, Chestnut

In a research programme monitoring 2,728 patients, white flour was the big 'nasty' and was associated with many skin problems, asthma, sinus, hay fever, arthritis and migraine.

Sugar Consumption up 6 times

100 years ago, the average intake of sugar in Western countries was about 20lbs. per head, per year. In the 1990's, the intake is 5 or 6 times that, i.e. well over 100lbs per head. No small wonder then that illnesses like Diabetes are on the increase when the body's over-worked pancreas struggles to keep the sugar levels right. When one considers the amount of sugar in food products and drinks to-day, it is nothing short of scandalous that it goes on, seemingly uncontrolled. Where on earth are the controls to govern it's use as a potentially harmful substance?

Are all Foods Bad Then?

No, of course not. Cow's milk, white flour and sugar are mentioned here, because they are so often implicated when a person has food allergy problems.

Foods nourish you, can heal you, but with certain predisposed individuals they can also harm you. It is a question of finding out the culprits.

Artificial additives, flavourings, colourings and preservatives all play their part and we have seen the recent evidence concerning the effects of additives on children with problems of hyperactivity and the actions of young criminal offenders.

What Can You Do?

Allergy has become an all embracing word and covers problems associated with:-

Asthma
Household Chemicals (Inhalants & Skin)
Cosmetics (Inhalants and Skin)
Metals (Skin, e.g. Nickel)
Environmental Chemicals (Inhalant & Skin, e.g. Insecticides)
Foods
Medicines, e.g. Aspirin reaction
Moulds, Plants, Pollens and Pets
Smoke, Fumes
Office Environmental Issues, e.g. cavity walls
The list is endless for indeed, allergy, in all its forms now affects 30/40% of the population.

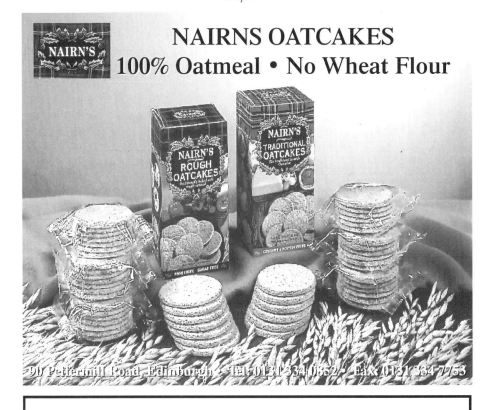

When it comes to Food Allergy, getting help is not easy. It is all very well to be advised to see your Doctor, only to find that when you do so, he or she dismisses the notion or simply says ...."If you think you have a problem with (say) milk, then don't drink it!"

Improving Slowly

To be fair to GPs, they are at last starting to respond to the demands coming in relating to allergic problems, but given the fact that for the most part a GP needs to spend most of his or her time attending to the immediate needs of the traditionally sick patient, the best you can expect is a referral to an Allergy Clinic which can often be miles away, just like the appointment date you will be given. You may also be referred to the local immunology department where a blood test or a skin-prick test will reveal if your body is producing anti-bodies to the things you are being tested for.

Case Not Proven

If there is no antibody reaction, then it could be assumed that you are not allergic to the thing(s) you are being tested for. But is that the case? You can still feel unwell if, for example, you are having dull, prolonged headaches, and coffee is found to be the activator. You would not have shown to be allergic to coffee on the hospital blood test or skin test for that.

Elimination

Your Doctor would have been right when he or she said ... "If you think you have a problem with (say) milk, then don't drink it!" This is by far and away the best advice, and in any case, why on earth put yourself through discomfort by continuing to eat something when you know jolly well it upsets you? That is the rationale of the heavy smoker!

However, the choice of which foods to eliminate is difficult. You can do some detective work yourself, but you could also get a test done.
Articles in magazines will advise you to see your GP first, but, as most people have reported this often does not give the person the feeling of satisfaction they are seeking.

Dangerous or Faddy Diets

Other articles in magazines will advise you to seek the help of a professional who is an expert on diet, because dietary manipulation is dangerous, etc. It certainly can be dangerous for people with extra special dietary needs but it is difficult to see how the elimination of crisps, or tomatoes, or oranges can be dangerous however! So where is the risk when changes to the diet are planned? It concerns the dangers of the re-introduction of a food, back into the diet, following an elimination period, where the food in question had previously given a violent reaction. That should not be attempted without medical help.

It's all a Question of Balance

Secondly, there are the nutritional implications of ensuring that we get the balance of proteins, carbohydrates, fats, vitamins and minerals right, just as we should be doing normally anyway. That is surely common sense? There are also special 'at risk' groups to be considered, e.g. anorexics, pregnant women, diabetics and others with rare dietary disorders. There is perhaps therefore, an unwritten piece of understanding which says that depending on how sick you are, decides whether you seek the advice/help of a medical professional or whether to do some detective work yourself if you have irritating, daily problems which your Doctor has not been

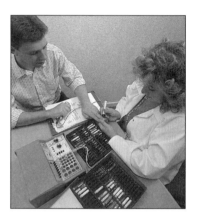
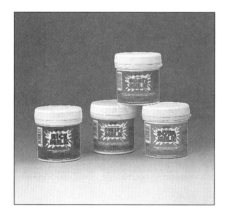

able to relieve. Things like headaches, migraine, fatigue, hyperactivity, aching muscles, irritable bowel, wind, joint pains, oedema (water retention), diarrhoea and so on. These problems will not show up on a hospital blood or skin prick test, so where do you go next?

Expensive Tests
There are several laboratories offering very good tests but, at £200 or so per test, the average person would find it difficult to fund it, and it is not available on the NHS anyway. One of the problem areas with Allergy Testing is that it is such a controversial subject. Experts disagree and each testing laboratory reckons that it's system is the only accurate one! It is true to say that if you deliberately set out to find faults with any system of allergy testing you will find them.

Elimination
The best route to follow is still the time-honoured way of eliminating the items which appear to be a problem for a period of one month, and then re-introduce those items one at a time so that you can monitor your symptoms. Now the problem is, that you can spend many hundreds of pounds and lost time on trying to get a 100% accurate 'test' done before you commence with your elimination programme. It is far better to get on and do something positive and at a price the average person can afford.

Scientific Proof
There are other tests of course, some of which have a controversial tag because they cannot be scientifically proven with an antibody response or because their competitors find it convenient to point out their failings! But you do not necessarily need to be 100% accurate in your test results to get started with an elimination diet, for the chances are that you will feel so much better once you have eliminated certain foods, even if the short-list you started with was not necessarily 100% accurate.

The Important Issues are:-

- Don't go hungry, eat less but more often
- Drink more water and less coffee and 'ordinary' tea
- Don't try and achieve 100% perfection in any test results before embarking on an elimination programme. You will drive yourself nuts and spend a lot of money in the process.
- The only real test if YOU! Your body will tell you if it doesn't like something when you re-introduce the items you eliminated to start with.
- You can get help with Tests which are easy and convenient to get done, and which will get you started at a price you can afford. Ask your local independent pharmacy or health food shop for details.
- If you feel so much better after having left something out of your diet then why bother to re-introduce it? There will be a suitable alternative to it anyway. Your local health shop has a large choice of alternative products which you can use. There is no need for anyone to go hungry or to follow an imbalanced diet.

Good luck in your endeavours.

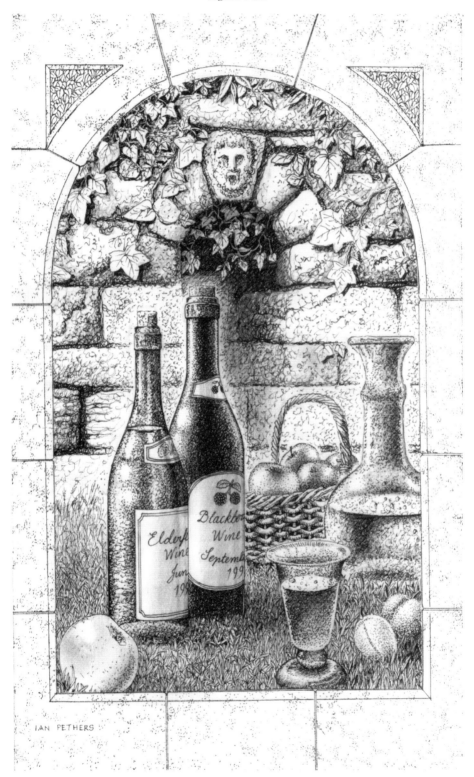

IAN PETHERS

ORGANIC WINES (Vine to Table)
by A G Williams

Wine is essentially nothing more than fermented grape juice. A perfectly natural product, it has been an integral part of civilisation since biblical times. During the twentieth century the demand for increased production and greater uniformity led many producers towards an industrialised form of viticulture, utilising chemicals both in the vineyard and in the winery. Since the early 1970's however, there has been a movement away from this commercially intensive form of wine - making towards more natural methods. In the first instance this involved only a handful of producers, mostly in France, and these were viewed with much scepticism by the mainstream industry. More recently the movement has become widespread, with huge numbers of producers adopting various degrees of organic production.

Identifying, or indeed defining, organic wine is not a simple matter. In order to be sold as organic a wine must satisfy certain criteria both in the growing of the grapes and in the vinification process. Organic viticulture is essentially a system of grape growing without recourse to synthetic chemical products. There has been much debate in the wine industry as to what exactly should and should not be allowed in an organic vineyard. While there is a proscriptive definition, which lists the things forbidden in organic viticulture, it is more useful to define the practise through its aims and practices. The prime motive for adopting organic practices is to increase the microbial activity in the soil and avoid adding any unnatural extraneous substances. This is done through the use of composts and manures, in preference to synthetic chemical cocktails. In fact vines produce the best wines under conditions which cause them stress. If planted on rich soils or if over fertilised they tend to produce too much foliage and low quality fruit. Organic fertilisers give a more gradual release of nutrients to the soil and maintain an equilibrium that chemical fertilisers cannot emulate. The argument in favour of the organic approach is simply that low intensity, organic farming is better suited to the needs of quality grape growing.

There are many wine-makers who believe that organic practices also promote the individuality, or terroir, of each site. The notion of terroir is that each individual vineyard or vineyard region has its own specific character. This is the basis of the French Appellation Controlee (AC) system. The terroir of a particular site is made up of a combination of factors, including micro-climate, geography, topology and soil. Most important of these is soil type. Under modern viticultural practices vineyards are treated with chemical fertilisers, these are all essentially the same and they encourage the creation of uniform conditions, and uniform wines. This lessens the effect of terroir. The use of natural fertilisers and compost will tend to cause greater diversity and underline the individuality of each vineyard site. The second consideration is the physical effect on the land. Organic practices give a more stable soil structure and make soil erosion less of a problem. This is particularly significant in steep vineyard sites such as those in Germany's Mosel Valley. Here vineyard owners are constantly working to restore soil to the hillside, as it slides down to the valley floor. Many have discovered that by adding organic matter to the site they are better able to create an element of stability.

Another environmental concern which organic producers are aware of is that their practices have a wider effect. Chemical sprays used on crops can eventually work their way into natural waterways and pollute rivers and streams. Gratuitous use of chemicals, used as a safety net, in case any problems occur can only add to this problem as the chemicals are gradually leached from the soils. Organic producers use natural sprays and even these are only used as necessary. This reduces the risk of harmful chemicals leaching into the water table and rivers.

Vineyards are necessarily monocultures, with grapes the only crop and no option of crop rotation. Organic producers try to overcome this by planting grass or other crops between the rows of vines. This helps to protect against soil erosion, while at the same time fixing nutrients in the soil and offering undergrowth for insects which prey on various pests in the vineyard. Indeed some organic vineyard owners have even hit on the idea of growing cash crops, such as strawberries under their vines during the early years when vines are unproductive.

The greatest problems for viticulturists are the fungal diseases which strike throughout the year. These are prevalent in warm, wet conditions, and are therefore most noticeable in the vineyard regions of northern Europe. The organic vineyard owner's principal protection against fungal and bacterial disease is the traditional Bordeaux Mixture, a blend of copper sulphate and lime which is sprayed on the vines when necessary. This substance was originally used as a deterrent to human grape thieves. Bordeaux Mixture turns the vine leaves, and grapes, blue and was thought to deter locals who were tempted to help themselves to a free meal of grapes. However, as each application of copper sulphate lengthens the ripening period by up to three days, it is not something to be used lightly. Conventional farmers may spray routinely, but organic farmers tend to use the treatment only as needed.

The risk of these infections diminishes in warmer climates and it is not surprising that the cradle for the organic renaissance in the 1970's and 80's was the south of France. The hot dry climate of regions such as Languedoc - Roussillon and Provence makes them ideally suited to organic viticulture. When organic wines were first marketed in the UK only French wines were available, and, for the most part, these came from the south of the country. At that time the pioneering work was being done by estates such as Mas de Daumas Gassac and Domaine Trevallon. These are comparatively expensive, hand crafted wines made by producers who believe passionately in the fact that organic viticulture is an integral part of quality wine production.

Producers such as these make small quantities of wine which are snapped up by aficionados. For those wine drinkers seeking out organic wines of more modest repute, it is important that there should be some recognisable and reliable sign on the bottle that this "vin biologique" is genuinely organic. This was achieved, in a less than perfect manner, by committed growers who joined one of a plethora of monitoring organisations. Any wine bearing the logo of **Nature et Progres** or **Lemaire-Boucher**, amongst others, was guaranteed an organic product. In July 1991 the European Union introduced legislation to define the parameters of organic production and these rules are overseen by the existing organisations within each member country. Thus any wine which bears the logo of an organisation such as the Soil Association is guaranteed as an organic product. However, increasingly, there are a number of wines on the market which do not announce their organic credentials. Major "conventional" producers such as Chapoutier in the Rhone, Domaine Leroy in Burgundy and Ernst Loosen in Germany have recently turned to organic methods, although none of them chooses to mention the fact on their labels. In a more commercial manner some of the larger wine producers have decided to join the organic movement. The Australian giants Penfolds produce a red and a white organic wine, as do Fetzer, one of California's larger producers.

Some of these producers have even embraced the most extreme form of organic production - biodynamics. Biodynamic methods are based on the teachings of Rudolph Steiner, and involve organic systems combined with a cosmic dimension. Viticultural and wine - making processes are undertaken in conjunction with certain phases of the astrological calendar. Part of the reason that this system has been so readily accepted in France is that it codifies many of the practices which French vignerons had always accepted on folkloric level. Terms such as "harvest moon" take on a new significance when viewed from a biodynamic standpoint. One of the prime proponents of biodynamic is James Millton of **Millton Vineyards** in New Zealand. His wines are an extremely good defence of biodynamic principles. He produces barrel fermented Chardonnays and Chenin Blancs of tremendous power and elegance, as well as stunning late harvest desert wines. Other adherents to the biodynamic line include Nicholas Joly of **Coulee de Serrant** in the Loire, **Nuova Cappelletta** in Piemonte and **Domaine Leflaive** in Burgundy.

During the 1980's a handful of specialist wine merchants appeared who concentrated exclusively on organically produced wines. Initially these were exclusively French wines but gradually the range of wines grew and availability became more widespread. Today France still dominates the lists of these merchants, but they are now as diverse and varied as the lists of more conventional wine companies. Every major region of France is represented, although the south remains dominant. Among the outstanding producers here are **Domaine Bassac**, who produce both red and white varietal wines. Particularly impressive is their Syrah which is bursting with ripe juicy berry flavours, with a serious backbone of tannins. Provence remains a centre for organic production. Nicolas Cartier, at **Mas de Gourgonnier**, produces excellent red wines, redolent of the herbs and heather of the garrigues. At **Domaine Richaume**, Henning Hoesch produces varietal wines of stunning power and intensity, rich in fruit and with great tannic structure. Further north, in the Rhone Valley, **Pierre Andre** makes superb red and white Chateauneuf du Pape. The white in particular is worthy of note both for its rarity and because it is an excellent fragrant blend of Marsanne and Roussane. If you are looking for real value for money the Cotes du Rhone from the co-operative **Cave la Vigneronne Villedieu**, in the southern Rhone, offers rich, succulent spicy fruit. Another property of note here is **Domaine de Grande Bellane** which is full-bodied with soft berry fruit and undertones of chocolate and coffee.

The classic region of Burgundy is well represented. In addition to the many producers such as Leflaive who use organic methods but are not approved by the monitoring organisations, there are numerous small producers making excellent Chardonnays and Pinot Noirs. **Jean Claude Rateau** owns vines in Beaune where he produces excellent Pinot Noir. His whites, which are outstanding, come from the village of Puligny Montrachet. **D'Heilly Huberdeau** and **Jean Musso** both produce excellent Bourgogne Passetoutgrain where juicy, jammy Gamay grapes are blended with lighter Pinot Noir to produce a fruity yet elegant wine. Look out too for **Paul Giboulot's** Bourgogne Rouge. Bordeaux is also well served by organic producers making wines ranging from everyday drinking to those for special occasions. **Chateau Le Rait** is a good simple Bordeaux. **Ch Coursou** is a Bordeaux Superieur produced from a blend of Merlot and Cabernet Sauvignon. Prolonged wood maturation gives this wine a cedary spiciness to overlay the ripe cassis fruit. One of the finest wines from the area is undoubtedly **Ch de Prade**. This comes from the area around Castillon la Bataille, in northern Bordeaux. Prade displays a cedary aroma, mixed with hints of tobacco leaf over ripe, supple fruit. This is classic Bordeaux. **Clos de la Perichere** is another classic, from the Graves district to the south of the river Garonne. Here winemaker Gabriel Guerin produces a silky smooth, elegant red using a high percentage of

Merlot. Excellent value for money is represented by **Ch Rocher du Puy**, the second wine of **Ch du Puy**, this is actually more elegant and better balanced than its more expensive big brother.

As you move further north, organic viticulture becomes increasingly difficult. Despite this **Guy Bossard** makes excellent organic Muscadet at the mouth of the Loire River. Another excellent Muscadet producer is **Domaine de la Parentiere**. Further inland **Gerard Leroux** produces wonderful sweet wines from the Chenin Blanc grape.

Far to the east ,Alsace is home to a thriving organic wine - making fraternity. This is home to the marvellous annual organic fair at Rouffach. One of the organisers of this show is **Jean-Pierre Frick**. He and his wife Chantale make a superb range of varietal wines on the family estate at Pfaffenheim using biodynamic methods. I have also been tremendously impressed by the wines of another biodynamic producer in Alsace, **Andre Stentz** , who makes a superb rich, mouthfilling Tokay d'Alsace and an excellent Gewurztraminer.

In addition to all these splendid still wines, the organic producers of France make a number of sparkling wines. One of my favourites is the **Cremant de Die** of **Achard Vincent**. Made from the Muscat grape this has a wonderful floral bouquet, and a zappy grapey taste with just a hint of sweetness balanced by fresh acidity. For those that want the real thing there are plenty of Champagnes on the market, the best of these come from **Jose Ardinat, Jean Bliard and Andre Beaufort**.

Organic principles have been adopted by a great many producers in Germany. Initially this was difficult as many vineyard areas are sprayed by helicopter and the problem of spray drift could affect organic vineyards. However, recently many growers have been alerted to the benefits of organic viticulture. The rising price of chemical sprays and the need to stabilise their steep vineyards has driven many towards greener methods. In fact the VDP, a grouping of the finest estates in the country has recently rewritten its constitution and now requires all its members to follow organic practices in the vineyard. **Ernst Loosen**, one of the finest winemakers in the Mosel Valley, started making organic wines in the early 1980's and his barrique fermented Muller Thurgau remains one of the finest, and oddest, wines on the market. Unfortunately English importers have largely ignored the excellent wines of Germany, but one or two have found their way on to the lists of the organic specialists. The **St Ursula Weinkellerei** in Rheinhessen makes an attractive quaffable wine from the greatly underestimated Scheurebe variety. The classic grape of Germany, the Riesling, is sadly under-represented here, but there is one excellent example to keep the classicists happy. **Weingut Klaus Knobloch** in the Rheinhessen produce an elegant, balanced Riesling Trocken, which shows great varietal character and true finesse.

You need a hair shirt mentality to make wine in England, but you need a perverse streak to try and make it organically. Despite all the drawbacks, Roy Cook has stuck to his guns and he is now producing excellent wines from his **Seddlescombe Vineyard** in deepest Sussex. Particularly impressive is his Dry White. Made from a blend of Reichensteiner and Bacchus grapes, it is packed with fruit, balanced by lively acidity and with a slight spritz giving a lift to the finish.

The warmer climes of the Mediterranean countries should be ideally suited to organic production, but, with a few exceptions, I have been unimpressed with the Italian and Spanish wines on the market. Too often good fruit is spoilt by sloppy wine - making. Fortunately some producers have got it right. **Guerrieri-Rizzardi** are large producers from the Veneto region. They are not certified as organic, but do follow organic principles in making their Soave, Bardolino and Valpolicella, all of which are excellent examples of their type. From the same region **Fasoli Gino** make a light, fresh melon flavoured Soave. The same producer makes an interesting Vino da Tavola called **Orgno**. This retails for around £13, and being a table wine this may seem excessive. However, it is made from 100% Merlot, and although this is one of the world's great grapes, it is not an approved variety in the Veneto, so the wine must be classified as a table wine irrespective of quality. Further south in Tuscany the **San Vito** estate of Roberto Drighi produce light, fresh Chianti packed with bitter cherry fruit. Another good, light Chianti is made by **Casale**, who also produce vin da tavolas from the Sangiovese grape.

In organic terms Spain is pretty much a vinous disaster area. However the Tempranillo of **Albet I Noya** shines out like a beacon, showing just what could be achieved if wine - making practices were brought up to date. It has wonderful plummy fruit, with a hint of chocolate and black cherries. Why can't they all be like this?

Increasingly, New World producers are moving over to organic methods. The dry, hot climates of Australia and South Africa are perfect for organic viticulture, and yet the winemakers here have been very slow to take up the challenge. One of the pioneers in Australia was Gil Wahlquist. A journalist from Sydney, Wahlquist decided he needed a change of life style, so he moved to Mudgee in New South Wales to make organic wines. His **Botobolar** wines rapidly made an impact and more than a few friends. Gil has now retired but the rich velvety smooth wines of Botobolar continue to charm, and occasionally bludgeon, drinkers throughout Australia and the UK. Wahlquist converted some of his neighbours in Mudgee to the organic cause, and the excellent **Thistle Hill Estate** now exports a powerful Cabernet Sauvignon. Adam Wynn's **Eden Ridge** wines are not certified as organic but Wynn has been following an organic regime on his Adelaide Hills estate since the mid eighties. He makes a number of varietal wines, but the ones that have impressed me the most are his splendidly understated, elegant Chardonnay, and his powerful spicy, vanillin flavoured Shiraz. The Australian wine industry is dominated by a handful of companies, but so far only one, **Penfolds**, has joined the organic bandwagon. The result, as might be expected, is excellent. They make a white from Chardonnay and Sauvignon Blanc, and a red from Cabernet Sauvignon and Shiraz. Both are benchmark wines showing both elegance and power, and illustrating just why Australian wines are so popular.

The New Zealand wine industry is decidedly small scale, and I know of only two organic producers. I have already mentioned **Millton Vineyards**, and I can only reiterate that James Millton is one of the best. His wines stand comparison with those produced anywhere, and the fact that he can do this using biodynamic methods in the damp conditions of the land of the low white clouds is even more remarkable. **Richmond Plains** is a new vineyard, planted in 1991 on the South Island of New Zealand. Winemaker Jane Cooper makes a Sauvignon Blanc which typifies the grassy New Zealand style, and an elegant, lightly oaked Chardonnay.

Undoubtedly the best organic wines in South Africa come from the **Buitenverwachting** estate in the Constantia district. These are not certified but the land is farmed organically. Outstanding here are the Rieslings and "Christine" - a Bordeaux blend of Cabernets, Franc and Sauvignon, and Merlot. The house style is for intense pure fruit and elegant structure. The only certified organic wine produced in South Africa comes from the **Sonop** winery in Paarl. The winery

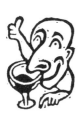
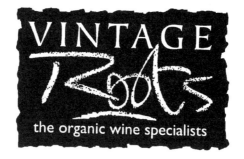

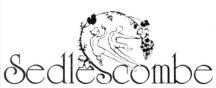
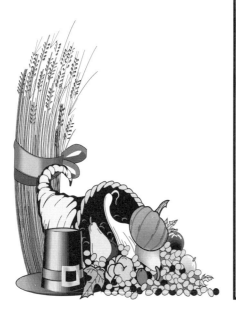

makes a number of wines, but only their Sauvignon Blanc is organic. However, this has proved so popular that the winery plans to extend biological farming practices to all it's sites.

Surely, ultra-hip California should be at the forefront of organic production. sadly this is not the case. What interest there is focused in the north of the state, in Mendocino County. Here the massive family operation of **Fetzer** has made quite an impact. Fetzer make a range of wines which are not organic, but some years ago they became interested in the concept of organic farming and set up an impressive organic market garden on their estate at Hopland. The results here encouraged them to experiment with organics in the vineyard, and they launched a red and a white organic wine in the early 90's. Both have proved tremendously successful, and both are worth tracking down. The other major producer in the region is **Frey Vineyards**. Paul Frey gave up work as a physician in order to move to Mendocino and become a "country gentleman". He then discovered that even country gentleman have to make a living. Frey turned to wine - making and today his extensive family make wines which are as distinctive and idiosyncratic as their originator. The family produce very rich, intense wines from their dry farmed estate, most notable amongst these is a big grunty Zinfandel. *Stockists;*

Importers (All of whom sell by mail order);

The Organic Wine Co, P.O.Box 81, High Wycombe, Bucks, HP13 5QN

Tel; 01494 446557

Vinceremos, 261 Upper Town St, Bramley, Leeds, LS13 3JT

Tel; 0113 257 7545

Vintage Roots, Sheeplands Farm, Wargrave, Berks, RG10 8DT

Tel; 0118 940 1222

Retail outlets;

Bumblebee Wholefoods, Brecknock Rd, London N 7

Out of this World, 52 Elswick Rd, Newcastle upon Tyne, NE4 6JH.

Tel; 0191 272 1601

Planet Organic, 42 Westbourne Grove, London W2 5SH.

Tel; 0171 221 7171

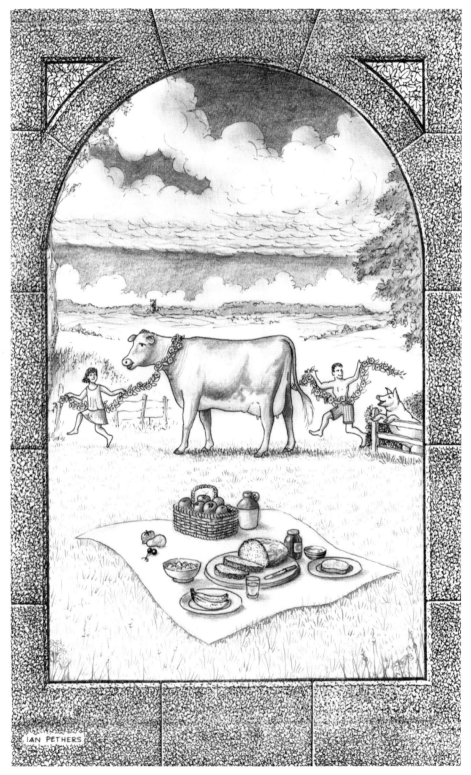

Vegetarian Issues - Revolution is the Solution

by Juliet Gellatley

If Earth was a hospital patient it would be in intensive care. So devastating has been the impact of humankind during its brief tenure that all its health indices are in free fall. Check the vital signs of the oceans, the atmosphere, the landmasses and their occupants and you will find they are all becoming more feeble by the day.

As a species we have set ourselves up as the arbiters of the globe in an act of such breathtaking arrogance that it usurps the role of gods and creates a monstrous imbalance in the natural order. We slaughter owls, hawks, crows, and magpies so that grouse or pheasant can be reared in large numbers. We then slaughter them by sending lead shot ripping through their flesh - and call it sport. We destroy rabbits as vermin and then demonise the foxes that live on them and hunt them to death. We gas badgers because they might have TB; we trap and kill rooks because we don't like their habits; chase hares with dogs for entertainment; do anything we like to rats and mice; shoot pigeons in their millions.

We determine which animals we will eat and deny them everything; we determine which will be labelled vermin and try to annihilate them; others we pamper and allow the comfort of our hearth. Across the globe we chase whales and harpoon them for cultural reasons. We destroy dolphins and seals because they dare to eat fish. There is hardly a species we will not exterminate if their interests and ours collide.

By selective breeding, genetic manipulation and dietary interference we are producing food animals which are increasingly incapable of life without our intervention. As factory farming intensifies so medical treatment with antibiotics and other powerful drugs increases and alongside the increase goes a resistance to the very drugs vital to the animal's survival. As a consequence we are producing creatures with a tenuous grip on life and at the same time are destroying the wild gene pool from which they evolved.

By so cavalierly playing with the fate of other animals we are risking our own. It seems we are incapable of understanding that every living creature has its part to play in maintaining the glorious fabric of our world. None of the animals we persecute pose any threat to the survival of the planet. It is not they which threaten it but us.

The only hope we have is to fundamentally reassess our role and our attitude to the planet and the living creatures which share it with us. Vegetarianism is integral to that reassessment and there is a gradual dawning of this fact.

There are many reasons why vegetarianism offers a way forward because at the heart of the world's major problems is our diet. However, this knowledge is still largely obscured and the current growth in vegetarianism is largely due to two factors - a growing awareness of the way in which farm animals are treated and the effect that meat has on human health.

It took two news stories in the mid 1990s to thrust the issue of animal welfare into the headlines. Pictures of terrified little calves and lambs, staring through the slits in the sides of lorries, were beamed into the nation's living rooms. As the story developed, images of bewildered and beaten animals, often desperate for food, rest and water were overlaid with scenes of the barbaric veal crates to which half a million calves were despatched from Britain every year.

Two and a half million sheep and lambs were exported annually simply to be slaughtered in the most brutal manner and their meat labelled as " home produced" by the importers. Unimaginable suffering simply for a five pound premium.

But no sooner had the Press become bored by live exports than mad cow disease (BSE) screamed into the top news spot and held it for weeks. People were genuinely shocked to find that this incurable and horrible degenerative disease was spread by feeding cattle ground up bits of other cows. Totally vegan animals had been turned into carnivorous cannibals in order to increase profit margins. There is now a sense of a nation holding its breath, waiting to see how severe and how widespread is the risk to humans.

These events started many people on a voyage of discovery which winds its way through the intensive factory farms, through the impoverishment of the developing world, opens up vistas of a degraded environment, sails over and under dying oceans and peers inside the human body. The conclusion to the journey is inescapable - we can no longer afford to eat meat. But it all starts with the animals.

The majority of meat eaten in the West is factory farmed, a phenomenon which first appeared after the Second World War. The systems have now been polished and honed to perfection in the pursuit of cheap meat. Every production question has been posed and answered except one - what about the animals?

Pigs are descendants of the wild creatures which inhabited the forests of Europe but were hunted to extinction in Britain in the 17th Century. They are intelligent and sociable and we have driven them mad. The means by which we have done it is the dry sow stall. The majority of pigs in Europe are kept for their whole five month pregnancy in metal barred stalls so small that they can take but a half-a-pace forward and the same backwards. They cannot turn or move sideways and are frequently further restricted by a tether around their middle or neck, secured to the ground with a shackle. The less they move the less food they consume.

The slatted floor on which they stand produces severe back and leg pain and the urine which it is supposed to allow through, frequently splashes back to cover the sows' legs and belly. No bedding, no social interaction, no contact even with other pigs The result of this sterility is stereotypic behaviour - the constant repetition of one particular movement, often the biting of the bars which imprison them. The same repetitive behaviour can be seen in patients in psychiatric hospitals.

The only break in the pig's sterile life is when she approaches full term and is transferred to the farrowing crate to give birth. Again there is no bedding and her instincts to build a nest for her young are denied. They are born onto bare, perforated metal. She is now forced to lie down, again restricted by metal bars which prevent her from nuzzling or nurturing her young - she is nothing more than a milk provider.

At only about three weeks old, the piglets are removed and placed in sterile, overcrowded boxes or "open deck" pens. It is commonplace for their teeth to be crushed with pliers and their tails to be cut off, both without anaesthetic, in order to avoid the "vice" of tail biting. They are eventually moved to equally overcrowded fattening pens before being killed at five or six months old for bacon, ham and pork.

Throughout their short and unnatural lives, these intelligent little creatures, as inquisitive as puppies, never see a piece of bedding, never feel wind, rain or sunshine and never discover what it is like to root for their own food.

And the sows? It is straight to the "rape rack" with no choice of partner and back into the sow stall for a further five months. When the tissues of her body eventually break down and the abscesses and ulcers start to appear, usually at around five years old, this baby machine faces an ironic fate - slaughter for use in low grade meat products including baby foods. Under other circumstances she would live into her twenties.

But the pinnacle of human intervention in the lives of animals is reached with broiler chickens, the type that account for almost all the chicken meat produced in Europe. In the space of only 25 years, producers have halved the time it takes them to grow to full size, from 84 days to 42. So fast do they now swell that they outstrip their heart's ability to cope.

It struggles to pump enough blood to feed the ballooning muscles - and frequently fails. Some 12 per cent of the national flock dies every year from heart disease - over 72 million birds - and if the remainder weren't slaughtered when they are, the number of fatalities would increase dramatically.

So much effort has gone into increasing the amount of edible flesh that other, less profitable, parts of the bird - incidentals such as the skeleton - fail to develop properly. As a consequence, foot, leg and other bone deformities are commonplace, as is the bizarre phenomenon of bones breaking under the bird's own weight. Even an industry quango, the Agriculture & Food Research Council, admits that four fifths of birds suffer in these ways.

But that isn't the limit of suffering. Up to 100,000 chicks are crammed into a windowless shed on deep litter of straw and woodchip. Over the 42 days of their life, the chicks expand and grow until they carpet the entire floor and there is little room to move. Their droppings saturate the flooring and the ammonia created frequently causes painful ulcers to the feet, legs and even breasts. There is no escape from it, no way to avoid the constant burning. These great "advances" have been achieved by genetic selection and dietary manipulation and quaint little devices such as keeping the lighting on for 23 hours a day. Why the one hour of darkness? So the birds won't panic at the unaccustomed gloom should there be a power cut!

Life for egg-laying chickens is no better. They face a life or death decision as one day old chicks. Males are too scrawny for meat and unable to lay eggs so they are dumped into a bin. The ones at the bottom struggle desperately to escape suffocation as others are piled in on top of them. When the bin is full with a mixture of dead and alive little birds it is transferred to the gas chamber where the killing is completed with CO2. Or the alternative might be a steel roller which crushes them. One fate or the other befalls 40 million chicks every year.

The females are transferred to holding cages, frequently being debeaked with a red-hot automatic knife first. Just a piece of hard tissue without feeling, is how the beak is usually described but in fact we know better. It is a highly sensitive organ and the pain of amputation is possibly felt throughout the bird's life. But some never survive that long, dying from shock or blood loss after the "trimming".

As they approach laying age at three months old, the birds are transferred to the battery cages where they will spend the rest of their 18 month to two year life span. Close descendants of restlessly wandering jungle fowl, they are crammed five to a cage little bigger than a domestic microwave oven. There is insufficient room for one hen to stretch her wings let alone five. And with cynical deception, producers tell the world the birds prefer it that way.

They are surrounded by wire mesh, including underfoot, something for which their feet were never designed. The 300 eggs they lay every year suck the calcium from their bodies, leaving behind brittle bones which snap like dry twigs.

It is hard to imagine a more nightmarish existence and although the system has been scientifically shown to be cruel and painful, even though government advisers have called for its banning, nothing has been done to end battery cages and they still account for 90 per cent of all egg production. What a monument to human domination of the planet!

As the pursuit of money turns into a fetish, there is an inexorable drive towards extracting the maximum possible from all animals, humans included. Sheep, traditionally seen as the most free range of farm animals, are not excluded and neither are cattle.

By tricking ewes with hormone implants and by using artificial insemination, farmers are able to force them to produce more lambs, more frequently and at times earlier than the traditional spring lambing. Even though ewes have evolved to bear a single lamb, it is now common for them to produce triplets, one of which will be sent to market at a few days old because the ewe can't feed it.

The outcome is that 20 per cent of all lambs born in the UK die from cold, hunger or disease shortly after birth. As production demands increase, all the usual high tech and pharmaceutical interventions begin to appear and lowland sheep are on the inexorable path towards a factory farmed existence.

Much the same has already happened to cattle in the USA where most spend their lives in grossly overcrowded pens called feedlots. Examples have started to appear in Europe and it won't be long before they are widespread. The first one in Britain outraged people who lived near it because of the stench caused by the chicken droppings, feathers and pieces of dead chicken which were present in the cattle feed.

Another outcome of the live export issue was to force both meat eaters and vegetarians to confront the cruelty inherent in the dairy industry. For many it has been an uncomfortable exercise. The seemingly idyllic life of dairy cattle has been exposed for what it is - an overworked, short and painful existence as cruel as that of any factory farmed animal.

It is hard to imagine anything more brutal than depriving a mother, any mother, of her offspring at a day or two old. When 450,000 of these babies annually faced the horrendous ordeal of long transportation to the veal crates of Europe, cruelty had been taken to new heights. Bewildered little orphans in boxes so small they can't turn round and can barely lie down; purposely diseased by being deprived of solid food and then driven uncomprehendingly to slaughter with electric goads, so weak they are almost incapable of walking. And the whole system defended by producers and governments alike. BSE has brought an end to calf exports from the UK for now but it is the fate still facing millions of calves in Europe.

If we survive long enough, people will one day look back on this abuse of innocence with the same abhorrence they now reserve for witch burnings and the slave trade.

Even before their offspring are bundled off to market or the slaughterhouse, the mothers are being milked. Selectively bred to produce ten times the amount her calf could ever drink, the dairy cow spends nine months of every year with a double burden - providing milk and pregnant with her next calf. She has been pushed beyond her ability to cope and at any one time, one third of the UK dairy herd is afflicted with the painful disease of mastitis. It is the same proportion that are forced to hobble with other painful diseases of the legs and feet. As her body tissues begin to break down, exhaustion and a combination of foot and udder diseases leads to dairy cows, which could live well into their twenties, being killed at between five and six years old - the equivalent to a woman's body having physically broken down in her teens.

The extraordinary fact is that this catalogue of acute suffering is for food products that humans don't even need. Even more surprising, they are healthier without them. There is no longer any argument about this as research from all over the world now points an unwavering finger at the fact that meat - and dairy products to some degree - are bad for health.

The evidence is overwhelming and even back in 1986, the British Medical Association, in its report on diet, nutrition and health, said: "Vegetarians have lower rates of obesity, coronary heart disease, high blood pressure, large bowel disorders and cancers and gall stones. Cholesterol levels tend to be lower in vegetarians and a number of components of the vegetarian diet have been noted to lower blood cholesterol."

In 1995, the US Physicians Committee for Responsible Medicine (PCRM), reviewed all the published literature on the subject and were able to put some percentages on it. Meat eaters' rate of high blood pressure is one third to one half greater than vegetarianism; for heart disease it is from a quarter to a half greater. This same increased rate of risk applies also to cancers - all types of cancers. Diabetes is about 90 per cent higher in meat-eating men and 40 per cent higher in women. Veggies stand only a quarter of the risk of developing gall bladder disease.

These are, quite simply, staggering figures. Why aren't they public knowledge? Well, why are you able to walk into any sweet shop in the country and buy a cheap drug which is linked to one in three of all deaths? The answer is that similar vested interests protect both the tobacco and meat industries. As the government's handling of BSE proved beyond doubt, protection of meat and dairy industry profits is far more important than public health.

One piece of information which does appear to have filtered through is that saturated animal fat and cholesterol are bad for you. What is not yet public knowledge is that far from being a good source of other nutrients, meat is extremely lacking. It contains no calcium, complex carbohydrates or fibre and little or no vitamins A, C, E, D or K. It is the lack of ACE vitamins which should tell us something.

In recent years a dramatic discovery was made which revealed that a particular process of the body's metabolism plays a part in causing disease. It is called oxidation, which happens when you perform almost any function such as breathing and digesting food. Unstable molecules called free radicals are produced which create a chain reaction by grabbing ions from other molecules in order to stabilise themselves. This process causes damage to cells and even DNA, the body's blueprint for repair and regeneration. Free radicals are believed to play a part in causing over 60 diseases.

The counter to these out-of-control molecules are substances called antioxidants, which have a neutralising effect. They are principally the vitamins A (not retinol, the animal form of vitamin A), C and E, present in a wide range of fruit and veg and almost totally absent from meat. The world's leading health authorities are now fully aware that a vegetarian diet is not just healthier but actually bestows protection against a whole range of diseases and their dietary recommendations reflect this.

Health and the treatment of animals are powerful reasons to reject animal protein but there is even further convincing evidence. A "catastrophe" is facing nine of the world's 16 main fishing areas as they teeter on the brink of environmental collapse. Even the remaining seven areas are being exploited to the full and are degrading at an alarming rate. This isn't my assessment but that of ICES (International Commission for Exploitation of the Seas) and it is fully supported by the UN. Quite simply, the seas are dying from over fishing.

The situation is much the same on the world's main land masses. Due to over grazing by food animals, deserts are expanding at an alarming rate - the Sahara 320 kilometres in 20 years. As they expand, weather patterns change ensuring there is no recovery. The semi arid regions of the world - a huge belt which girdles the earth and makes up one third of its land surface - is on the point of turning to desert for similar reasons. Rain forests are still being felled in their millions of acres in order to provide grazing for hamburger cattle. In a few years, the thin soil will cease to be productive and turn to dust. The greatest reservoirs of biodiversity destroyed for short-term profit for a few.

The 20 or so gallons of water it takes to produce one pound of vegetables is dwarfed by the 3,000 gallons it takes to produce a pound of beef and as a consequence the great acquifers of the US are drying out and will take centuries to replenish, if at all. Just as frightening, the great rivers of Africa are also drying as the ravages of livestock production begin to degrade whole continents. Acid rain, ozone depletion, water pollution, global warming - they are all accelerated because of animal rearing.

Those who suffer the most are humans themselves and one nation's addiction is another's starvation. In Britain, 90 per cent of all agricultural land is used to graze animals or grow fodder for them. The proportions are similar throughout the Western world. But so voracious are their appetites that even more fodder is required and so the elites of developing countries, anxious to pay off their external debts, grow animal feed for us while their own children starve to death.

The EC alone imports feed produced on land equivalent to the area of the UK, France, Italy and New Zealand.

Why so much animal food? It is that extraordinary ratio of 10 to 1. It takes about 10 kg of vegetable protein to produce 1kg of animal protein. It leads to the obscenity of US cattle consuming, and largely wasting, enough protein to feed two billion people.

The population of the world stands at around 5.4 billion. On a typical western, meat-based diet there is sufficient food to feed less than half of them. On a plant-based diet the world could feed some six billion people.

It is against this catalogue of cruelty and insanity that vegetarians are beginning to react in increasing numbers. They have always traditionally straddled the moral high ground but they now also command the scientific heights. But it is not science nor morality which is the problem but politics. So long as the dominant philosophy is one of greed and the supremacy of profit, all animals, humans included, will be viewed merely as commodities to be exploited. That is something we all have to tackle.

Juliet Gellatley is Founder & Director of the vegetarian and vegan charity, Viva! It campaigns on all the vegetarian issues with a concentration on youth education. Juliet is author of the book the Silent ark (Thorsons), the first book to explore all the vegetarian issues. She is also author of The Livewire Guide to Going, Being and Staying Veggie (Women's Press), aimed specifically at teenagers.

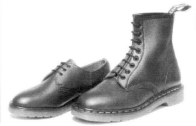

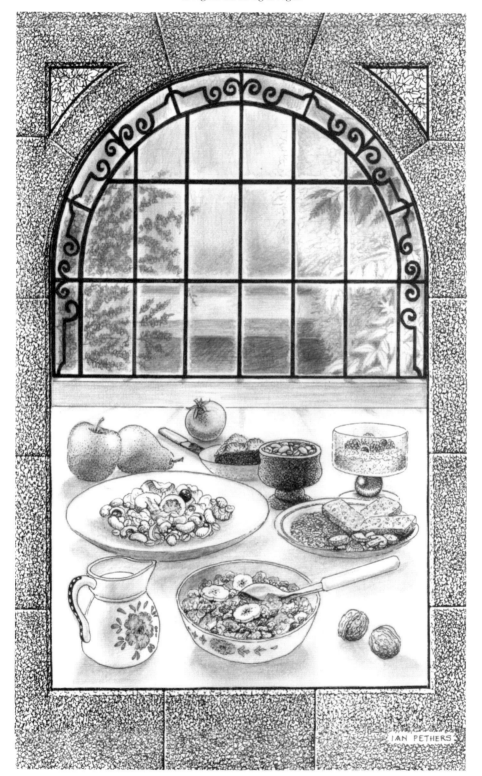

IAN PETHERS

In a current survey 60 vegan volunteers are being asked if they were omnivore or vegetarian before becoming vegan. The following summary of answers on their previous diet shows that today's vegetarian is tomorrow's vegan. (Vegan is pronounced vee-gan).

GENERAL OBSERVATIONS AND COMMENTS

MALE/FEMALE
Of the 60 vegans who completed the questionnaire 20 were male and 40 were female.

AGE GROUP

No. of males	under 25 years	1
	25-35 years	5
	35-45 years	8
	over 45 years	7

No. of females	under 25 years	8
	25-35 years	15
	35-45 years	9
	over 45 years	7

LENGTH OF TIME VEGAN

No. vegan for	1 year or less	17
	2-5 years	18
	6-10 years	14
	over 10 years	10
	No reply given	1

PREVIOUS DIET
59 of the 60 respondents had been vegetarian prior to becoming vegan. One made no reply to this question.

STATE OF HEALTH SINCE BECOMING VEGAN

Not known (not been vegan long enough or no comment made)	6
Health remained constant	24
Health improved	30

Many respondents commented on improved health, either generally   or regarding a specific health condition. Listed below are some of the remarks made.

"...improved health...especially in old age compared with nearly everyone else."
"I was a weakling child - too weak to be vaccinated. Turned vegetarian at age 14 and never looked back!... I have never used any medicines ... never been ill! Now nearly 85 without a trace of rheumatism or other disease."

"...improved health ... more energy, less tired."

"...dermatitis has cleared since becoming vegan."

"There is a lot of sickness at work,(amongst the meat-eaters)but I am very rarely off sick, and never off with 'upset stomach' like many others."

"Improved health...always full of energy."

"Improved health...less viruses, less sinus trouble."

"Improved health...nasal allergy has much improved."

OTHER VEGANS AT SAME ADDRESS

Of some 60 respondents, 8 had at least one other vegan at the same address. of these 8, 7 stated that the other vegans were either partners and/or children.

REASONS FOR BECOMING VEGAN

Below are some of the remarks made by respondents concerning their reasons for becoming vegan.

From a mother - "...I realised about milk whilst I was breastfeeding."

"...cannot bear to be responsible for the separation of mother cow and calf."

"I realised I was not going far enough (being vegetarian), I was hypocritical."

"...realised how cruel the dairy industry was - that really decided me."

"I did not want to exploit any animal or cause it suffering."

"I create in my own little way a more compassionate society in which to live in."

"...mainly because it's not natural to be any other way."

It is interesting to note that there were far more females than males taking part in the survey and further that the majority were in the 25/35 age group.

The moral of this is that vegetarian restaurants, guest houses and caterers in general need to provide vegan alternatives in their menu and may also like to bear in mind that whereas 2/3 decades ago at vegetarian functions very little or no vegan fare was provided, these days at all vegetarian functions, including the Vegetarian Society (UK) Ltd AGM, vegan fare is used exclusively.

MANUFACTURERS' LABELS

Where manufacturers of vegan products are concerned, attention needs to be given both to labels and any recipes provided e.g. vegans shy off buying products which just state vitamin D as an ingredient knowing that vitamin D2 is from a vegetable source, but the cheaper D3 is animal based, so that ingredients section should state clearly 2 or 3. Some manufacturers say on their labels "suitable for vegetarians" and in many cases could equally say "suitable for vegans" but appear ignorant of the fact that there are an ever increasing number of vegan prospective purchasers who don't bother to look at the ingredient section when it only says on the front label "suitable for vegetarians" because they readily assume it is not formulated for the vegan purchaser. Indeed ambiguity is rife where some manufacturers labels are concerned i.e. they just provide the mandatory requirements but their marketing is abysmal when it comes to detail. To cite one example, where lecithin is included in the ingredient section without specifying whether it is soya lecithin or egg lecithin. Also where margarine is one of the ingredients it is misleading to print merely "vegetable margarine" forgetting that some so-called "vegetable margarines" are not 100% vegetable. (Ipso facto not vegan).

Yes labelling needs to be tided up considerably and much more attention needs to be given to the ingredient section.

DEFINITIONS
It would seem appropriate to define a vegetarian and a vegan as follows:-

The definition of a vegetarian, is one who does not eat the flesh of any animal that once lived, nor products derived from its corpse. This includes the obvious products such as flesh, fish and fowl, and also those by-products hidden in modern convenience foods (which may be of animal origin in only some cases) such as; calcium stearate, charcoal, cochineal, enzymes, fatty acids, gelatine, glycerol, lard, rennet, shellac, vitamin D3, E120, E124, E422, E470, E471, E472a, E472b, E472c, E472d, E472e, E473, E474, E475, 476, E477, E478, 542, 904 and 920.

A vegan is one who also abstains from dairy products, eggs and honey, and has to be aware of more additives (which again may be of animal origin in only some cases), E131, E270, E322, E325, E326, E408, 901, and whey - a by-product, of the cheese making process.

The Vegan Society's definition may be defined as a way of living which seeks to exclude, as far as possible and practical, all forms of exploitation of, and cruelty to, animals for food, clothing or any other purpose. In dietry terms it refers to the practise of dispensing with all animal produce - including meat, fish, poultry, eggs, animal milks, honey, and their derivatives. Abhorrence of the cruel practices inherent in dairy, livestock and poultry farming is probably the single most common reason for the adoption of veganism, but many people are drawn to it for health, ecological, resource, spiritual, and other reasons.

These definitions are accepted all over the world, and it is interesting to note that the largest vegan society outside the UK is in the USA and the Swedish one is the largest in the European community. It will be seen that the above definitions go beyond dietary factors. The vegan one particularly more so and this includes clothing and utensils of all kinds. To put it simply a vegetarian is a lacto vegetarian, but a vegan is one who has followed through the principles logically in so far as it affects all facets of life. Some may consider this too restrictive and difficult but to a practising vegan this is being practical and does not impose any difficulty. 50 years ago because there were then fewer alternatives available, and it was a case of overcoming one difficulty after another; these days there are no problems whatsoever. Space does not permit me to go into the questions as to why vegans do not resort to the consumption of honey nor the use of wool, but there are useful leaflets on these subjects from the HQ of the national Vegan Society at Donald Watson House, 7 Battle Road, St Leonards on sea, East Sussex, TN37 7AA.

PHILOSOPHY
A vegan is a person who believes that cow's milk was never meant for humans.

Milk is a food secreted by female mammals to ensure that their offspring adjust from the womb to the outside world. The milk of each species of mammal is nutritionally tailored to its particular developmental needs. The early development of cows and humans is quite different. When a calf is born it must quickly build a strong bone structure in order to stand and move about. Cow's milk, richer in protein, minerals and fats than human milk, is designed to promote this. The greatest early development in humans, however, is not in bone and muscle but in the nervous system. Human milk is therefore rich in easily digestible fats intended to build up the nervous system. It contains lighter, more digestible protein than cow's milk, and is sweeter and more alkaline. Although cow's milk may build strong bones, no one ever makes claims for what it does to intelligence. Human milk varies in composition during the first few weeks of infancy according to the baby's changing needs. It also transfers from mother to babe a degree of immunity to disease. Cow's milk, because it lacks all these properties, is not suitable for human infants.

Milk of any species of mammal is only intended as a food for their young. No other mammal uses milk after infancy. In fact we humans tend to lose the ability to digest milk properly as we grow older. About 80% of the adults in the world lack the enzyme lactase needed to digest lactose (the sugar in milk). Undigested milk forms mucus, which can clog the system and cause disease.

Advertisers often claim that milk is an excellent food because it contains large quantities of essential nutrients, particularly protein and calcium. In fact milk contains only about 3% protein by weight, compared with about 10% for grains, 20-25% for beans, and about 50% for some soyabean products. Moreover the protein of cow's milk is the insoluble substance caseinogen, Which forms a dense curd in the stomach that is difficult to digest. Milk is also by no means as high in calcium as we are led to believe. Sunflower seeds contain at least as much, kale leaves more than twice as much, sesame seeds about eleven times as much, and wakame and hijiki sea vegetables over thirteen times as much calcium as milk (per 100 grams edible protein). A good balanced diet based on whole grains, beans, vegetables, seeds and sea vegetables therefore provides more protein and calcium, not to mention other nutrients, than dairy products. Such a diet can be health promoting, delicious and easy on the pocket.

ETHICS

A vegan is a person who finds the whole system of the dairy industry abhorrent, so just pause and think for a moment, and you will soon realise that dairy milk is based on a principle of cruelty and inhumane practise. Within a few days of birth the majority of calves are sold through auctions or dealers and a few are slaughtered almost immediately. Some calves go (mostly for export with horrendous journeying) to be reared for veal or baby beef. The rest are reared for a year or longer after marketing as young calves to be killed for beef. Rennet comes from the stomach of a newly born calf which is slaughtered. Constant births are brought on by artificial insemination and higher and higher milk yields (for profit) are induced. All forms of exploitation without regard to the pain, anguish and distress of the animals. All this in order that so-called civilised man may have ('steal' would be a better word) the milk which unquestionably was meant for the calf and no other species.

This is explained in more detail. The heifer (female cow) will give birth to her first calf when she is approximately two years of age. Her calf is then taken away from her a day or two after birth. About 10% of calves die before they are six months old. The heifer, developed for high milk yields, is then milked to capacity - up to 45/50 litres (10/11/gallons) a day - 10 times the amount a calf would drink. The heifer is milked for ten months after her calf's birth. During this time she is already pregnant, having been artificially inseminated, and she is only rested for a scant few weeks before her next calf is born. The heifer is put in calf about 12 weeks after the birth of her calf so she gives birth to a calf every year. The dual burden of pregnancy and lactation makes the heifer susceptible to disease - mastitus (infection of the udder) occurs in 1/3 of cows. Every year over 17 million shots of antibiotics go up the teats of our cows!

Dairy cows are slaughtered at an early age - 25% before they are 3 years old. Only 25% live for more than 7 years; a cow's natural life-span is twenty years.

Approximately 30%/40% of British beef comes from specialist beef herds. The remainder comes from our dairy herds. The dairy cow's meat is tough and is used for burgers, pies and in other processed foods.

Heifer (female) calves are kept for dairy herd replacement and bull (male) calves are mainly reared for veal. Whilst some may be reared for beef, generally, calves from dairy cattle are unsuitable for beef.

Around 500,000 calves are exported live usually to France, Belgium and the Netherlands to be reared for veal.

ECONOMICS/PROTECTIONISM

According to the Official Journal of the 1996 European Communities Chapter B1-20 the total subsidy budget on milk and milk products in 1995 amounted to £52.5 billion (yes billion). Efforts are being made to find out how much this is costing you and I as UK tax payers. However not satisfied with the huge subsidies handed out to it, the milk lobby has sought "protection" from competition despite the single market being supposedly for free trade. It was instrumental in having a Council Regulation (EEC) number 1898/87 brought out on 2 July 1987 "ON THE PROTECTION OF DESIGNATIONS USED IN MARKETING OF MILK AND MILK PRODUCTS". There was a clause under its Article 3.1 saying "this provision shall not apply to the designations of products the exact nature of which is clear from traditional usage". The UK Government accordingly interpreted this clause as not ruling out the title "soya milk" because it had become a traditional name long before the UK entered the common Market. However the EU put added pressure on the UK Government to force a label change in place of the UK traditional one of soya milk, when in June 1994 its Management Committee for Milk and Milk Products ruled that the name soya milk must discontinue. Regrettably, in December 1994, the UK Government meekly caved in and said there was nothing more that it could do to save the name. However the soya milk industry was not prepared to be kicked around in this fashion and Plamil Foods (pioneers of British made soya milk in 1965) on behalf of the Soya Milk Alliance, consulted Mark Watts its constituency MEP who convened a seminar for MEPs in Brussels Parliament in February 1995 to brief them on the issue leading to over 70 of the 87 UK MEPs signing a petition which was presented to Franz Fischler the EU Agriculture Commissioner in Strasbourg European Parliament in July 1995, which had the backing of Angela Browning in her capacity as Food Minister and Parliamentary Secretary to MAFF. He promised to review the ruling. However in October 1995 he advised Douglas Hogg, Minister of Agriculture that there was no framework in place to overturn the decision of the Management Committee for Milk and Milk Products.

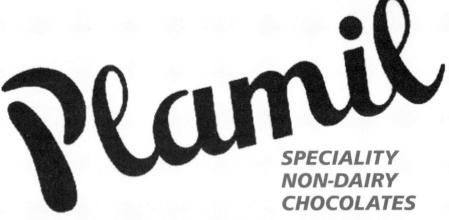

Plamil

SPECIALITY NON-DAIRY CHOCOLATES

3 rich dark chocolate bars plus Martello – 'milkier' in taste

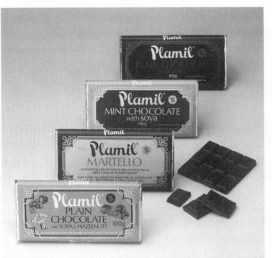

Plamil's expertise in making chocolates ensures they are sumptuous tasting with a superfine texture that just melts in the mouth.

Plamil confections do not contain any unacceptable milk content, artificial flavours, colours, animal-based emulsifiers or release agents

IN ADDITION PLAMIL PROVIDES A RANGE OF ORGANIC CHOCOLATE BARS AND IS THE WORLD'S ONLY MANUFACTURER OF ORGANIC CHOCOLATE DROPS

AVAILABLE from your HEALTH STORE

No genetically modified ingredients

DID YOU KNOW MOST 'ORDINARY' SO-CALLED PLAIN CHOCOLATES CONTAIN BUTTERFAT AND LACTOSE. NOT SO WITH PLAMIL!

Please send me

☐ FREE informative literature & recipes

☐ Booklet on healthy vegan Infants/children £1.00

Name .... (BLOCK CAPITALS)

Address ....

....

SAE please to Plamil Foods Ltd, Folkestone CT19 6PQ

NEW NAME

A vegan is a person who uses soya milk instead of cow's milk, he will therefore, need to call it "SOYA - non-dairy alternative to milk". This is because the Soya Milk Alliance refused all along to call it "soya drink" as the EU Commission would have liked. The terminology "soya drink" would not have conveyed the versatile uses for which the product is ideally suitable i.e. for all uses in the kitchen. Labels bearing the name "soya milk" will, with Government consensus, still be around well into 1997, but each manufacturer will bring in the new title as a particular print run is undertaken. Doubtless authors of cookery books and the media will, for years to come, continue to call the product soya milk, instead of the more cumbersome, but Government approved title of "SOYA - non dairy alternative to milk". Coincidentally by referring to it as an "alternative", it links it to alternative therapies so that alternative therapies now embrace alternative foods!

INFANTS/CHILDREN

A vegan naturally wishes its offspring to have a good start in life with vegan fare and a "Healthy Vegan Infants/Children" booklet has been printed. It contains a foreword from a medical doctor, background information on a brand of soya milk in relation to supplementary feeding, guidance for later infancy, and nutritional data. This booklet provides case histories of a number of children, together with updates on children from a previous booklet. It gives details of their diets written by their parents and contains a wealth of useful information for prospective parents, or parents of infants/children. Among the many comments on the previous edition was; "The booklet was really helpful and supportive - when I was unsure if it was possible to bring up a child as a vegan and faced much opposition from friends, family and authorities. No-one doubts it any more".

A questionnaire is put in each booklet to solicit salient comments, and these comments have revealed the usefulness of the booklet such as; "I found the information reassuring. There is so little really practical information around regarding vegan infant babies and their diets. The practical tips and experiences of others was good to read". "We are planning to have a baby within the next year or two and want to bring it up vegan". From an expectant mother "information is needed to combat the panorama and misinformation from the medical profession. I don't want to be harassed. I am vegan and my baby will be vegan". This booklet is available priced £1 from Plamil Foods Ltd., Bowles Well Gardens, Folkestone, Kent, CT19 6PQ.

BOOKS

There are a range of books on the market on a vegan diet and it would cover many pages to list them. However the following are the ones which stand out as useful reading and I particularly recommend.

VEGAN HEALTH PLAN by Amanda Sweet - A source book of information of interest to anyone concerned with healthy living. Contains over 300 inspiring recipes, together with a comprehensive nutritional guide covering every aspect of diet, from proteins and carbohydrate, to vitamins and minerals set out in easy to follow charts showing their different functions in the body and vegan source, in effect a vegan's bible.

VEGAN COOKERY by Eva Batt - this cookery book is most comprehensive and advises on the preparation of nutritious, appetising meals without meat, fish, eggs or dairy produce. Essential

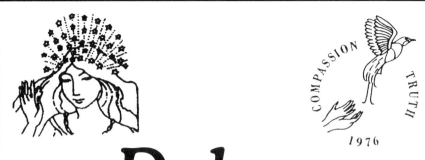

Dolma

Dolma offer an exclusive range of high quality vegan perfumes, toiletries and skin care based on pure essential oils, herbal extracts, aromatic waters and vegetable oils. All products are carefully blended from safe, long established animal free ingredients and a fixed cut-off date of 1976 applies.

The range includes original perfumes, aromatic shampoos for the body, hair, face and feet, lip salves, cleansers, toners, moisturisers, facial scrubs and masks, aromatherapy facial and massage oils, hair treatments and conditioners, shaving fluid, aftershave balm and cologne, pre-shave, hand creams, soaps and essential oils etc.

Send an S.A..E. for free mail order brochure and price list or £14.25 for a set of ten trial perfumes to:

DOLMA
19 Royce Avenue, Hucknall, Nottingham NG15 6FU

A Member of the Cosmetics Industry Coalition for Animal Welfare

nutrients from vegetable sources, planning meals for best food value, savoury dishes, snacks, desserts, cakes, bread, biscuits, sauces, garnishes etc.

THE ANIMAL FREE SHOPPER published by The Vegan Society - a shopping guide for those wishing to buy goods which are entirely free of animal ingredients and involve no animal testing. The Shopper lists thousands of products under the following categories: Food, drink, toiletries & cosmetics, remedies & supplements, baby & infant care, footwear & clothing, home & office, animal care and garden & leisure.

CRUELTY FREE GUIDE TO LONDON by Alex Bourke and Paul Gaynor - this is the definitive guide to compassionate living in the metropolis. Also gives nearest tube stations, opening times of restaurants, museums and entrance fees where applicable. This cruelty free Guide to London is equally good for tourists, day trippers and Londoners. Mainly dealing with London, it also lists a selection of useful data on Bath, Bristol, Brighton and Cambridge. This is the most comprehensive and helpful guide of its kind.

These are available from either the Vegan Society, Donald Watson House, 7 Battle Road, St Leonards on sea, East Sussex, TN37 7AA or from Plamil Foods Ltd., Bowles Well Gardens, Folkestone, Kent, CT19 6PQ.

CJD

It would seem appropriate to close on a somewhat chilling note with a very significant message. It relates to a book by Professor Richard Lacey entitled 'Mad Cow Disease', published in 1994 by Cypsela Publications. Lacey is an acknowledged expert on food safety and an internationally acclaimed scientist. He is Professor of Clinical Microbiology at the University of Leeds and a consultant on Microbiology to the World Health Organisation. He served on the UK Government's Veterinary Products Committee (1986/89) but resigned from it because of his opposition to the idea of injecting cows with BST (bovine somatotrophin) to increase milk yields, which he declared would aggravate BSE.

The significant message is that he relates the case of a LIFELONG lacto vegetarian who had become a victim of the human form of BSE, Creutzfeldt Jacob Disease (CJD). This surely leaves little to the imagination that affected cow's milk is responsible. This means in reality only vegans can be assured of not succumbing to CJD.

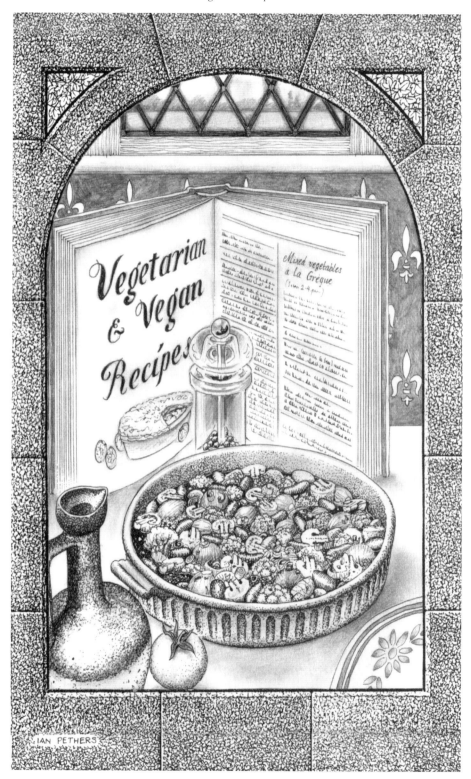

Vegetarian Recipes

This collection of recipes, all tried and tested by the originators has been gathered together to give you the opportunity to try out at home some of the excellent and exciting dishes you will have enjoyed in restaurants. I hope that in the second edition of this book in 1998 you will have written to me asking me to include your favourite recipes as well as new ones you have discovered when eating out.

This is not meant to be a cook book and is therefore not divided into sections for each course of a meal. Where it is applicable I have shown the origin of the recipe so you can try it when you visit the appropriate eaterie.

From Miss Val Maccomell, The Moon Restaurant, Kendal, Cumbria

MUSHROOM, BROADBEAN & OKRA KORMA

6ozs Chopped onion
A little oil
1oz Butter
1 Clove Garlic (crushed)
½ tsp Ground Ginger
1 tsp Ground Coriander
1 tsp Ground Cumin
2ozs Creamed Coconut
4ozs Okra (sliced into 1/4 inches diagonally)
6ozs Mushrooms (quartered)
2floz Double Cream
1floz Natural Yoghurt
Salt and Pepper

Method
Saute the onion, oil and butter together with the garlic and spices, until the onion is soft. Add the mushrooms and okra and the chopped creamed coconut. Bring to the boil then turn down. Once the cream coconut has melted, take off the heat and then add the yoghurt, double cream, salt and pepper. Serve with brown rice.

MUSHROOM, GARLIC & DILL STROGANOFF

2ozs Butter
4 Large Cloves Garlic (crushed)
2 tps Dill
1lb Mushrooms (quartered)
2ozs Plain Flour
3floz Water
2floz Double Cream

Method
Gently saute the butter and garlic until soft. Add the mushrooms and dill. Bring to the boil. Add mixture of water and flour to thicken. Continue to cook for another two minutes until the mixture has thickened. Take off the heat and stir in the cream. Season to taste.

CURRIED LENTIL, APRICOT AND CASHEW NUT ROAST

4oz sliced onion
2ozs Red Lentils
2ozs Brown Lentils
2ozs Grated Carrot
2ozs Chopped Leeks
2 Sticks Celery, chopped
8floz Orange Juice
2 tsp Madras Curry Paste
4ozs Chopped Apricots
2 tbsp Double Cream
2ozs Cashew Nuts
1/4 tsp Salt

Method
Wash the brown and red lentils separately and drain. Put brown lentils, onion and orange juice into a large pan. Cook until the brown lentils start to soften. Add the red lentils, leeks, carrots and celery and the madras curry paste. When the red lentils are soft add the apricots, cream and salt. Stir in the cashew nuts. Empty the pan into a large casserole dish. Cook on Gas 6 until the top is browned. Serve with pacific chilli and apple sauce.

TOMATO APPLE CHILLI & THYME SAUCE

4ozs Chopped Onion
4ozs Chopped prepared Onion
1 tsp Dried Thyme
½ tsp Chilli Powder
Little Oil
5 tsp Creamed Coconut
1 tbsp Tomato Puree
400 gram Tin Chopped Tomatoes
2floz Red Wine

Method
Saute onion, oil, apple, chilli and thyme until the onion is soft. Add tomatoes, creamed coconut, tomato puree and red wine, simmer until the creamed coconut is melted into the sauce. Liquidize. Season to taste.

BROCCOLI, SWEETCORN & TARRAGON SOUP

8ozs Onion
8ozs Broccoli
326 gram Tin of Sweetcorn
1 pt Milk
½ pt Water
1/4 pt Single Cream
Heaped tsp Freeze Dried Tarragon

Method
Coarsely chop the onion and broccoli.
Put onion, broccoli, butter, water and tarragon in a large pan. Bring to the boil, turn down the heat, cover and simmer until   the vegetables are soft.
Add the sweetcorn, milk and cream, then liquidize. Season to taste. Go easy when using tarragon it is powerful stuff especially dried. Fresh or freeze dried is subtler.

COURGETTE, CAULIFLOWER & PESTO SOUP
Serves 6
8ozs Onion
8ozs Courgette
8ozs Cauliflower Florets
1 tbsp Pesto Sauce
½ pt Water
½ pt Milk
1/4 Pt Single Cream

Method
Coarsely chop all the vegetables.
Put all the ingredients, except the milk, cream and pesto sauce into a large pan.
Bring to the boil, turn the heat down and leave simmering until all the vegetables are soft.
Add the milk, pesto sauce and cream, then liquidize. Season to taste.

FENNEL, RICE, MOZARRELLA & SWEETCORN FILLED CABBAGE DOLMAS
8ozs Brown Rice
8ozs Diced Fennel
1 tsp Dill
1 tsp Fennel Seeds
5floz Water
5floz Orange Juice
6ozs Grated Mozarrella
5floz Double Cream
2 Diced Red Peppers
1 Small Tin Sweetcorn
1 White Cabbage
Salt & Pepper

Method
Cook the rice with the water, fennel and orange juice, dill and fennel seeds. As the fennel is softening add the sweetcorn and diced peppers. When the rice is 'al dente', turn off the heat and stir in the cream and mozarrella. Allow to cool. To prepare the cabbage leaves - bring a pan of water to the boil. Add 12 cabbage leaves separately. When the leaves have softened, remove from the water. Trim the stalks with a sharp knife and fill the 12 leaves with the rice filling to make a parcel. Serve on the lemon couscous with the tomato and garlic sauce.

TOMATO, GARLIC AND ALLSPICE SAUCE
1oz Butter
15oz Tin Chopped Tomatoes
4ozs Diced Onion
1 tbsp Tomato Puree
½ tsp Ground Allspice
3 Cloves Garlic (crushed)
3floz Red Wine
Salt & Pepper

Method
Saute the onion and allspice with the butter until soft. Add tomatoes, tomato puree with the red wine. Bring to the boil, take off the heat and liquidize. Add salt and pepper.

MAIN COURSE 1

LENTIL, MUSHROOM & TOMATO FILLED AUBERGINE CANNELLONI WITH GRUYERE & GINGER SAUCE
1 Leek
4ozs Red Lentils
4floz Water
4floz White Wine
4 Cloves Garlic (crushed)
Olive Oil
1oz Butter
8ozs Mushrooms, finely sliced
2ozs Onion, finely diced
14ozs Grated Carrot
2ozs Sundried Tomatoes in strips
2 Aubergine

Method
Saute the onions, leek and lentils in the butter and a little oil. Once well coated add the water, wine and carrots. Simmer gently until the lentils are soft, stir regularly. The mixture needs to be thick so don't be tempted to add water, keep the lid on the pan to retain the moisture. When the lentils are nearly ready, ie becoming mushy add the mushrooms and sundried tomatoes. Allow the mushrooms to start to soften, then remove from the heat. Cover and leave to rest. Slice the aubergines lengthways 1cm thick. Fry on both sides in oil until golden brown. Leave to drain and cool in the colander.

GRUYERE AND GINGER CHEESE SAUCE
½ Pt Milk
½ Pt Single Cream
1oz Plain Flour
11/2oz Butter
2ozs Grated Gruyere Cheese
1oz Fresh Ginger, finely chopped
Pinch of Cayenne Pepper
Salt & Pepper

Gently melt the buttter and stir in the flour. Gradually stir in the milk, stirring continuously. Bring to the boil, cook for a further 2 minutes until the sauce thickens. Take off the heat and stir in the cheese and fresh ginger. Season to taste.

PUTTING IT ALL TOGETHER
Pre-heat the oven to 200c. Place one tablespoon of the lentil mixture at one end of a slice of aubergine roll to form a filled tube. Repeat until all the mixture and aubergine slices are used. Place rolls in a large shallow oven-proof dish. Pour the sauce over the aubergines. Bake in a hot oven until golden top has formed.

MAIN COURSE 2

CAJUN SPICED VEGETABLES IN FLOUR TORTILLAS
4ozs Small diced Aubergine
2ozs Chopped Onion
4ozs Small Cauliflower Florets, sliced

4ozs Courgettes, sliced
1 Red Pepper, finely sliced
1 198gram Tin Sweetcorn
1 400gram Tin Chopped Tomatoes
1 tbsp Tomato Puree
A Little Water
½ 400gram Tin Kidney Beans, washed
1 tbsp Cajun Spices
2 tbsp Olive Oil
1 Packet Flour Tortillas

Method
Saute the aubergine, onion, oil and cajun spices in a large pan for 4 minutes. Add the tomatoes and cauliflower. On medium heat cook until the aubergine is very soft. Add the courgettes, pepper and sweetcorn cook until the courgettes are slightly 'al dente'. If the mixture becomes dry and sticky add a little water, but keep the mixture quite thick. Stir in the tomato puree and kidney beans and season.

GUACAMOLE
1 Very Soft Ripe Avocado, not black
2ozs Onion
2 Ripe Tomatoes
Juice of ½ Lemon
1/4 tsp Chilli Powder
Salt & Pepper

Method
Put all the ingredients, except the lemon in a food processor. Process until you have a creamy smooth sauce. Add the lemon juice and adjust seasoning.

SOUR CREAM
Either buy already made sour cream or mix equal quantities of cream and low fat yoghurt together. 2floz of each will be enough for 4 servings of tortillas.

CAJUN SPICES
It is possible to buy cajun blends, but just in case you cannot here's the mix.
1 Clove Garlic, crushed
1 tsp Paprika
1/4 tsp Ground Black Pepper
½ tsp Ground Cumin
½ tsp Colmans Mustard Powder
½ tsp Cayenne
½ tsp Dried Thyme
½ tsp Oregano
1 tsp Salt

PUTTING IT ALL TOGETHER
Divide the spiced vegetable mixture between the 8 tortillas. Wrap or roll as shown on the packet. Place without overlapping in a shallow oven-proof dish. Heat through in pre-heated oven 200c until the tortillas are just colouring. Serve with guacamole, sour cream, brown rice, salad and jalapeno chillies.

SUMMERFRUIT KISSELLE

4ozs Gooseberries
4ozs Baking Apples, peeled, cored and chopped
4ozs Blackberries
4ozs Strawberries
4ozs Raspberries
1 Pear peeled and chopped

Topping
1oz Toasted Porridge Oats
1/4 pt Whipped Cream
Little Demerara Sugar

Method
Cook the apple in a little water until mushy. Add the rest of the fruit, cover and simmer for 5 minutes. Gradually bring to the boil. Then leave to cool. This should produce a thick fruity consistency. Gently stir the oats into the cream (a touch of whisky can be added). When the fruit is cool, spoon into glass dishes and sprinkle the top with a little sugar. Top with the cream.
Use whatever fruit is in season. It is just as good with frozen fruit or half and half. When using frozen add the fresh fruit as you take the fruit from the high heat to keep its texture.

RASPBERRY AND ELDERFLOWER CHEESECAKE

BISCUIT BASE
2ozs Butter
4ozs Crushed Digestive Biscuits

CHEESECAKE
1/3 pt Double Cream
10ozs Low fat Cream Cheese
2ozs Caster Sugar
4floz Elderflower Cordial
1 dessertspoon Lemon Juice

TOPPING
2 15oz Tins Raspberries
1 dessertspoon Arrowroot, mixed with a little cold water

8" Loose Bottom Shallow Cake Tin

Method
Melt the butter and stir in the biscuit crumbs. Press the mixture evenly over the base of the tin and leave to cool. Using a hand mixer, beat together all the ingredients for the cheesecake mixture until smooth. Spread over the biscuit base. For the topping, bring the raspberries quickly to the boil, stir in the arrowroot. Take off the heat. Divide into 8 portions and spoon over the raspberries.

FROM THE OLD POST OFFICE,LLANIGAN, HEREFORD

VEGETABLE HOT POT

1lb onions
1lb carrots
1lb potatoes
1/2lb courgettes
1/2lb parsnips
1/2lb aubergine
1 Green Pepper
Any other vegetable in season
Seasoning
Worcester or Tabasco
1/2lb cheese

Method:
Warm 2 tbs oil in ovenproof casserole. Peel and slice vegetables. Arrange in layers starting with onions, Season as you go. Put on lid and cook in moderate oven for at least one hour. Remove lid. Top with cheese and brown under grill.

PARSNIP AND WALNUT LOAF

1lb parsnips
2onions
2oz butter
4oz breadcrumbs
6oz chopped walnuts
2 beaten eggs
7fl oz milk
2tbls parsley
large pinch of Basil and oregano
½ tsp grated nutmeg
Seasoning

Method:
Peel and dice parsnips. Cook 5 min in boiling salted water. Finely chop onion and cook gently in melted butter. Add parsnips and rest of ingredients. Mix well and place in greased mould or loaf tin, cover with greased foil and bake at 350F for 1 hour. Cool slightly and turn out for serving.

From Merefield House, East Street, Crewkerne

BUTTER BEAN AND GINGER STEW COOKED IN CIDER

12oz butterbeans (cooked weight)
Medium onion chopped
1 large courgette thickly sliced
1 large carrot thickly sliced
2 sticks celery sliced
1 small red pepper cut in chunks
8oz mushrooms quartered
1/2 inch piece fresh ginger finely chopped
2 cloves garlic crushed
8ozs fresh tomatoes roughly chopped
1 tbsp tomato puree
1 tbsp flour
2 vegetable stock cubes
15 fluid ozs medium cider
Black pepper to taste

Method
Saute onions, garlic and ginger in a little oil. Add all other vegetables and cook for few minutes. Gradually add flour, stirring to coat vegetables, then add cider while continuing to stir. Add all other ingredients and cook until the vegetables are just to your liking. Serve with brown rice or jacket potato and salad.

STEAMED CINNAMON APPLE PUDDING

8 ozs 81% self raising flour
4 ozs vegan margarine
4 ozs soft brown sugar
2tsp cinnamon
1 large cooking apple peeled and grated
5 fluid ozs soya milk.

Method
Cream together sugar and margarine, fold in grated apple. Add dry ingredients alternating with the soya milk. Turn into a greased basin cover with foil and steam for approx 11/2 hours. Serve with soya custard.

From Crispins Restaurant, Dulverton, Somerset

BAKED AVOCADOS WITH SOMERSET BLUE CHEESE & WALNUTS

(Serves 4 as a starter, 2 as a main course)
2tbsp soya oil
1 onion thinly sliced
100 grams mushrooms, thinly sliced
2tbsp low-fat fromage frais
30zs Somerset Blue Cheese
1oz walnut halves
2 large Avocados

Method
Heat oven to 150c/300F/Gas 3. Heat oil in a pan, saute onions & mushrooms for about 5 minutes until soft. Add fromage frais, crumble in cheese, add walnuts and season with salt and freshly milled black pepper. Halve avocados & scoop out most of the flesh. Mash avocado flesh and add to cheese mixture. Pile into avocado shells and bake for 10 minutes until warmed through. Serve with salad and good bread.

FROM BRIEF ENCOUNTER, GREAT MALVERN STATION, MALVERN, WORCESTERSHIRE

CREAM OF LETTUCE AND PEA SOUP
Serves 6
12oz spring onions
1lb peas
6 lettuce leaves
2 tbsp olive oil
2 tsp plain flour
21/2 pints vegetable stock
Salt and pepper
5oz single cream
2oz mange tout for garnish
Croutons

Method
Chop spring onions and lettuce leaves. Saute with the peas in the olive oil, until peas are tender. Stir in the plain flour. Add the vegetable stock, bring to the boil, simmer for 5 minutes. Liquidize and season. Heat to serve, adding a swirl of cream, a few mange tout and croutons.

CARAMELISED APPLES WITH CREME FRAICHE
Serves 4
4oz unsalted butter
4   firm apples
1/4 tsp ground cardoman
Pinch ground cinnamon
Pinch ground cloves
5oz castor sugar
3tbsp flaked almonds
2tbsp chopped walnuts

Method:
Peel, core and slice the apples. Melt the butter in saucepan, add apples, spices, caster sugar and nuts. Cook over medium heat for 2-3 minutes, then on high heat for 8 mins, stirring, until apples are caramelised. Serve with creme fraiche

SUMMER VEGETABLES WITH SATE SAUCE
Serves 8
4 tbsp sunflower oil
1lb baby sweetcorn
1lb baby carrots
2 stems of lemon grass finely chopped
8oz small button mushrooms
1lb summer cabbage shredded
12 spring onions, trimmed and chopped

Sauce
8 tbsp crunchy peanut butter
4 tbsp soy sauce
4oz creamed coconut
Juice of 1 lemon
4 tsp soft brown sugar
2tsp ground coriander
2tsp ground cumin
6 fl.oz boiling water

Method
Stir fry the sweetcorn and carrots in the oil for 5 minutes. Add lemon grass, mushrooms, cabbage and onions and fry for 10 minutes, stirring. Mix all the ingredients for the sauce together. Add to the vegetables and stir well. Serve with rice.

FROM THE AMADEUS VEGETARIAN HOTEL, HARROGATE, YORKSHIRE HG1 5EN

YORKSHIRE RHUBARB CRUMBLE CAKE
For Sponge Base
4oz Butter or Margarine
4oz Caster Sugar
2 medium eggs beaten
4oz Self Raising Flour

For Crumble Topping
4oz Plain Wholemeal Flour
2oz Butter or Margarine
2tbsp Brown Sugar
1 tsp Cinnamon
11/2lbs Rhubarb chopped

Method
Stew Rhubarb with 4 tbsps brown sugar until soft. Drain off about half of the excess juice. Make sponge base by beating butter and sugar until smooth, then beat in eggs, a little at a time. Add flour 1oz at a time and fold in until well blended. Make Crumble Topping by rubbing butter into flour. Then add sugar and cinnamon. Take an 8-9 inch loose bottomed tin which has been well oiled. Put half of sponge mixture in base, spreading it out to the edges. Then spoon cooked rhubarb juice on top, followed by rest of sponge mixture. Finally spread crumble topping over mixture and bake at 180c for 45 minutes to one hour until

centre of sponge is set and springy. Dust with icing sugar if desired. Serve warm with cream or ice cream. Substitute rhubarb for plums or summer fruits when in season.

LEMON AND BANANA TOFU CHEESECAKE ON A GINGER BASE
Ingredients
2x250g Tofu (Silken is best)
Juice of half a lemon
2 or 3 large ripe bananas
2-3 drops vanilla essence
2oz sultanas (optional)
Runny honey or concentrated apple juice to taste

Base
5oz Ginger biscuits
5oz Digestive biscuits
4oz Margarine or butter

Method
Process biscuits into crumbs (or crush with a rolling pin) Melt margarine/butter and mix in biscuit crumbs. Press mixture into base and sides of an 8-9 inch loose bottomed tin. Chill in Fridge. Blend all ingredients for topping (excluding sultanas) until smooth. You can taste at this stage and add more lemon juice or honey/apple juice as required. Then stir in the sultanas and pour mixture onto chilled base. Bake in oven at 170c for approx one hour until set. Then chill until needed. Decorate with slices of Kiwi Fruit or Grapes.

FROM BURRASTOW HOUSE, WALLS, SHETLAND, SCOTLAND

WILD MUSHROOMS WITH A SAFFRON AND WALNUT SAUCE
TO SERVE WITH HOMEMADE PASTA
3/4lb Mushrooms (mixture of all local ones)
2 small onions, finely chopped
2ozs walnuts
1oz butter or vegoil
1 glass of white wine
A few strands of Saffron
Salt and Pepper
125grms Creme fraiche

Method
Sweat onion in butter or oil, add mushroom coarsely chopped, saffron and white wine. Simmer 2-5 minutes, season. Add creme fraiche and broken walnuts, bubble and pour over cooked spaghetti. Serve immediately

CHOCOLATE PANCAKES WITH CHESTNUT CREAM AND CHOCOLATE SAUCE

Batter
3ozs flour 1 oz cocoa
2 eggs   1/2-3/4pt milk
Pinch of salt.

Filling
6ozs chestnut pureed
1/2pt single cream or half cream and half yoghurt
2-3 drops vanilla essence
2-3 tsps castor sugar

Sauce
6ozs Dark chocolate
1/4pt water
1oz caster sugar
1oz butter
2tbls rum

Method
 Mix and whisk all batter ingredients and leave to stand for 20 minutes. Make filling. Fold cream, essence and sugar into pureed chestnuts (it needs to be firm but not too stiff) Put all sauce ingredients into a heavy based pan, melt slowly, bubble for 2 minutes, ready to serve. Make small thin pancakes spread in a little chestnut cream (it is very rich) to 2 pancakes, then pour over a little chococlate sauce - and it's heaven!

FROM N.KIMBER ENTERPRISES, CREAG-NA-MARA, EAST MEY, CAITHNESS

SOUP
Take any vegetable of your choice cook with onions and maybe if you like it a little garlic, puree, sieve if necessary (tomato particularly) add seasoning. I frequently use fruit juices to add flavour as vegetable stock is rather strong. Nutmeg, cinnamon, mace are good flavourings also. Serve with or without cream. For tomato soup, use italian plum tomatoes they give excellent colour and flavour whereas other varieties tend to be insipid.

FRENCH MUSHROOM
Slice mushrooms,onion and garlic saute, then simmer with water and tomato juice for 15 minutes add seasoning and 1 teaspoon French mustard. Serve as for French onion with French bread topped with cheese.

POTATOES
Thinly slice potatoes and layer in a dish dotted with butter or marg and bake for 1-1 ½ hours at 200c
or sprinkle some cheese between layers then bake
or sprinkle some onions between layers then bake
or sprinkle some leeks between layers then bake
or cover with cream
or layer with coxs apples

Mash together potatoes and turnip/swedes or potatoes and celeriac or potatoes and onion. Cook small new potatoes and toss in cheese and pine nuts. Boil new potatoes and for each

1lb, melt 2ozs butter and 1oz sugar, stir gently and don't allow to burn, add potatoes and coat evenly. Using washed and sweet potatoes boil for 15-20 minutes drain, peel and slice thickly, arrange in layers dotting with butter or marg and sprinkling of soft brown sugar. Cover with foil and bake for 20 minutes.

VEGETABLES

All root vegetables and squashes will roast, simply place in a pan with olive oil and a few herbs and cook until tender 45-60 minutes at 200c. Place sliced aubergines, courgettes, thinly sliced peppers and asparagus drizzled with olive oil and mint under the grill for 15 minutes. Chop red cabbage, onion and cooking apples, place in a casserole with cider, water and brown sugar (juniper berries optional) cook until tender. Gently simmer root vegetables in apple juice. Cook a medley of vegetables and coat with sweet and sour sauce to serve. Slice mushrooms with onions, garlic, oregano and celery, season and place in pan with small amount of water and cook until tender. Gently poach avocado slices and apple in either apple juice or white wine, place in gratin dish top with oatmeal and grated cheese, place under grill to brown, use as a starter or a main course.

PIRATES PASTIES
makes about 10

Pastry
1lb plain flour
6ozs margarine
water
salt

Sauce
1 large tin tomatoes
2 large onions, chopped
2 chillies, chopped
Root ginger, chopped
2 tbls tomato puree
2 tbls rum (optional)
Mixed herbs

Lightly fry onions, chillies and ginger, add herbs, add tomatoes and tomato puree, boil until thickened then add rum.

For the Nut Roasts
Olive oil
4 carrots, chopped(optional)
2 onions, chopped
1 stick celery, chopped
½ bulb of fennel, chopped
1lb mixed nuts, chopped
½ pint marmite stock
1 or 2 beaten eggs to bind
1 clove garlic
4ozs wholemeal breadcrumbs
salt
pepper

Method
Lightly fry onions and garlic in olive oil, add celery, fennel and carrots cook gently for 10 minutes. Meanwhile mix nuts, breadcrumbs and stock together, combine nut mixture with vegetable mixture and bind together with beaten egg, season to taste.

Roll out pastry and cut out around a tea plate place soup spoon full of tomato sauce in centre and the same of nut roast on the top, moisten edge of pastry and close together to form a pasty, glaze with egg or milk and bake at 200c for 35 minutes.

These can be frozen and cooked later, or cooked and reheated, they keep very well. Serve with more tomato sauce over the top. Goes well with any vegetables and can be eaten cold with a salad and either new boiled minted or jacket potatoes.

The nut roast of course can be used on its own by baking it in a loaf tin for 45 minutes at 200c and again eaten either hot or cold, served with the same sauce or an apricot relish.

8ozs dried apricots poached overnight
1 onion, chopped
½ red pepper, chopped
1 tps salt
1 tps ground cinnamon
½ pt white wine vinegar
8ozs soft light brown sugar
4ozs sultanas

Method
Place apricots in a heavy based pan, add all the ingredients except the sugar, cook for 10 minutes then add the sugar and cook until pulpy, do not cover whilst cooking. Will store in a jar in the fridge or can be frozen.

BAKED CHEESECAKE
6ozs digestive biscuits, crushed
3ozs butter or margarine
12ozs cottage cheese
12ozs cream cheese
Rind of 1 lemon, grated
5ozs caster sugar
2 eggs
1/4 pint double cream
4ozs raisins
Syrup
4ozs sugar
8 fl ozs water
1 large lemon or 2 limes

Method
Melt butter and combine with biscuits and line an 8 inch loose bottomed spring loaded tin, pressing up sides , I find this easier with a metal dessert spoon rather that a wooden one. Beat together the cheeses and then add lemon rind, sugar,eggs and cream, add raisins. Spoon into the tin and bake at 180c for about 1 hour until firm. It will rise whilst cooking and sink back whilst cooling. Heat 4ozs sugar and 8 flozs water to boiling add lemon or lime slices, simmer for 25 minutes. Arrange on cake and brush with the syrup.

Alternatively you can leave out the lemon and raisins and just make a plain cheesecake. Top with any fruit of your choice, if you leave the topping off until you serve it you can have a variety of toppings. Serve either plain or with cream.

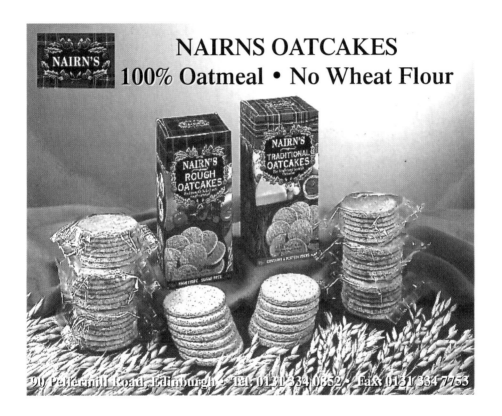

BUTTERBEAN SLICE
Either 3ozs cooked butterbeans or canned butterbeans
1 onion, chopped
2 sticks celery
½ bulb of fennel
2 eggs
½ tsp salt
Black pepper
6ozs cheese, grated
1 tbls fresh chopped parsley or 2 tps dried
2ozs white breadcrumbs

Method
Place drained butterbeans in a processor with the onion, celery, fennel, eggs, salt and pepper and process until smooth, add the cheese, parsley and breadcrumbs. Line and grease a 2lb loaf tin and fill with the mixture. Bake at 180c for 50-60 minutes until firm. Serve with the tomato sauce as for the nut roast, or mix natural yogurt and mint together for a sauce.
Use as a starter or as a main course, serve hot or cold but with a tossed salad and jacket potato.

GATEAU PITHIVIERS
1lb puff pastry
4ozs butter or veg marg
4ozs caster sugar
3 egg yolks
1½ozs cornflour
1 tbls icing sugar
4ozs ground almonds
1 tbls brandy (optional)
You could use walnuts instead of almonds

Method
Cream the butter and sugar until light and fluffy, beat the egg yolks in one at a time then add the cornflour, almonds and brandy.
Divide the pastry into two with one piece slightly larger, roll out the small piece to a 9 inch circle and the larger one to a 10 inch circle. Place the small one on a wetted baking sheet, spread the filling in the centre, glaze the edge with milk or egg, place the large circle on top, press edges down well. Using a round bladed knife to scallop the edges, every two inches press thumb and fore finger onto edge and draw knife towards the centre between your thumb and finger, using a sharp knife mark crescents on top of pastry but do not cut through. Bake at 225c for 25-30 minutes. Sieve icing sugar over top and grill for 2-3 minutes to caramelise. For a savoury version omit the icing sugar on top, and glaze with beaten egg. Use cream cheese and broccoli to fill the centre, or blue cheese, tomato and walnuts, or celery, cottage cheese and pineapple. You can make one large one or 2 small ones.

Allergycare™

Food Sensitivity Testing

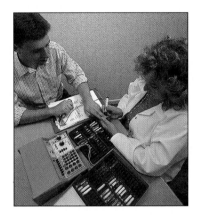

- Now in our 8th Year, we have a network of 30 qualified Testers providing our Food Sensitivity Testing Programme in 700 convenient locations in the UK.

- Our Test costs just £29 and covers 60 items, plus nutrients and dietary information on what not to eat and what you can eat.

- This low-cost, local service is immediate, convenient and does not invade your body at all. Test results are instant and our Free Nutritional Support Phone Line is open throughout the week.

- For details of your nearest Testing Centre and dates please phone 01823 325022

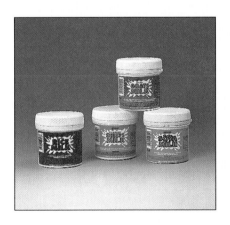

Allergycare Products

If you are eliminating or have eliminated certain foods from your diet, and need to put back something similar (but without incurring the same problems), Allergycare has a wide range of staple foods from which to choose. Available at your local health food store or independent pharmacist or direct from Allergycare. Please phone us for a Free Catalogue on 01823 325023.

Allergycare

Pollards Yard, Wood Street, Taunton, Somerset TA1 1UP
Telephone: 01823 325023 Fax: 01823 325024

FROM GRAIANFRYN, PENISARWALLN, CAERNARFON, WALES

GARDEN SPINACH AND PINE KERNEL BALLS
WITH A ROAST PEPPER AND TOMATO COULIS

1lb Garden spinach
Grated nutmeg
zest of 1 lemon
31/2 oz wheatgerm
3 1/2 oz pinenuts
2 1/4 oz raisins
Black pepper
2 beaten eggs.

Method
Stir fry spinach and nutmeg in a little olive oil until wilted. Squeeze any excess moisture and puree in processor. Combine wheatgerm, pine nuts and raisins. Add spinach, then eggs and pepper. Form into ping-pong size balls and roll in wheatgerm. Drizzle with a few drops of olive oil and bake at 170.c for 20minutes.

ROAST PEPPER AND TOMATO COULIS
1 red pepper
1lb tomatoes (fresh or tinned)
1 chopped onion
1 clove garlic, peeled and crushed
1 tsp dried basil
1 tsp dried marjoram
Black pepper.

Method
Roast red pepper in oven at 200.c for half and hour until skin is charred. Leave to cool. Peel and remove seeds. Saute onion in olive oil till tender, add garlic. After 1 minute add tomatoes and herbs. Bring to boil and simmer for 30minutes. Puree in processor and serve with balls.

FROM TREMEIFION VEGETARIAN COUNTRY HOTEL, TALSARNU, NR HARLECH, GWYNEDD

BROCCOLI PATE WITH BARA BRITH

Broccoli Pate
250 gram Broccoli
150 gram Cream Cheese
1 clove garlic (crushed)
3tsp Mixed Herbs
Seasoning & little single cream

Method:
1) break broccoli into florets
2) put all ingredients into blender
3) Whiz together. Thin the mixture with single cream to a spreadable consistency

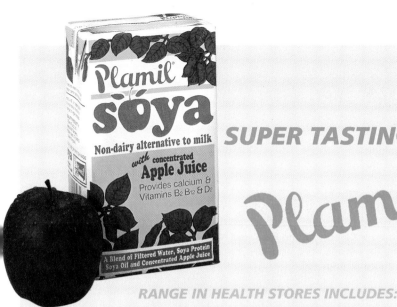

SUPER TASTING

Plamil

RANGE IN HEALTH STORES INCLUDES:

Soya 'milks'
Rice puddings
Carob bars
Carob spreads
Carob drops

Egg-free mayonnaise
Chocolate bars
Organic chocolates
Organic chocolate drops
Veeze

BENJAMIN ZEPHANIAH PREFERS *Plamil* TO UDDER MILK

The EC Management Committee for Milk and
Milk products has ruled that the name soya
milk must discontinue and the Government
new approved name "Soya non dairy alternative to milk" will be gradually phased in
(the name Soya milk will still
be around in 1997)

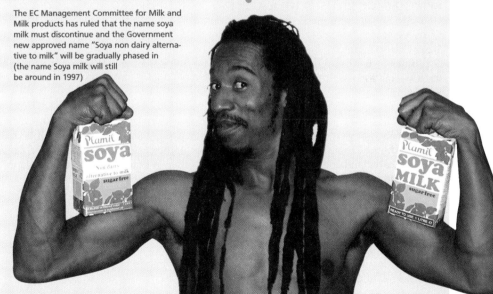

Please send me

☐ FREE informative literature & recipes,
☐ Booklet on healthy vegan Infants/children £1.00

Name   (BLOCK CAPITALS)

Address

SAE please to Plamil Foods Ltd. Folkestone CT19 6PQ

BARA BRITH

300 gram dried fruit, currants, raisins, sultanas
75 gram brown sugar
350 gram Self raising wholemeal flour
2tsp mixed spice
1 free range egg
Juice of half a lemon

Method:
1) Soak fruit in hot tea overnight
2) Next day put all ingredients into bowl adding enough liquid from fruit to make a dropping consistency
3) Grease and line a 900gram loaf tin. Bake on 190c, 375/Mark 5 for approx 45 mins. If the loaf is cooking on the outside too quickly lower heat half way throughout to 180c. It should feel firm to the touch when ready.

To Serve:
When the Bara Brith is cold, slice into fairly thin slices. Allow two slices per person. Put a mound of Broccoli Pate onto a plate along with the Bara Brith. Sprinkle a little paprika over pate to give a little contrast colour. Decorate the plate with either lemon slices, cucumber or just a sprig of fresh herb.

FROM THE OLD POST OFFICE LLANIGAN

RED CABBAGE BRAISED WITH APPLE
1lb Red Cabbage shredded
5fl oz Vinegar
1/2oz Castor Sugar
2oz butter
6oz Cooking Apples
Seasoning

Method
Place cabbage in well buttered casserole. Add vinegar and sugar and cover with buttered paper and lid or foil. Cook in moderate oven for approx 1 ½ hours. Add peeled Apples diced. Recover and cook until tender (approx another ½ hour) If more cooking liquor is needed add a little vegetable stock.

WELSH TOFFEE
Preparation time 30 minutes
Cooling time 1 hour

4oz unsalted butter - melt
1lb granulated sugar - add and stir into butter

2tbs warm water   )
2tbs white vinegar   )   Add & stir until dissolved
4tbs golden syrup   )   (or ½ & ½ treacle & syrup))

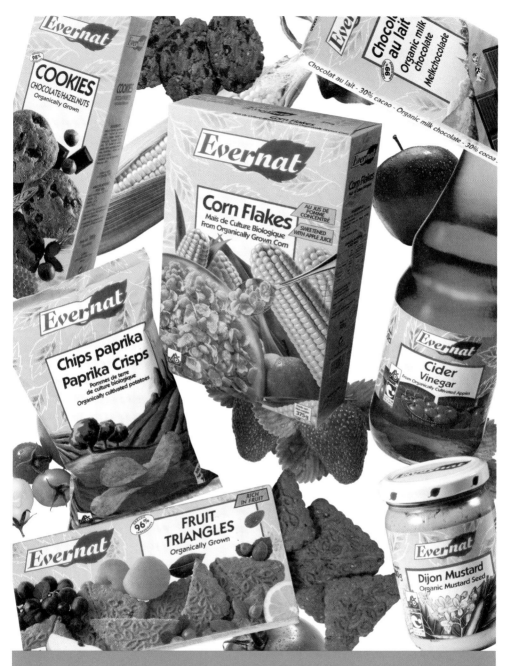

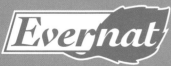

Method
Bring to boiling point. Boil for 15-20minutes or until a little toffee put into a bowl of cold water will snap. Temperature should be 152c. Pour into well buttered rectangular tin 11" x 7". Leave to cool. As soon as it begins to set mark out squares. When cold break into pieces and wrap in cellophane. Store in airtight tin or jar.

LEEK TURVEY - MAIN COURSE
1lb Leeks sliced
1 small red pepper chopped
1/4 tsp coriander
1oz margarine
2 eggs
4fl oz milk
3oz brown bread crumbs
3oz cream cheese
1oz grated cheese
Pepper to taste

Method
Sweat vegetables in margarine, place in 8" Pyrex dish Scatter half the breadcrumbs on top and dabs of cream cheese. Whip eggs and milk put in grated cheese and remaining breadcrumbs. Pour over mixture in dish. Bake at 325F Gas 3 for 35 mnutes or until set.

SPECKLED MUSHROOM SOUP
3oz melted butter
2 medium onions chopped
12oz mushrooms roughly chopped
1pt vegetable stock
1tbs flour
½ pint milk or soy milk
2tbs Soy Sauce
Salt and Pepper

Method
Gently fry onions and mushrooms in butter for 5 minutes. Add flour and stir in for 1 minute. Add stock and simmer for 30mins. Add milk, Soy Sauce and salt and pepper. Heat for 10minutes, liquidize, check seasoning.
Optional - lots of chopped parsley or watercress may be added.

TROPICAL CITRUS SQUASH
'Tangy, Sharp and Sweet - all at the same time'
This can be used to brighten up home-made lemonade, squashes or to greatly enhance a cheap lemon squash bought from the shops.

1 jug home-made or shop lemonade
1 tin pineapple slices
1 grapefruit

Method
Once your lemonade is ready in the jug, scoop out the fruit of the grapefruit, and add it along with some of the grapefruit peel, to the lemonade. Add 1-3 pineapple slices and leave overnight. An excellent summer cooler!

Free Food

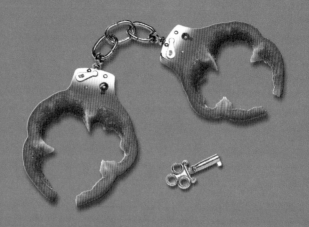

Liberate yourself from punishing slimming regimes and diets with a built-in failure factor. At our friendly weekly classes you'll discover how to eat unlimited "Free Foods" including pasta, rice and potatoes! Our famous "Sin-a-Day" Eating Plans mean no more hunger and you choose what weight you would like to be. Slimming World is simply a revelation for slimmers everywhere. Telephone the number below for details of a class near you, where warmth and support mean such a lot.

With our money back guarantee, what have you got to lose?

Slimming WORLD

0 1 7 7 3 5 2 1 1 1 1

TROPICAL FRUIT SALAD
2 tins pineapple or 1 fresh pineapple
2 mangoes
1 Paw Paw
2 Grapefruits
3 Bananas
1 litre carton of apple juice

Method
Prepare, pip and stone each fruit and place in a bowl with the apple juice. Leave to soak overnight in fridge. The apple juice blends well with the taste of the mango

ENGLISH FRUIT SALAD
10 grapes
3 plums
2 large oranges
1 tin Peach slices or 3 fresh peaches
1 tin pineapple or ½ fresh pineapple
2 medium pears
1 red apple
2 small bananas
1 tub glace cherries or 10 fresh cherries
1 litre carton of orange juice

Method
Slice and dice all of the ingredients except for the oranges. Break the oranges into segments. Remove stones and pips from any of the fruit.
Place stone/pipped fruits into a large fruit bowl and pour on the fruit juice. Place in the fridge and leave to soak and chill overnight.

OYSTER MUSHROOM STIR FRY
An accompaniment to pasta or rice

Oyster mushrooms
3 green chillies
soy sauce/veg oil
Beansprouts
Frozen peas
Rice or Pasta Courgette

Method
Slice the mushrooms, chilli peppers and courgette into thin strips. Place in a colander with beansprouts and wash with cold water. Place frozen peas in a saucepan of water and boil. Do the same for your Pasta or Rice. Place a few tablespoons of soy sauce or 4 tablespoons of vegetable oil in a wok or frying pan, and heat at a low temperature for a very short time. Now add your sliced ingredients to the frying pan or wok and keep at a fairly low temperature, stirring and shifting now and again to ensure ingredients do not stick to pan. Once pasta is ready, take it out of the water and put on a plate. Add boiled peas to frying pan or wok and increase the temperature to med/high, depending on how well the mixture has been cooked. Once ready, put the mixture of vegetables through a colander and shake off the excess sauce/oil. Serve with the pasta/rice, hot or cold.

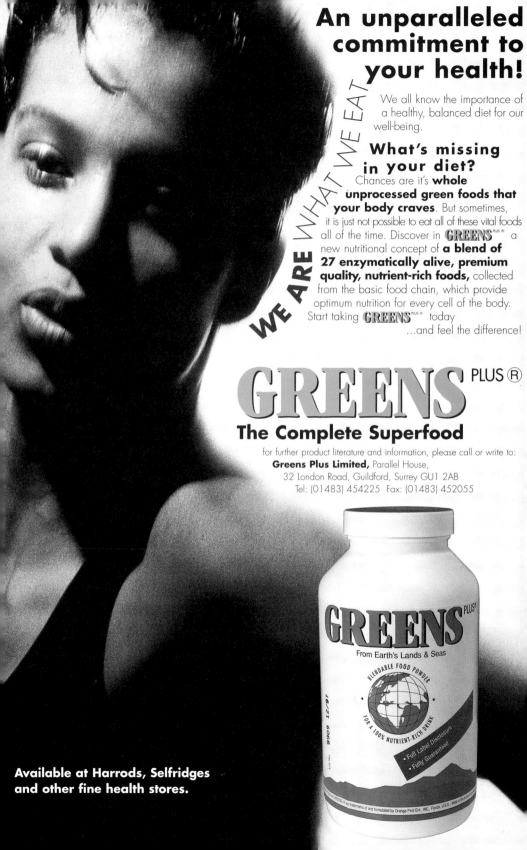

An unparalleled commitment to your health!

WE ARE WHAT WE EAT

We all know the importance of a healthy, balanced diet for our well-being.

What's missing in your diet?

Chances are it's **whole unprocessed green foods that your body craves**. But sometimes, it is just not possible to eat all of these vital foods all of the time. Discover in **GREENS** PLUS ® a new nutritional concept of **a blend of 27 enzymatically alive, premium quality, nutrient-rich foods,** collected from the basic food chain, which provide optimum nutrition for every cell of the body. Start taking **GREENS** PLUS ® today ...and feel the difference!

GREENS PLUS ®

The Complete Superfood

for further product literature and information, please call or write to:
Greens Plus Limited, Parallel House,
32 London Road, Guildford, Surrey GU1 2AB
Tel: (01483) 454225 Fax: (01483) 452055

Available at Harrods, Selfridges and other fine health stores.

FROM MIKE BRIDGE, THE OLD COFFEE HOUSE, ASHBURTON, DEVON

MIXED BEAN AND WHEAT CASSEROLE
serves 4

1lb Mixed Beans (tinned or dried), Haricot, Conneloni, Black Eye
Chick Peas, Kidney Beans, Flageleot - all or any other mixture
1 Large Onion chopped
Red, Green & Yellow Peppers - roughly chopped
2 Carrots sliced
2 large cloves of garlic - crushed
3 sticks celery - sliced
10oz Bulgar Wheat
1 x 14oz tin tomatoes + same quantity of Passatta
1 tsp tomato puree
½ tsp chilli powder and/or tabasco to taste
Salt and fresh ground peper
1tsp each of cumin and fennel seed
2 bay leaves
3 tbsp of oil

Method
Heat a large saucepan, add oil, bay leaves, cumin and fennel seeds and stir for 30seconds. Add onion, peppers, carrots, celery and garlic and fry until onion is transparent. Add chilli powder and/or tabasco, stir and cook for 1 minute. Add tomatoes, passatta, tomato puree, stir and simmer for 5 minutes. Add bulgar wheat, stir in and simmer for a further 5 minutes stirring occasionally. Add drained beans, salt and pepper and stir. Cover and cook very low, stirring occasionally for 30 minutes or until all ingredients are cooked to taste. You can then, if desired, place in individual or one large dish, dot with butter, breadcrumbs and/or cheese and brown under the grill.

CHICK PEA AND RED BEAN CASSEROLE
8oz/225g Red Kidney Beans
8oz/225g Chick Peas (cooked)
2 medium onions - sliced
4 sticks celery - sliced
4 carrots - sliced
4 large potatoes cut into cubes
2tsp curry powder
2tsp mixed herbs (English,Italian or French)
1tbsp Soy Sauce
1/2pt passata
1tsp tomato puree
1/4 pint of water
Salt and pepper

Method
Fry the onion until just browning. Add the curry powder and stir whilst cooking for 1 minute. Add all other ingredients - except soy sauce and herbs - and simmer, stirring occasionally for 25 minutes. Add soy sauce and herbs and cook for another 15 minutes. Adjust seasoning. Serve with rice.

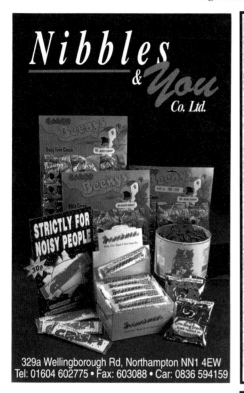
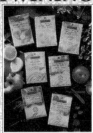
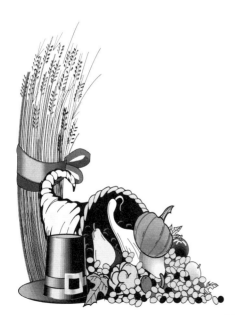

FROM GREENS HEALTH FOODS 175 HIGH STREET, LINCOLN LN5 7AF

NUT ROAST RECIPE
6oz Ground Mixed Nuts,
6oz WholemealBreadcrumbs
6oz finely chopped onions
2tsp mixed sweet herbs,
1 large tsp Yeast Extract
1/2pt of water
1 Egg
2oz Vegetable Oil
1oz Wholemeal plain flour
Ground black pepper or seasoning to taste

Method
Use some oil to lightly grease an oven proof dish or bread tin, the bottom may be lined with grease proof paper. Fry the chopped onions with the rest of the oil. Boil the water and pour it into a jug with the Yeast Extract. Stir until dissolved. Mix Ground Nut, Bread crumbs and Herbs in a bowl, together with any seasoning. When the onions are soft and transparent, add the flour and stir. Then add the water and Yeast Extract from the Jug and stir until thickened. Pour this mixture into the bowl with the dry ingredients, and mix well together. After a few minutes add the beaten egg, and mix well again. Pour this mixture into the greased dish or tin and cover with foil. Bake at 200'C or 400'F for 1 hour. If required, the foil may be removed and the dish left to cook for a further 10 minutes to crisp the top. Use a knife round the edge and turn out carefully onto a plate. Garnish as required and serve with vegetables and gravy.

FROM TAIGH-NA-MARA, SCOTLAND

WILD VEGETARIAN HAGGIS PIE
4oz Toasted organic Jumbo Oats
2oz Chopped walnuts
Small tin (200g) Red Kidney Beans (drained)
1 Medium Onion finely chopped
4oz Oyster mushrooms finely chopped
1 organically grown carrot - finely chopped
3 tsp of Marmite, yeast extract or vegetable extract
1 teaspoon Black Pepper
½ teaspoon Cayenne pepper
Small sprigs of Thyme, Parsley and Sage finely chopped
½ teaspoon nutmeg
Juice of one small lime
Tablespoon of nut oil
A nip of whisky
2oz Vegan margarine
1lb shortcrust pastry (or use 6oz margarine to 15oz S.R flour, salt & cold water)

Method
Toast the oats in a frying pan with 1oz of margarine until golden brown - put to one side. Fry the onions and mushrooms in the oil and 1oz of margarine until starting to crisp. Add

A Magik Offer from the Dead Sea

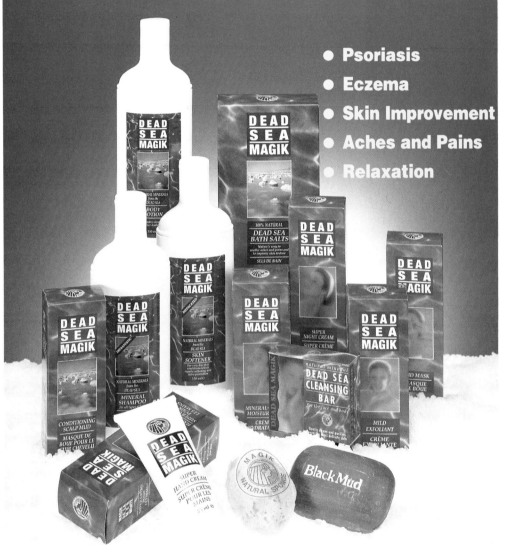

- Psoriasis
- Eczema
- Skin Improvement
- Aches and Pains
- Relaxation

- Helps Improve and Soften the Skin
- Helps Dry and Flaky Skin Conditions
- Relaxes and Soothes the Body

FINDERS INTERNATIONAL LIMITED
Orchard House, Winchet Hill, Goudhurst, Kent, TN17 1JY, England.
Tel: 01580 211055. Fax: 01580 212062.

remaining ingredients and cook for 5-10minutes whilst stirring on a med Heat. Line oiled pie dish with pastry and fill with Haggis mixture. Cut remaining pastry into strips and place on top of pie in Lattice fashion. Paint with oil or soya milk and bake for 30-40 minutes in 200' oven or until golden brown. Serve accompanied with rich thyme or whisky and mustard gravy, mashed potatoes with rosemary, orangedcarrots, stir fried parsnips, and mashed neeps (swede)

HIGHLAND BANOFFEE SLICE WITH WHISKY & CHOCOLATE SAUCE
(This receipe is suitable for Vegans)
Serves 8 covers

4 small ripe Bananas (2 for decoration)
4oz Chopped Dates
1pt Soya Milk (Apple sweetened or vanilla)
5oz Vegan Margarine
6 tbsp Maple Syrup
3tsps Arrowroot
2tsps Agar Agar powder
2oz Porridge Oats
Pinch of Salt
1/2oz walnuts crushed
1pt Orange juice
Dram of Whisky
8oz Dark Cooking Chocolate
(no whey or skimmed milk)
Tbsp polenta or semolina
Chocolate covered coffee beans

Method
For the Custard
Heat 1pt of soya milk, 2oz vegan marge, till it starts to simmer. Mix arrowroot, Agar Agar powder, 5 tablespoons of maple syrup and one tablespoon of orange juice until blended in a cup. Remove milk from heat and slowly blend in mixture. Return to heat till it starts to simmer again then leave to cool.

For the Toffee
Simmer chopped dates in ½ pint of orange juice for about 20 minutes till reduced by about 20%. Liquidize with 2oz Vegan Margarine and leave to cool.

For the crispy oaty base
Toast Oats and walnuts in a pan with 1oz Vegan margarine, pinch of salt. When golden brown add 1 tablespoon of maple syrup and leave to cool.

Put it all together
Oil a 1lb loaf tin, line with greaseproof paper and oil again. Spread the oats on the bottom. Liquidize the custard, one banana and half the toffee mixture together. Chop another banana into chunks stir it in, then pour half this mixture onto the oats. Then pour a layer of the remaining toffee mixture followed by a layer of the remaining banana custard mixture. Cover with foil and freeze for 2-3 hours. Serve with Chocolate Sauce (melt chocolate in ½ pint of orange juice and whisky) and decorate with chocolate covered coffee beans and slices of banana.

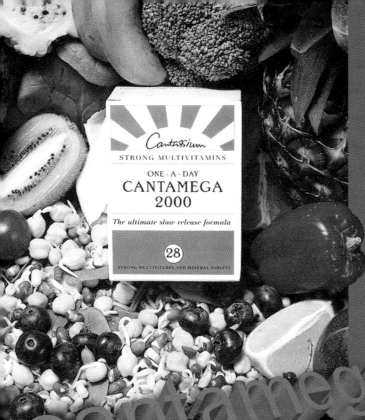

Unbeatable

After 15 years it is still the most comprehensive and best value multi-nutrient supplement on the market.

Vitamins:	per tablet	%RDA
Vitamin A (7500iu)	1250µg	156.3
Vitamin B1	80mg	5710
Vitamin B2	100mg	6250
Vitamin B6	83.8mg	4190
Vitamin B12	100µg	10000
Biotin	0.1mg	66.7
Folacin (folic acid)	400µg	200
Niacin	100mg	556
Pantothenic Acid	100mg	1667
Vitamin C	300mg	500
Vitamin D (400iu)	10µg	200
Vitamin E (200iu)	136mg	1360
Vitamin K	10µg	-
PABA	50mg	-
Choline Bitartrate	100mg	-
Inositol	100mg	-

Minerals:	per tablet	%RDA
Boron	100µg	-
Calcium	108.4mg	13.5
Chromium	40µg	-
Copper	0.3mg	-
Iodine	232µg	154.7
Iron	3.9mg	28.2
Magnesium	39.5mg	13.2
Manganese	1mg	-
Molybdenum	100µg	-
Potassium	2.3mg	-
Selenium	10µg	-
Silica	1mg	-
Zinc	7.5mg	50

	per tablet
Energy	1.1kJ/0.3kcal
Protein	21.1mg
Fat	6.2mg
Carbohydrate	29.6mg

Herbs	
Alfalfa	10mg
Kelp	10mg
Horsetail Grass	3mg
Golden Seal Root	5mg

Enzymes/Assimilators	
Bromelain	5mg
Papain	5mg
Betaine Hydrochloride	25mg
Glutamic Acid Hydrochloride	25mg
Lecithin	10mg

Bioflavonoid Group	
Citrus Bioflavonoids	50mg
Hesperidin	10mg
Rutin	25mg

Fibre Sources	
Acacia	20mg
Guar Gum	10mg
Apple Pectin	5mg

artificial additives FREE · salt FREE · refined sugar FREE · milk FREE · vegan · egg FREE · vegetarian · yeast FREE · calorie counted · grain FREE · GLUTEN FREE (wheat, rye, barley, oats) · British Made © Rita Greer

Cantamega 2000 provides an exceptional range of vitamins, minerals and enzymes, in a timed release, one-a-day tablet. Many years of research have provided the experience needed to produce this special, state-of-the-art formula, which provides essential nutrients and their important co-factors in the most easily utilised form, continuously over 6-8 hours. For those who find larger tablets hard to swallow, we also offer the formula in a divided dose of four small tablets.

The Cantamega 2000 Challenge

We are so confident that Cantamega 2000 is unbeatable that we offer a challenge to anyone who has bought this supplement. Just compare the formula (as printed on the carton) with that of any other manufacturer. If their product is better value than ours, then we will give you your money back – and you can keep your Cantamega 2000!

Cantamega 2000 is available from health stores and selected chemists nationwide.

For further information & free nutritional advice please contact one of our nutritionists at:
Larkhall Green Farm
225 Putney Bridge Road, London SW15 2PY

Tel: 0181-874 1130

PINEAPPLE AND COCONUT COLESLAW

1lb finely chopped cabbage
2oz toasted dessicated coconut
1 small tin pineapple cubes
1 jar (approx 250ml) mayonnaise

Method
In a salad bowl mix 3/4 of the mayonnaise with the juice from the tinned pineapple. Add the toasted coconut, cabbage and pineapple cubes. Mix well. Add remaining 1/4 jar mayonnaise if a creamier coleslaw is desired.

LENTIL FRITTERS AND YOGHURT SAUCE (makes 10)

3/4lb red split lentils
1tsp salt
1 heaped dessertspoon curry powder

Method
Check lentils removing any small stones. Place in a heavy based saucepan with the curry powder and salt. Cover with water (approx 1" above lentils). Bring to boil, then turn to a very low simmer, stirring frequently. Add water gradually as lentils cook to produce a very thick paste. This takes about 40 minutes. When cold form into rissoles, coat with flour and shallow fry in oil for five minutes each side. Cook's tip:- If too much water is added the mixture will be too sloppy and it will be difficult to form into fritters.

Yoghurt Sauce
Mix ½ pint natural yoghurt with 1 tsp dried mixed herbs/parsley and one clove of crushed garlic. Thin the sauce to a pouring consistency with a little milk.

THE WATERMILL RESTAURANT,PRIESTS MILL, CALDBECK, WIGTON, CUMBRIA

CHERRY CHOCOLATE CHIP AND COCONUT MACAROONS

Delicious, melt in the mouth macaroons, a firm favourite at the restaurant especially with customers on a gluten free diet.

2 Free range egg white
4oz castor sugar (unrefined if possible)
2oz chopped flaked Almonds
2oz Dessicated coconut
2oz real chocolated chips
2oz Natural Glace Cherries - cut into quarters

Method
Whisk egg whites until they form soft peaks. Gradually add sugar a little at a time. Fold in remaining ingredients. Place in small moulds the size of a tablespoon, on oiled greaseproof paper on a flat baking tray 12"x16" (or on two Swiss Roll tins). Bake in oven for 10-12 minutes at 180'C, 350"F. Mark 4. Do not overcook, the centre of the macaroon should remain soft. When cooked remove carefully from the tray with a palette knife onto a cooling rack. Store in airtight container once cold.

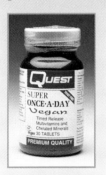
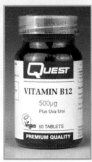 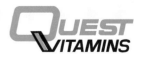

SPICY PARSNIP AND COCONUT SOUP

2 tbsp Sunflower oil
3 tsp Madras curry powder or paste
2 tsp Ground Cumin
2 tsp Tumeric
2 tsp Crushed Chillis
2 Medium Onions finely chopped
2lb Parsnips peeled and sliced - preferably organic
1 large potato peeled and chopped
21/2 pints water
Salt and pepper to taste
2oz Creamed Coconut - grated
Fresh Coriander to garnish

Method
Heat oil in large saucepan. Add spices, cook gently for 2-3 minutes stirring occasionally. Add vegetables, 3tsps of salt and some freshly ground black pepper, continue stirring frequently to prevent vegetables sticking. Cook for a further 5 minutes. Add water, bring to the boil, reduce heat, cover saucepan with lid and simmer for 45 minutes allowing vegetables to cook and flavours to mingle. Add grated coconut 5 minutes before the end of cooking time. Blend until smooth in a food processor or liquidizer. Adjust seasoning if necessary. NOTE - If soup is too thick add a small amount of boiling water during blending. Garnish with fresh Coriander.

OLIVE AND PEANUT PATE
Serves 4 generously

6oz Green Olives de-stoned (use olives stuffed with pimento for a different taste and colour
4oz Peanut Butter - Crunch or smooth
2tbs Olive Oil
2tbs Lemon Juice
5fl oz Water
Parsley - optional

Method
Keep back a few olives for decoration, blend the rest of the olives with olive oil, lemon juice and water. Chop most of the parsley. Mix everything together. Serve at room temperature, decorated with the remaining olives and with peanuts and a sprig of parsley.

AVOCADO WITH ROAST WALNUTS
As either a snack, a starter or a main item with salad, this version of guacomole looks and tastes exciting.

2 Avocados
4 Tbs Lemon Juice
4 tsp Sugar
2 Tbs Walnut Oil
1 tsp Mint (preferably fresh but dry is acceptable)
8oz Walnuts

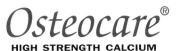

Method

Keep four good walnut halves and chop the rest reasonably small. Roast the pieces and the whole halves on a baking tray in a reasonably low oven, turning frequently, until dark brown.

Cut the avocados in half lengthways and scoop out the flesh (keeping skins for later). Mix it with everything except the walnuts in a blender, to a smooth cream. Fold in the roast walnut pieces. Fill each avocado skin, either with a spoon or by piping the mixture in, place the half walnuts on the top.

FROM AROMA, 36A ST MARTINS LANE, LONDON WC2N 4ET

MUSHROOM, PINE KERNEL, ASPARAGUS AND WALNUT CREAM CHEESE ROLL
From Aroma's innovative Sandwich menu

1/2lb Wild Mushrooms
2oz Butter
2oz Toasted Pine Kernels
Several large leaves Oak Leaf Lettuce
4oz (6 spears) Fresh Asparagus
4oz Cream Cheese
2oz Crushed Walnuts,
Sun dried Tomato Ciabatta

Method

Saute the washed mushrooms with butter in a frying pan with a little salt and freshly ground pepper (and garlic if you wish). Put the pine kernels into a hot oven for about 8 minutes, or until slightly brown. Wash the lettuce leaves and leave to dry. Cook the Asparagus in salted boiling water for 2 minutes (or until cooked but yet very firm). Immediately place under running cold water. Mix crushed walnuts thoroughly with cream cheese. Cut the Ciabatta loaf in half lengthways and spread both sides with the walnut cream cheese. Place the sauteed mushrooms on Ciabatta, then sprinkle with the toasted pine kernels. Place the cooked asparagus on top and then add the lettuce. Close sandwich and cut into three.

SPICED LEMON STRAWBERRIES
Summer strawberries have more flavour, but this is a useful recipe for imported strawberries out of season. Very impressive for Christmas as an alternative light dessert. Oranges can be used instead of lemons for a sweeter dessert. Serve with shortbread and scented cream (cream with rosewater and icing sugar added then whipped)
Serves 4-6

2lb Strawberries
3 Lemons (unwaxed preferably)
1 tbsCinnamon
1 tbsMixed Spice
Sugar

Method

Hull and wash the strawberries. With a zester or grater take off long strands of the lemon rind. Squeeze the lemon juice. Thoroughly mix the juice and the spices, adding sugar to taste, or even more spice if wanted. Gently coat the strawberries in the spiced juice and chill for at least 30 minutes to allow the flavours to mingle. Cover with the lemon rind to serve.

Thursday Plantation
Tea Tree Oil

The most powerful natural antiseptic known to man

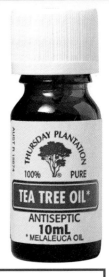

Thursday Plantation, the worldwide brand leader and original Tea Tree Oil Company has created the ultimate skin and hair care system. Utilising the powerful natural antiseptic properties of Tea Tree Oil, Thursday Plantation have produced deep penetrating cleansers that kill surface bacteria yet are totally mild and gentle to the skin.

The Tea Tree Body Care Range includes vegetable French milled soap, herbal skin wash, deep cleansing shampoo, moisturising hand and body lotion plus aluminium-free deodorant.

For full details of the widest range of Tea Tree products available in the UK, please call **01274-488511** and ask for our free brochure.

Thursday Plantation products are available from Boots, Holland & Barrett, Superdrug, all good health food stores plus selected pharmacies nationwide.

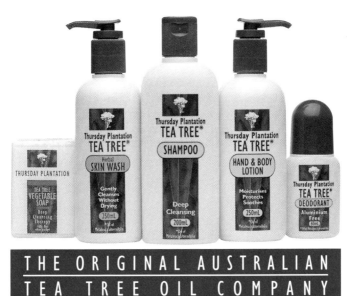

THE ORIGINAL AUSTRALIAN TEA TREE OIL COMPANY

BROCCOLI AND CHESTNUT SOUP

Cauliflower can be used instead of broccoli, but although the taste may be no less pleasing the colour certainly will be. For the broccoli version, the addition of a little spinach further enhances the colour.

Serves 4
1 head Broccoli   (Or bunch of smaller pieces)
1 tin Chestnut Puree (unsweetened)
2oz Spinach-optional (frozen is acceptable)
1/4pt Double Cream   (Or soya milk with less of the water)
1 Tbs Grainy Mustard
Salt & Pepper
Water

Method
Cut the very tops of the broccoli into small florets, and trim the stalks as they are also used in this recipe. Roughly chop the stalks and place them in shallow water below a steamer containing the florets. Steam the florets lightly and boil the stalks until soft. Blanch the spinach if using fresh, or defrost frozen spinach. Blend the stalks and the spinach with the cooking water to reduce it all to a fine pulp. Blend in the chestnut puree, cream and seasonings, and transfer the mixture to a saucepan. As the soup heats up add the broccoli florets and as much water as wanted to create either a thin or thick soup.

COURGETTE FILLED COURGETTE FLOWERS

Courgette flowers can sometimes be bought with tiny courgettes still attached, but better still grow your own. Serve either as a main item with salad, or as an accompaniment at a barbecue, for an outdoor summer lunch.

Serves 4
8 Courgette Flowers
8 baby Courgettes
4oz Wholegrain rice
4oz Pine Kernels
Fresh Herbs
Mayonnaise

Method
Cook the rice. Dice and lightly saute the courgettes. Toast the pine kernels in a moderate oven or under a grill until brown. Chop the herbs. Mix the stuffing ingredients when cold with just enough mayonnaise to hold together. Having ensured the flowers are clear of insects (but do not wash them), fill with stuffing mixture

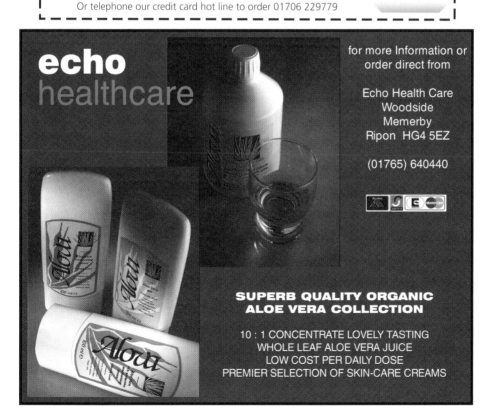

SWEET AND SOUR PASTA SAUCE
Many different vegetables could be added to the basic sauce to make a light or substantial dish.
Serves 4

8oz   Lentils
4oz   Crystallised Ginger
5 floz White Wine Vinegar
10 floz Orange Juice
4 tbs Lemon Juice
1 tbs Mustard Seeds
Dried Apricots
Celery
Baby Sweetcorn Cobs
Peas
Carrots

Method
Cook the lentils in just enough water until completely soft. In a processor with a sharp blade blend the ginger to form a smooth paste. Add the cooked lentils, the vinegar, and the orange and lemon juice and blend again until completely smooth.
Cut the vegetables as required into small neat pieces. In a shallow pan fry the mustard seeds until popping then add the vegetables and stir fry until cooked but still crunchy. Add the chopped apricots and the lentil mixture, and heat through

NUTEREE
A version of kedgeree. A simple dish suitable for either a light lunch or supper, or more particularly for breakfast. Serve hot on toast or with crusty bread, and accompany with something like sage and apple jelly.
Serves 4

80z   Rice (white or wholegrain)
2   Rosehip teabags
1/2tsp Turmeric
1lb   Mixed Nuts
1Tbs   Sage
1Tbs   Olive Oil
Water

Method
Using the amount of water required to cook the rice (quantity depends on the cooking method used) pour boiling water onto the teabags and turmeric and leave to stand for 5 minutes. Use the tea to cook the rice. Chop the nuts so that some of them are well ground, some in large pieces and a few still whole. Into the rice mix the nuts, sage and olive oil and just enough water to allow the whole thing to cook through without sticking and hold lightly together. Top with fresh herbs for serving.

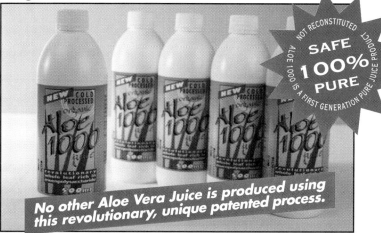
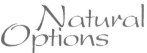

SWEETCORN CREAM HORNS

A dish that looks like a dessert but is actually a savoury!

Serves 4

Puff Pastry
1 Egg
1lb Sweetcorn (frozen)
8oz Cream cheese
1tsp Rogan Josh Curry Paste
Alfalfa Seeds
Poppy Seeds
Dessicated Coconut etc

Roll out puff pastry (ready made or your own) and cut strips 2cm wide. Wrap around conical cream horns (available from cake shops), brush with egg and bake. Allow two horns per person.
Defrost sweetcorn and in a processor blend it to a cream. Add the cream cheese and curry paste and combine to blend until as smooth as possible. When the horns are cool fill them with the cream and dip the open end in the mixed seeds and coconut.

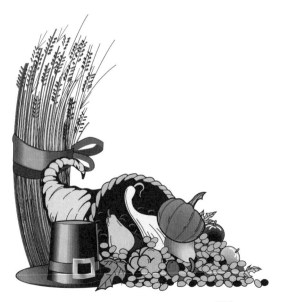

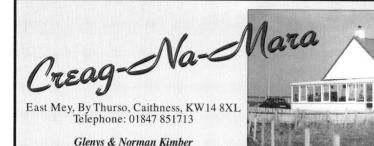
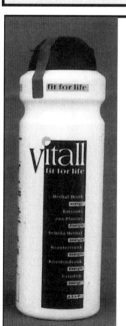

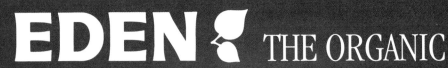

EDEN

THE ORGANIC VEGETABLE JUICE RANGE

- Beta carotene-rich Carrot Juice, Vegetable Cocktail and lactic-fermented Beetroot Juice

- Cold pressed raw from mature organic vegetables

- Soil Association approved

- Available through health stores or all leading health food wholesalers

For further information contact Harry Stead at Sandoz Nutrition Ltd. 01923 271565.

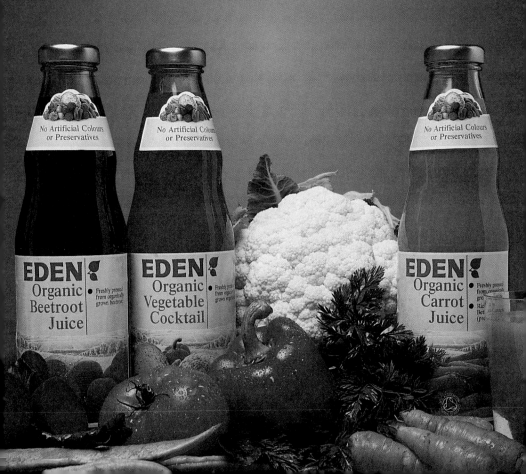

EDEN JUICES FOR HEALTH

Germany's leading range of fresh vegetable juices is now available in the UK. Eden Organic Vegetable Juices are produced using an organic gardening method developed by a group of vegetarian German farmers who started the company in the 1890s.

There are three pure juices to choose from, each free from artificial colours and preservatives and rich in nutrients – Eden Organic Carrot Juice, Vegetable Cocktail and Beetroot Juice.

Eden Organic Vegetable Juices are cold pressed raw from freshly grown organic vegetables, picked when they are mature, ensuring that the nutrient levels are at their peak. The juice is flash pasteurised once bottled to maintain shelf life for maximum freshness, without loss of vitamins and minerals.

Approved by the Soil Association in meeting it's organic standard, Eden Organic Vegetable Juices are packaged in 750ml bottles and available in health food stores or through all leading health food wholesalers.

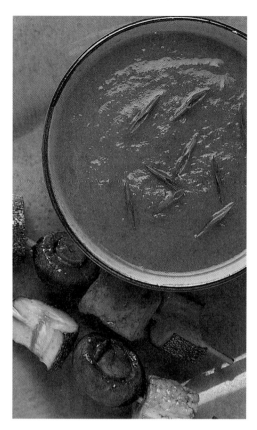

Above: *Eden Tofu Kebabs with Carrot and Pepper Sauce.*

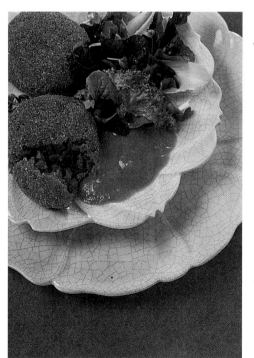

JUICE UP YOUR COOKING WITH EDEN

Eden Juices are excellent when used as ingredients in cookery. JUICE UP FAMILY MEALTIME is Eden's latest recipe booklet featuring eight vegetarian dishes created by leading home economist Roz Denny with both adults and children in mind.

Copies are available free from CBPR, PO Box 1089, Pulborough, West Sussex. RH20 2YX.

Left: *Eden Beanburgers with Brown Rice and Beetroot Juice.*

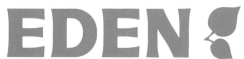

A SWING TO A
HEALTHY LIFESTYLE

by
Bob Mann

A SWING TO A HEALTHY LIFESTYLE
by
Bob Mann (author and journalist)

INTO THE NEW AGE? As countless people have discovered, the decision to adopt a healthier and more natural diet, or the experience of healing by unorthodox means, is unlikely to remain an isolated event in one's life. Often it is just the beginning of an exciting and open-ended process of personal re-evaluation and discovery, resulting in far-reaching changes of philosophy and lifestyle. Once your mind has been opened to the possibilities and implications of natural healing, in whatever form, you seem to be lead inevitably to a deepening interest in a whole constellation of diverse but related subjects, all of which are linked by the concept of 'healing' in the broadest sense. These include the exploration of different ways of personal growth and development, the many varieties of psychotherapy and the million paths to spiritual experience.

There is also a vital recognition that healing is needed on a wider, social and planetary scale. A new, more immediate and personal concern for the environment is thus likely to be part of the process. Having experienced for yourself that there is obviously 'something in it', you may feel a strong compulsion to become a healer or therapist yourself. Almost before you realise it, you can find yourself absorbed into that highly eclectic, colourful, bewildering and creative world which is, in common parlance, contained within the phrase 'New Age'. It is only necessary to read the cards and posters on the notice board of your local wholefood store, or take a look around one of those shops, now to be found in most large towns, which sell crystals, scented candles, self-help manuals, Buddhist scriptures, tarot cards and tapes of gentle, soporific synthesised music designed as a background to meditation, in order to see that, like it or not, the New Age is a significant element in late 20th century culture.

Many are of the opinion that it represents the true current of the times, and that eventually it will be the dominant mode of life for society as a whole. Whether this idea appals or inspires you, the phenomenon has been with us for quite a long time now, and is clearly not going to be dismissed or ridiculed out of existence.

WHAT IS THE NEW AGE?

The expression 'New Age' means many different things, according to your point of view. To most people with any knowledge or sympathy towards it, the term would certainly be used to cover the numerous alternative medical systems and techniques, and all forms of psychotherapy except the most orthodox. It would include any kind of meditative practice or spiritual path where the emphasis is on personal experience and autonomy, rather than the passive acceptance of dogma. The 'environment' in the broadest sense of the word, and our relationship with it, is an essential element, as well as a belief that probably the best thing an individual can do for the planet as a whole is to look after the well-being of his or her immediate neighbourhood - one of the best-known slogans to have arisen from this way of thinking is 'think globally, act locally.' Key words are 'green', holistic and 'alternative', all of them used as much as, if not more than, 'New Age', at least by the people involved. They all imply an attitude of reverence and respect for life and a desire to interfere with natural processes as little as possible, as well as a recognition

227

that nothing can adequately be viewed in isolation, but must be seen as inextricably interconnected. Sometimes people talk of a resurgence of 'feminine' values, meaning gentler, uninvasive and nurturing ways of relating to life, but many feminists consider this is itself a restricting, male attitude towards what constitutes femininity.

The New Age is therefore not so much a single movement as a convergence of many diverse streams, not all of them particularly comfortable bedfellows, but which tend to see themselves as having more in common with each other than they have with what is perceived as the mainstream of society and its relentlessly materialistic worldview. Homoeopaths, permaculturalists, green activists, Steiner educationalists, astrological counsellors, biodynamic farmers, neo-pagans and those who dowse for the shape of the goddess in the configurations of the landscape, all recognise each other, despite their great differences of style and philosophy, as companions on the road towards what they hope is a saner, wiser, more spiritually aware and environmentally sound way of life.

To astrologers, the New Age is specifically the 2000 year-long Age of Aquarius. Whether it really did begin in the summer of 1967 or whether it has not quite started yet is unclear, but it is commonly agreed to be characterised by idealism and the fusion of rational with intuitive ways of thinking. It is, according to astrological teaching, a period in which humankind can, if it chooses, finally learn to live peacefully and harmoniously with itself and the universe around it, and rediscover lost or undeveloped potential. The rigid systems and heirarchies of the past will, we are told, be broken up and transformed, and all aspects of life will be viewed holistically, as a single, indivisible whole, rather than as separate, unconnected elements. People will achieve their own unique 'personhood', while at the same time recognising their oneness with each other and all life.

Although the idealism concerning the Aquarian Age which used to be so apparent in the late 1960s and 70s has been tempered, somewhat, by the hardships and gross materialism of the 1980s and 90s, these elements are still alive in many people's hearts, and add up to a vision well worth pursuing, whether you literally accept the theories of astrology or not. There are, of course, other ways of responding to the term New Age. To many local councillors it immediately conjures up a picture of homeless, unemployed layabouts, high on 'magic mushrooms', living squalidly in ancient caravans, buses and ambulances with rainbows painted on the sides.

With their scrawny dogs and vulnerable children, these 'New Age Travellers' are an unlikely threat to society, but the fear and anger they can inspire is extraordinary. They are often compared unfavourably with 'genuine travellers and real gypsies' whom the same councillors, under other circumstances, would be equally hostile towards. To Fundamentalist Christians the New Age and everything pertaining to it is the work of the Devil, and its practitioners will burn in Hell for all eternity. To old-fashioned rationalist humanists it represents a bizarre, immature escape into the comforts of magic and superstition when what we should be doing, surely, is working to solve the dire problems facing humanity with the means provided by science and technology. This last view is usually the one adopted by the media, overtly or implicitly, in their inevitably shallow investigations of the alternative scene.

In recent years the British public has gained, from newspapers and television, a clear view of the typically 'New Age' lifestyle as being that of an affluent middle class couple who, to assuage

Europe's First Certified Aloe Vera Range

Aloe Vera Capsules
One a day Double Strength Aloe Vera Capsules 60mg - equivalent to 12ml/12000mg of Juice. For ease of use, ESI have developed a unique formulation of Organic Aloe Vera whole leaf and inner gel to maximise the natural beneficial properties of the juice in a high potency, one a day capsule. Available in 30's and 90's.

Aloe Vera Gel Skin Care System
ESI Aloe Vera Gel Skin Care System is produced from 100% pure gel capturing the maximum nutritional activity of the Aloe Vera Barbadensis plant. This bio active treatment gel moisturises, softens and helps restore dry and damaged skin, sun burn, skin irritations and minor burns. Economical 200g tube.

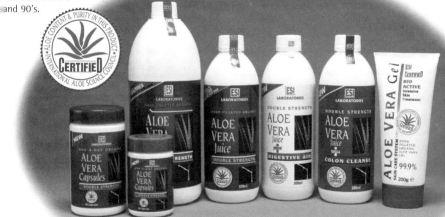

Pioneers in Aloe Vera Research
The Natural Choice

Aloe Vera Plus
Digestive Aid
Using our original double strength formulation we have added Peppermint oil, papaya, camomile and slippery elm, herbs used widely for their digestive and soothing properties.

Aloe Vera Plus Colon Cleanse
Using double strength organic Aloe Vera we have added Aloe Vera pulp- the natural fibre found in the plant; F.O.S.- used to promote friendly intestinal bacteria; Milk Thistle, Dandelion and Liquorice- herbs used widely for their cleansing properties. This unique combination is aimed at maintaining digestive regularity and helping to promote intestinal well being.

Aloe Vera Double Strength Juice
A unique blend of both whole leaf and inner gel providing twice the level of enzymes and nutrients to maximise beneficial activity.

ESI Laboratories
38/39 St Mary Street, Cardiff CF1 2AD
Telephone (01222) 388422 Fax (01222) 233010

ESI

their guilt at having had so much, have given up their successful, 'outer-directed' careers in the city in order to settle in a converted barn in Wales or the Westcountry. Here they can become 'inner-directed' and live in rhythm with the forces of nature, growing their own organic vegetables, dabbling in every kind of therapy and meditative practice, educating their children at home or in a suitably alternative school, and recycling absolutely everything.

They drive a beaten up Morris Traveller covered in anti-nuclear stickers and imprecations to save the whale. Glastonbury, in Somerset, and Totnes, in Devon, have become especially well known for their supposed concentration of New Age activity, although it is not always clear why these places in particular have been singled out. It is true that many people are drawn to Glastonbury, as they have been for at least a century, by the strange, powerful topography and sense of something mysterious and regenerative in the landscape, while in and around Totnes there are, indeed, large numbers of people who advertise themselves as healers. But anyone visiting either town in the hope of finding a community genuinely based on spiritual values or ecologically sound principles will find them disappointingly conventional, and as politically conservative (if not Conservative) as small towns everywhere.

All this can give an impression that the whole New Age scene is somehow insincere, ineffective and of minimal importance. Certainly the cliches associated with it - endless talk of the self, navel-gazing, psycho-babble, self-congratulation, arrogance - are, like all such external signs and trappings, easy to demolish and ridicule. This has been done most cleverly by two books a decade apart: Martin Stottis Spilling the Beans (1986) and Gerry Thompson's Astral Sex to Zen Teabags (1996). Both authors are, in fact, sympathetic, and are laughing not at the desire for healing and wholeness, which they treat with respect, but simpy the mindless use of jargon, and the predictable uniformity of style and appearance, which often go with them (as they go with most human activities). But jokes about ex-hippies, self-indulgence and escapism can make the 'ordinary person', for whom this book is intended, and who has perhaps just tried dipping a toe into this strange and intriguing stream, understandably cautious of stepping any further. After all, it is a stream which encompasses beliefs and approaches that are markedly different from the ones most of us have been brought up with. It is also the case, of course, that there are some dubious practices and unqualified practitioners around, which we need to be wary of.

SEEKING A PHILOSOPHY OF LIFE

I believe, however, that a clear path can be steered through the many therapies and systems on offer in the brightly coloured bazaar of the New Age, and that much of value can be found amongst its stalls. The rich medley of ideas which it brings together, drawn from such different sources as quantum physics and eastern mysticism, embracing elements from almost every cultural and spiritual tradition, does have sense behind it, and is not as unscientific and absurd as the more conservative rationalists may suggest.

Thinkers like Theodore Roszak in Unfinished Animal (1976), Person/Planet (1977) and The Voice of the Earth (1992), Fritjof Capra in The Tao of Physics (1975) and The Turning Point (1982), Marilyn Ferguson in The Aquarian Conspiracy (1981) and Peter Russell in The Awakening Earth (1982), have, very lucidly, put the whole movement into its historical and philosophical perspective. Each of these books is a marvel of clarity and erudition, and should be read by anyone with a desire to understand the deeper implications of the period we are living in (they

Shape up to another busy day

Like many people constantly on the go today, you would like your diet to include all the vitamins and minerals you need. But in practice it's never easy to be sure of your intake, which is why FSC Liquid Gel Multi-Vits can be a good safeguard.

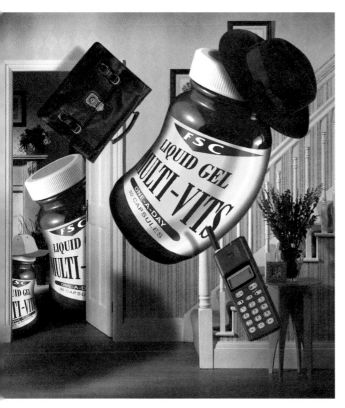

Each capsule contains a comprehensive variety of nutrients including vitamins, minerals and anti-oxidants in a carefully selected form-ulation which, as part of a healthy diet, helps to ensure that your body is getting everything it needs.

Being in Liquid Gel form they're more easily digestible, without the risk of reflux of the B vitamin content which can bring back an unpleasant aftertaste.

So start each busy day fresh, with FSC Multi-Vits.

A healthier approach to life that you can build on with the full range of FSC vitamin and mineral daily supplements, available from leading health stores.

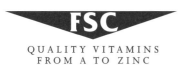

FSC

QUALITY VITAMINS
FROM A TO ZINC

FSC Quality Vitamins, Europa Park, Radcliffe, Manchester M26 1GG. Telephone 01204 707420.
Available from General Nutrition Centres (GNC), Health & Diet Centres and all good health food stores.

will also help you to understand the subtler jokes in the two books mentioned above). On a more fundamental level, the desire to be healed and to heal which so many people, of all ages and backgrounds, are feeling, is to be trusted.

The impulse towards a more natural, spiritually aware way of life is sound. The sense that the well-being of the planet is our responsibility and that how we choose to live on it makes a difference, is, on the deepest level, correct. No ridicule can alter these deep-seated convictions, which more and more people are beginning to share. Few would now argue with the statement that material progress is not, in itself, going to make us happy and at ease in our environment, however good and desirable it may be. Some of the wares on display in the New Age bazaar might look eccentric when viewed in isolation, but together they present quite a compelling response to the crises of our times, and the presence of so many of them in the market is reason for hope.

Whatever the media may say, significant numbers of people are finding through these therapies, techniques and paths a more meaningful, creative and healthy way of life, which inevitably ripples outwards to affect the society around them. What is becoming increasingly apparent is that people everywhere are seeking a comprehensive philosophy of life. For the last two or three hundred years, the dominant philosophy of the west has been based on scientific materialism. This has enabled us to literally transform the world, and has brought levels of comfort, control over the environment and freedom from pain which are miracles of ingenuity and intellect. We should not denigrate these achievements or glibly reject them.

But the limitations of this view of the world, and the activities based upon it, are becoming clearer every day. Despite the power of modern medicine, for example, its reliance on drugs and technology leaves people profoundly unhealed, and the possibilities opening up for genetic engineering are morally dubious, to say the least. It is most noticeably in health care and medicine that people are turning to alternatives, and expressing their deep longing to find the right relationship with themselves, the society around them and the planet on which we live. This chapter is not a consumer's guide to the range of therapies, medical systems and spiritual paths which are on offer.

Many excellent guides of this nature are readily available: one of the best, which also includes much of the scientific and philosophical background, is The Arkana Dictionary of New Perspectives by Stuart Holroyd (1989). Instead, I wish to pick out a number of ideas which are common to many of them, and which I believe offer an approach to life which does help to satisfy the need for a living philosophy that so many are seeking.

THE ULTIMATE POWER IS WITHIN OURSELVES

We have become used to thinking of ourselves in reductionist terms, as being small, insignificant bundles of impulses, memories and mainly negative desires. Modern psychology has a severely limited model of what it is to be human and what constitues mental or spiritual health. The most striking thing about so many of the more alternative systems is that they start from the basic assumption that, beneath the illness or conditioning, we are fundamentally all right. There is a state or condition of life within us that has immense potential for health and wholeness, and the aim of the therapy is to reveal and draw this state out, rather than to put it there from outside.

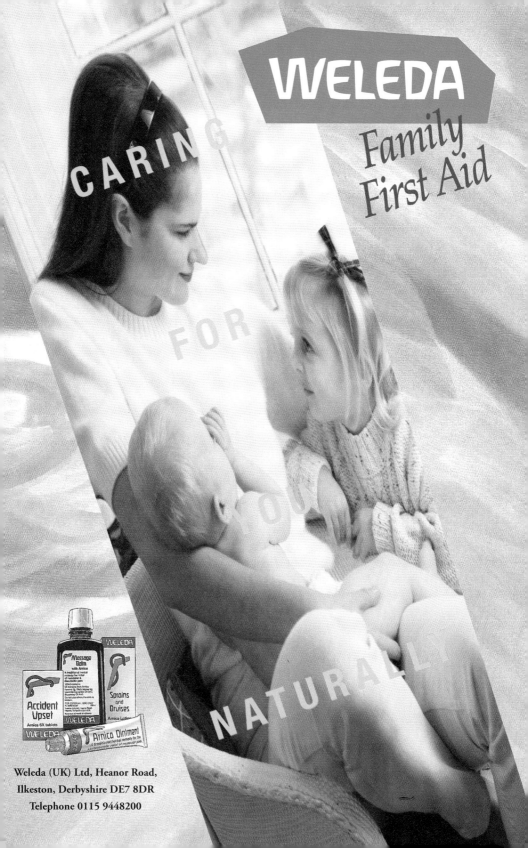

WELEDA

Family First Aid

CARING

FOR

YOU

NATURALLY

Weleda (UK) Ltd, Heanor Road,
Ilkeston, Derbyshire DE7 8DR
Telephone 0115 9448200

Hence the emphasis on allowing the body's natural healing ability to work with as little interference as possible. From this follows the idea that WE ARE IN CONTROL OF OUR LIVES

This is a stumbling block for many, who imagine it as meaning that everything that happens to us is our fault, and therefore we deserve no sympathy when things go wrong. Put like that, it does seem a callous and unhelpful doctrine. But accepting responsibility for our lives, our health and the quality of our surroundings does not have to mean that we beat ourselves up with guilt when something negative happens. It is simply giving us the dignity of being in control, rather than being passive victims. There is no doubt that such a positive, responsible attitude does have beneficial effects, and can make a great difference to the process of healing.

THE ONENESS OF BODY AND MIND

Philosophies and religions throughout history have pondered the nature of the relationship between the physical, tangible, measurable aspects of life and the unseen, mental or spiritual aspects. Most have emphasised one or the other. What is becoming clear, however, is that they are most usefully seen as two equally essential sides of the same coin, inseperable and continually influencing each other.

ONENESS OF LIFE AND ITS ENVIRONMENT

Even more complex is the nature of our relationship with our surroundings, but ancient philosophies and modern physics are coming to agree on the fact that everything in the universe is, in a sense, a single system, constantly interracting. 'The environment' is best understood not as a space 'out there' which we do things to, but an extension of our own life. Our state of being is mirrored by our environment. We have all had the experience of being angry and irritable and having this reflected by everyone and everything around us. Likewise, when we are happy and in rhythm, things and people react positively. American Indian teachings are commonly invoked to express this understanding of the connection between ourselves and the land, but it is found in every culture.

All these principles, if pondered and examined with an open mind, can, I think, help us to take from the diverse stalls and booths on offer in the New Age market the particular systems and therapies which can be most useful to us.

REAL

Here's Health
NATURAL PRODUCT
AWARDS
1997
WINNER
OVERALL PRODUCT
ESSENTIAL OIL
PRODUCTS

aromatherapy

TISSERAND

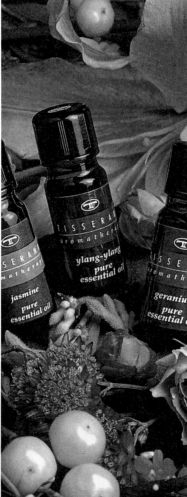

PURE ESSENTIAL OILS

VAPORISERS

BODY OILS & LOTIONS

SHOWER GELS & SOAPS

BATH OILS & SOAKS

HAIRCARE

HAND & NAIL CREAM

FOOTCARE

TEA TREE RANGE

LAVENDER RANGE

MOIST TISSUES

CRUELTY FREE

Purity and Quality

CALL 01273 325666 FOR STOCKISTS DETAILS

235

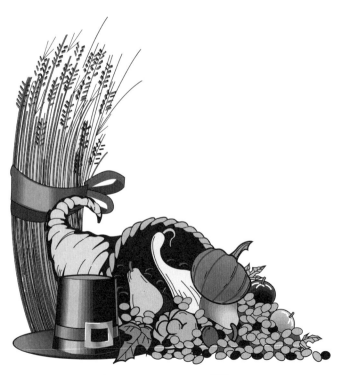

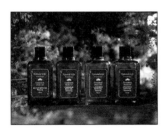

List of Advertisers

A & N Health Foods
Allergycare
Alternatives
Arbonne
Ayurvedic Herbal Laboratories
Bean Bag Wholefoods
Beanfreaks
Bethany
Bideford Health Food
Bodytreats
Bran Tub (The)
Brewhurst
C.W.Daniel
Cotswold Health Products
Country Fayre
Courtyard
Dolma
Doves Farm Foods
Easternbase Ltd
Echo Essential Oils
Echo Health
Eden Organic Co.
Energos
EOTA
ESI
Essential Oil Co
Eve Taylor
Ferrosan Health Care
Finders International
Fit As A Fiddle
Freshlands
Frome Wholefoods
FSC
Goat House (The)
Good Health
Good Nature
Goodness Wholefoods
Grayshott Health Stores
Green People Company
Greens Plus Ltd
Harvest Natural Foods
Hazel Nut Health Foods
Health Imports Ltd
Healthy Pulses
Healthy Hampers
Herbal Remedies
Holbeach Wholefoods
Holistic Healing Centre
HSW
Impulse Foods
Kingsley Company

Larkhall Green Farm
Libra Wholefoods
London School of Aromatherapy
Lyme Regis Fine Foods
Lyn Hicks
Martha Hill
Meadows
Michael's Wholefoods
Natural Life Aromatherapy
Natural Options
Natural Store (The)
Natural Wheat Bag Co.
Nature's Gate
Newlife Products Ltd
Nibbles & You
Olive Tree (The)
Orchard Foods
Peppercorn Natural Foods
Phoenix Natural Products
Plamil
Quest Vitamins
R.A.H.
Richards
SDF
Secopra
Sedlescombe Vineyard
Shambala
Sheldon Press
Simmers
Slimming World
Solgar Vitamins
Spatone
Spice Of Life
Stratford Health Foods
Sukar
Suma Wholefoods
Summerbee Products
Thursday Cottage Ltd
Time For Change
Tisserand
Totnes Health Shop
Tuppenny Rice Wholefoods
Twinings
Vegetarian Shoes
Vintage Roots
Vittal
Vitabiotics
Weleda
Westmill Foods
Westwight Wholefoods
Wild Oats

Chapter 15

Where to Shop

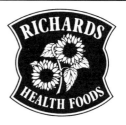
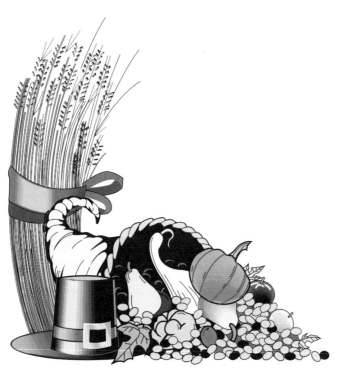

SCOTLAND

EDINBURGH

NATURE'S GATE, 83 Clerk Street, Edinburgh EH8 9JG Tel/Fax 0131 668 2067
Wholefood shop with a wide range of vegetarian, vegan, macrobiotic and organic food and
wines, plus related products. **OPEN;** 10.00am-7pm Monday to Saturday

ENGLAND

AVON

THE GOAT HOUSE, Bristol Road, Brent Knoll, Somerset TA9 4HJ Tel: 01278 760995
WILD OATS 9-11 Lower Redland Road', Bristol BS6 6TB Tel: 01179 731967

CHESHIRE

FIT AS A FIDDLE 108 Mill Street, Macclesfield, Cheshire SK11 6NR Tel: 01645 612555

CORNWALL

GOOD NATURE 2, The Esplanade, Fowey, Cornwall PL23 1HY Tel: 01726 832110
THE NATURAL STORE, 3, The Parade, Helston TR13 8RT Tel: 01326 564226
A&N HEALTH FOODS 62 Fore Street, Saltash, Cornwall PL12 6JW Tel: 01752 844926
Suppliers of Homeopathic, Herbal remedies, Vitamin Supplements, Wholefoods, Frozen and
Chilled Foods, Organic Bread and Distribute Organic Vegetable Boxes.
GOOD HEALTH 10 Tregenna Hill, St Ives, Cornwall TR26 1SF Tel: 01736 794726
Wholefood Health Products. Extremely well stocked shop carrying most of the latest lines in
Health Foods. Specialises in Gluten free diets, Non-alcoholic wines, Organics, Bach Flower
Remedies, Oils, Books and Tapes. Mrs Sutcliffe, the proprietor very willing to advise and
obtain most items if they are not stocked.

DEVON

BIDEFORD HEALTH FOOD 14 Mill Street, Bideford, Devon EX39 2JT Tel: 01237 472715
Interesting store selling health food and dietary supplements at competitive prices. Owned
and run by Mr and Mrs Noblet who provide a friendly and informed service which makes
shopping here a pleasure.
ORCHARD FOODS 5a Mill Street, Ottery St Mary, Devon EX11 1AB Tel: 01404 812109
HEALTHY PULSES 49-51 Eastlake Street, Plymouth PL1 1BT 01752 261669. Wide range
of wholefoods
THURSDAY COTTAGE Carswell Farm, Uplyme, Devon DT7 3XQ - Tel: 01297 445555
Fax: 10297 445059 International +44 1297 445555
This small family owned and run jam business is based on a farm in the Devon countryside.
The best possible jams, marmalades and curds. Purchase either direct from Thursday Cottage
or find them in good quality grocers and delicatessens, farm shops, health food shops, food
halls ... anywhere discerning fod lovers buy their special foods.

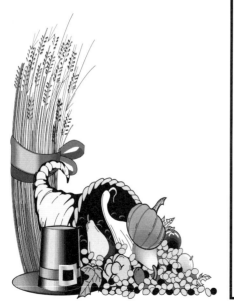

GREATER MANCHESTER

HAZEL NUT HEALTH FOODS
207 London Road, Hazel Grove, Stockport SL7 4PS Tel: 0161 483 1576

HAMPSHIRE

THE BRAN TUB 20 Lavant Street, Petersfield GU32 3EW Tel: 01730 267043
Independent family owned. Open 17 years. Probably the widest range of vegetarian foods, cruelty free cosmetics, vitamins, special diet foods. Visit our friendly shop soon!
TIME FOR CHANGE
167 Fawcett Road, Southsea, Portsmouth PO4 0DH Tel: 01705 818786
PEPPERCORN NATURAL FOODS
11 Latimer Street, Romsey SO51 8DF Tel:01794 513499

ISLE OF WIGHT

WESTWIGHT WHOLEFOODS
3 Clarence Building, Avenue Road, Freshwater PO40 9UU Tel: 01983 754891

LINCOLNSHIRE

TUPPENNY RICE WHOLEFOODS, 1 & 2 Castle Street, Stamford, PE9 2RA Tel: 01780 62739. Cafe established for 5 years, is within well stocked shop. Wide range delicious food prepared on premises. Mon-Fri from 8am for Veggie Breakfasts. Saturday evening a set 3-course menu is served with live music. Bring your own wine. V/VG.NS. Children welcome. Disabled access. **(Also in Travel section)**
SPICE OF LIFE 4 Burghley Centre, Bourne PE10 9EG Tel: 01778 394735
HOLBEACH WHOLEFOODS Tel:01406 422149. Two large Natural Food Stores with Self Serve Loose Wholefoods. All welcome! Mail Order.

LONDON

ALTERNATIVES
1369 High Road, Whetstone N20 9LD Tel: 0181 445 2675 Advice on alternative food.
ALTERNATIVES
339 Ballards Lane, North Finchley, London N12 Tel: 0181 445 4397 Advice on alternative food
THE OLIVE TREE 84 Willesden Lane, London NW6 7TA Tel; 0171 328 9078

NORFOLK

LIBRA WHOLEFOODS 50 Market Place, Swaffham. Tel: 01760 724704
Well stocked with a range of products. The owners, Mr and Mrs Clarke have a breadth of knowledge which is available to all customers in this friendly store. You will find everything needed for a Vegetarian or special diet. Homeopathic medicines, Bach flower remedies, Vitamins and Supplements, Herbal Teas, Coffee, freshly ground or beans, Aromatherapy, Jams, Pickles, Honey, Norfolk Punch.

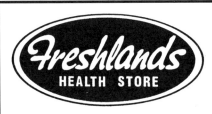

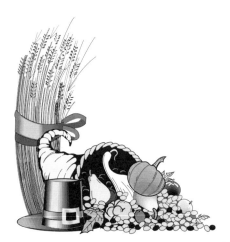

NORTHAMPTONSHIRE

GOODNESS FOODS WHOLESALE - South March, Daventry, Northants NN11 4PH - Tel: 01327 704474 Fax: 01327 300436. A well established company that specialises in own brand labelling, and has complete range of stock for all your needs. This company is happy to deliver nationally.

OXFORD

BEAN BAG WHOLEFOODS 48 High Street, Witney OX8 6HQ Tel: 01993 773922

SOMERSET

FROME WHOLEFOODS 8 Cheap Street, Frome BA11 1BN Tel: 01373 473334
HARVEST NATURAL FOODS - 37 Walcott Street, Bath BA1 5BN - Tel: 01225 465519 Now celebrating its 25th Birthday. Harvest is a name known by vegetarians and vegans from all over the country and is warmly supported by local people playing an important role in developing the health and whoilefood markets. Harvest provies consumers with a diverse choice of vegetarian, vegan and organic foods from around the world. Harvest can also be found in Bristol in New Bond Street under the name of Nova, this branch of the company is also a wholesaler. Please ring the Bath office for more information

SURREY

GRAYSHOTT HEALTH STORES, Grove House, Headley Road, Grayshott, Hindhead GU26 6LE Tel: 01428 604046

WARWICKSHIRE

STRATFORD HEALTH FOODS + WHOLEFOOD & VEGETARIAN CAFE Unit 1, Greenhill Street, Stratford-upon-Avon CU37 6LF Tel: 01789 292353/01789 415741 (Cafe situated at rear of shop). We supply Wholefood Takeaway, Bach Flower Remedies, Organic Produce and the complete range of Food Supplements.

La Verja

100% pure juice available in all good health food shops - made with the pulp of the fruit, using sun-ripened local crops to preserve the genuine taste and nutrition of the fruit - see inside front cover.

ORGANiCO

The new name in delicious organic food - pasta, tomato sauce, soups, juices, biscuits - totally natural, totally organic. Our products are all certified and controlled by EC recognised bodies - your guarantee of our organic credentials. ORGANiCO - for food that does not cost the earth.

Vitalia

Pure pressed organic juices from the South of France - apple, orange, white and red grape, carrot, vegetable, prune and more! Certified by Ecocert - see inside back cover.

Babynat

Organic infant formula milk made with organic skimmed milk and first cold pressed vegetable oil - formulated according to strict pediatric guidelines to provide a balanced nutritional diet.

SdF Limited, 125 Parkway, London NW1 7PS
Tel: 0171 380 0906, Fax: 0171 380 0907

SHOP IN CONFIDENCE
WHERE YOU SEE THIS SIGN

HSW is the buying society which is owned and run by its members who are proprietors of Health and Wholefood Shops.

For over 60 years its members have offered a friendly and knowledgeable service to the community. They and their predecessors have observed and promulgated the high standards and principles set by the forward thinking pioneers of the Health movement. Their concepts and beliefs are today being acknowledged and accepted by many in the field of medicine and nutrition, and people in all walks of life are seeking a more natural diet.

The range of ETHOS Health Products is made to meet these high standards and principles. They can only be found in shops who are members of the buying group HSW.

Retail members are expected to hold at least the certificate in Health Food Retailing, which can now include the Royal Society of Health Certificate in Hygiene, Food and Health.

The majority of members also hold the diploma in Health Food Retailing and are members of, and answerable to, the national professional body, The Institute of Health Food Retailing.

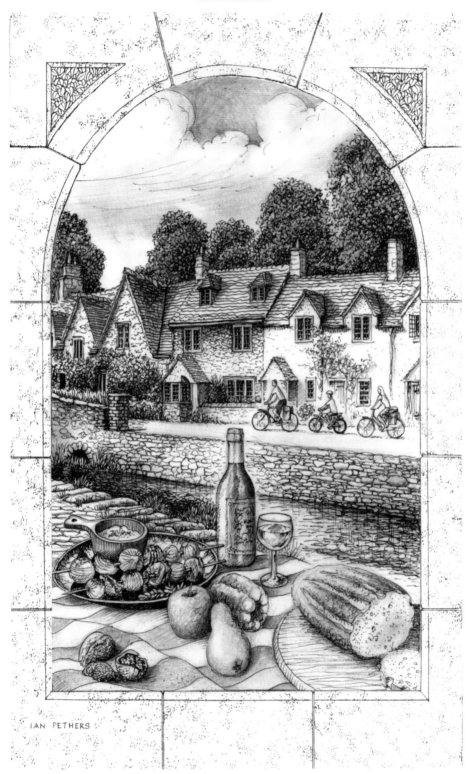

IAN PETHERS

Chapter One

The Westcountry

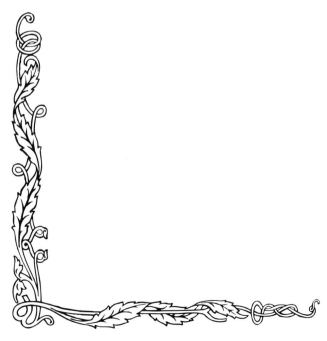

Chapter One
THE WEST COUNTRY
Cornwall, Devon, the Isles of Scilly & Avon

INCLUDES

THE WEST COUNTRY
Devon, Cornwall, the Isles of Scilly, Somerset and Avon

T hose of us lucky enough to live in this fabulous part of the world in which everyone of God's ingredients seems to have been made into a perfect cake, sometimes forget to look around us and see the stunning beauty of the coastline, the awesome and sometimes bleak grandeur of the moors -**Dartmoor, Exmoor and Bodmin Moor** -which all come within this Baileywick. The visitor does not make this mistake and as a result sometimes suffers from mental indigestion and the indecision that comes when the choice is great. I hope in this chapter to whet your appetite and encourage you to discover the West Country and all it has to offer.

Because you will inevitably reach **Bristol** first lets take a look at this fascinating city which owes much of it's prosperity to navigation, the Avon estuary just before it reaches the sheltered Bristol Channel acting as a harbour, and a wide river to take cargoes inland. Trade was active from the early days of sail when ships left port for many parts of the world, bringing back exotic and unusual goods. The medieval woollen trade to Portugal, Spain and Ireland was at the beginning of a long period of importance for fine woollens in the region. More recent industries which have been at the centre of Bristol's success are papermaking, printing, flour milling, tobacco, engineering, chemical processing, and aircraft production. The city's wealth reached out into the surrounding area and can be seen in the status of buildings in many of the towns and villages..

One of the most impressive sights in Bristol is the **Clifton Suspension Bridge** built by Isambard Kingdom Brunel and completed in 1864, which crosses the Avon Gorge at a staggering 245 feet above the high water level. Brunel's work is much in evidence in this area, often associated with the Great Western Railway which was a feat of elegant engineering. His ship 'Great Britain', the world's first ocean-going, propellor-driven iron ship was built at Bristol in 1843 and following restoration after being marooned in the Falklands, is now on display here at the **Great Western Dock**.

Bristol has it's own Cathedral and some of the oldest churches in the country. It also has a fabulous shopping centre which, in addition to the nationally known shops and department stores, are a wealth of small shops of all kinds selling antiques, designer clothes, books and many others.If you have some serious shopping to do the **Broadmead** shopping centre is the place to visit. There was an element of resistence to this project initially. Many believed that some of the buildings planned for demolition should be spared, however there comes a time when new and innovative schemes have to be introduced to prevent a place stagnating. Broadmead is a success, it contains virtually every major department store and literally hundreds of smaller shops, many of which are housed undercover in the **Galleries**. It is mainly pedestrianised which makes shopping so much safer and easier especially for families with young children and the less able-bodied. Bristol is blessed with two good theatres, a thriving university and dozens of important art galleries and the exhibitions range from Old Masters to contemporary artists, ceramics, jewellery, sculpture, the list is infinite. So too is the variety of music which can be enjoyed throughout the city. **Colston Hall** offers performances which cannot fail to appeal to the most catholic of tastes. Where else could one expect to find The Bristol Bach Choir and Cambridge Baroque Camerata one week and Shirley Bassey the next?

You will find Bristol full of interesting old pubs, good eateries which, even if they are not entirely Vegetarian, will always have a choice for the non-meat eater. The hotels range from five star to the more modest Guest House but always with a good standard. Bristol makes a wonderful base from which to explore the surrounding countryside which has been carefully preserved and nurtured and it is still possible to find places where wild flowers grow undisturbed and the best of these is the **Avon Gorge Nature Reserve**. This haven stretches along the West side of the Avon and it is one of the most important lowland limestone reserves in the country. Archeologists among you can see the Iron Age hill fort of Stockleigh camp which lies within the boundary.

There are many other attractions for nature lovers. It is possible to arrange a guided tour around the lovely Long Ashton Cider orchards near Abbots Leigh and be reminded of the golden days of apple orchards and farmhouse cider in stone jars. The English Nature Warden will accompany you on seasonal walks through Leigh Woods and you are recommended to wear stout shoes and bring binoculars for an ornithological tour of Blaise.

Bath, a frisson of excitement courses through me whenever I think about this wonderful city. I treat it like an old friend but always with a decorum and an awareness that Beau Nash, together with the Master of Ceremonies at the assembly and pump room, insisted on the highest degree of civility and manners. It is always with a certain amount of impatience and eager anticipation that I seek out this incomparable city. I prefer to behave in the manner of an ostrich and bury my head in the sand when it comes to the outskirts, or the 'new'Bath, which arose because of indifferent planning. Thankfully, Georgian Bath still remains. It is not the individual buildings that make this city so wonderful but the whole architectural assembly.

Take a walk down through Laura Place looking at the houses in which society used to dwell in it's heyday when Bath was a fashionable watering hole, cross Argyle Street and so to Pulteney Bridge which spans the Avon. You could be forgiven for thinking you were in Florence as you cross this enchanting bridge which has small shops on either side of it not unlike the Ponte Vecchio. The Abbey must come high on your list of places to see. It is probably the most beautiful place in the city. There is more glass than stone in the walls which fill it with light. It is sometimes called the Lantern of the West. It is the West front that is it's greatest glory. It looks down on the square where all the visitors gather outside the Roman Baths. The West door it'self is heavily carved with heraldic shields set in a triple arch, and on each side are wonderful stone canopies covering ancient figures of St Peter and St Paul.

In Broad Street there is **The Bath Postal Museum**. The first known posting of a Penny Black, the world's first stamp took place from this historic building on the 2nd May 1840. The ground floor displays introduce the story of the letter writing and the carriage of mail throughout the ages. There are working machines and a life-size Victorian post office as well as children's activities room. The Museum opens every day from 11-5pm throughout the year and on Sundays from April to October 2-5pm. **The Victoria Art Gallery** in Bridge Street is a major venue for touring exhibitions of national importance. It also has a fine permanent display of European Masters, 18-20th century British paintings and drawings together with decorative art.

The Bath Boating Station in Forester Road, is a unique surviving Victorian boating station with tea gardens and licensed restaurant, a living museum with traditional wooden skiffs, punts and canoes for hire by hour or by day. A pleasant way for a family to spend a summers day on the river Avon. Abundant wildlife, kingfishers, heron, wild geese, moorhens, cormorants etc excites and delights birdwatchers. Punting is a speciality and you need have no fear if this demanding science is foreign to you; there is tuition! You can find bed and breakfast here and somewhere to park your car - no easy matter in Bath.

If you have ever thought of viewing Bath from the air, may I suggest **Heritage Balloons**. The magic is inescapable and I promise that a trip in a hot-air balloon offers the adventure of a lifetime. From the air, the city of Bath and the surrounding countryside takes on an entirely new dimension. Only from the air can you truly appreciate the beauty of the designs of John Wood, the architect and his son, whose vision came to life in the shape of the **Royal Crescent** and **The Circus**. Flights take place early in the morning and early evening and the whole exercise lasts about three hours. In the oldest tradition of ballooning, each flight is celebrated with a glass or two of chilled champagne. The take off site is Victoria Park and to book your flight which must be between March and October please ring 01225 318747.

The list is endless of exciting things to see and do. There is **The Roman Bath Museum** in the Pump Room, Abbey Churchyard. **Beckford's Tower and Museum** stands on the summit of Lansdown, with extensive views from it's Belevedere, reached by 156 easy steps. **The Museum of Costume and Assembly Rooms** in Bennett Street tells the story of fashion over the last 400 years and is brought alive with one of the finest collections of it's kind in the world. The displays include 200 dressed figures and up to a thousand other items of costume, accessories and jewellery to illustrate the changing styles in fashionable men's women's and children's clothes from the late 16th century to the present day. **Royal Crescent** which is popularly regarded as the climax of the **Palladian** achievment in this most classical of English cities is epitomised in **No 1 Royal Crescent** which provides one with an opportunity to see how a house in this wonderful crescent might have appeared when it was first built. **The American Museum** at **Claverton** has 18 period furnished rooms from the 17-19th centuries. The building of **Bath Museum** in the Countess of Huntingdon Chapel, The Vineyards, The Paragon is somewhere in which you will discover how one of the architectural masterpieces of Europe was created. At the same address is **The Museum of English Naive Art (1750-1900)**. This is the first museum of English folk painting, by travelling artists of the 18th and 19th century.

Without doubt one of the best ways of seeing Bath is on the splendid **Kennet and Avon Canal**. Run by the Bath and Dundas Canal Company you can join a boat at Brass Knocker Bottom, opposite the Viaduct Inn in Warminster Road, Monkton Combe. From this historic base near the famous Dundas Aqueduct in the beautiful Limpley Stoke Valley, five miles from Bath, attractive self-drive electric boats are available for the hour, day or evening hire. Picnicking becomes a delight or you can visit the canalside pubs and tea gardens along the delightful stretch between Bath and Bradford-on-Avon. You will find a number of these pubs also have bed and breakfast accommodation. The normal availability is from Easter until the end of September from 9am-5.30pm. Advance booking is advisable. At Sydney Wharf you can join the **John Rennie**, named after the architect and engineer who designed the 87 mile long canal which joins the River Avon at Bath with the River Thames at Reading. This really is a magical cruise with the opportunity of dining on board. If you become addicted to travelling on the, canal as many do, you will see that there are stretches where it is obvious that work still needs to be done and more time and money spent, especially on the width and dredging, but one has to remember that in the 1950s and 60s parts of the 'cut' were merely wet ditches and but for the totally voluntary work of the Kennet and Avon Canal Trust, would still remain un-navigable.

There are various places that I enjoy visiting within easy reach of Bristol. **Badminton** is one of them. It is here on the Duke of Beaufort's estate that one of the great equestrian occasions of the year, the horse trials are held. People come from all around the world to spectate and to take part. It is also one of the rare times in the year when the great house is open to the public and the opportunity to see it should not be missed. It has always been a jealously guarded house by the Dukes of Beaufort and is hardly visible from the village. The trials are always held in April and frequently attended by members of the Royal Family. Indeed the Princess Royal was a winner here one year.

Chipping Sodbury was a 12th century property speculation! It lies on the edge of Old Sodbury parish and was primarily a market centre. The property developers laid out the plots in a regular pattern on each side of the road and so it has remained. It has some wonderful street names - Hatters Lane, Horse Street, Rouncival Street, Hounds Lane and Shoutinge Lane. It really is an attractive place in which to wander and while the population has grown, little has been built to it's detriment.

The M4 with it's unceasing traffic crosses the county a little to the south of Chipping Sodbury and just below that is **Marshfield**, surrounded by cornfields and at one time a place that supplied malt to Bristol and Bath. Those days have long gone but not so the attractive malthouses. The town thrived on the wool trade and many of the fine 17th and 18th century houses reflect the wealth of the citizens in that era. It's ancient traditions are carried on by the Marshfield Mummers, whose play is performed on Boxing Day each year. The play never varies in it's presentation of the traditional conflict between Good and Evil.

Radstock will not please everybody but it is of great interest to the industrial archaeologist and to railway historians. Both of these industries were for many years the main providers of work and money in the town. The last coal mine closed in 1973 but well before that, great thought had been given to grassing and planting the batches - spoil tips for those who have not heard this word used in this context before - I always associate it with cooking and baking!

Here **The Radstock, Midsomer Norton & District Museum** at Barton Meade House, Haydon, is an 18th century converted barn and outbuildings standing in beautiful countryside in the former North Somerset Coalfield. You can see how a Victorian miner lived and worked with a re-constructed coalface and cottage. You can see where the colliery children went to school and where the family shopped at the co-op. There are displays covering 200 years of farming and railways, complete with a model layout. Everywhere there are reminders of the past including an early Methodist meeting room, blacksmith shop, and Saxon artefacts. Temporary exhibitions relating to local themes are held throughout the year. The tea room produces an excellent cup of tea but on a fine day you may prefer the picnic area. There is a souvenir shop and free car parking. It is only open at weekends on Saturdays from 10-4pm and Sundays and Bank Holidays from 2-5pm.

Going westwards you come to the **Chew Valley Lake**, a place of infinite beauty. It is a great place for anglers and for those who just want to stroll along it's banks. Chew Valley has two villages worthy of note. **Chew Magna** and **Chew Stoke**. At Chew Magna you enter it by traversing one medieval bridge and leaving it by another.

Back on the main A368 you will come to **Blagdon** which also has a beautiful lake attracting tourists from afar for it's trout fishing. It is also lucky enough to have a cosy and typically English village inn, **The Seymour Arms**.

You will either love or hate **Weston-Super-Mare**. There seem to be very few people who feel indifferently about it. There is no doubt that it has much to offer the visitor in every conceivable way. The question is where to start. I read one of the promotional brochures put out by the local Tourist Board and it describes the town as 'Miles of Smiles'. It is true that as a good family resort it has something to put a smile on every face whether young or not so young, with it's attractive setting and choice of things to do and places to visit. The two miles of clean, golden sandy beach and the Grand Pier, with it's large amusement centre and Blizzard white knuckle ride, certainly delight people. For those who enjoy leisure complexes you will not find a better one than **Tropicana Pleasure Beach** with it's heated swimming pool, wave machine, water chutes and children's adventure equipment, based on a tropical fruit theme.

The Marine Lake should not be forgotten, here there is always shallow water for children to bathe and splash around in complete safety. I am not sure who is responsible for the flower displays in Weston but whoever it is does the town proud. The spacious beach lawns add a touch of charm to the seafront and the attractive parks and gardens around the resort have superb colourful displays. Just sitting and looking at them is joyous and therapeutic. You can ride in style along the Marine Parade daily during the season in a horse drawn Landau. It makes you feel very important and is quite delightful. If you have small children with you it will take them some time to be lured away from the land train which services the whole length of the promenade from April to September, weather permitting.

For those who want to walk with a purpose I would suggest collecting a series of leaflets published by the Civic Society which will help you follow trails around the town at your own pace. You will find them on sale at both the Tourist Information Centre and the Heritage Centre.

Three interesting museums should not be missed. **The International Helicopter Museum** at Weston Airport holds the world's largest collection of helicopters and autogyros, unique to Britain. You can see restoration work in progress and nobody seems to mind your asking questions in this friendly place. It is open from March-October daily from 10am-6pm and from November to March 10am-4pm. It is closed on Christmas Day, Boxing Day and New Years Day. **Woodspring Museum** is right in the town centre and is a re-creation of everyday life at the turnof the century. Having recently been to the dentist and suffered hardly at all, thank heavens, for I am a miserable coward, I was more than appreciative of the techniques used today when I saw a replica of an Edwardian dentist's surgery complete with the most horrendous implements. There are many displays and if you ever wondered what our Victorian ancestors did when they went to the seaside you can soon find out by examining one area of the museum which is devoted to this very subject. The Museum is open all the year round.

Clara's Cottage is another museum in it's own way. This time it is a restored Weston seaside landlady's lodging of the 1890's which also includes the Peggy Nesbitt doll collection. It is open daily except Sundays from 10am-5pm and admission is free.

There are a host of delightful villages to be discovered and with the advent of the motorways, which in many ways has been a blessing you can travel more easily from one place to another and they do not prevent you from slipping off at various junctions to explore. **Winterbourne** is one such place, although really it has become part of Bristol today. It's oldest part has managed to stay untouched. In the quiet area around the church are a few cottages, and the adjoining Winterbourne Court Farm. I like to think of Winterbourne when hat-making was a cottage industry and between 1770 and 1870 the whole place flourished with the trade brought to them because fashion dictated the wearing of beaver hats.

The church too has a romantic story surrounding a knight whose effigy lies by the north wall. The knight is thought to be Hugo de Struden who eloped with a fair lady but was a bit of a rogue. He made a pact with the devil in return for certain favours. He agreed that when he died he would not be carried into the church, buried in the churchyard, feet or head forward. He managed to cheat even on that and gave instructions that his coffin be carried in sideways and be buried in the wall. On one wall is a brass which I found fascinating. It is about 1370 and one of the Bardestone ladies whose family were lords of the manor. Her dress has pocket holes which show part of the girdle beneath. It is thought to be the oldest brass in the county.

And now for Somerset. The geology of Somerset is very noticeable: the low-lying and flat **Somerset Levels** in the centre of the county dotted with small round hills, through the middle of it running the Polden Hills, to the north the flat-topped Mendip Hills, to the south west the Blackdown Hills and to the west the Quantocks beyond which is Exmoor.

The miles of wet willow-lined Levels are some of the last surviving water meadows in Britain to be left undisturbed by modern farming. Once under the sea, the silt has provided rich soil and peat. Although much has been cut and used in garden composts, where it remains it provides a rare sight of endangered species of flora. Peat is a great preservative and many important finds of Neolithic, Bronze and Iron Age man have been made in the area. Many of the roads that cross this water-logged landscape are on timber Bronze Age causeway and medieval embankments, the suddenly rising hills in the flat landscape once islands in the water. **The Willows and Wetland Visitors Centre** which is at **Stoke Gregory** in the Sedgemoor area tells the story of the district and of traditional Somerset basket making from withies.

On the Levels, the fenland isle of **Athelney** is where King Alfred took refuge from the Vikings in the 9th century. Living as an outlaw he was hiding out in the hut of a herdsman's family when the cakes on the open hearth were burned. The wife, not knowing who he was, blamed the King for not keeping an eye on the cooking! Thus came into being the story of Alfred burning the cakes.

Another story relating to food is that of 'Little Jack Horner'. The Abbot of Glastonbury, wishing to placate Henry VIII, sent him a pie containing the deeds of the manor house at **Mells**. The emissary was one Thomas Horner who opened the pie, put in his thumb and pulled out a plum.

Driving south west down the M5 from the Mendips towards Devon, every junction will lead you to attractive and interesting places.**Brent Knoll** can clearly be seen rising from the Levels. Likewise out of the levels, **Cadbury Hill**, with it's Iron Age hill fort considered by some to be Arthur's Camelot. Not far from Brent Knoll is the pleasant town of **Burnham-on-Sea**, these days lived in by many commuters to Bristol. It has a laid back feel about it, no one seems to be in a hurry. You can walk for miles along the beach, enjoy the shops and find one or two very good hostelries. It's only drawback is it's nearness to the less than pleasant site of **Hinckley Point**.

The high ground of **Exmoor** to the west (part Somerset and part Devon) has a great variety of birds, rare plants and flowers, shaggy ponies and large herds of deer. This was at one time a royal hunting forest and still today the deer are hunted, but given refuge on land owned by Paul and Linda McCartney for that purpose as well as the sanctuary land owned by the League Against Cruel Sports. The moorland plateau rises to around 1,700 feet at Dunkery Beacon and terminates with the tallest cliffs in England, overlooking the Bristol Channel, designated as 'Heritage Coast'.

The subterranean rivers of the **Mendips**, have resulted in wonderful caves, potholes and gorges. At first sight of the spectacular **Cheddar Gorge** and **Wookey Hole** with the many caves full of magnificent stalactites and stalagmites, it must have been a wonderful experience for visitors. Now sadly it is marred by the sheer volume of people who come here - some 1.5million a year - which has resulted in overcrowding and too many tacky tourist trappings. However, the surrounding scenery of the Gorge is wondrous. It can be seen at it's best from the vantage point on the **West Mendip Way**, a walk that starts at Wells Cathedral and concludes after 30 breathtaking miles at the Bristol Channel.

If you are a keen walker you will enjoy the 28 miles of the **Leland Trail** following in the footsteps of the 16th century John Leland, starting on the National Trust's Stourhead estate and crossing the quiet, southern Somerset countryside to another National Trust Property , Montacute House, and on to the high viewpoint of Ham Hill. The Gardens at **Stourhead** (just into Wiltshire) are best visited in the early summer, but at any time of the year the lake surrounded by classical temples and monuments are serenely beautiful. One of the loveliest evenings I have ever spent was at Stourhead on a summer's evening, listening to a concert whilst sitting by the lake enjoying a champagne picnic.These concerts are held quite regularly and are almost always with a theme. For example this year it was Chinese and one was expected to dress suitably for the occasion. **Montacute House**, not far from **Yeovil** is another of my favourite places. It is a fine example of Tudor domestic architecture which, although huge, is on a comfortable scale, set within early Jacobean gardens.

Montacute lies on the route of the Roman Fosse Way, one of the four Royal Roads, running from the south west to Lincolnshire. From this point you can follow the Fosse Way to another of the many fine houses in the region at **Cricket St Thomas Wildlife Park** now more associated with Noel Edmunds and Mr Blobby than the television programme with Penelope Keith, Peter Bowles and Angela Thorne, To the Manor Born. It is home to many rare and exotic species of animal and bird and recently also to a Heavy Horse Centre as well as being a place of enormous fun for children with an adventure park etc. At **Rode** is a 17 acre **Tropical Bird Garden.**

Who could resist turning off for Glastonbury and Wells with their wealth of history and beauty. **Glastonbury** is thought of as the cradle of English Christianity, but for me it is a place of legend, history, mystery and an overworked imagination. It may well have been the earliest Christian shrine but it is certainly the site of the richest monastery, and to this day still a place of pilgrimage. The Glastonbury legends are told again and again, and over the centuries have no doubt been embellished, but I never fail to feel excited by the thought of a visit here.

Towering over the town is **Glastonbury Tor**, possibly Arthur's Isle of Avalon, some 521 feet above sea level, and a landmark visible for miles around. St Michael's Tower on the summit is the remains of a 15th century church, the effort of climbing to which is rewarded by stunning views. First the home of primitive man, then a place of Christian pilgrimage, the Tor is still visited by thousands every year. I would advise you to walk up the Tor if it is possible because of the restricted availability of car parking nearby.

One of the legends told is of Christ coming here as a child with his merchant uncle, Joseph of Arimathea. Another is of Joseph coming here with the Holy Grail and yet another of the Apostle Philip sending missionaries from Gaul to establish a church, and one of those missionaries finding a church already here, dedicated by Christ himself. The undoubted Irish influence here is traced back to St Patrick who came first as an Abbot and to whom the lower church in Glastonbury is dedicated. Then there is the story of St Bridget from Kildare, Ireland, who left her bell and wallet behind at **Beckery** just one mile south west.

Glastonbury is so full of history. It was St Dunstan who laid the foundation of it's spiritual and economic power. By the time of Domesday, Glastonbury owned an eighth of the county of Somerset covering much of the Somerset Levels, large parts of which were almost immediately drained to bring gain to the Abbot. It was Henry of Blois, Bishop of Winchester who built himself lodgings on such a grand scale that they would have made Buckingham Palace look small, who invited William of Malmesbury to write the history which has helped us develop the legends of Glastonbury over the centuries. In 1189 when Royal support dried up and monks were thrown back on their own resources, they felt the Lord was smiling upon them when, as legend says, they were digging a grave for a monk, they found between the shafts of two ancient crosses, 16ft down in a wooden sarcophagus, the bones of a large man and a woman who must have been very beautiful; she certainly had long tresses - the story said these locks were totally preserved until one monk with straying hands touched them and they fell to dust. The monks were in no doubt that here were the remains of King Arthur and Queen Guinevere. Strangely however, William of Malmesbury had never mentioned Arthur in his 'History of Glastonbury' but the monks were adamant, and for them their acute need for money was immediately alleviated by this lovely, romantic idea. They never looked back!

Places to visit should include **The Somerset Rural Life Museum** with it's relics from Somerset's past.**The Chalice Well** at the foot of the Tor. Set in attractive gardens, the waters of the well are claimed to have curative powers, and legend has it that Joseph of Arimathea hid the Chalice of the Holy Grail here. **The Lake Village Museum**, in the High Street, which displays many of the artefacts from an Iron Age settlement near Glastonbury. At **Westhay** is the **Peat Moors Visitor Centre**, where you can learn about the extraordinary history and natural history of the Somerset Levels. At the nearby village of **Meare** you can see the **Abbot's Fish House** dating back to the 14th century. This is where fish caught in the former Meare pool was dried, salted and stored by the monks of Glastonbury Abbey.

To the east of Glastonbury lies the village of **Boltonsborough**, the birthplace of St Dunstan. It was said that it was he who diverted the River Brue, sending it along the course of the little southward stream so that the village might have more power for it's mill.

Godney to the north west of Glastonbury is somewhere the monks used to call the Island of God; one of their seals has been found among the ruins of Glastonbury Abbey. It is older than any monk, older than christianity and in a field is Lake Village dating back to 250BC.

Wells is outstandingly beautiful and very special. A place that delights the eye and makes the heart beat faster. It is the smallest city in England with a population of just 9,400 but it is it's Cathedral which gives it city standing. It is in fact Somerset's only city. It lies sheltered beneath the southern slopes of the Mendip Hills, and combines a wealth of historic interest and beautiful architecture with it's role as a thriving market centre.

The swans at the **Bishop's Palace** have learnt to ring a bell when they are ready for lunch. The Palace is within the inner walls of the city which also enclose the Chapter House and Deanery as well as the **Cathedral.** What an enchanting place the city is with it's narrow streets and lovely buildings. A place in which to spend many happy hours.

To me the little town of **Bruton** is one of the loveliest in Somerset.It has two parts, divided by the River Brue which meanders gently over stones and under a packhorse bridge. The part to the south which runs beneath and beyond the church is the oldest in Bruton, a Saxon religious centre which once had two churches, one founded by St Aldhelm. There was a mint here in the 10th century which opened up the way for the growth of a small town by the 11th century growing beyond the river around a market place near the present Patwell and Quaperlake streets. What attracts me most about this pretty place is the way in which the red roofed houses cling to each other in the winding and narrow streets. Standing on the little pack horse bridge sights of the past evoke all sorts of memories and the bonus is the entrancing peep across the valleys. The architecture of the town shows a rare continuity, through six centuries, of styles and techniques used where stone meets timber in Wessex. The regular form of the High Street is medieval town planning at it's best. It includes the former Abbey Court House of the mid-15th century and Sexey's Hospital. Believe it or not this was established by a local stable lad who made his name and fortune and returned to Bruton to found this fine school. The school stands in a suburb called Lusty! Education is now the biggest business in Bruton.

One of England's smallest churches lies hidden in a wooded combe overlooking the Bristol Channel at **Culbone**, away from roads and cars. Nearby in a farmhouse Coleridge wrote 'Kubla Khan'.

Coleridge lived at **Stowey** on the Quantocks at the end of the 18th century and his home is now open to the public. Here he wrote 'The Ancient Mariner'. The 'Rock of Ages'immortalised by Augustus Toplady in his hymn, was written at **Burrington Combe** on the Mendips.

Near to **Dulverton** on Exmoor the river Barle is crossed at **Tarr Steps** with huge, closely fitting stone slabs each weighing up to five tons. The age of the bridge is unknown but it was certainly used by packhorses during the height of the successful cloth trade. The woods and hills of Exmoor close around Dulverton on three sides, the Barle flows past it's front doorsteps. It is a place steeped in history and one of tranquillity. In the church are two memorials to the Sydenhams who lived from 1540 to 1874 at Combe, a beautiful Tudor House. The life of the moor has made great literature and Dulverton is a name often found in books. Here Jan Ridd met Lorna Doone. Richard Jefferies watched the red deer. If you come to Dulverton in the spring take a walk in Burridge Woods which becomes totally carpeted with bluebells.

Winsford is arguably the prettiest village on Exmoor and it certainly has one of the most charming inns, **The Royal Oak Inn**, with an immaculately thatched roof, soft cream washed walls and a profusion of colourful hanging baskets on the outside. The pub dates from the 12th century and it's open fireplaces and oak beams have been subtly combined with the modern facilities we all expect today. Winsford it'self was described by W.H. Hudson in 1909 as 'fragrant, cool, grey green - immemorial peace - second to no English village in beauty, running waters, stone thatched cottages, hoary church tower.' Little has changed over the centuries. I believe there is still one lady in the village who has seen aeroplanes and cars but never a ship or a train because she has never left the village.

Dunster is charming with it's impressive 17th century octagonal market hall by a wide main street, originally used for the sale of locally woven cloth. Here the **Gallox Bridge** which again used to carry pack-horses, has two ribbed arches, spanning the old mill stream in a picture-book setting. The medieval **Butter Cross** once stood in the high street but is now some way from the centre.

Yeovil does not draw the visitor in the normal way but it should not be ignored. It has an excellent shopping centre, some good hostelries and is a good base from which to strike out into Dorset if one wishes - it is right on the boundary. One might say much the same of **Street** which was home to Clark's Shoes but now it has **The Shoe Museum** showing the history of shoes from Roman times to the present day. Housed in the oldest part of the original Clark's factory, the exhibit's include documents and photographs, shoe buckles, fashion plates, hand tools and shoe machinery, as well of course, as shoes. There are also shoe-making demonstrations and 20 factory shops set within this small town made handsome by the Quaker Clark family who landscaped the factory buildings and built a school, a Quaker meeting house and even a temperance inn.

Not so far from Yeovil, **Crewkerne** is a town whose streets converge in the market square. It has many old stone houses and four groups of almshouses but the church is the magnet. It is a grand cruciform church with glorious windows. The west front is almost cathedral like. Inside it is a little disappointing but the width of the windows brings light to the lovely panelled roofs. Thirteen great stone angels stand holding up the enchanting nave roof. At Crewkerne is one of Somerset's most interesting and beautiful gardens, **Clapton Court**. It has ten acres with formal terraces, spacious lawns, rockery and water gardens. Recently designed is the gorgeous rose garden with arbors.Open March to October, Mondays to Fridays 10.30-5pm and Sundays from 2-5pm.

Taunton is the county town of Somerset and a very busy place with so much to recommend it. Cricket lovers will know that it is Somerset's ground. There is horse-racing at regular intervals, It is a town of wide streets, a sprinking of medieval buildings even in the centre of the town, notably the timber-framed and gabled houses in Fore Street. It has super shops in well laid out areas, much of it pedestrianised. Several old churches to visit including St Mary's which is a sure reflection of the town's prosperity, and many hostelries and restaurants. It is a place in which to mooch. At least three times in it's history Taunton has supported the dissenter; in 1497 it proclaimed Perkin Warbeck king, and in the Civil War, Taunton backed Parliament and many of it's population were killed or wounded in the Battle of Sedgemoor fighting for the Duke of Monmouth in 1685. The small team of professionals who run **The Brewhouse Theatre** will tell you that the theatre exists to present a wide range of arts and activities of the highest standard. The range is varied, drama, dance, opera, jazz and films make up the repertoire. It is recognised as one of the country's leading theatres and art centres. It provides hundreds of people with the opportunity to participate in the arts; either through workshops and courses or by joining forces with the hundreds of volunteers who help out.

The Somerset coast is a must for anyone visiting the county. There is one corner of **Minehead** where a steep flight of steps takes you to the church of St Michael. It is quite charming and reminds me so much of **Clovelly**. Until you have been to Minehead you cannot appreciate what a delightful place it is. Protected by the hills which rise behind it, the houses have flowers climbing over their doors and walls. It is still a little old-fashioned which is part of it's charm. It is the home of the **West Somerset Railway** where steam trains will take you on 20 miles of scenic delights. From the vale of Taunton Deane through the rolling Quantock Hills. Past the beaches of Blue Anchor Bay to Minehead or the reverse journey. There are nine restored stations at which you may break your journey, museums, displays and steam locos.

The little port of **Watchet** is somewhere that has a harbour so small that you wonder how any ship could safely manoeuvre in and out. The 15th century church stands above this miniature seaside town and has a 600 year old cross beside it. A family called Wyndham lived at Kentisford Farm near the church and a square 17th century pew bears their arms. One brass honours Florence Wyndham, an Elizabethan about whom a strange story is told. Whilst she was lying in her coffin in the church awaiting burial, a greedy sexton saw her rings and coveted them. He broke open her coffin and did it so roughly that she woke from her trance, went home and soon after gave birth to a child. History does not relate what happened to the sexton, was he a life saver or hung for being a thief?

Finally in this brief tour of Somerset we come to **Monksilver**, the home of that wonderful house **Combe Sydenham** with it's fine Country Park. You must make sure you allow time to spend a day here. It was at Combe Sydenham that Francis Drake courted the beautiful daughter of the house, Elizabeth Sydenham, who finally agreed to marry him. The dashing Sir Francis then sailed away to fight more battles and chase the Spaniards. His voyages were so long and arduous that the lovely Elizabeth became despondent believing that he would never return. Encouraged by her father she finally agreed to wed another suitor. The day of her wedding arrived and she was driven to **Stogumber** church for her marriage. As she alighted from her carriage a cannon ball fell at her feet. Her heart leapt in excitement. It had to be a sign that Drake was back in harbour. She abandoned her unfortunate bridegroom and went home to await Drake. Drake came and they were married probably in this church. The cannon ball can be seen even today at Combe Sydenham, which experts believe to be a meteorite, in fact. It has become a symbol of good fortune for all those who touch it. It was this marriage that brought Buckland Abbey at Yelverton in Devon into Drake's possession. Their marriage lasted until Drake's death ten years later. Soon after she married Sir William Courtenay and became mistress of Powderham Castle in Devon. Her happiness lasted only a few months, until she too died.

Devon is a county of extremes. It has more roads than any other county in England which will lead you through highways and byways, sometimes amid leafy hedgerows teeming with plant and wildlife, sometimes along a coastline that is breathtaking or on the busy A38 which traverses the county to the borders of Cornwall and beyond. The roads will take you to the romantic and stark beauty of Dartmoor and Exmoor, the lush glory of the South Hams, the attractive resorts in Torbay, the spectacular coastline of North Devon, countless pretty villages tucked away and to the two cities of Exeter and Plymouth whose history goes back hundreds of years. It is a county that begs to be explored and will reward anyone who takes the time. It offers an abundance of stately homes, wildlife parks, museums, glorious sandy beaches, safe bathing, water sports and enough golf courses to inspire even the most ardent golfer. Fishing has always been part of Devonian life whether it be along the banks of flowing rivers or from a boat that will take you out from a sheltered harbour to spend hours of pleasure surrounded by the sparkling blue sea with the backdrop of the coast - it almost makes the catch unimportant!

Plymouth tucked away and separated from Cornwall by the River Tamar is a super centre for anyone wanting to tour the county and maybe pop over the border into Cornwall. It is a city which rose from the ashes after the German bombing in World War II. The bombing, horrific as it was, made way for a new city centre to grow, dispensing with the colourful old narrow streets that would have crucified modern commerce. There is no finer vantage point than Plymouth Hoe to take in the brilliance of Plymouth Sound on a sunlit day, it's waters dotted with the white and often brightly coloured sails of the innumerable boating enthusiasts who flock to the Marinas and the Yacht Clubs here. Plymouth has been host to many people over the centuries. Catherine of Aragon first stepped ashore in Plymouth when she came to marry the unfortunate Prince Arthur and later Henry VIII. She would have seen a very different city from the one we know today. The narrow winding streets of the Barbican would have been unpaved. I doubt if any of the buildings now exist. Southside Street, now the main thoroughfare of the busy Barbican is first recorded in 1591. What an exciting place this city must have been in the time of Drake and Hawkins. It was from Plymouth that Drake sailed on the 19th July 1588 to defeat the Spanish Armada, and it was on Plymouth Hoe that he played his famous game of bowls. The construction of the Breakwater by Rennie (1812-1840) gave Plymouth one of the largest and safest harbours in Britain. Plymouth is blessed with many attractions. **The Theatre Royal** is one of the finest in the country and provides theatrical entertainment from drama to comedy, ballet to opera. **The Pavilions**, a complex which offers ice skating, a swimming pool and a venue for concerts of all kinds from Shirley Bassey to the Bournemouth Symphony Orchestra is comparatively new. **Plymouth Dome** on **The Hoe** should be high on any visitors list and then there is the National Trust's **Saltram House** and across the river **Mount Edgcumbe**, given by the family to the city of Plymouth for the benefit of it's people. A superb house and wonderful grounds stretching right round the coast to **Cawsand, Rame Head and Whit'sand Bay**.

In the last twenty years Plymouth has grown almost out of recognition and taken under it's wing several places which were at one time quiet villages. **Ivybridge** is a prime example. Here a rather sleepy community has found it'self woken to life in the 20th century and the influx of massive new housing developments. Oddly this has not destroyed the village but allowed it to develop a community spirit that has found expression in the main street, now pedestrianised, where everyone seems to congregate from time to time either to shop or enjoy the various hostelries and restaurants. This main street now has major food stores and a big branch of Boots for example.

Another small place that is just outside Plymouth but likes to be thought of as part of the South Hams, is **Noss Mayo** nestling on the opposite side of the River Yealm from **Newton Ferrers.** It is a different kettle of fish here because the river and the hinterland prevent either village from growing too large. Both are charming places offering pretty walks along the river, plenty of boating and yachting opportunities and a very pleasant way of life.

Plymouth not only has it's magnificent Plymouth Sound but in the hinterland lies **Dartmoor National Park**. Only a short drive from the city and you are up on the moor adapting your eyes from the blue of the sea to the haze and wondrous purple, green and brown colouring of the moor which seems to stretch endlessly with great beauty but at the same time is awesome. **Yelverton** would be your first stop outside Plymouth. A small community, with a nice church and tucked away at **Leg O'Mutton Corner, The Paperweight Centre** which has given me hours of pleasure over the years. No charge for going in there and certainly worth a visit.

There are many counties who envy Devon's good fortune in having **Exeter** as it's county town. It has everything. The River Exe wends it's gracious way through the heart of the city, stopping every now and again to prepare it'self for the opening of the swing bridge which lets small coasters upstream for unloading. The jewel in the crown is the magnificent cathedral which dominates the city centre and dictates much of the lifestyle immediately around it. Exeter is Roman, Saxon and Norman; it has walls and a tower built by Athelstan, the first King of England, but most of all it is medieval. There are still miles of quaint streets and passageways, rambling walls, a plethora of churches and of course the cathedral bequeathed to us by many generations of the finest builders, apart from it's Norman walls and towers. Of course the 20th century has crept in and much has had to be changed, but on the whole it has been done with the greatest care and dedication to the preservation of all that is good. Shopping is a pleasure, with the big stores living comfortably alongside medieval buildings. As in most county towns there are innumerable small shops which entice - most of them hidden away in enchanting alleyways. All the time you are wandering in and out of these alleyways you are probably getting closer and closer to the cathedral. Such is the dimension of it's beauty that I find it hard to do it justice on paper. Gazing at the outside will give you hours of pleasure and probably an aching neck!

I love walking along the little Cathedral Close and Southernhay with it's beautiful buildings, almost entirely occupied by professional people rather than residents. Perhaps I will walk in the garden of the 14th century Bishop's Palace, with it's fine trees taking shade from the great walls of the cathedral. Certainly I will look at the Deanery where Catherine of Aragon stayed. Once inside the cathedral I am always mesmerised by the beauty around me. It is almost like being in a heaven in which modern man is allowed to go about in a peaceful, ordered existence which in no way lacks purpose. There is no strife, no threat of war, no anger, just a great sense of the presence of God in the most wonderful surroundings. If there is any cry for help at all it comes from the need to keep this treasure safe. The years are telling on it and constant war is waged against decay. It takes an immense amount of money which is mainly raised by the public. It is not only money that is needed, craftsmen are continually at work and some of them are getting very old. Finding replacements becomes quite a battle in it'self.

Exeter is blessed with many fine churches, some of which are never used but most have stories attached to them. One entrance into the Close is by the tiny church of St Martin with it's porch looking across to the Cathedral. It is quite easy to disregard this little gem because of the stunning beauty of the Elizabethan structure alongside, which was known as Moll's Coffee House. The tiers of windows lean out and are crowned by a little gallery. It's front reminds one of an old ship - not surprising because it was here that Drake used to meet his captains. Nothing much has changed since his time. The panelling is oak, almost black with age, and there is an intriguing gallery painted with 46 different coats of arms. The most fascinating sight though is the whole front of the low room, which is glass. I am told that there are no less than 230 panes and no two the same size.

Apart from the Cathedral, nothing can compare to the **Guildhall**, whose walls have stood for 650 years. It makes sure you will not miss it for it thrusts it'self out into the busy main street, in amongst all the 20th century buildings. I can almost hear it saying 'I bet I will be here still when you are long gone.' Quite right too. Can you imagine C & A or Marks and Spencers still being there in 600 odd years? Inside it is quite lovely. The hall has a superb roof with gilded beams, from which hang dazzling candelabra. Displayed elsewhere are royal and other gifts that have been collected over the years, including a sword used by Nelson and some of the rarest seals in the land. One dates back to 1175 and is believed to be the oldest in the country.

From Exeter one can take a drive of about ten miles to **Exmouth**, the oldest seaside town in Devon. It is a cheerful resort with a good beach. Not the most attractive place architecutrally, apart from the rather distinguished houses on the Beacon, where Lady Nelson lived at No.6 and Lady Byron at No 19. **Ottery St Mary** has an annual carnival. Nothing strange about that except here the young men rush through the main street carrying barrels of flaming tar, a sight worth beholding. **Otterton** has in it's midst the **Domesday Mill**, somewhere every visitor should go. It is a collection of old buildings with a flour mill still working. There are a lot of craft shops there and a very good wholefood restaurant.

Budleigh Salterton always makes me think of retired colonels! It is one of Devon's most charming and unspoilt places. There is a gentle brook running right through the street that houses the shops. The brook starts it's run at Squabmoor, a drab name for such a beautiful spot adjoining Woodbury Common where Nigel Mansell owns the Woodbury Park Golf and Country Club. Enter the foyer there and you will see his famous Williams Renault Car as well as a McClaren. Like many beaches along this part of the coast, Budleigh Salterton is not blessed with golden sand but with pebbles that do not entice you to walk barefooted - but it is of no importance, the scenery makes up for any minor inconvenience.

Further along the coast you will come to one of my favourite parts of the Devon coast. Seemingly not quite of the 20th century, **Seaton, Sidmouth** and **Beer** have altered little since coming to prominence in Victorian times. Sheltered in Lyme Bay, all sharing shingle and pebble beaches and the dignity of yesteryears. These are not places to visit if you want a sophisticated life. Sidmouth springs to life for the annual Folk Festival which has become the Mecca for entrants from all over the world. The first time I saw it I could not believe that there were so many variations of Morris Dancing and Folk Singing, let alone the clacking Clog Dancers. Seaton has that rare item today, a tramway. It is even more of a rarity to find a tramway working on an old railway line. Once run along the promenade at Eastbourne, and doomed when the promenade's extension was planned, the tram was rescued by the enthusiasts who care for it today - a considerable benefit for Devon. The hour's journey travelling the three miles aboard the double-decked tram, through the Axe and Coly valleys along the route of the old railway, will take you to **Colyton** one of the prettiest small towns in Devon. **Beer** is little more than a fishing village which attracts an influx of visitors in the summer, but unlike many similar seaside haunts, it does not die in winter. The community get together and a hundred and one activities spring up to occupy the winter months.

Axminster has a curiously shaped town centre dominated by the parish church of St Mary's. Inside the church you will be astounded by the magnificent carpeting. The pews are set well back so that one can admire this unexpected beauty. Then you realise that it is really quite natural as Axminster is the home of the carpet industry. One of the earliest Axminsters made in 1775, can ben seen in the Guildhall in which is also housed the original market charter dated 1210. Thomas Witty pioneered the carpet industry in Axminster having discovered the techniques from the Turks. His first carpets were produced in a little building alongside the church, and so important was the completion of each carpet that the church bells were rung in celebration.

Wandering about Devon is one of the pleasures of my life and I find myself equally enchanted with every corner. For those who like a resort atmosphere **Torbay** has to be the answer. It always gives one the feel of being on the French Riviera. The sea is a brilliant Mediterrannean blue coming ashore to sandy beaches and row upon row of sparkling white buildings which range from high class hotels to the many small guest houses. Torbay is made up of Torquay, Paignton and the old fishing port of Brixham. It welcomes visitors all the year round and most people who come out of season seem to prefer it when it is quieter.

Paignton is renowned for having one of the best Zoos in the country. The town and sea front are gentle places generally. Flowers and rockeries along the promenade and a wonderful park, man-made out of marsh this century, are the outstanding features. Paignton is the sort of place that people of my age enjoy in the spring, autumn and even winter but who will probably avoid it like the plague in the height of the season.

Brixham has always been the home of fishermen, whose houses perch on the side of the hills leading to Higher Brixham. Some are close to the harbour or open onto little streets or steps bringing their occupants to the seafront. Whilst tourism is not ignored it has always had to take a second place to the fishing industry and so the character of the town has changed little over the centuries. For me Brixham will always stay in my mind whenever I hear Henry Francis Lyte's wonderful hymn 'Abide with Me'. He was the vicar for over a quarter of a century of the 19th century All Saints Church. It is a hymn that has been sung throughout the Christian world by people in times of great emotion.

My father told me that in World War I it was sung by the men in the trenches and when they had finished the Germans would take it up from their dugouts. It has brought peace to thousands. Henry Lyte wrote it in the dusk after evening service. He did not know he had taken his last service in the church. He died not long afterwards. If you listen you will hear the bells of All Saints ring out his hymn every night.

No one comes to Torquay without seeing **Cockington**. If you want to see it at it's best go early in the morning, soon after sunrise, when it is still. Later it will be swamped with visitors and all you will remember will be the crowds and perhaps the thatched cottages. Seen early it is as if you were back in the 16th-17th century when Cockington was first built.

Newton Abbot thankfully is by-passed today which makes it pleasanter to look at the town and much easier to reach other places such as **Ipplepen**, a village as old as time. Conan Doyle spent many a happy visit here with his friend Bertie Robinson who lived at Parkhill House. Exploring Dartmoor was one of his great pleasures and he used to be driven in a horse and carriage by the Robinson groom, one Harry Baskerville. Did you ever wonder where the title 'Hound of the Baskervilles' originated ? Now you know. No one ever denies the beauty of **Broadhempston** reached through a network of small lanes. It's church is 15th century with graceful arcades, old carved beams and bosses in the porch and roofs.

If you take the coastal road out of Torquay you will come to **Teignmouth** and **Dawlish** two unashamedly Victorian resorts of great charm. On the approach road to Teignmouth a turning off at **Shaldon** just before the bridge will take you to **Stoke-in-Teignhead**. It lies in one of Devon's combes by the mouth of the Teign. Full of pretty cottages and an old church which must have been here in Norman times. When you look at the mosaics in the sanctuary, you will wonder how so many years ago, such work was done by Italian craftsmen. Where did they stay, how did they cope with the language barrier and how long did their journey take?

Dawlish is close to **Powderham Castle**, one of the quiet glories of Devon, built between 1390 and 1420. It has been the home of the Courtenay family ever since. Sir Philip Courtenay was the first occupant, the sixth son of the second Earl of Devon, from whom the present Earl is directly descended. If you look at the castle you will see that every generation has made some form of alteration in order to keep up with the changes of their time. None of this has detracted from it's beauty. A visit to Powderham will always remain in your mind as a red letter day.

The South Hams is one of the prettiest areas in the whole of Devon. **Modbury** built on the slopes of a valley with four main streets intersecting at right angles is full of nice buildings and many enchanting shops plus a sprinkling of good hostelries and the bonus of a free car park. The road from Modbury towards the sea winds it's way towards **Kingsbridge** which rises sharply from the Salcombe estuary. It is a charming place with a church that stands on massive 13th century arches. Apart from the excellent shopping facilities in the main street take a look at the **Cookworthy Museum of Rural Life**. The A381 takes you from Kingsbridge to **Dartmouth**, the undoubted 'show-stopper' of the South Hams. You approach the town from the top of a steep hill and if traffic permit's I suggest you stop for a moment or two to catch the stunning panoramic view of the town and the river. The dramatic scenery is heightened by the tiers of houses which cling for dear life to the hillside overlooking the River Dart. It is always a busy and delightful place to be. You will see constant passenger and car ferries crossing the busy river to **Kingswear** on the other side.

Salcombe delights every one who goes there with it's colourful streets, vibrant river estuary and lively life style. It is full of good places to stay, places to eat, ferries to take you across the estuary to **East Portlemouth** where there are wonderful beaches. It is a paradise for anyone who enjoys being waterborne.

Totnes, first mentioned in the reign of Edgar about 959AD, was probably a small settlement. Today it is a busy, attractive town which is not much more than one beautiful street climbing up a hill by the River Dart. You will find a lot to entertain and interest you here.

For me exploring the South Hams is a never ending treasure hunt with constantly different and unexpected clues to it's beauty.

Changing route entirely, it is time to take a look at some of the places on **Dartmoor** which, when you are in Devon, is never far away. **Tavistock** one of the Stannary towns, is a favourite haunt of mine. I love the sense of pride and stability. It has so much history which started a hundred years before the Conqueror, and was originally controlled by it's Abbey. You can seek out a great deal of the past in the fine medieval parish church, with it's pinnacled tower, it's wide nave, and countless gables that dominate the streets. It may well have been here that Francis Drake was taken to worship as a child for Tavistock was his home town, something one is never allowed to forget.

Many small villages surround Tavistock, all of which are worth seeing. On the Okehampton road there are two **Tavys, Mary and Peter**, the twins grew out of the settlement on either side of the River Tavy. Each has a church linked together by a bridle path and a little bridge over the river known as 'The Clam', an old name for a bridge. In **Mary Tavy** there is an excellent Vegetarian Restaurant,**The Stannary,** probably one of the best in the country. No one should miss seeing **Lydford Gorge**. Water pours off the moor onto the boulders of the gorge with a ferocity which would overshadow a witches cauldron. A mile or so away is **Lewtrenchard Manor**, the composer of great hymns, Sabine Baring-Gould's old home which is now a stunning country house hotel.

To the north of the moor is **Okehampton** with it's romantic Castle, Okehampton seldom gets the recognition it deserves and is well worth taking a look at. **Chagford** is a sleepy market town that should also be on your list. It has grown up around the village square. Do visit **James Bowden & Sons**. It is an experience. Founded in 1862 it can only be called an emporium. This is a Stannary Town where tinners would come from miles around to have their precious metal weighed and given the King's Stamp before it was sold. Farmers too would come to sell their cattle and sheep and, in particular, their fleeces, for wool was an important industry. All this activity was watched over by the most distinctive of the town's many historic buildings: the old market house in the middle of the square.

Drewsteignton in addition to having a remarkable hostelry and charming thatched cottages, is home to the amazing **Castle Drogo**, the last castle to be built in this country. Julius Drewe was responsible for it and he got Sir Edward Lutyens to design it. The enchanted world of **Fingle Bridge** is just below Drewsteignton. You do not just simply arrive here, you have to seek it out. It is hidden away at the end of a long winding leafy lane that seems to descend forever, until suddenly there it is; a low pack horse bridge which dates back to Elizabethan times, if not earlier, straddling a river dancing and cavorting as it plays with the boulders strewn in the path. The paths leading away from the bridge were probably the way that merchants came with their laden pack-horses and the terrain was too difficult to develop further. We can count ourselves lucky that this was so, otherwise Fingle Bridge might not have survived the wear and tear of men and vehicles over the years. There are three Iron Age hill forts around Fingle Gorge. **Prestonbury** you can see clearly from the bridge. **Wooston** is down river and if you see it on a spring morning with the sun behind you, it is breathtaking. The third, **Cranbrook**, is higher up. At **Shilston** to the west is the best known of the cromlech or dolmens in Devon, with the odd name of **Spinster's Rock**. Legend has it that three spinsters put it in place, but fact says it is the remains of a Bronze Age megalithic tomb.

Moretonhampstead holds the key to so much that is beautiful. Within my lifetime it has changed considerably. Forty years ago it was a shopping centre for farmers and people living in outlying hamlets. It had everything a community needed. Today the butcher is still here and the chemist but the general store is no more and it is only recently that the baker has returned. It gets it's livelihood mainly from tourists. The 'hampstead' part of it's name has been added in the last century or so and most local people ignore it, calling the little town Moreton, derived from the Saxon Mor Tun. The 15th century church of St Andrew standing on high ground has tombstones in the porch in memory of two French officers who lived at Moreton during the Napoleonic Wars when they were on parole from their prison at Princetown. Four other villages in the vicinity should be looked at. **Doccombe, Dunsford, Bridford** and **Christow**, each has it's own merit's and all are part of the Dartmoor scene.

Close to Moreton is **Becky Falls.** High up in the solitude of Dartmoor you approach it through glorious woods. On one side of the road there is a car park, where, if you have any sense, you will don stout shoes or wellies, before making the descent alongside Becka brook, where the water cascades over and between massive boulders until with a roar it reaches it's peak, and falls in sparkling torrents on it's way to the sea. This enchanted world is at it's best in November after the mid-winter rains.

Moments up the road is the isolated village of **Manaton**, with it's green nestling beside the church. Mentioned in the Domesday book it seems to have been there for ever. Away to the south the great rocks known as **Bowerman's Nose** look like a petrified sentinel guarding the rugged hills, or a man with a sense of humour wearing a cardinal's hat playing God.

Bovey Tracey is one of the Gateways to Dartmoor and has been important since the days of the Normans. It has charming, narrow streets and sit's sedately overlooking the River Bovey. Perhaps not as peaceful as it once was, it is still a delightful place to visit.

To describe the routes that one can take on the moor to get the greatest pleasure out of walking takes more space than I am permitted in this book. The Dartmoor Visitors Centre at **Princetown** will provide you with a comprehensive choice of books and pamphlets on the subject. The sort of things I look for are the old guide posts which are no more than pieces of granite standing on end. Each is marked with a letter. From Two Bridges one would be marked 'P' showing the direction of Princetown or 'M' for Moretonhampstead. It is primitive but effective. Frequently you will come across the remains of Bronze Age dwellings, just circles of stones which once were a hut. Sometimes you will see the remains of beehive huts. Not that they ever housed bees! They were used by medieval tinners for hiding their unsold tin, and other bit's and pieces.

The clapper bridges are to be seen quite regularly over the streams that run through Dartmoor. **Postbridge** has one of the best examples. It is a tribute to the skill of the 14th century builders. You will see that all the bridges are made of huge slabs of granite balanced one upon the other. Built so well that they have withstood the onslaught of human feet, the insistent hammering of the river and the Dartmoor climate, for centuries.

Then there are the Dartmoor 'Letter Boxes'. If you know nothing about them; it is purely a fun thing that has developed over the years into quite a serious hobby. You seek out the position of the boxes, usually tucked away in a crag somewhere, quite well hidden. You then post your own cards and take out any that are already there, which then become your duty to post on. Inside the hiding place you will find a visitor's book for you to sign, a rubber stamp, and an indelible pad, and you have to stamp your cards with the Dartmoor Letter Boxes' own crest. One for instance, is to be found at Cranmere Pool, south west of Okehampton, another at Crow Tor.

Princetown is always an attraction, albeit a macabre one because of the infamous Dartmoor Prison, built by French Prisoners of War. It is a threatening place and dominates this small village. Even on the sunniest of days it still looks formidable and extremely depressing. There is nothing depressing however about the lively **Plume of Feathers** where mine host is James Langton. This is a favourite watering hole for people from miles around and is equally popular with visitors who find the informality and fun infectious.

I am addicted to the road that runs from Two Bridges to Ashburton which has endless places of enchantment that run off it. Past **Dartmeet** and on to **Poundsgate, Widecombe-in-the-Moor** can be seen from miles away with it's tall church tower built 400 years ago, by tin miners in thanksgiving for the thriving industry. It is dedicated to St Pancras and known as 'The Cathedral; on the Moor'. For centuries the village remained almost unknown and it was not until 1850, when the vicar decided to hold an annual fair and Sabine Baring-Gould popularised an old folk tune that made Widecombe become world famous. There will be few who do not know the old song 'As I was going to Widecombe Fair wi' Bill Brewer, Jan Stewer, Peter Davy, Uncle Tom Cobleigh an all.' If you are one of the few you may rest assured that someone in Widecombe will tell you the story of Uncle Tom Cobleigh and his grey mare. Whether he was fact or fiction is strenuously argued. What is a fact is that a Thomas Cobleigh was born in the nearby village of **Spreyton** in 1762 and died there in 1884. It could be that he brought his grey mare and his motley crew to Widecombe for the fair.

Buckland-in-the-Moor is enchanting with some of the loveliest thatched cottages I have ever seen. On a hill stands the 15th century church with carved bosses in the porch and old tiles under the tower. When you look up at the clock you will note that it does not have numerals. In their places are the words 'My Dear Mother' and it's bells chime out 'All things bright and beautiful'. There is no official explanation for this curiosity but legend has it that it was placed there by a man in memory of his mother. This remarkable lady, when told the news that her son had drowned at sea, refused to believe it. Every night she placed a candle in her window to guide him home. Her faith was rewarded. When she died this is how he repaid her constancy.

Holne is a little village of no more than 300 people. A busy community who have great links with **Ashburton**, a town of contrasts and beauty. In 1305 it was designated a Stannary Town. Tin mining and the wool industry brought it great wealth and with it the building of some fine houses. **Buckfast Abbey** must be one of your ports of call. Not during the day, although it is beautiful then, but at night. Buckfast Abbey during Compline is magical. The monks come silently down the aisle, the only sound the swish of their long robes as they pass by, the only light, the bidding one high over the altar. As they reach their stalls, they push back the cowls from their heads and the service begins. It's simple message is chanted and reaches out to every corner of this great building. One cannot doubt that God is present.

In Mid-Devon **Tiverton** is a place that grows on you. The prettiest way to approach this very old town is by the Exe valley road. It goes back to Saxon days when it had fords across the Exe and the Loman, and it is where these two meet that the town looks down from it's high ground between the rivers. Right by the medieval gateway of Tiverton Castle is the 15th-century St Peter's Church. It's spacious windows glisten in the afternoon sunlight highlighting it's pinnacles and battlemented parapets. The centuries have not destroyed the wonder of the carving on the outside walls. Look for a bear that creeps along a hollowed wall, a monkey holding fast to it's baby and the proud lions which crouch on the buttresses. **Tiverton Castle** built by the Normans is still important to the town but it was the wool merchants who provided Tiverton with many of it's finest buildings.

The rivers are not the only waterways in Tiverton. The reach of the **Grand Western Canal** has been lovingly and carefully restored and is now open to the public who can enjoy the gentle trip by horse drawn boat along this beautiful canal as far as **East Manley**.

The road that takes you from the very old town of **Crediton** with it's ancient and very beautiful cathedral like church, to Tiverton takes you close to **Cadbury**, a small village amongst the hills, with wonderful views over the Exe valley. The tall church tower which has stood for over 500 years dominates all around it at first sight, until you realise that it, in turn, is overshadowed by the mighty **Cadbury Castle**. Standing 700ft up, it is a fort of the ancient Britons. Nothing much left there now other than two ramparts enclosing a great space. It was here that General Fairfax pitched his camp in the Civil War.

So much beauty and history is crammed into the scenic village of **Bickleigh**. It has everything; a castle, a river flowing under a superb bridge, thatched cottages, an award-winning mill and two very good hostelries. Two other villages should not escape your attention. **Bampton** about 8 miles north of Tiverton should be visited if only to discover it's ducks! **Holcombe Rogus** south of Bampton is the other. It is mentioned in the Domesday Book and has Holcombe Court where the lords of the manor from Tudor times were the Bluetts. Supposedly haunted it is said that tough American servicemen during World War II were frightened out of their wit's by the persistent presence of an unknown ghost. Worth a nosey, I think.

North Devon is different again, wonderful countryside and a spectacular coast. Starting inland, the quiet market town of **Holsworthy** has two striking viaducts and a good pub. **Black Torrington** got it's name because the stones in the nearby river turn black with iron oxide in the water. **Sheepwash** is a great base for anyone wanting to walk along the Torridge valley. Game fishing attracts keen anglers with salmon, sea trout and brown trout all providing excellent sport at different times of the season. Pony trekking and riding are available nearby. There are good golf courses and it is heaven for eager ornithologists. From here it is easy to visit **Rosemoor Garden** only a short journey from Sheepwash and one mile south of **Great Torrington.** Before moving on one should take a look at the sleepy village of **Hatherleigh** with the excellent **George Hotel** which is Heritage at it's best.

In Great Torrington I am always reminded of it's past. It was literally blown into history by the great explosion of eighty barrels of gunpowder. It happened in the Civil War, when General Fairfax marching from the east, took the Royalists by surprise, and captured the town. The prisoners were shut off for safety in the tower of the church. They were held in complete darkness and had no idea that they were scrambling about in what had been the arsenal of the Royalists. Somehow the powder was set alight and the ensuing explosion shattered the church, killed 200 men and nearly killed the General as well. Today Great Torrington is the home of the world famous **Dartington Glass**.

North west of Torrington is **South Molton**. This ancient sheep and cattle market town is on the edge of Exmoor. It dates back to the 12th century and until the middle of the 19th-century thrived as a centre of the wool trade.

Now for the coast. **Lynton** and **Lynmouth** are linked together by a remarkable Cliff Railway which opened in 1890. It climbs 500ft above sea level along a 900ft track and allows you to enjoy both villages without having the severe climb from one to the other. Both are attractive places and especially Lynmouth. The Napoleonic Wars were responsible for the rising popularity of the two villages. Restrictions on travelling abroad made people look for alternatives and here they found comfort and beauty. Shelley and Coleridge were regular visitors. The River Lyn runs through Lynton and tumbles over moss strewn rocks and boulders, through thickly wooded hills as it falls to the sea at Lynmouth.

The main road from Lynton will take you to **Combe Martin**, but there are some spectacular walks in between which should not be missed, nor should you leave out the little village of **Parracombe** which lies between steep hills and must have been one of the first places in Devon to have a Christian church, for 1450 years ago, St Petrock came here and built a little chapel of cob and wattles, with a roof of straw.

Combe Martin has one of the longest village streets in the whole of the country. It became part of history over 750 years ago when it's silver mines produced the wherewithal to pay for the Hundred Years War. **Ilfracombe** is the next stop and as you drive from Combe Martin you will be bewitched by the panoramic and stunning views glimpsed only occasionally over the cliff to the sea. Wonderful scenery, a good beach and friendly pubs are good reasons for coming here.

The winding coast road takes you to the seaside villages of **Mortehoe, Woolacombe** and **Croyde** with their magnificent beaches beloved by surfers and families. They are all just big enough to have a life style of their own but small enough to remain intimate. From Woolacombe you can just see, far out to sea, **Lundy Island,** the granite haunt of pirates long ago and now chiefly the haunt of sea birds; the island stands out 400ft above the sea.

Baggy Point offers some outstanding walks and this may attract you to **Croyde** which is tucked away on the southern flank of the peninsula. **Saunton** three miles away is renowned for it's Championship Golf Course.

A busy main road will lead you from here through **Braunton** and into **Barnstaple** which claims to be the oldest borough in England. Whilst it remains an interesting town, much of the old has given way to the new to allow it to develop as the business centre of North Devon. It has an excellent theatre. From Barnstaple to Bideford you have the choice of two roads. The main A339 or the small B3233. The latter allows you to take a look at the villages of **Fremlingham** and **Instow** on the banks of the River Taw as it comes out of the sea at **Bideford Bay**. From Instow a ferry trip across the river to **Appledore** is rewarding. It is here that the two great estuaries of the Taw and the Torridge meet. Appledore is charming and picturesque. The little street running up from the quay is nothing short of beautiful.

Bideford is an excellent base for anyone who wants to explore the coast and villages between it'self and **Hartland Point**. It is a friendly town looking over the river. Nothing ever changes in **Clovelly**. It is an artist's paradise. Cars are taboo. You leave your vehicle in the car park at the top of the village and descend down the cobbled street which tumbles for half a mile to the sea. On either side are old cottages with flowers and creepers climbing up their walls. The scenery is unforgettable. High above you trees reach for the skies whilst way below the sea sparkles in the sunshine. It is divorced from this world.

Hartland is a place that goes nowhere and makes a good place in which to end this rather hotch potch tour of Devon. Here we have **Hartland Abbey** which stirs the heart and soul of everyone who visit's. It dates from the 12th century, is situated near the wild, desolate coastline, has monastic origins and has been lived in by the same family, although frequently inherited through the female line, since the Dissolution, when Henry VIII gave it to William Abbot, the Sergeant of his royal wine cellars. There are many lovely rooms and the grounds are outstanding. The Valley is still as beautiful as it must have been in the days of the Abbots. It is open to the public from May-September on Wednesdays, Bank Holiday Sundays and Mondays from 2-5.30pm. Dogs on leads are allowed in the grounds.

I have an unashamed love for Cornwall from whence my family stemmed. It is an incredible mixture of glorious coastline running up either side of the peninsula until it joins Devon across the Tamar, the Atlantic and the English Channel. In the middle of this sandwich are the mining villages which frankly would not be out of place in a sci-fi film and have frequently been used for this purpose. Mineral wealth below ground, shaped the destiny of Cornwall and the Cornish for hundreds of years, changing the landscape and creating these unique villages, harbours and quays.The National Trust now owns a third of the coastline of Cornwall, more than 100 miles of magificent walking country including many spectacular stretches and popular holiday resorts.

The coastal villages have always been among the most picturesque and sought after for film makers and artists, some liking the softer south side and others the incredible, harsh beauty of North Cornwall. Whichever way you go you are never far from the sea and for this part of the chapter I am going to take you across the North Devon border into Cornwall at **Bude**. John Betjeman described this place of endless golden sands, 'the least rowdy resort in the county'. People come here to enjoy family holidays in the traditional manner, revelling in the sun, sea and sand. Surfers flock here because the Atlantic rollers rise to great heights and provide them with some superb rides. It is only in recent years that Bude hs come to prominence. At the end of the last century it was not even on the map. Next door **Stratton** was the established market town where the famous Battle of Stamford Hill took place in 1643 when Sir Bevil Grenville defeated the Parliamentary forces led by the Earl of Stamford. Every year in May this battle is re-enacted by members of the Sealed Knot Society.

Drive down the A38 and turn off towards the coast on a signposted B road and you will come to **Boscastle** which must have been known to sailors since men first sailed the English seas. If you have a choice of roads, then to see Boscastle at it's most spectacular, approach from **Camelford** on the B3266 where the road rises until you suddenly see the most glorious prospect over the Valency Valley and the Atlantic Ocean before you drive down the twisting road into the village. There is no doubt that the little harbour is one of the oddest in the country. It has a medieval breakwater, a long greasy slipwater and a huge dog leg opening into the ocean. For those who pass the stone jetty and clamber over the slippery rocks, the sea opens out in front of them to a sight that is unforgettable. If the tide is right you will not be able to miss the famous blow-hole working and rumbling. It is a natural curiosity throwing out a cloud of spray with a deep rumble like a tiny volcano. I have heard it called the Devil's Bellows.

Thomas Hardy came here as a young architect to help in the restoration of the church where he met his wife, Emma Gifford. This was not a marriage made in heaven although it lasted over 30 years. Oddly enough after her death in 1912 Hardy returned to Cornwall and the memory of their early romance at Boscastle inspired him to write some of the greatest love poems ever.

There are some magical walks around here. You can walk inland or take the coastal path from the harbour to **Penally** and on to **Pentargen** or climb the lane linking Boscastle with **Lesnewth** and nearby **Minster** with it's church in an almost theatrical setting with not a house in sight and tall trees forming a backdrop. In spring the whole of the floor of this imaginary stage is covered with a carpet of bluebells and daffodils. The walk along the coast from **Boscastle** to **Tintagel** is nothing short of stunning. When the sun is shining, the sea is unbelievably blue and laps the rocks with such gentleness that it is hard to visualise the fury that is whipped up on a stormy day when the wind drives the sea in. So powerful is the wind that it is difficult to stand upright but the sight is awesome.

I lived in the village of **Tintagel** for a while in 1950 and I used to walk up the long hill to the 14th century church which is the oldest in Cornwall. It is set high on the Clebe Cliff exposed to the ravages of the Atlantic storms. Take a look at the gravestones and you will see that the force of the wind has bent them all in the same direction and some have had to be supported by little buttresses. One really does not know whether King Arthur ever set foot here but there is no doubt that Tintagel's most famous attraction is his castle. It is a romantic place identifiable as a settlement from AD400 in the time of the Celts. In the 12th century it became a royal castle but by the 1500s the central portion had been washed away by the erosion of the sea. Edward, the Black Prince is supposed to have stayed here and if you climb down the path that leads to the shingle beach you will find Merlin's cave where it is alleged King Arthur spent his childhood.

Soft golden sand is to be found at **Bosinney Cove** and **Benoath Cove** - havens for the bather and sun-worshipper. **Trebarwith Strand** with it's sandy beach is a popular place for surfers. One needs to take care, the tide roars in here and it is not always safe.

Another castle that is worth seeing is **Launceston Castle** which dominates the market town of **Launceston**, and is an easy drive from either Tintagel or Boscastle. It is a small, busy town with friendly people and a wonderful parish church. **Camelford,** closer to the coast and **Wadebridge** should both be on your visiting list. Between them they form the base of the triangle that takes in so many pretty places. I always enjoy the small village of **Port Isaac** with it's charming, irregular steep streets with cottages that lead down to the harbour. It is a village that is the essence of a Cornish fishing port. The estuary of the River Camel divides **Rock** from **Padstow**. Each side of the estuary has it's afficionados. One of the strange things about Rock is that it lost it's church in the sand! Sand dunes on the banks of **Padstow Harbour** engulfed an ancient chapel and it was out of use for ages until the middle of the 19th century when it was restored. You can see it now as it stands on the sand with a fine view across to Padstow. **Padstow** has a charm of it's own. It is a little town that has clung to it's own ways and traditions for centuries. For most people Padstow will be synonymous with it's curious May Day custom of welcoming summer with songs and dancing in the streets while a man in a mask dances in front of a **Hobby Horse.**

The National Trust own **Bedruthan Steps**. The climb down the steps is definitely demanding and worse on the way back but the reward far and away outweighs the puffing and panting of those of us more used to driving than walking.

It's not that I dislike **Newquay** that I am bypassing it this time. Purely a lack of space and this busy resort is known by everyone. I like some of the places nearby like **Trerice,** one of the few Elizabethan manor houses in Cornwall which have escaped extensive alterations. For 400 years the home of the Cornish Royalist Arundell family, this glorious house still retains most of it's 16th century glass in the great hall window of twenty four lights, comprising 576 panes. It was acquired by the National Trust in 1953. **Perranporth** to the south with it's sand dunes and vast beaches is always popular in the summer for family holidays and for day visitors, especially at weekends.

St Ives provides a different vista and a different feel from the towns and villages we have just covered. It is the home of so many artists that it does not need me to paint in words how very attractive it is. It was much frequented by Whistler and Sickert who delighted in the light which has a high ultra violet content. The whole reach of **St Ives Bay** from **Navax Point** to **St Ives** is glorious. The sea always seems to be bluer here than anywhere else in Cornwall. The streets are narrow and it is the worst possible scenario for drivers. You are well advised to leave your car at **Lelant** and use the excellent Park and Ride service which operates with stops all along the bay. As you wander round the centre of St Ives you will find pretty aspects at every turn. Little houses jut out at funny angles and lead to other houses, until you have climbed steadily to **St Ives Head** under which the town snuggles, safely sheltered.

Now we are approaching **Lands End** and the coast and hinterland change again. There are small villages like **Zennor** clinging to the cliff and further down **St Just** next, not to be confused with St Just in Roseland to which we will come shortly. Spring comes early here with the beauty of the hedgerows ablaze with wild flowers - autumn lingers and in winter, frost and snow are rare visitors. But the exhiliration of facing up to the Atlantic gales is an experience you are unlikely to forget!

Sennen is America's nearest neighbour! It stands high above the sea with a deep cove into which the sun hardly ever shines in winter. There is an odd story about the little medieval church. A great stone stands outside and round it seven Saxon Kings dined and wined, so the story goes, and then continues to say that when another seven kings dine here the end of the world will come!

Once I used to be filled with an enormous excitement when I stood at **Land's End**, the very end of Britain. There was nothing there then except the land and the sea beyond. Now it has a smart hotel, endless attractions and restaurants - not the same at all.

If you take to the lanes from Penzance and drive to the coast a few miles away you will reach **Porthcurno, St Levan** and **Lamorna** right by the sea and so beautiful. Take a look at **Paul**, the last village in Cornwall to speak the Cornish language back in the early 1700's. Winding roads lead to the fishing village of **Newlyn**, beloved by artists and then to **Penzance**. This is a nice old town with a busy port and wide promenade. **The Scillonian** sails daily for the **Scilly Isles**, twenty eight miles south west of Lands End. Directly in front of the fishing village of **Marazion** is **St Michaels Mount** rising out of the sea in **Mounts Bay**. Originally the site of a Benedictine Chapel established by Edward the Confessor, this spectacular castle dates from the 14th-century. To get there you can walk across from Marazion when the tide is out, or during the summer months take the ferry at high tide. It is a wonderful experience and the gardens which seem to grow out of the rock, are unique. Because of the narrow passages within the castle, it is necessary to limit the number of visitors at any one time.

The Lizard will be our next port of call but en route one should take a look at **Helston**, famous for the annual Floral Dance which is performed through the town rather like the Hobby Horse in Padstow on the north coast. The Royal Navy have a presence at Helston. The air station at **Culdrose** is home to several squadrons of helicopters and it is a rare day when you do not see these ungainly creatures of the air, landing and taking off. The skill of the pilots is unmatched. Many a sailor and visitor has been saved from certain death by the efficiency of their rescue skills and their bravery.

It would be sad not to visit the remote and wildly beautiful villages of **Manaccan, St Keverne,** and **Coverack.** Manaccan hides itelf in it's hilly slopes. No matter which way you approach it you have to come down or climb up hills. Indeed the whole coastline of The Lizard is on the descent. One incline goes to St Keverne, another down the pretty valley to **Gillian Creek** and yet another to the **Helford River.**

The sea has never been kind to St Keverne and if you wander in the churchyard you will see graves of 400 people who have drowned off this shore in ships brought to their doom on the dreaded **Manacles.** On a calm summer's day when the sea is a brilliant blue and the little church surrounded by palms and hydrangeas, it is hard to conjure up the harshness of this piece of the coast in the height of a storm. But be there when a storm is raging and you will never again doubt the power of the ocean. **Coverack** is more sheltered and is charming. From there you need to go inland a bit to pick up the lanes that will lead you down to **Ruan Minor** and **Cadgwith**, two delightful spots. I almost forgot **Mullion** which has graves of some Ancient Britons on the downs above the cove. The cove it'self is enchanting and has an impressive cavern and the striking **Lion Rock.**

Falmouth and **Truro** have not always seen eye to eye. In 1663 Truro was punished for it's role in the Civil War and the whole river from **Tregothan Boathouse** was given to the new Co-operative of Falmouth. It was hard on Truro and it took from then until 1709 to assert it's rights over Falmouth harbour, a claim strongly contested by Falmouth, which was by then a port of some consequence and saw no reason for Truro to have any say in the matter. It took the courts to settle the matter. Each today is a delightful place in it's own right. **Truro** is the county town of Cornwall and with it's fine cathedral attracts many a visitor. The cathedral is not all that old, it celebrated it's centenary only in the last decade. It gives the appearance of having been there for ever and certainly creates a focal point for the city. If you can take a short while to sit within it's walls, taking stock of life, you will find it rewarding. You may be lucky enough to have chosen a time when evensong is being sung by the splendid choir. The music soars into the rafters and the whole church is uplifted.

From Truro, the rivers leading to the great **Carrick Roads** wander through some of the most beautiful scenery in the world. There are pleasure boats that will take you on a voyage of discovery that is a never ending delight, right the way down to **Falmouth** and **St Mawes**.

Inland the road from Truro to St Mawes is almost like trying to find the pot of gold at the end of a rainbow. You seem to drive forever, sometimes through sumptuous scenery. And at others indifferent, in the way that Cornwall has of teasing those who seek to know all about her. Finally, less than twelve miles from Truro you are rewarded by sought for treasure, **St Mawes**. Everything is beautiful here, the glory of the sea, the majesty of **St Mawes Castle**, and it is surrounded by the villages of **The Roseland**. No nothing to do with roses. In this instance Roseland means promontory or commonland.

St Just in Roseland is a famous beauty spot with it's pretty church nestling against the banks of the river. It has curious stones inscribed with slightly mawkish sentiments lining the steep path through the churchyard down to the church. I heard it described once as 'the sort of churchyard one would be happy to be buried in'. The church is open daily and I would list it as a must for visitors.

On the other side of the Fal, **Pendennis Castle** guards the entrance to the Carrick Roads as it has done, together with **St Mawes Castle**, for hundreds of years. Both castles can be visited. The easy way to get across the river to **Falmouth** is to take the little passenger ferry or go further up the river and take your car across on the King Harry Ferry. The road from there will take you via **Perranorworthal** to Falmouth. From here you are within easy reach of the enchanting inlets of **Feock, Mylor,** and **Restronguet**. Wonderful places in which to wander and spend the most contented of days.

En route for Falmouth you will come to **Penryn**, now by-passed but it does not like being missed out. It always seems to me that it is resentful of Falmouth and puts on a sombre forbidding air. It is far older than Falmouth, whom it considers a modern upstart, but the problem really lies in the fact that Falmouth became the chosen port and they would not be far wrong, a fact only denied by the seafarers who have used the haven of the Carrick Roads for centuries. Tourism is clearly very important to **Falmouth** but for all that the town is a very busy port with ship repairing facilities and a dry dock which is capable of taking vessels up to 90,000 tons. It is a pleasant town with lovely gardens, beautiful beaches and a climate which permit's palm trees to grow.

Before we go inland and take a look at **Camborne** and **Redruth**, lets take the A30 a little north of Redruth and seek the turning for **Chacewater**. It lies in the heart of the Cornish mines - most no longer working - and had the richest vein of copper in the world. It can boast the first steam pumping engine in a Cornish mine, made by James Watt. Today Chacewater is a pleasant rural village with some nice houses and a fine old pub **The Rambling Miner** in Fore Street. From the village it is simple to visit the famous **Wheal Jane** mine and the entrancing **Blissoe Valley**.

Camborne is famous world wide for it's School of Mines but apart from that it is a busy market town. The fine medieval church is well worth visiting with a churchyard crammed full of interesting gravestones, many with entertaining epitaphs. Near Camborne is **Magor Farm** where in this century, ruins of a Roman villa were found.

Redruth is almost joined to Camborne these days but it still has it's separate existence. William Murdoch lived in one of the plain little houses here. It was he who gave us gas light and invented the locomotive. A Scot by birth he married a Redruth girl and it was their house which had the very first gaslight in the whole of the country.

If you find the tin-mining industry interesting, you will not want to miss **Cornish Engines** at **East Pool.** Here there are impressive relics of these great beam engines which were used for pumping water from over 2,000ft deep, and for winding men and ore. The engines exemplify the use of high pressure steam patented by the Cornish engineer, Richard Trevithick of Camborne in 1802. It is open Good Friday to the end of October, daily from 11-6pm or sunset if earlier.

High above Redruth stands **Carn Brea Castle,** silhouetted against the sky, and near it is a great column in memory of Francis Basset who did so much for Cornish miners. It is worthwhile making the effort to climb up the inside stairway of this monument which stands 90ft high. From the top you get the most amazing view of the whole of this mining area and the sight of more coastline than anywhere in the county.

Where did miners go if they had free time? **Gwennap Pit**. This was the place where they would listen to the stirring oratory of John Wesley preaching in this naturally tiered open-aired ampitheatre. In my imagination I can hear the great sound of the Wesley hymns resounding around the place from the glorious Cornish voices. John Wesley converted the Cornish to Methodism in their thousands.

St Austell is one of the busiest towns in Cornwall. It does not have a great deal to offer the visitor other than it's fine church which stands among palm trees, rising from a beautifully manicured lawn, right in the heart of the town opposite the premier hostelry **The White Hart**. It has a tower well over five centuries old but the church's rarest possession is it's massive Norman font with a bowl carved with extraordinary creatures and resting on columns ending in human faces.

As a base for a holiday St Austell is excellent because there are so many stunning places within easy reach. **Mevagissey** in **St Austell Bay**, is the largest fishing port in the bay and probably one of the most photographed harbours in Cornwall. Colourful fishing boats still sail out from here and nothing can take away the charm of the whitewashed cottages as they cling to the steep sides of the roads to Fore Street, where attractive shops flank the inner harbour. **Gorran Churchtown** should not be missed. Just one and a half miles from Mevagissey. It has a pub, **The Barleysheaf**, built in 1837 by a Mr Kendall who, hearsay states, had it erected for his own use because he was barred from every other hostelry in the area! You are close here to the wild headland that sailors call **The Dodman** with it's 550 year old tower, a massive structure rising 110ft; a famous landmark from the sea.

Fowey with it's spectacular harbour is a place of discovery; narrow winding streets where flower decked houses and cottages jostle side by side with quaint little shops and pubs on the hillside that slopes down to the glory of the Fowey river. From the days of pirates and smugglers with their barges and brigantines brazenly at moorings, to the hundreds of colourful craft that now fill what is undoubtedly one of the most enchanting harbours in this country, time has changed very little.

Rising in Bodmin Moor, the River Fowey has always been the life-blood of those towns and villages through which it flows on it's way to the open sea at St Austell Bay. Directly opposite Fowey and reached by a ferry is **Bodinnick** and at it's heart is **The Old Ferry Inn** which has one of the world's most picturesque views from it's lounge right over the estuary, past Fowey and Polruan to the sea. It is a great place to stay and full of the atmosphere built up over the four hundred years of it's existence.

I am always drawn to the small, and so far unspoilt, harbour village of **Charlestown** where the tiny entrance to the harbour defies belief that any vessel of size, let alone the big clay carrying ships, can enter it's sheltering arms, but they do and demonstrate this every day. It is the home of the **Shipwreck Museum** which is Britain's biggest exhibition of shipwreck artefacts.

Lostwithiel may not appeal to you because of it's rather uninteresting main street but do not judge it by this. Explore this little town on foot and you will find much to please you. The majesty of the ruins of **Restormel Castle** watch over the town. The Castle is a delightful place to be, the ruins enhanced by magnificent rhododendrons, trees and shrubs. Built in the 13th century it was a ruin by the 16th. Lostwithiel was strongly Royalist in the Civil War and legend has it that Charles II was hidden in an oak at **Boconnoc**, hence the name of the excellent pub in Duke Street, **The Royal Oak**. Lostwithiel was once the capital of Cornwall. It is an ancient borough with a working community who will tell you that they do not put on a special face for holiday makers for a few weeks in the year, but aim to give the same friendly welcome all year round. It is an excellent centre for fishing, walking or just relaxing and enjoying the Cornish countryside. The 13th century church of St Bartholomew is worth a visit.

From Lostwithiel the river continues meandering past the lovely little church of **St Winnow** on the east bank, which dates mainly from the 15th century, although there are some remains of Norman and 13th century architecture. A little further on is the creek that leads up to the pretty waterside village of **Lerryn**, where once sailing ships came to discharge their cargoes of road-stone from the quarries at **St Germans**. Now it is so silted up that you must keep a watchful eye on the tide if you are water-borne. It might be worth being stranded if it gave you the opportunity to visit **The Ship Inn**, a delightful hostelry with good food, good beer and good company.

On the west bank is an even smaller village, **Golant**, much beloved by small boat owners. They come to enjoy the sailing but also to visit **The Fisherman's Arms** which you will find at the end of a road marked 'Road liable to flooding at high tide'. The pub overlooks the water but it is outof harm's way - even the pavement is 2ft high!

Almost in the centre of Cornwall is the old county town of **Bodmin** and if you take the road from St Austell to the town you will go through English China Clay country. Go via **Nanpean** and **Carthew** and you will come to **Wheal Martyn Museum**. This will give you an unforgettable insight into Cornwall's single largest industry. Great white, eerie mountains appear on all sides, evidence of the industry that has provided so much of Cornwall's employment. In Bodmin, the handsome church of **St Petrock** delights all who see it. It is the biggest in the county, 151ft long and 65ft wide. Mainly 15th century it has been much restored. On **Beacon Hill**, looking down on the town, is a column of granite rising 144ft high. It is in memory of Sir Walter Raleigh Gilbert, a brave soldier, and belonging to the family of Sir Humphrey Gilbert who was the step-brother of Sir Walter Raleigh. Bodmin has a lot to offer including **The Bodmin and Wenford**

Railway which allows you to explore some of Cornwall's finest countryside from a steam-hauled Branch Line train. **The Light Infantry Museum** is opposite the station and **Bodmin Town Museum** is a short walk away from the town centre. **The Camel Trail** paths to Wadebridge and Padstow start near the historic Bodmin Goal.

Just outside Bodmin is **Washaway** where you will find **Pencarrow House**, the home of the Molesworth family and has been so since it was completed by Sir John Molesworth, the 5th baronet in about 1770. Essentially a family home, it is a delight to explore. For Gilbert and Sullivan fans it is interesting to know that Sir Arthur Sullivan composed the music for Iolanthe here. The Pencarrow Gardens cover some 50 acres. Huge rhododendrons and camellias provide a wonderful display every Spring. There are several gardens within striking distance from here which should not be missed. At **Prideaux Place, Padstow**, there is a deer park and a newly restored garden overlooking the Camel estuary. **Lanhydrock** has rare trees and shrubs, the unique circular herbaceous garden and exceptional magnolias. **Lancarffe** at Bodmin has four and a half acres of sheer beauty and then there is the fabulous **Longcross Victorian Gardens** at **Trelights**, near Port Isaac, which is open all the year round from 10.30am until dusk. It has fascinating maze type walkways and one of the best cream teas anywhere.

Had we started this tour of Cornwall from **Plymouth** crossing by the **Torpoint Ferry** we would have had a pleasant run through the small town of **Torpoint** and then on to **Anthony**, a small hamlet really which has a pub, **The Ring of Bells** in which the Duke of Edinburgh used to play skittles before his marriage. It also has one of the nicest, small stately homes, **Anthony House**, now belonging to the National Trust but also the family home of the Pole-Carews. Open to the public it is a pleasure to spend time there both in the house and the gardens which reach down to the River Tamar.

The traffic from the ferry and from the **Tamar Bridge** which has made entering Cornwall so much easier, meet at **Trerulefoot**, where maybe you would have decided to carry on deeper into the county but for our journey we are cutting off to the east and through the pretty **Hessenford Valley** until you reach the quaint fishing villages of **East** and **West Looe**. Here the river meets the sea, picturesque houses climb the steep hills, fishermen set sail every day in their colourful boats and visitors set out with some of them to go shark fishing. For the less adventurous Looe it'self is fascinating, full of good pubs, sandy beaches and a plethora of hotels from which to choose if you should decide to stay.

Across the old bridge which divides East and West Looe you will find the road that will lead you to **Talland Bay**, surely the most beautiful stretch of smuggling coast in Cornwall! And from thereon to the little fishing village of **Polperro** which is a visitor's dream come true. So small are the streets that you have to leave your car at the top but the reward is a journey that will take you between houses that almost touch each other. They are quaint as are the shops and the pubs. Every road leads to the harbour and if one had to talk about somewhere that paints the picture of what the visitor imagines Cornwall is all about then **Polperro** has to be that place.

Farmhouse Guest House - **HUXTABLE FARM**
West Buckland, Barnstaple, Devon EX32 OSR
Tel/Fax 01598 760254

In a secluded position on the edge of Exmoor, 'Huxtable' is surrounded by traditional stone farm buildings, open fields, woods and a stream. The house it'self dates back to 1520 and has many original features such as oak beams, screen panelling, open fireplaces with bread ovens, uneven floors and low doorways. It is the comfortable home of Jackie and Antony Payne and Antony's well travelled parents, Barbara and Freddie. South Molton is 10 minutes away and there are a range of activities within easy distance from clay and pigeon shooting on the farm to surfing at Croyde. Six golf courses are within 35 minutes away. Huxtable has it's own sauna, fitness room, tennis court and games room with a dartboard and table tennis table.

To end your day, relax in the Medieval Dining room over a four course candle lit dinner served with a complimentary glass of homemade wine. Whilst the dishes on offer also cater for non-vegetarians, there are delicious choices across the board for the vegetarian. The 5 ensuite bedrooms and one with private bathroom are warm and comfortable. Huxtable is ideal for a break at any time of the year. Telephone for informative brochure.

USEFUL INFORMATION

OPEN; All year
CREDIT CARDS; None taken

CHILDREN; Welcome.Outside
              play area

ON THE MENU; Home-cooked fare using
fresh local and farmland produce
and Devonian cheeses
VEGETARIAN; Made to order
DISABLED ACCESS; No.

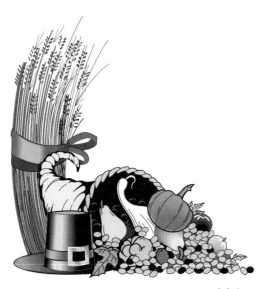

Vegetarian Restaurant - **DEMUTHS VEGETARIAN RESTAURANT**
2 North Parade Passage, Abbey Green, Bath BA1 1NX
Tel: 01225 446059
Fax: 01225 314308

This bright, spacious, strictly non-smoking restaurant is to be found in a Grade II building in which the lower floor is medieval and has a Saxon cross in the wall. Upstairs there is fine Georgian panelling. What strikes one most is the air of happiness and contentment which has a lot to do with the decor but mainly stems from the welcoming attitude of the owners, Rachel Demuth and Nick Troup. Demuths is well established in Bath and needs little introduction to local people, but for the visitor, especially the vegetarian visitor, it is an oasis in a city which is renowned for it's good eating places. The secret of it's success gastronomically is the creativity that goes into the dishes. One cannot pin the cuisine down to any particular style. To describe it overall as 'flavours of the world' would be most appropriate. Preparation, which is half the battle in any vegetarian dish , is carried out using only the best ingredients and the finished result is nothing short of amazing.

In addition to the main menu there are always daily specials and vegans, diabetics and lacta diets come within the scope of this accomplished establishment. Breakfast, coffee, lunch, tea or dinner at Demuths, with jazz or world music playing in the background, art posters on brightly painted walls, banquettes and potted palms, intimate alcoves, make the occasion memorable. For the sweet tooth there is a fine selection of cakes and puddings, many of them supplied by the award winning Hobbs House Bakery. Demuths is licensed and you will find organic wines on the list. Bottled beers and cider are also available plus a comprehensive range of juices and soft drinks, speciality teas and coffee. Demuths lives up to it's reputation and has the added bonus of one of the finest locations in the city with it's ground floor windows overlooking Ralph Allen's Townhouse and the towering majesty of Bath Abbey.

USEFUL INFORMATION

OPEN; Mon-Sat: 9am-10pm,
       Sun: 10am-9pm
CREDIT CARDS; Access/
   Visa/Mastercard/Switch
CHILDREN; Welcome
LICENSED; Yes

ON THE MENU; Exciting vegetarian dishes plus organic wines and beers
DISABLED ACCESS; No
GARDEN; Courtyard with tables
ACCOMMODATION; Not applicable

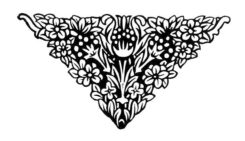

Hotel - **ARCHES HOTEL**

132 Cotham Brow, Cotham, Bristol BS6 6AE

Tel/Fax 0117 9247398

Set off the road, this early Victorian house provides quiet, comfortable surroundings and a friendly welcome whether on holiday or business. The hotel is situated approximately 100 yards from the main A38 and so, is accessible by both private and public transport. The main commercial centre, theatres, exhibition centres and waterfront are all within approximately one mile. The hotel has an English Tourist Board One Crown rating and a Commended Quality Grading. All ten bedrooms are centrally heated, have a wash basin, hair dryer, colour television and tea and coffee making facilities (with herb teas on request). Two bedrooms are ensuite. All bedrooms are equipped with an ioniser, which removes dust, smoke and pollen, to aid a good night's sleep. Guests are asked not to smoke in the diningroom and other public areas. Included in the tariff is a continental breakfast, which consists of a large selection of beverages, fruit juices, cereal, warm croissants with jam and as much toast as you can eat. In addition there is a choice of six cooked breakfasts with traditional, vegetarian and vegan tastes catered for. No evening meals but there are many traditional and vegetarian restaurants within a 2 to 10 minute walk.

USEFUL INFORMATION

OPEN; All year except Xmas & New Year
CHILDREN; Welcome
CREDIT CARDS; Master/Visa/Amex/Switch
LICENSED; No
ACCOMMODATION; 10bedrooms 2ensuite

DINING ROOM; Continental or cooked with 6 choices
VEGETARIAN; Yes + Vegan choice
DISABLED ACCESS; No facilities

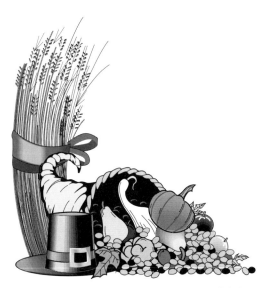

Restaurant - **BOUBOULINA'S**
9 Portland Street,
Clifton, Bristol
Tel: 0117 973 1192 Fax: 0117 9738387

This delightful restaurant concentrates on providing healthy and enjoyable food providing both dishes for vegetarians and carnivores. Free range eggs, organic produce and an insistance on quality in every ingredient used ensures the very best of food. Essentially Greek in character, the restaurant is a lively, happy place in which regulars know they will not only be well fed but made extremely welcome. For newcomers the welcome is enthusiastic and Bouboulina's will always be remembered by anyone who has been there. In addition to the printed menu there is also a blackboard which displays the daily 'Chef's Specials'. If you have never tried a Vegetarian Meze now is your chance. Meze is one of the specialities of the house. This dish beloved of Greeks and of those who have become acquainted with it, is a feast of vegetarian hors-d'oeuvres and main dishes.

Bouboulina's is an ideal venue for Birthdays, Celebrations and Weddings. There are private rooms available in which you can have a wonderful time enjoying the food, the wine and the ambience. Although the restaurant is licensed you are very welcome to bring your own wine and Champagne. The restaurant is fully air-conditioned and the smoking of cigars and pipes is not allowed.

USEFUL INFORMATION

OPEN;Tues-Sat 10am-11,30pm
Sun-Mon 5pm-11,30pm
CHILDREN; Welcome
CREDIT CARDS; All major cards

RESTAURANT; Wonderful Greek food
BAR FOOD; Meze bar menu available
VEGETARIAN; Extensive selection
DISABLED ACCESS; No special facilities

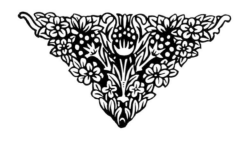

Restaurant - **MILLWARDS**
40, Alfred Place, Kingsdown, Bristol, Avon BS2 8HD
Tel:0117 9245026

Just round the corner from the Kingsdown Sports Centre and near the University and main hospital. Millwards has become a name synonymous with excellent Vegetarian fare. For nine years Patricia and John Millward have striven to make their attractive, intimate restaurant in a mid-Victorian building complete with the very high and ornate ceilings of that period, a place on which a Vegetarian can rely. That they have succeeded is apparent when you realise that they are former winners of the Vegetarian Restaurant of the Year UK and have an entry in many National and International Food Guides.

You dine at beautifully appointed tables in a totally non-smoking atmosphere with the sound of unobtrusive classical music in the background. The menu is imaginative and highly recommended is 'The Millward's Platter' of two or three courses offering a taste of three dishes at each course. There is a set price for two or three courses. Where dishes are suitable for vegans you will find a V after the entry. Imagine a meal which might be Warm Tabbouleh with Toasted Almonds followed by Aubergine Fritters in a Guinness Batter on a bed of spiced Cous Cous with red peppers and pine kernels. There are also some scrumptious and innovative desserts such as Poppyseed Parfait with Passion Fruit sauce or Millward's brown sugar meringues with ice cream and cream. Delicious.

Millwards is proud of it's wine list which features many small growers and also a good selection of half bottles. There is a choice of 70 wines including some from Europe, Mexico, Australia, New Zealand, Chile, USA and England. 12 wines are vegetarian and 15 are organic.

USEFUL INFORMATION

OPEN; Tues-Sat from 7pm.
Closed 1 week at Xmas, Easter & 2 weeks
In October
CREDIT CARDS; Visa/Master
CHILDREN; Welcome

ON THE MENU; Vegetarian with vegan options.
Other dishes on request
DISABLED ACCESS; Wheelchair access but no
suitable toilets
LICENSED; Yes

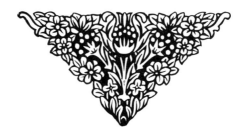

Bed and Breakfast/Self Catering **- TREFFRY FARM**
Lanhydrock,Bodmin,Cornwall PL30 5AF
Tel/Fax: 01208 74405

Treffry Farm reminds one of everything that is good about Cornwall. The historic old farmstead was once the Home Farm of the Lanhydrock estate which is now owned by the National Trust and the estate now provides guests with a perfect location for peaceful country walks. The house is centrally heated and with it's thick walls is as cool in summer as it is warm in winter. All the rooms are delightfully furnished in traditional country style and there is a particularly charming wood panelled lounge for your relaxation. There are 3 pretty, ensuite bedrooms. Breakfast taken in the dining room, offers a varied selection of cooked or Continental and vegetarians are well catered for. Pat Smith has researched and organised four different activities in depth: Golfing, Fishing, Cycling and Walking based on her sound local knowledge. Several pubs and restaurants nearby serve evening meals. Also available are well equipped self-catering farm cottages.

USEFUL INFORMATION

OPEN; All year.	**DISABLED ACCESS;** No
CHILDREN; Welcome.	**LICENSED;** No
CREDIT CARDS; Yes	

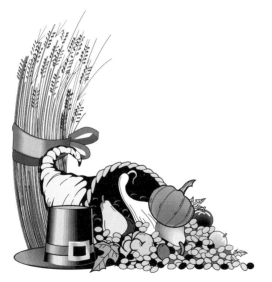

Hotel - **THE BULSTONE**

Higher Bulstone, Branscombe, Nr Seaton, Devon EX12 3BL

Tel: 01297 680446

The Bulstone is especially designed and equipped for those with young children. In the beautiful old world village of Branscombe where badgers outnumber people, much of which is National Trust property and being on the Heritage Coast there are many well signposted footpaths and spectacular views. It provides a wonderful opportunity for every member of the family to relax and enjoy themselves. There is a large well-stocked Playroom and outside there is an enclosed play area with swings, climbing frame, and other toys where children can play safely. Parents and children alike can enjoy an informative stroll along the woodland paths and through the flower meadow of the hotel's wildlife garden. For the very young there are all the facilities needed to maintain family routines. Children's tea is fun and the food is great. After the children have gone to bed enjoy a candlelit dinner with home-cuisine prepared to a very high standard. The fully licensed bar carries a wide range of wines, spirit's and local beers. This is a non-smoking establishment.

USEFUL INFORMATION

OPEN; All year
CHILDREN; Specially designed
CREDIT CARDS; All major cards
NON-SMOKING ESTABLISHMENT

ON THE MENU; Good home-cooking
for the vegetarian and others
DISABLED ACCESS; Yes

Guest House - **CAMES BARTON**

Stockland Bristol, Bridgwater, Somerset, TA5 2QA

Tel:01278 653453

Cames Barton is a comfortable home that has been achieved out of a remarkable and skilful barn conversion. It is the epitome of comfort and Pat Curtis is a charming and welcoming hostess. Stockland Bristol is in a peaceful and secluded corner of Somerset - a wonderful place to regain peace and tranquillity before facing once again the rigours of modern day life. From here you can walk to Steart Bird Sanctuary and a short drive will take you to the beautiful Quantock Hills. There are stately homes, pretty villages, interesting old hostelries and a wealth of wonderful countryside to explore.

Pat Curtis will always meet individual requirements if it is at all possible and she is only too pleased to cater for Vegetarians. The prettily furnished bedrooms all have tea/coffee facilities and sharing bathrooms is minimal. Pat will tell you that people who enjoy the countryside, and a relaxed atmosphere, good food and comfort, enjoy themselves at Cames Barton.

USEFUL INFORMATION

OPEN; All year
CHILDREN; Welcome
CREDIT CARDS; None taken
GARDEN; Yes

ON THE MENU; Good food
VEGETARIAN; Catered for
DISABLED ACCESS; No special
facilities
ACCOMMODATION; Well appointed rooms

Farmhouse - **TREWORGIE BARTON**

Crackington Haven, Bude, Cornwall EX23 0NL

Tel/Fax: 01840 230233

Treworgie once belonged to the Prior of Launceston and was annexed to the Duchy of Cornwall by Henry VIII in 1540, illegally sold by Elizabeth I in 1601 and repossessed by James I a few years later. The house has the atmosphere that only the centuries can bring; the beauty of it has been enhanced by the owners Pam and Tony Mount over the last twenty years. It is a happy house, full of friendliness and just the place to unwind, have fun and enjoy rural Cornwall at it's best. So much pleasure has been given to guests over the years that something in the order of 65% is now repeat business which in it'self speaks for the high reputation the Mounts have achieved.

The four pretty bedrooms are all with private bathrooms or shower room, attractively furnished, comfortable and welcoming with their freshly picked posies of flowers. Breakfast is whatever you wish it to be and the four course dinner is memorable. Pam Mount is a superb, imaginative cook who uses, where possible, local produce and her own fresh herbs. The menu changes daily and she caters for vegetarians with an equal flair. Both breakfast and dinner are served in the traditional, antique-furnished dining room, complete with granite fireplace and original cloam oven. Treworgie Barton is not licensed but guests are welcome to bring their own wine to complement their dinner. From Treworgie Barton you can set out to explore the magic of both Devon and Cornwall.

USEFUL INFORMATION

OPEN; Apr-Sept (Feb, Mar, Nov Advanced bookings)

CHILDREN; Over 10 years

CREDIT CARDS; None taken

LICENSED; No - bring your own

ACCOMMODATION; 4 en-suite rooms

A NON SMOKING HOUSE

DINING ROOM; Superb home-made fare

VEGETARIAN; Dishes across the Board

DISABLED ACCESS; No

GARDEN; Yes

PETS; No

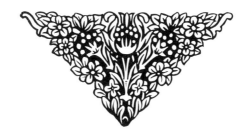

Restaurant - **CRISPINS**

26 High Street, Dulverton, Somerset, TA22 9DJ

Tel: 01398 323397

Once a row of cottages, Crispins is now a charming and atmospheric restaurant with two rooms serving the restaurant. The front and main restaurant is bistro style and seats 22. The centre room has a fine oak fireplace and oak beams, seating up to 20. It is used for family groups or small parties. In summer the delightful vine covered garden sets the scene for open-air lunch or candlelit dinner. Margaret Grimes, who with her husband Tony owns Crispins, is a talented chef who has always been attentive to the needs of vegetarians and also adds a percentage of Vegan options. 55% of the starters are vegetarian and 33% of the main courses. The Wine List is small, but sensibly chosen with wines from France, Spain, Germany and Bulgaria. The average price is about £8 per bottle. Somerset Cider Brandy and local Farmhouse Cider are two of the interesting drinks on offer. For anyone wanting to stay in Dulverton, close to the Exmoor National Park, Crispins has Bed and Breakfast Accommodation.

USEFUL INFORMATION

OPEN; Summer: closed Sun eve. Monday Lunch. Winter: open Tues eve to Sunday Lunch. Closed throughout February

CHILDREN; Welcome

LICENSED; Yes

ACCOMMODATION; Bed & Breakfast

ON THE MENU; High percentage of vegetarian starters, maincourses & puddings.

DISABLED ACCESS; Yes but not the toiltes

GARDEN; Yes

Farmhouse - **WHITEMOOR FARM**

Doddiscombeleigh, Nr Exeter, Devon EX6 7PU

Tel: 01647 252423

Charming listed 16th century thatched farmhouse, set in seclusion of own garden and farmland, within easy reach of Exeter, the Coast, Dartmoor and Forest Walks. It is a relaxed and friendly establishment, where children and pets are welcome. Vegetarian evening meals on request which are also available at the well known inn nearby. Swimming pool with solar heating available for guests

USEFUL INFORMATION

OPEN; All year

CHILDREN; Very welcome

CREDIT CARDS; None taken

ON THE MENU; Good choice of Vegetarian food as wel! as traditional

DISABLED ACCESS; No

Hotel - **TRESILLIAN HOUSE HOTEL**

Stracey Road, Falmouth, Cornwall TR11 4DW

Tel;01326 312425/31115

If you require a relaxing holiday where you can forget what is going on in the rest of the world and completely unwind, then the Tresillian House Hotel is the place to stay. This very friendly hotel owned and run by Robert and Jane Brown, is the perfect holiday location. The ensuite bedrooms are very comfortable indeed with colour television, radio/intercom, hair dryers, central heating, direct dial telephone and tea and coffee making facilities. There are lounges for you to sit and plan your day or read the papers. There is a well-stocked bar where you can enjoy a drink before dinner and meet other guests. The food is excellent with a wide and varied choice, a vegetarian menu is available on request. It is a pleasure to dine and stay here.

USEFUL INFORMATION

OPEN: March to October

CHILDREN; Welcome with reductions according to age

CREDIT CARDS; Visa/Master/Amex

LICENSED; Yes

ACCOMMODATION;12 en-suite rooms

DINING ROOM: Excellent home-cooked fare, varied choice & generous portions

VEGETARIAN; Menu available on request

DISABLED ACCESS; No

GARDEN; Yes

Hotel - **COMBE LODGE HOTEL**

Chambercombe Park Road, Ilfracombe, Devon EX34 9QW

Tel: 01271 864518 Fax: 01271 867628

Combe Lodge Hotel offers you and your family a welcoming, quiet and enjoyable holiday with a difference. They will take you from the hotel to the start of all sorts of wonderful walks and cycle rides and pick you up at the end of the day at a prearranged time. This allows you to explore without the nuisance value of driving. A service for which the hotel has won awards. This small, licensed Victorian property is just on the outskirts of Ilfracombe overlooking the picturesque harbour and sea, and only a 15 minute walk to the shops, theatre, cinema, promenade and harbour. There is a large car park - something very necessary in Ilfracombe. Most of the bedrooms have their own ensuite facilities. Some enjoy the picturesque view of the harbour and, on a clear day, the Welsh coast in the distance. Combe Lodge is non-smoking throughout and has a reputation for good food and plenty of it, served in their licensed dining room. The meals are imaginative and typically English with a hint of something special, made up of three courses followed by a good selection of cheese and biscuit's, coffee or tea. Most importantly there is a full and interesting vegetarian menu. The hotel is quite happy to comply with any special diets and to make packed lunches on request.

USEFUL INFORMATION

OPEN; All year round.

CHILDREN; 10 years and over

CREDIT CARDS; Visa/Mastercard Eurocard/ Amex

LICENSED; Yes

ACCOMMODATION; 4 dbl 1sgl 3family.

ON THE MENU; Imaginative vegetarian menu

DISABLED ACCESS; No

GARDEN; Overlooking the sea

PETS; elcome

Farmhouse Guest House - **BURTON FARM**
Galmpton, Kingsbridge,South Devon TQ7 3EY
Tel: 01548 561210

You and your family can be assured of a warm welcome from Anne Rossiter at Burton Farm. The farm is a large working unit situated in the South Huish valley, 1 mile from the picturesque old fishing village of Hope Cove and 3 miles from the famous sailing haunt of Salcombe. The beautiful surrounding area is ideal for walking (National Trust) and the many nearby sandy coves and beaches are perfect for sailing, windsurfing, bathing, diving or fishing. Guests are welcome to look around and take part in farm activity, with supervision when appropriate. The centrally heated accommodation is either en-suite or with private facilities. There are also 2 self-catering cottages 1 sleeping 4 + cot and the other 5+ cot,a few minutes walk from the farm. The Menu consists of traditional farmhouse cooking using as much home produce as possible. Four course dinner with choices across the board for vegetarians and special diets. Childrens teas can be served between 5-5.30pm. Fully Licensed. English Tourist Board 2 Crowns Highly Commended.

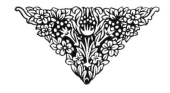

Guest House - **START HOUSE**
Start, Slapton, Kingsbridge, Devon TQ7 2QD
Tel: 01548 580254

Comfortable family house in the hamlet of Start, one mile from Slapton village. It faces south and overlooks a valley running south-east to the sea at Slapton Ley. Large elegant sitting room with open log fire, a conservatory from which with your binoculars you can watch the birds against a background of the valley which extends from a glimpse of the sea and the Ley at one end to a typical Devon farm nestling amongst it's fields at the other. The attractive bedrooms have delightful views. They are all centrally heated and have wash basins, electric shaver points and tea/coffee making facilities, and two have a shower room ensuite. Cots available. Meals are served in the Georgian dining room with it's Adam-type fireplace. Breakfasts are cooked to order. Vegetarians will be provided with their own menu.

USEFUL INFORMATION

OPEN: All year
CHILDREN: Welcome
CREDIT CARDS: No
LICENSED: No but please bring your own

DISABLED ACCESS: No
PETS: Dogs welcome £1 charge if sleeping in the house

Hotel - **THE BEAR HOTEL**

Lydiate Lane, Lynton, North Devon EX35 6AJ

Tel: 01598 753391

This hotel which won the Sanatogen Vegetarian Award in 1995 for 'Best in the West', is a delightful Georgian building found in England's own 'little Switzerland' - a truly beautiful area. To be found in the old village of Lynton off the main road, it is able to combine the spirit of the early 19th century - in which it has it's origins - with all the comforts of modern day. Historically it is one of the oldest, original lodging houses in all of Lynton, it's renovations and exquisite decor have created a unique, gracious and warmly welcoming hotel. A log fire is always lit on chilly days.

All rooms have private en-suite facilities and all are centrally heated, with colour television and beverage making facilities - and each has it's own resident teddy bear. The elegant dining room features imaginative and tempting menus. The evening meal is a candle lit dinner of four courses, complemented by a varied wine list. Breakfast is the full English traditional, vegetarian or continental should you prefer. The Bear Hotel prides it'self on it's flexibility and will always prepare special diets and interesting menus to suit vegetarian guests. The hotel has been awarded an RAC Highly Acclaimed, ETB 3 Crowns Commended and the AA QQQQ Selected Award for high standards of comfort, hospitality and cooking.

USEFUL INFORMATION

OPEN; All year
CREDIT CARDS; None taken
DISABLED ACCESS; No
Bargain breaks available

ON THE MENU; Freshly prepared
Produce. Vegetarian and Vegan
options always available

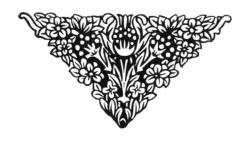

Farmhouse - **ENNYS**

St Hilary, Penzance, Cornwall TR20 9BZ

Tel/Fax: 01736 740262

Ennys is a beautiful 17th Century Cornish manor situated at the end of a long tree-lined drive with sheltered gardens which guests are welcome to use. The emphasis here is on an idyllically peaceful holiday within easy reach of all the popular holiday haunts of the Penwith peninsula. This small working farm has fields that stretch to the River Hayle, along which there are many lovely walks and picnic sites. Many guests have returned year after year to enjoy what Ennys has to offer. The food is especially good cooked in an imaginative way to a very high standard, and makes use of the many fresh herbs and organically grown vegetables from it's own kitchen garden. Home-made bread is baked daily. Dinner, preceded by a glass of sherry in the cosy sitting room, is served by candlelight on separate tables and guests are very welcome to bring their own wine. On warm mornings, guests may breakfast on the patio overlooking the walled garden if they so wish. There are three, large, stylish bedrooms, two with four-posters and all en-suite, and in a converted barn two family suites. Altogether delightful. Vegetarians are given particular attention. Open all the year, there are excellent value Winter Breaks. Luxury self-catering for two in the Well Studio.

USEFUL INFORMATION

OPEN; All the year

CHILDREN; Welcome
CREDIT CARDS; All major cards
LICENSED; No
ACCOMMODATION; 5 ensuite
PETS; By arrangement
No smoking in bedrooms and bathrooms

DINING ROOM;
Delicious,imaginative
Traditional fare. Organic herbs
& vegetables
VEGETARIAN;Choice across the board
DISABLED ACCESS; No
GARDEN; Sheltered gardens.Patio

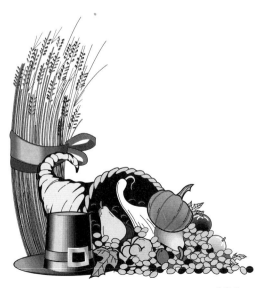

Restaurant - **PLYMOUTH ARTS CENTRE**

38, Looe Street, Plymouth, Devon PL4 OEB

Tel: 01752 660060

The Plymouth Arts Centre has so much to offer including films that are either not shown in the main cinemas or ones that you have missed the first time around. There are exhibitions of all kinds, workshops, music, poetry and that boon, a Vegetarian Restaurant. Here in the Arts Centre you can combine a meal and a cinema ticket, enjoy a two course meal or coffee in the restaurant followed by an evening enjoying a film. The combined ticket not only gives you a first class evening out but also saves you money! Children's portions are available. Special nights are occasions to remember, for example it might be Flavours from the Middle East, Food from Gambia, or simply Festive Fayre. Whatever the destination the Vegetarian food, music and entertainment will be authentic.

The building dates back to Elizabethan times when it was reputed to be the largest coaching house in England, and has a splendid atmosphere. The Restaurant is surrounded by galleries, the cinema and studios and has a special ambience of it's own. It is a peaceful place with no music to disturb one, is partly non-smoking, seats 55 and is self-service. You will find all the food very acceptable and inexpensive. The most expensive dish is a Mushroom Biriani, Dhal and Yoghurt Sauce at less than £3.50. There is a very good Spinach and Courgette Filo Pie, a Spicy Vegetable Crumble, a selection of Quiches and many more good things. Bread rolls and some ice cream from Salcombe Dairies are the only ready-made food bought in. The restaurant is licensed and has a small number of wines plus canned lagers, beers and ciders and a variety of country wines.

USEFUL INFORMATION

OPEN; Mon-Sat 12-2pm. Lunch
Evening Tues-Sun: 5-8pm.
Tues-Sat: 10-8pm. Mon 10-3pm.
Closed Bank Holidays
CREDIT CARDS; None taken
LICENSED; Yes. Restaurant
GARDEN; No

ON THE MENU; Entirely Vegetarian
Light refreshments
CHILDREN; Welcome
DISABLED ACCESS; No.
The old building is not suitable for
wheelchairs. There are toilets
for the not so active.

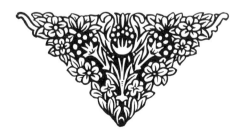

Country Guest House - **SEAPOINT**
Upway, Porlock, Somerset TA24 8QE
Tel: 01643 862289

This Edwardian country guest house situated on the fringe of the pretty village of Porlock with it's narrow, winding streets and thatched cottages, is a truly delightful place in which to stay. The views across the bay to the distant coast of Wales are spectacular and the house is surrounded by the beautiful wooded hills of Exmoor. Porlock offers much to the visitor and Seapoint, in the capable and friendly hands of Christine and Stephen Fitzgerald provides comfort, warmth, and excellent vegetarian, vegan or traditional meals. The atmosphere is relaxed and unfussy and in chilly weather the already warm welcome is enchanced by the pleasure of an open log fire. The tastefully furnished bedrooms are all ensuite and equipped with colour television together with tea, coffee and herbal tea making facilities.

The reputation for good food has been richly deserved. There is a wide choice of starters available for breakfast followed by a selection of cooked main courses including Seapoint's renowned Vegetarian breakfast. To round off breakfast there is a range of coffees, teas and herbal teas together with a selection of delicious home-made marmalade or locally produced honey. All the evening meals are home-made using wholefood ingredients. There is also an interesting selection of wines.

The Fitzgerald's specialise in walking holidays on Exmoor - either moorland or coastal routes and can arrange daily rambles from Seapoint. Simply choose your walk and you will be supplied with maps amd walking instructions at no extra charge. Weekend Breaks offer a two day walking weekend at Seapoint rounded off by a high tea on Sunday afternoon prior to your departure. Exmoor is wonderful at anytime of the year and so too is the hospitality at Seapoint.

USEFUL INFORMATION

OPEN; All year
CHILDREN; Welcome
PETS; No

ON THE MENU; Excellent vegetarian
DISABLED ACCESS; No special facilities
ACCOMMODATION; En suite rooms

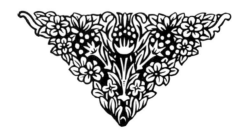

Hotel - **LYDGATE HOUSE HOTEL**

Postbridge,Devon PL20 6TJ

Tel: 01822 880209 Fax: 01822 880202

Looking at the charm of Lydgate House Hotel it is hard to imagine that in the middle of the 17th century it was a squatters' cottage. The main part of the house was built in 1895 as a farmhouse; recently a conservatory has been added and is used as the dining room.

Set in it's own 36 acres with the East Dart River running through, the location is very peaceful. Staying here is much like being part of an informal well-managed house-party. All rooms have their own bathrooms and are furnished in keeping with the house. There is an imaginative but not elaborate menu which has Mediterranean and Eastern influences. All meat comes from a local farm co-operative and has been naturally reared. Local and home-grown organically produced vegetables are used whenever possible. The menu changes daily and there is a vegetarian dish at every course. Vegans and other diets can be catered for with prior notice. Lydgate House is licensed.

USEFUL INFORMATION

OPEN; Dinner is served at 7.30pm
Cream teas served Apr-Oct. 3pm-5.30pm
Closed 3rd Jan-3rd March
CREDIT CARDS;
Amex, Visa, Euro

ON THE MENU; Traditional and vegetarian choice from the small menu. Reservations for non-residents is required
DISABLED ACCESS; Yes, but no special toilet facilities.

Inn - **THE PLUME OF FEATHERS**

The Square, Princetown, Devon PL20 6QG

Tel: 01822 890240

Situated in the moorland village of Princetown, Dartmoor's main village, and also the site of the world renowned Dartmoor Prison. Completed in 1809, it was originally built to house the French and American prisoners of war. The Plume of Feathers started it's life before that in 1785. It is warm, friendly, has copper bars, log fires, oil lamps and plenty of atmosphere. Owned and run by James Langton this is a pub beloved by people who come from quite a distance to join the fun and hospitality. With live music on Sunday lunchtime and something happening all the time, it attracts all age groups throughout the week and the standard is excellent. There are bar snacks of all kinds. You can stay in the Inn in comfortable rooms, pitch your tent or park your caravanette in the space behind the pub which has a toilet block and free showers. The 'Alpine Bunkhouse' provides 42 comfortable beds arranged in dormitories of 10, 4 or 2 bunks, with showers, hot and cold, toilets, excellent facilities and a day room. The Plume serves breakfast for those on the camp site or in the bunkhouses. Good value, good fun, The Plume is there to be enjoyed.

USEFUL INFORMATION

OPEN; Mon-Sat 11-11pm Sun:12-3pm & 5-10pm
CHILDREN; Families room & menu
CREDIT CARDS; Visa/Master/Switch
LICENSED; Full Licence. Real Ale
ACCOMMODATION; Yes + bunkhouse & campsite

RESTAURANT;Large selection Inn food
BAR FOOD; Wide variety
VEGETARIAN;Special menu
DISABLED ACCESS; Ramps & toilets

Farm Guest House - **MOUNT PLEASANT FARM**

Gorran High Lanes, St Austell, Cornwall PL26 6lR

Tel: 01726 843918

Jill and Nick Bayly, the Vegetarian Proprietors of Mount Pleasant Farm do not keep animals on their Small Holding but it is nonetheless a farm on which bees thrive and vegetables are grown organically. The aim is to be environmentally friendly. Organic food and free range eggs are used wherever possible. Mount Pleasant was originally built as a farm in the 17th century. It is a supremely quiet and peaceful location situated in typical rural Cornish countryside, enjoying fine views over traditional stone walled fields with woodlands and the sea beyond. The spectacular cliffs and coastline of South Cornwall are only one mile away featuring some of the finest beaches in Cornwall including Porthluney Cove with it's fairly wide sandy beach, a mile away, Vault Beach, secluded but a bit of a climb, three miles and Gorran Haven, a small sandy beach approached directly from the village, just 2 miles distant.

Mount Pleasant is a relaxed and friendly house ideal for families - one bedroom on the first floor has a double bed, two single beds and a cot is available if required. Each of the three bedrooms is comfortably furnished and has a TV and a beverage tray. The rooms are not ensuite but that does not pose a problem as the bathroom facilities are adequate. The house is centrally heated and there is a separate guest lounge with an open log fire. Vegetarian and vegan food is a speciality and other special diets are catered for with prior notice. A full range of herb teas and other alternative beverages are also on offer.

USEFUL INFORMATION

OPEN; All year

CHILDREN; Welcome

CREDIT CARDS; None taken

LICENSED; No. Welcome to bring your own. Free corkage

ON THE MENU; Good organic food wherever possible. Evening meals 24 hour notice

DISABLED ACCESS; No

GARDEN; Yes. Small Holding

ACCOMMODATION; 3 rooms not en-suite

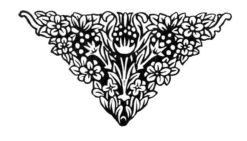

Hotel - **THE BELYARS CROFT HOTEL**

The Belyars, St Ives, Cornwall TR26 2BZ

Tel: 01736 796304

Owned by Rita and Trevor Coop for the last twenty years, The Belyars Croft Hotel reflects their personalities and offers an abundant welcome in a relaxed, informal and convivial atmosphere. Your wishes are of paramount importance and whether you are a vegetarian or not, the menus are designed to tempt your tastebuds. Every ensuite bedroom has been furnished with an eye to comfort and includes both a beverage tray and colour television. There is a spacious and well appointed lounge bar serving a wide selection of both alcoholic and non-alcoholic drinks - a favourite place in the evenings to chat over the day with newly made friends.

The hotel is located in one of the loveliest gardens in the area, and has a commanding position overlooking St Ives Bay and the safe, sandy beach of Porthminster. Less than five minutes away from the Town centre it is equally accessible to the solitude and grandeur of cliff walks or the many sporting recreations available. Ample free car parking is available at the hotel.

USEFUL INFORMATION

OPEN; Easter to October
CHILDREN; Welcome
CREDIT CARDS; None taken
LICENSED; For residents
ACCOMMODATION; All en suite rooms
PETS; By arrangement only

DINING ROOM; Caters for all tastes and diets especially vegetarians.
DISABLED ACCESS; Yes
GARDEN; One of the loveliest in St Ives. Ample free car parking

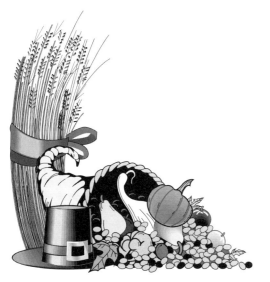

Bed and Breakfast Hotel - **THE OLD FORGE AT TOTNES**
Seymour Place, Totnes, Devon TQ9 5AY
Tel: 01803 862174

Just out of the centre of Totnes, one of the most delightful Tudor towns in England, is the Old Forge, owned and run by Jeannie Allnutt. This fine stone building was converted from a 600 year old forge, wheelwright's workshop, coach houses and stables, which served Berry Pomeroy Castle and it's estate in the old days. The buildings have been lovingly restored since 1985 by Jeannie and her late husband to provide what is now reputed to be the best accommodation in the Totnes area. Open all year, this small hotel provides great comfort with a warm welcome for travellers, holiday visitors and business people. There are 10 pretty colour-themed ensuite bedrooms, two of these and a 'cottage suite' being on the ground floor - ideal for the elderly, partially disabled or young families with children. Each guest room has numerous extras to make it a home-from-home.

Breakfast is served in the Tudor-style dining room, with an extensive choice menu - vegetarian and special diets well catered for. Cream teas and daytime snacks are available in season. No evening meals but excellent inns and restaurants in Totnes (and nearby villages) are in plentiful supply. A coach arch through the building gives access to a delightful walled garden. The Old Forge is an environmentally friendly zone where everything - especially the garden - has been created to be as aesthetically pleasing as possible, and where the owner is very conscientious about recycling and other green issues - but without compromising the very high standards. The latest addition for your comfort is a delightful conservatory -style leisure lounge with the luxury of a whirlpool spa (jacuzzi) for guest use.

USEFUL INFORMATION

OPEN; All year
CHILDREN; Welcome
CREDIT CARDS; Visa/Master/Euro
PETS; In cars only
GARDEN; Delightful
NO SMOKING INDOORS

ON THE MENU; Excellent breakfast
extensive choice. Cream teas &
daytime snacks in season
DISABLED ACCESS; Partially disabled
and elderly

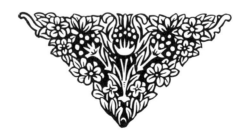

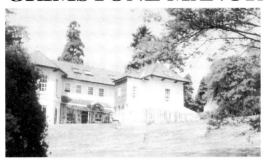

MIDDLE RYLANDS

Redmoor, Nr. Bodmin, Cornwall PL30 5AR Tel/Fax: 01208 872316

Charming Cornish Cottage with duck pond in quiet rural location. Central all coasts, moors, nature reserves. TV and Kettle in rooms. No smoking in cottage. VG. PETS ESR CP Cooked vegan breakfast.

TREGATHERALL FARM

Boscastle PL35 0EQ Tel: 01840 250277.

Working farm offering a great welcome. On the North Cornwall Coast 16 miles from Bodmin and Launceston. 3 miles from the main A30 Atlantic Highway. Panoramic views. On Brown Circular Ramblers Route and 12 miles from Camel Trail for Cyclists. Attractive house with pretty garden complete with furniture. Comfortable accommodation and excellent food. Uses own Spring Water. Open all year. Children very welcome. Pets welcome. No Credit cards. No disabled access.

TREHANE FARM

Trevalga, Boscastle PL35 0EB Tel: 01840 250510

A family dairy farm set in a magnificent position with extensive views over the Atlantic and rugged coastline, close to the coastal path and many unspoilt beaches and coves. Peaceful and secluded, you will find Trehane relaxed and welcoming with comfortable accommodation and plenty of wholesome, nourishing food, home-made bread and exciting vegetarian concoctions. Three pretty bedrooms overlook the sea. Individual spinning lessons are available. Cream of Cornwall member. OPEN; All year including Christmas. Packed lunches available. Walks from selected points and collection arranged. 17 miles from Bodmin and Launceston. Children welcome.

WOODCOTE HOTEL

The Saltings, Lelant, Cornwall TR26 3DL Tel: 01736 753147

Established in the early 1920's Woodcote is the oldest vegetarian hotel in the United Kingdom. Family run, in a beautiful setting overlooking the tidal estuary and bird sanctuary of Hayle. A great base for a holiday, the atmosphere is relaxed and informal. All rooms are comfortable. Bedrooms have hot and cold water, central heating, shaver points and complimentary tea making facilities. Additionally some rooms have ensuite shower/WC, plus colour television. Not licensed - welcome to bring your own. Open all year. Children welcome.

THE TREMARNE HOTEL Polkirt

Mevagissey, PL26 6UY   Tel: 01726 842213 Fax: 01726 843420

This charming, peaceful hotel on the outskirts of the picturesque coastal village of Mevagissey offers superb accommodation, imaginative cuisine and everything that a visitor to the heart of Cornwall could require. Surrounded by beaches, fascinating countryside redolent of the history of the county, The Tremarne is an ideal base for anyone wanting a wonderful holiday or a short relaxing break. Open all year. Credit Cards taken. Children welcome. Traditional & Vegetarian food. B&B £24.50-£29.50. 4 course dinner £14.50.

THE PORTAFINO HOTEL

Penhallow road, Porth, Newquay, Cornwall TR7 3BY   Tel: 01637 875589

When you pull up outside the Portafino, just look back for a minute. You are a seagull's cry off Porth's sandy beach and Porth Island. This small 10 bedroom hotel is beautifully run. You will be extremely well cared for and you will eat well for sure. Guests from all over Europe praise the high standard and the good value of the food. If you are wanting peace this is ideal. No very young children, a Beauty Therapist on the premises. Comfortable Lounge Bar. Log fires in winter. Full central heating. Mostly ensuite bedrooms. No pets. Credit Cards accepted. Short breaks. Open all year.

THE CAFE, Island Square, St Ives, Cornwall. Tel: 01736 793621.

A charming Vegetarian Restaurant, now in it's seventh year, where the Chef/Patron, Carol Gibbs, delights not only vegetarians but others who find her interesting and varied vegetarian menu delicious. The menu changes daily but try the Mushroom Stroganoff if you get the opportunity - it is exceptionally good. Licensed with a small but select wine list. You will find the Cafe in a quiet location adjacent to the Tate Gallery. OPEN; All year. Children welcome. No Credit Cards. Disabled access but no special facilities. Licensed.

BOSWEDNACK MANOR

Zennor, St Ives, Cornwall TR26 3DD   Tel: 01736 794183

Peaceful guesthouse in wildest Cornwall overlooking the sea and moors. Organic garden. Meditation room. Guided wildlife walks, birdwatching and wildflower weeks. Bed and Breakfast, Vegetarian evening meals. No smoking throughout. Self catering cottage also available.

MAKING WAVES

3 Richmond Place, St Ives, Cornwall TR26 1JN Tel: 01736 793895

Vegan guest House in a beautiful Victorian building in a quiet cul de sac overlooking sub-tropical gardens and St Ives Bay. 2 minutes walk from the town centre, 5 minutes from beaches, Tate Gallery and coast path. The delicious home-made food is 100% animal free, with emphasis on health and nutrition. Organic products are used extensively, including locally grown fruit and vegetables. Making Waves caters for special diets, including gluten free, sugar free etc. Children, hikers & cyclists most welcome. Whether you are coming to relax, recuperate, adventure or let your hair down, you will enjoy this friendly and comfortable household. Call Simon or Sue for more Information.

TREGERAINT HOUSE, Zennor, St Ives, Tel/Fax: 01736 797061.

Comfortable and friendly guest house in the picturesque village of Zennor. Offering a relaxed holiday excellent food and comfortable beds.

CUDDYFORD VEGETARIAN BED AND BREAKFAST

Rew Road, Ashburton TQ13 7EN Tel: 01364 653325

To reach Cuddyford go through the main street until you reach the Golden Lion. Opposite the hotel you will find Roborough Lane. After half a mile turn left at crossroads into Rew Road. Cuddyford is the fourth house on the right. The house stands in a rural setting within Dartmoor National Park and is ideally situated for exploring the moor, Dart Valley, and South Devon coastline. Wholesome cookery: home-baked bread, free range eggs, honey from their own hives and organically grown fruit and vegetables. Special diets catered for. Children welcome. Open all year except Christmas.

THE MOUNT HOTEL

Northdown Road, Bideford, Devon EX39 3LP Tel: 01237 473748.

The English Tourist Board has awarded The Mount Hotel 3 Crowns and the AA QQQ and you can see why. It is a warm and welcoming Georgian house, set in peaceful surroundings. The owners take great pride in their home cooked dishes. Children are welcome, by arrangement. Smoking is allowed only in the Bar. Sorry but pets are not allowed. The Mount is close to the historic town centre of Bideford, with it's Quay and medieval Long Bridge. It is ideally suited for touring North Devon and Tarka Country (made famous by the author Henry Williamson in his book 'Tarka the Otter'). Why not take a cruise to the remote, romantic and inspiring Lundy Island. Keep fit and healthy by cycling or walking the Tarka Trail. With it's mixture of sandy beaches, secluded coves, rugged cliffs, moorland and tranquil wooded river valleys, North Devon is a great place in which to relax and unwind.

THE GNOME RESERVE

Wild Flower Garden and Pixie Kiln.

West Putford, Nr. Bradworthy. North Devon EX22 7XE

Tel/Fax: 01409 241435.

Do you like magic and enchanted woodland, herb gardens and wild flower meadows? Yes? Good, then let the 1000 gnomes weave their elfin spell and take you into wonderland - regardless of whether you are a child, an adult or a re-cycled teenager. They promise to return you to normal before you leave. However some people are unable to stop laughing!!! OPEN; 21st March-31st October 10.00am-6.00pm. 7 Days a week. (1st November-20th March 10.00am-4.00pm Shop only.)

DODBROOKE FARM

Michelcombe, Holne, Devon TQ13 7SP Tel:01364 631461.

A delightful home offering Vegetarians and others comfortable and friendly accommodation. Dodbrooke Farm is a 17th century former long house in an idyllic valley at the edge of Dartmoor. Food is home-produced from the farm and kitchen garden and the rooms are warm and comfortable.

Complete with it's own filtered moorland spring water, Dodbrooke Farm has a cobbled yard, old stone barns, a beautiful cottage garden, woods, meadows and streams beyond. Holne Gorge is magnificent. The sea is 3/4 hour drive away and there is easy access to the sights of the South Hams and Torbay.

OPEN; All year except Christmas. 5 miles from Ashburton and the A38. Children welcome. Evening meal available.

MILL LEAT FARM, Holne, Ashburton TQ13 7RZ Tel: 01364 631283

A traditionally run family farm set into the foothills of Dartmoor, comprising of 120 acres of unspoilt farmland. It is a country lovers haven with the open moorland just five minutes drive away. Buckfast Abbey is only two and a half miles, horse riding, carriage driving, fishing and other sporting activities are all available within the locality. The 18th century farmhouse supplies comfortable accommodation with plenty of good wholesome home-cooking on the menu - ideal for vegetarians and special diets can be catered for if known in advance. Some bedrooms are ensuite. Evening meals available and served at a time to suit you. Children welcome. OPEN; All year except Christmas

SOUTH WORDEN FARM

Bradworthy, Holsworthy EX22 7TW Tel: 01409 241827

South Worden is a delightful oasis in which to stay for coast and country walking in North Devon. Conservation policies can be seen in practice. The wool from the sheep is uncontaminated by harmful chemicals and is used for hand spinning and the production of garments. The food presented is as far as possible home produced with a number of dishes specifically for vegetarians. NO SMOKING. Open all year. Children welcome. Bed and Breakfast and Evening Meal £44 for 2 nights.

VENN FARM

Ugborough, Ivybridge PL21 0PE Tel: 01364 73240. Friendly home-from-home

SLADE BARN & NETTON FARM HOLIDAY COTTAGES

Noss Mayo, Nr. Plymouth, Devon PL8 1HA Tel: 01752 872235.

Tucked away in a corner of Devon unspoilt by time, B & B or S.C. complimented by an indoor swimming pool, private gardens, tennis court, games room, and professional Reflexology by appointment, if so desired. Superb walks, sandy beaches, many local attractions and picturesque local villages. Alternatively, Dartmoor is only half an hour away. This is a relaxing holiday - where you can still enjoy all that is best of the simple quality of life. Sandy Cherrington will be pleased to hear from you.

TRELUSWELL HOUSE
Treluswell, Penryn, Cornwall 01326 375053

TRILLIUM HOUSE HOTEL
4 Alfred Street, The Hoe, Plymouth Tel:01752 670452
Family owned Hotel with a homely, friendly atmosphere close to the City Centre, Seafront, historic Hoe and Barbican. Situated in a quiet area. Imaginative home-cooked food to your requirements with vegan and vegetarian options. Reservation for car park required. En suite rooms. TV/radio/alarm clock. Hospitality tray. Residents lounge. Licenced. Children welcome. Credit Cards accepted. Sorry no pets.

GEORGIAN TEAROOM AND RESTAURANT
Broadway House, 35 High Street,
Topsham, Devon EX3 0ED Tel: 01392 873465.
The elegant pre-Georgian High Street is full of beautiful buildings and none more so than Broadway House. Built by a Dutch merchant for three thousand pounds in 1777, it is now a delightful Tea Room and Restaurant. Heather and Gerald Knee are the owners, and it is Heather who cooks the delicious food with a menu that concentrates on freshness. All fresh vegetables are used and Vegetarians can count on a choice of meals daily as well as the excellent home-made cakes and jams. The 'Heartbeat Award', an achievement awarded by the local Environmental Health Authority has been given to the Tea Rooms several years running. OPEN; 7 days a week 9.30-5pm. Children welcome. Disabled access from side entrance.

WILD ROSE.
Cornwall Women's Holidays.
Small group special interest holidays eg. Walking, Singing, Drumming, Writing.
Ring 01752 822609 for Brochure.

PEEK HILL FARM
Dousland, Yelverton, Devon PL20 6PD Tel: 01822 852908
Built in the late 19th century, replacing a 16th century longhouse, this is a typical working Dartmoor hill farm. The ensuite bedrooms offer a good standard of comfort with spacious family and double rooms providing outstanding views of Cornwall. Good traditional farmhouse or vegetarian breakfast. Ideal base for touring South West.

MEREFIELD HOUSE
East Street, Crewkerne TA18 7AB Tel:01460 73112
Spacious Grade II listed house in historic town, serving imaginative vegetarian cuisine with seasonal home grown produce. Walled gardens, large lounge with books and videos. Open all year. No Children. No Disabled accommodation. Not Licensed. No smoking in Public rooms.

HERBIES
15 North Street, Exeter EX4 3QS Tel: 01392 58473
Restaurant. V/VG. LIC. Children welcome. Wheelchair access but not to toilet. No smoking area

EXMOOR LODGE

Chapel Street, Exford TA24 7PY Tel:01643 831694

In the heart of Exmoor National Park, overlooking Exford village green. Exmoor Lodge operates on cruelty free principles, along with healthy food. '95 Heartbeat award for healthy food. Exclusively V/VG/NS ESR/ 1 ground floor room. No credit cards.

Chapter Two

Southern England

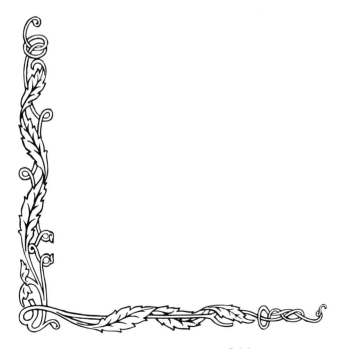

Chapter 2

SOUTHERN ENGLAND

Dorset, Wiltshire, Hampshire & Sussex

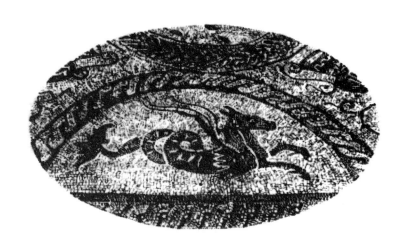

INCLUDES

SOUTHERN ENGLAND
Dorset, Wiltshire, Hampshire & Sussex

Southern England covers many counties and each has it's own characteristics and charm. If you asked me to name my favourite I would be hard put to choose and in fact I find that wherever I happen to be at the time means the most to me. My journey through these counties must be fleeting and you will have to forgive me if I leave out some of your favourite places. Each county would make a book in it'self.

The whole of the region is crammed with history, from the abundant fossils on the Dorset coastline, to the hundreds of stone circles and monuments of early man. The Bronze Age settlements and Iron Age forts, and later sites of events so momentous that they have marked the course of history it'self.

Dorset has that lovely sleepy feeling about it. It is both comforting and timeless with it's smoothly-rounded hills and convexities which have a passive and ancient solidity that soothes and reassures. 'Here I stand and here I be' might well be the motto of a landscape that has sustained Man since his earliest days, from the cliffs, coves and shingle of the coast, the whin-clad heaths, the hills and dales and woodlands of the hinterland. The configuration is so attractive and so varied that it might almost be taken as an epitome of the scenery of Southern England.

It is an intensely rural county, averaging rather more than one acre per inhabitant and is not disturbed by motorways or major road works. There is only one major conurbation, that of **Poole** and **Bournemouth** with the remainder of the population residing mainly in the numerous small market towns and countless villages and hamlets whose names have a resounding ring out of all proportion to their size and present day standing: Rime Intrinsica, Melbury Osmond, Toller Porcorum, Chaldon Herring and Tarrant Gunville. The names, the people and the scenery have inspired writers and artists over the centuries.

In common with many other such rural areas, early settlements seem to have proliferated along the banks of streams and rivers, hence the numerous Winterbournes, Piddles, Puddles, Tarrants, Cernes, Chars and Weys. The great expanse of enclosed water that is Poole Harbour provided the county's earliest sheltered part, and one that remains of great economic importance to this day.

My journey this time started in the extreme south-west in the delightful little town of **Lyme Regis** close to the boundary with Devonshire. Once an important harbour and protected from prevailing south-westerly winds by the massive breakwater known as the Cobb, Lyme Regis was granted it's royal status by Edward I in 1284 during his wars against the French.

The town is enchanting, set on the shore surrounded by a backcloth of high steep hills and with houses and shops set around narrow winding streets. It is a deservedly popular seaside resort, a role that replaced smuggling as a local, and profitable, pastime in the late 18th century. Jane Austen gives a vivid portrayal of the town in her novel 'Persuasion' written in 1815:

'..as there is nothing to admire in the buildings themselves, the remarkable situation of the town, the principal street almost hurrying into the water, the wall to the Cobb, skirting round the pleasant little bay, which in the season is animated with bathing machines and company, the Cobb it'self, it's old wonders and new improvements, with the very beautiful line of cliffs stretching out to the east of the town, are what the stranger's eye will seek; and a very strange stranger it must be, who does not see charms in the immediate environs of Lyme, to make him wish to know it better.'

I disagree with the eminent novelist's opinion of the local architecture, but wholeheartedly endorse the rest.

The wide main road through the village of **Charmouth** was first laid by the Romans on the foundations of an ancient pack-horse trail and after their departure it was favoured by the Saxons. The ancient highway became of increasing importance, linking the county towns of Exeter and Dorchester and the handsome Georgian and Regency buildings bear witness both to the popularity of the village as a coaching stop, and to the attractions of the area as a resort. Some of this history can be seen reflected in the displays at the **Charmouth Heritage Coast Centre**, together with exhibitions of fossils, geology and wildlife.

The lovely coast and inland scenery, combined with these small seaside communities, offers the holidaymaker a glimpse of more certain and simple pleasures and it is hardly surprising that families return year after year. Neighbouring **Chideock** has much the same atmosphere, albeit on a small scale; the houses here also line the hillside but the thatched cottage, rather than the grander Georgian and Victorian buildings of Charmouth, predominates. The happily named Duck Street leads to the tiny sea-side hamlet of **Seatown**, where the small River Winniford flows into the sea. The little beach is dominated by the highest cliff of the South Coast, **Golden Cap**, 618 feet above sea level. Now under the stewardship of the National Trust, the gorse clad cliff was the look-out post for an 18th century smuggling gang based in Chideock.

Apart from the obvious enjoyment to be had beside the sea, this western-most area of Dorset has a multitude of attractions inland; historic sites, lovely walks, pretty villages, friendly pubs and stately homes. **Whitchurch Canonicorum**, two miles inland from Charmouth has a link with those Viking raiders of long ago; the 13th century Church of St Candida and the Holy Cross contains the tomb of the saint, also known as St Wita, and who is thought to have been a Saxon woman slain in a raid.

Pilsdon Pen also bears evidence of an earlier culture with Iron Age earthworks to be found on the bare top of the highest hill in Dorset, at 909 feet a landmark for half the county and one that offers the most wonderful views.

Further north, **Thorncombe** clings to a steep hillside close to the border with Devon and Somerset, and between the village and the Somerset town of **Chard,** lie the lovely buildings of **Forde Abbey.** Started at the beginning of the 12th century, the Cistercian monastery was not fully completed for another 300 years. To avoid destruction at the Dissolution, the Abbot handed the Abbey over to the King. It has been a family home since the 17th century when Sir Edmund Prideaux, Attorney General to Cromwell, commissioned Inigo Jones to convert it into a private house. Set beside the River Axe in some 30 acres of beautiful gardens, the house and monastic buildings contain remarkable tapestries and furniture and pictures.

To the east, across the high rolling hills, lies the rambling village of **Broadwindsor**, reputedly the highest in Dorset, and close to the lovely wooded crest of **Lewesdon Hill**. Charles II stayed the night here after his failure to set sail from Charmouth; once again he had a narrow escape as the Parliamentarian soldiers were diverted by the site of one of their own camp-followers giving birth.

The principal market town for the area is **Beaminster**, a pleasant place which has had more than it's share of bad luck, having been virtually destroyed by fire in 1644, 1684 and 1781; nevertheless it is a cheerful place where the little River Brit runs beside the main street with it's handsome 18th century buildings.

Parnham House is world renowned as the home of John Makepeace furniture workshops, where innovative use of wood and the highest standards of woodworking skill reign supreme. The house dates from the Middle Ages, was rebuilt in Tudor times and further altered by the great Regency architect, John Nash. For 500 years it was the home of the Strode family, who are remembered in the church at Beaminster and within the park there is the grave of Lieutenant Rhodes-Moorhouse, the first airman to be awarded the Victoria Cross. The Makepeace family have restored both house and gardens and the result is superb.

Not far away is another house with lovely grounds, **Mapperton House** is perhaps the most beautiful manor house in Dorset and is set beside terraced gardens through which water gently flows. It is serene and timeless; qualities to be found throughout the county, but particularly in this region where the hills seemingly enfold and enclose minute communities guarding themselves against the intrusion of the modern world.

Now that **Bridport** has been by-passed it is much easier to enjoy this nice town with it's very wide and handsome main street where no two buildings are quite alike, and the brick and stone Town Hall, complete with stately cupola, presides over all. To the east **Burton Bradstock**, a pretty village tucked away from the sea by a low ridge, lies close to the beginnings of the extraordinary **Chesil Beach.** One of the great wonders of England's coastline, the Beach is some 15 miles of blue-clay reef covered with an immense coating of shingle, more than 40 feet high in parts. No expert has yet produced a convincing theory as to why the pebbles get progressively smaller the further west along the Beach one goes. Behind Chesil Beach is The Fleet, a brackish and reed-filled lagoon. North-east of Bridport, the narrow roads lead over the hills to **Powerstock**, a delightful village nestling beneath the 800foot high **Eggardon Hill**, where, from the massive earthen ramparts of an Iron Age fort on the top, excellent views are to be had of the surrounding countryside.

Returning southwards towards the fascination of Chesil Beach, the hilly country bounded by the A35 to the north and the Beach to the south has much to offer. **Kingston Russell** was the birthplace of Admiral Sir Thomas Masterman Hardy, Nelson's flag-captain at Trafalgar, and in whose arms Nelson died. A great seaman in his own right and passionately fond of his native county, particularly the village of **Portesham** where he spent much of his early life. The Hardy monument on neighbouring **Blackdown**, should not be confused with any memorial to Dorset's greatest author. The solid chimney like structure was erected to the memory of a great sailor and is still a notable landmark for those ships of the Royal Navy going about their lawful occasions in the Channel waters far below.

The gorse-laden heights overlooking the Beach are studded with reminders of far earlier civilisations; barrows, standing stones and circles mark the last resting places of forgotten tribal chieftains. **Abbotsbury** has a reminder of those pagan times in the survival of the ancient custom, Garland Day, held on May 13th. Thought to be a survival of sea-god worship, two garlands are carried through the village and one cast into the sea.

The village is one of the loveliest in the county, it's narrow streets lined with mellow stone cottages, many of them thatched. Abbotsbury has had but three owners in it's long history. First there was Orc, a steward of King Canute, and it was he and his wife Thola who established the Abbey. After the Dissolution, the village passed from the Church to the Strangways, Earls of Ilchester. The village suffered grievously during the Civil War; cottages were set alight, the Royalist Strangways' mansion was burnt to the ground and the pulpit of the parish church still bears bullet-holes received during a short but bloody battle, described by the Parliamentarian commander as being a 'hot bickering'. A masterful understatement

The Abbotsbury Sub Tropical Gardens have a wonderful display of rare and tender plants laid out around a walled garden with the added protection of a shelter-belt of trees. They were first laid out in 1760 and provide a stunning display of exotic blooms. **The Abbotsbury Swannery** dates back to the days when the monks reared swans for meat. Now the swanherd cares for around 1,000 mute swans, plus innumerable wildfowl, and his concern is that of a naturalist rather than that of an epicure.

Chesil Beach has long had a deserved reputation as a graveyard of ships and, together with the Fleet, as a haven for smugglers. This reputation was enhanced by the classic story of 'Moonfleet', which was written at the turn of the century by Meade Faulkner. It featured Fleet House, of Tudor origin and which is now the splendid **Moonfleet Manor Hotel.**

The eastern end of Chesil Beach runs into the massive rocky outcrop of **Portland**, the **'Gibraltar of Dorset'**, with it's great harbour until recently one of the main bases for the Royal Navy, and narrow isthmus connecting to the ancient town and port of **Weymouth**. A seaport since Roman times, the small harbour is still busy with fishing boats, yachts and cross-channel ferries, . It is also a cheerful seaside resort, with a beautifully protected sandy beach and a fine esplanade, where the variety and irregularity of the buildings make for a view that is both comforting and good looking.

Portland has been a fortress since Roman times but it is perhaps best known for the high quality of the stone that has been quarried there since the 1700's. From this rocky hump, some four miles long and less than two miles wide, came stone for buildings as diverse as St Paul's Cathedral, London University and the United Nations Building.

The southern tip of Portland is known as **The Bill,** and is marked by a lighthouse which warns shipping not only of rocks but also the presence of a dangerous tidal race, where currents of up to seven knots flow.

Economically, Portland's future is questionable. Stone is no longer a principal building material and the naval presence has gone. There are many plans for it's future and one hopes that the final outcome will be a happy and prosperous future for it's friendly people.

Just north of Weymouth, to the west of the road to Dorchester lies the immense Stone Age hill fort of **Maiden Castle**, one of the largest in Europe. Dating back to 2000BC, the earthworks are truly impressive, covering some 47 acres, and stand as a still, silent tribute to the energies of the simple military engineers of long ago. **Dorchester,** the county town is fascinating. It has a colourful and sometimes violent past and it's Roman origins are indicated by the layout of it's main street, the square outlines of the town wall which ran where there are now tree-lined walks, and the remains of a magnificent villa behind County Hall, which reveals some of the original mosaics and the hypocaust, or central heating system. Just south of the town, at **Maumbury Rings**, an ancient 'henge' type monument of the stone circle variety was adapted by the Romans as an amphitheatre; it is a gruesome fact that the public gallows stood here until well into the 18th century. Judge Jeffreys opened his Bloody Assizes here trying those who were involved in the disastrous Monmouth Rebellion in 1685. The victims were involved frequently for no greater crime than being absent from their habitations from and at the time of the Rebellion. Those executed were hung, drawn and quartered, and their butchered bodies exhibited throughout the county as a grim warning.

Nearly 250 years later, the town was the scene of another famous 'trial' when six farm labourers from **Tolpuddle** were sentenced to seven years transportation for attempting to form a trade union.

It has to be said that today's town is far more just and friendly and wears it's status as the county's capital far more lightly than many of it's contemporaries. I feel this is partly to do with the character of Dorset and the fact that Dorchester is not a cathedral city; there is a light-hearted market town atmosphere with little of the dignity of the diocese. There is plenty to do and see including the excellent **Dorset County Museum** in West Street which has a section devoted to Dorset's most famous literary son, Thomas Hardy. Hardy was to Dorset as Wordsworth was to the Lakes, with much of their writing inextricably bound to their place of birth. Wessex was a long forgotten Saxon Kingdom until Hardy revived the title for use in his novel 'Far from the Madding Crowd' and many of the fictitious names in his writings refer to actual places. For instance, Dorchester is 'Casterbridge', Weymouth is 'Budmouth' and Sherborne 'Sherton Abbas'.

Part of the charm of Dorchester is the fact that it is totally surrounded by the lovely rolling countryside. Nearby **Charminster** provides a link with the enterprising Spanish-speaking farmer, Squire Russell, for it was at **Wolferton House** that the future King of Castile stayed after his ship was driven into Weymouth by foul weather.

The modern traveller heads north along the A352, passing through the old and delightful village of **Cerne Abbas**. Lying in a chalk-lined valley and once more of a town than a village, the community's wealth was originally derived from the Benedictine Abbey, first established by the Saxon Ethelmaer, Earl of Cornwall, in 987 AD. The Dissolution brought the usual destruction and the only obvious remains are the handsome gatehouse, guest-house and tithe barns. The lovely 15th century church has a buttressed tower, a later Norman chancel and some early heraldic glass.

Cerne Abbas is probably best known for the enormous pagan figure of a priapic giant carved into the turf on the chalk hillside. His origins are unknown; local legend has a David and Goliath account of a local shepherd boy killing the giant while he slept on the hill, whereupon the villagers immediately rushed up and marked the outline of the massive corpse, some 180feet from head to toe. He may be Neolithic or he may be the god, Hercules, carved by Roman Soldiers; no-one seems quite certain, although there is a strong belief that fertility is assured by spending the night on the giant phallus! Whatever the truth, the giant's outline still lies on the hillside, surrounded for miles around, by the stone pillars and earthen mounds of earlier and more superstitious times. In this rounded and hilly landscape, a turn away from the main road brings the traveller, by way of narrow twisting lanes, to tiny settlements and hamlets and one has the feeling that even in the 20th century, the ancient ways are given more than passing acknowledgment.

Mintern Gardens, at **Minterne Magna**, are a series of beautifully landscaped gardens which utilises lakes, cascades, streams and pools to show off a wonderful array of trees, shrubs and plants. Before reaching Sherborne, the road runs down to what Hardy called 'The Vale of Little Dairies' Blackmoor Vale. In comparison with the chalk downland grazing, this is rich, lush countryside and many dairies still survive, albeit somewhat larger than in Hardy's day.

Who could not be enchanted by **Sherborne** which is rightly claimed as Dorset's loveliest town. It has charm, character, it abounds with fine buildings set beside curving little streets. The learned St Aldhelm founded the Abbey and School in the 8th century, and to our good fortune both have survived to this day, the school being re-founded by Royal Charter after the Dissolution. Sherborne Abbey as seen today dates principally from the 15th century although evidence of it's Saxon and Norman Predecessors clearly remain. The delicate stone fan-vaulting is beautiful and intricate and the local yellow stone from which the building is constructed lends to a feeling of warmth and mellowness to the magnificent interior. The people of Sherborne showed great far sightedness when they bought 'the Abbey, the grounds about it, the lead, the bells and other fittings' for the sum of three hundred pounds. Many of the abbey's old monastic buildings have been incorporated into the school, which rambles around much of the southern half of the town with it's numerous halls, houses and playing fields.

The town and the surroundings are full of the most marvellous treasures and attractions. **Sherborne Museum**, in the old Abbey gatehouse holds items of local interest, including Roman remains, a splendid 15th century wall-painting and a model of the town's original Norman castle. The actual castle was built between 1107 and 1135 by Roger, Bishop of Salisbury, and if the construction of a fortress seems a somewhat un-ecclesiastical act, it should be remembered that Bishops in those days were not 'all gas and gaiters'. Between 871 and 933AD three Bishops of Sherborne fell in battle against the Danes.

The castle passed into the ownership of Sir Walter Raleigh in 1597, but he was not to enjoy ownership for long, being indicted for treason in 1603. Nevertheless, he left his mark; evidently deciding that the massively-built stone castle offered little in the way of home comforts, he therefore initiated the building of a more suitable abode almost immediately adjacent to the grim fortress. Thus Sherborne has not one, but two 'castles'. **Sherborne Old Castle** and later **Sherborne Castle**. The old castle remained as a defensive position until the Civil War, when it was stormed by Parliamentarians under General Fairfax and destroyed. The new castle, originally known as The Lodge, is owned by the Digby family who have been there since Sir John Digby was awarded the estate by James I in recognition for his services as Ambassador to Spain - another Spanish-speaker made good! The Digbys utilised much of the ruins of the old castle to enlarge and enhance the house, and later employed Capability Brown to landscape the area around the two castles. The lake, waterfall and lovely gardens are the result, while the interior of the house is in restrained elegance, with notable collections of furniture and porcelain.

To the west of the town, close to the border with Somerset, lies another lovely home, **Compton House.** This 16th-century building is at the heart of a unique enterprise; for thirty years it has been the home of **Worldwide Butterflies,** where a variety of habitats provide the settings for butterflies and moths from all over the world. In conjunction with this amazing programme of conservation and breeding is **Lullingstone Silk Farm,** which has provided the silk used on many Royal occasions.

Just to the south is the intriguingly-named village of **Purse Caundle.** Amazingly this delightful community was described at the beginning of the century as a 'poor village... where most thatched roofs of the cottages have been replaced by corrugated iron, the churchyard of a ruinous condition...' All is now well, with the lovely 15th-century church possessed of an unusual panelled chancel arch, and the beautiful Elizabethan **Purse Caundle Manor** lying close beside the 'clear stream' that goes on to feed Sherborne lake. The manor has a most attractive garden, a great hall with minstrel's gallery, and an interior well, dug in case of siege!

Continuing eastwards, the road leads on to Shaftesbury, but the unhurried traveller will find it well worth turning off and exploring the area around **Gillingham,** the county's most northerly town. Centuries ago there was a forest around these parts and at the time of Elizabeth I, it was recorded as being 'Her Majesty's Park and Forest of Gillingham', and Sir Walter Raleigh once held the honorary post of Forest Ranger.

South east of Gillingham, the land rises steeply to a 700foot plateau where stands the Saxon town of **Shaftesbury.** It is claimed that this ancient town contains more history in one square mile than any other settlement in ancient Wessex; a claim the visitor can well believe. For all that, it is far from being a fusty old museum of a town, being bright, lively and cheerful. Today, as it has ever been, it is an important market centre and has expanded to take advantage of it's position and the talents of it's population. Nevertheless, from both the physical and historical viewpoint it is extremely attractive and, in places like the steep cobbled Gold Hill with it's wonderful views and varied architecture, quite enchanting. It has to be said though that particular view is oddly familiar to many since it is a favourite with art directors and has been used in television drama as well as numerous advertising campaigns.

The handsome Georgian appearance of **Blandford** owes everything to a great fire and two Bastards; the town was almost completely destroyed in 1731 and restored by two talented architects with that unfortunate name. **Stourpaine** nestles at the foot of the great chalk hills, guarding what was once an important crossing of the River Stour. The country lanes meander to the south-west, climbing along the side of the steep chalk downs. Tucked into the lee, small villages and hamlets huddle against the hillside, which rises to it's peak at **Bulbarrow Hill,** at 902 feet, the second highest in Dorset. It is alleged that both the Bristol Channel and the Isle of Wight are visible from this point.

Some three miles to the south-east, along a large tree-clad ridge, the road runs down into a steep narrow combe containing what must be the most unique village in Dorset, **Milton Abbas.**

Essentially it is little more than a grass-lined street flanked on either side by twenty identical thatched cottages. There is a lake, a school and a pub, **The Hambro Arms**. The story behind this extraordinarily neat litle community begins with the founding of the Abbey in 932AD by King Athelstan. Later it became a Benedictine Monastery and was surrounded by a small market town that contained a famous brewery, a grammar school and numerous pubs. This was the state of affairs until 1786 when one, Joseph Damer, acquired the Abbey and it's estates from the descendants of Henry VIII's lawyer who was awarded the Abbey (for a small consideration) at the time of the Dissolution for his servces in securing the said Monarch's divorce from Catherine of Aragon. Damer, afterwards Earl of Dorchester, proposed to build a great house on the site and objected to the rowdy presence of the small town. His solution was to buy up the entire town, lock, stock and barrel . This he accomplished over a period of twenty years demolishing each property as it fell vacant. Those who wished to stay in his employ were removed to the new village, built to a plan by the ever industrious Capability Brown. The house that Lord Dorchester built from the monastic buildings is now a school, but the Abbey Church remains and is a superb Gothic building dating from the 12th and 14th centuries.

The adjacent villages such as **Melcombe Bingham**, are every bit as attractive but rather more conventional; the 'toy town' effect of Milton Abbas takes a little time to get used to, but there is no denying it's charm and fascination.

The River Piddle lends it's name to the villages east of Dorchester known collectively as the Piddles and Puddles. **Tolpuddle** is celebrated for it's association with the ill-treated farm workers of 1831. Public outcry forced the Government to pardon six men, but it took time for the message to reach Australia and one of the Martyrs only found out by sheer luck; four years later on a remote sheep station, he read of his pardon in an old and discarded newspaper!

Piddlehinton has a good Perpendicular church and two fine houses in **Glebe Court** and **Marston Manor**, while **Piddletrenthide's** church is of Norman origin with the village school sporting gates that once graced Westminster Abbey; the gift of a local man who became a famous London jeweller. **Puddletown** has a superb medieval church with box pews, a musician's gallery and tombs and memorials of the Martyn family.

Bovington Heath has been the site of an army camp since the First World War, and the **Tank Museum** must be the most complete collection of armoured fighting vehicles in existence, containing over 260 such vehicles from 23 countries. The narrow chalk ridge that divides the sea from heath has many notable beauty spots, the best known being the nearly circular **Lulworth Cove**. The coastline here has been carved into fantastic shapes by the ceaseless motion of the sea, and just to the west, a great natural arch of limestone projects out into the water at **Durdle Door.**

Corfe Castle was begun in the 1080's and expanded over the centuries. King John made much of the place, which is understandable given his undoubted unpopularity, any large, remote and easily defended castle must have been immensely appealing. He kept his crown, his ill-gotten treasure and his unfortunate prisoners at **Corfe**, few of whom were ever seen again.

The great white cliffs of **Durlston** guard the attractive little resort of **Swanage**, once the principal port for the shipping of Purbeck stone and marble. The sandy beach and sheltered waters of the

Bay and that of neighbouring **Studland** make the area ideal for family holidays. Swanage is justly popular and the town is attractive and welcoming; apart from water-sports of every variety and the obvious attractions of the area, there is a fine parish church, built in the 13th century and sited next to the Millpond, the steam engines of **The Swanage Railway**, the **Tithe Barn Museum** and numerous pubs, hotels and restaurants.

The northern side of **Purbeck** is bounded by the huge natural expanse of **Poole Harbour**, whose perimeter, laid in a straight line , would stretch for some 95 miles.! The oldest community on the shores of this great lake-like harbour is **Wareham**, at the western end. The town suffered a terminal decline due to the silting up of the River Frome, attacks by pirates, plague and a succession of fires, the worst destroying over 140 buildings in 1762. The town fared no better in the Monmouth Rebellion with some of the citizens being brutally despatched by the dreadful Judge Jeffreys. It is hard to see what this most attractive and friendly little town ever did to encourage such a catalogue of disasters. It has two fine churches, plenty of interesting buildings, wonderful surroundings and in spite of the past, a remarkably cheerful atmosphere.

Poole has become almost as one with it's neighbour to the east, **Bournemouth,** but still retains a strong streak of individuality; besides being a port it is a major residential centre, a light industrial centre and a recreational centre. There are two excellent museums, **The Waterfront Museum** and the **Guildhall Museum** and the delightfully restored **Scaplen's Court**, a medieval merchant's house. On the Quay, **Poole Pottery** has an international reputation, while the revamped and pedestrianised High Street has a modern indoor shopping centre and a wide variety of shops, pubs and restaurants.

Within the harbour, boat trips are available to such attractions as **Brownsea Island**, a nature reserve and bird sanctuary where Baden Powell held his first scout camp. If the weather is unkind then the **Tower Park** is a vast indoor complex housing such diverse activities as bowling and ice-skating, together with water-slides, cinema, shops and restaurants.

Bournemouth is a town full of hotels and places to stay which concentrates on caring for tourists and business people. It is many things to many people depending on what you are looking for. Wonderful place for a quiet holiday with excellent beaches, pleasant walks along the cliffs and good entertainment in the theatre and concert hall. It has several attractive places around it including **Southbourne**.

Wimborne Minster is where the great twin towers of St Cuthberga stand on the site of an 8th century monastery. The church is a splendid amalgamation of ecclesiastical styles, from Norman to late Gothic, and contains many treasures, including an 800 year old font, a chained library, an Orrery or astronomical clock, and many interesting tombs and memorials. The town is an attraction in it'self with an award winning local museum to tell it's story in **The Priest's House Museum**. Other places of interest are the lovely **Knoll Gardens**, a six acre site of rare and exotic plants, and, to the south of the town, the Georgian **Merley House,** with it's fascinating model toy collection, and **Merley Bird Gardens**, with avians ranging from parrots to penguins.

Kingston Lacy, a National Trust property has wonderful pictures and grounds and should be visited. Some half a dozen miles north of Wimborne lies **Wimborne St Giles**, on the edge of the old royal hunting grounds of **Cranborne Chase**. The Ashleys, Earls of Shaftesbury, have their seat here and the pleasant but ornate little church is full of their memorials. Many of the family were noted political reformers and philanthropists and the welcoming **Bull Inn** was built for workers on the estate. Another great political family are the Cecils, Marquesses of Salisbury, who's home has been at neighouring **Cranborne** since 1603. The fact that there was once a great Saxon Abbey on the site of the 13th century church and that William the Conqueror gave the manor to his Queen, Matilda, shows the esteem that this attractive little village was once held in; perhaps because from 908AD to 1120, it was the seat of the Chase Court, which administered the hunting rights.

The deer that were once so prized by Saxon and Norman nobility still graze among the woods and coverts in this lovely part of the county. In the neat village which delights in the enchanting name of **Sixpenny Handley**, the cheerful **Roebuck Inn** is a reminder that the descendants of those noble animals are around; as too are the descendants of those who hunted them so long ago. Somehow, this seems only right in an ancient county possessed of timeless charm.

WILTSHIRE

The true inhabitants of South Wiltshire are unhurried rather than slow, thoughtful rather than thick. Their character has been shaped by the countryman's compromising attitude to the seasons and the weather, yet they don't lack for native wit. True Wiltshiremen are known as 'Moonrakers' after two of their number were challenged one moonlit night, raking the surface of a village pond with hay-rakes. Their explanation for this strange activity was that they were trying to retrieve 'they gurt yaller cheese' pointing to the reflection of the moon in the water. The interrogators rode away laughing and tapping their heads: but the last laugh was on them, for they were excisemen and unknown to them, the pond contained smuggled casks of brandy! There 'bain't no flies' on a Moonraker, as the over confident outsider can find to his cost. The story has echoes in other counties associated with the free-traders, but in Wiltshire it rings the truest.

My journey in Dorset ended on the edge of **Cranbourne Chase** which runs into the south-west of Wiltshire towards Salisbury. In medieval times much of this area was heavily afforested but now it is a region of chalkland divided by the valleys of the Ebble and the Nadder. The clearwaters flow by some of the most lovely little villages and hamlets in the county, often settlements of great antiquity that lie tucked into folds of the hills and protected by woodland. This is delightful country and an area that repays the peripatetic wanderer in full.

Ebbesbourne Wake is a rambling village to the south of **White Sheet Hill** (incidentally, there are two hills of this name in the area - this one is south of the Shaftesbury-Salisbury road and the other is near Mere, to the north). Thatched cottages cluster around what was once an important cattle drover's trail. Continuing eastwards via **Fifield Bavant** with it's miniature Norman church, the valley floor begins to broaden by the time one reaches the 'capital' of the stream-set villages, **Broadchalke**. The Ebble provides nourishment for watercress beds and is splendid for trout fishing and brewing! On the northern side of White Sheet Hill where the bridleways are still a favourite with local riders, are the neighbouring villages of **Ansty** and **Swallowcliffe** close to which are two castles with the name of Wardour. Strictly speaking neither are true castles; **Old**

Wardour Castle was more akin to the fortified chateaux of France and was a tower house of octagonal shape. It's defensive capability was proven in 1634, when the elderly Lady Blanche Arundell, commanding a force of twenty five men and some dozen or so womenfolk, held out against a besieging Parliamentarian force of 1,300. The siege lasted five days and nights and was ended when Lady Blanche negotiated an honourable surrender. The Parliamentarians reneged on the conditions, imprisoned the gallant defenders and looted the castle. When her son Lord Arundell heard the news, he became the besieger but at great cost: in order to force a conclusion to the siege, he was forced to blow up his own inheritance. In 1776, the family built a new house within sight of the romantic ruins of the old. **Wardour Castle** is a rather austere Palladian mansion designed by James Paine for the eighth Lord Arundell, which became a school after the Arundell family's tenure came to an end.

The surrounding countryside and villages are a delight to the curious visitor. **Chilmark**, where the best of the beautiful creamy limestone was quarried, has a wealth of lovely houses built of the same material; the stone being first utilised by the Romans and later in the construction of Salisbury Cathedral and then Wilton House. A stream running through the village is spanned by a delightful little stone bridge and the Early English church has a broad spire. The Teffonts, **Teffont Magna** and **Teffont Evias**, are charming. Many of the cottages in the latter have their own little stone bridges giving access across the stream from front door to street. To the south of the A30, at **Fovant**, there are some moving examples of 20th century graffiti; the huge regimental crests carved into the hillside by soldiers undergoing training during the First World War. Sad to reflect on how few returned to see their handiwork, and how few of those regiments have survived. **East Knoyle's** chief claim to fame is that it was the birthplace of Sir Christopher Wren who was far from being the only talented member of that family; the ornate plaster-work in the chancel of the parish church was designed by his father, the rector of the parish.

Close to the Somerset border, at **Mere**, is one of the finest churches in Wiltshire. St Michael the Archangel is an elegant blend of 13th and 15th century styles with fine decorative work and a 100foot tower which dominates the handsome small town. The undulating downlands to the north contain two of Wiltshire's most famous stately homes. The first is **Stourhead** where the famous gardens contain the source of the meandering River Stour. In 1714 the estate was sold to the Hoare family, goldsmiths and bankers, the old house was demolished and a handome Palladian mansion built in it's place. However the chief glory of Stourhead are the grounds; the talented Henry Hoare was inspired by a Grand Tour of Europe and devised a delightful series of romantic gardens surrounding the lake, complete with temples and a grotto sheltering amongst the magnificent specimen trees.

The Hoare family continued to enhance both house and estate until, following the loss of their only son in the First World War, the late Sir Henry Hoare generously donated it to the National Trust. There is a sad but touching postcript to this story when Sir Henry and his wife, having given away their beloved home to which they had devoted most of their lives, died within two hours of each other.

The second great stately home stands just to the north and close to the Somerset border. **Longleat**, a palatial Elizabethan mansion set in wonderful grounds landscaped by the inimitable Capability Brown, is perhaps the best known such house in the country. Until the Dissolution it was the site of a medieval priory; the great house that replaced it was built by Sir John Thynne and has remained in the hands of the same family ever since. During the late 19th century it was redecorated in Italian Renaissance style with elaborately painted ceilings. Some idea of the scale of the house can be gained by the fact that it has seven libraries housing over 40,000 volumes! The late Marquess of Bath, faced with the horrendous problems of maintaining such a huge and elaborate building was the first peer to open his house on a business basis to the public, and as an added attraction, turned much of the surrounding estate into a fine Safari Park. Other entertainments, rallies and events have meant that these radical and pioneering measures have produced one of the country's premier tourist attractions.

Warminster is an appropriate name for the old town that plays host to a number of military establishments who exercise on the great open spaces of **Salisbury Plain**, immediately to the west. It is near the head of the third of the river valleys that run from the western county boundary back towards Salisbury. The river is the Wylye, one of the loveliest of the gin-clear chalk streams so beloved by trout fisherman and it's valley was described in 1824 by William Cobbett as being 'Fine, very fine.'

Roughly halfway between Warminster and Salisbury is **Wylye** it'self now thankfully by-passed. The river runs past an old mill and many of the cottages feature the checker-work stone and flint to be found throughout this part of Wiltshire.

Wiltshire takes it's name from the West Saxons who settled in the valley at **Wilton**, the 'farmstead beside the banks of the Wylye'. Although now a small well-to-do town, Wilton was once capital of Saxon Wessex: Alfred founded an abbey here and there was also a royal palace. The Dissolution saw the Abbey in the hands of Sir William Herbert, first Earl of Pembroke, and the estates have remained in the possession of that family ever since. Sir William demolished the Abbey and asked his friend Hans Holbein to design him a house utilising much of the remains. It was a wonderful house. Elizabeth I held court here, Shakespeare's company first performed 'As You Like It' before James I, and Charles I declared that he did 'love Wilton above all places, and did come here every summer.' Sadly a great fire destroyed much of the house in 1647, but happily the great Inigo Jones was on hand to rebuild. The result is one of the most magnificent and dignified stately homes in the country.

The Pembrokes have a strong entrepreneurial streak and although Wilton has long been the centre for weaving, it was the eighth earl who established the famous Wilton reputation for carpets. He combined the local assets of plentiful wool from the sheep of Salisbury Plain with the talents and skills of French weavers, then renowned throughout the world for the superb quality of their work. Unfortunately, Louis XIV of France regarded his weavers as a national asset and guarded them accordingly; the earl was forced to adopt some underhand methods and smuggled a number of the coveted craftsmen out of France in a giant barrel of wine! **The Wilton Carpet Company** was established in 1655 and is still going strong. It has an excellent museum and shop.

There is a triumvirate of ancient and important dwelling-places close to where the three valleys of the Wylye, Nadder and Ebble meet, and their histories are all intertwined. The oldest recorded site is that of **Old Sarum**, a 56 acre earthwork on a rise to the north of Salisbury. Of Iron Age origin, it was appropriated by the Romans and later became a Saxon fortified town, important enough for King Edgar to hold a Parliament there in 960AD and to have a mint. The Normans, probably by virtue of it's raised and protected position, made a great to-do about the place, using it as an administrative headquarters and building a citadel and cathedral. It was here, in 1086, that William held council to establish the feudal system and to initiate the compilation of the Domesday Book. However, by the beginning of the 13th century all was not well within the ancient ramparts; friction between the soldiers and the clergy, coupled with cramped conditions and shortage of water led to Bishop Richard Poore seeking a new site for the cathedral. Naturally, he went first to Wilton, since it was the nearest community of size and importance, but the Abbess objected strongly to the thought of a rival religious foundation. Eventually Bishop Poore selected a site where the Wylye, Nadder and Avon met amongst lush green meadows. Legend has it that the spot was chosen by loosing an arrow from the ramparts of Old Sarum. The archer must have been an exceptional man, doubtless aided by a northerly gale, for the new site is some two miles from the old!

Under the direction of one Elias Dereham, rightly described as an 'incomparable artificer', building proceeded apace. The stone which has weathered over the centuries to a lovely greeny-grey was quarried and carted over the rutted lanes from Chilmark to New Sarum, or **Salisbury**, where the master-masons gave it it's final shaping before it was hoisted into position. The building was completed in the remarkably short time of 40 years and is consequently an almost perfect example of Early English throughout. Almost certainly, Elias was aware of the problems that beset another cathedral, Winchester, which was also built on marshy ground and whose central tower had collapsed in 1107, for he left the construction of the elegant spire to his successors in the next century. By the time the people of Old Sarum, who appeared to have sided with the Bishop against the uncouth soldiers, had deserted the old hill-fort and settled around the new cathedral. There was nothing haphazard about this settlement; the new town was carefully planned from the start with the streets neatly laid out in a grid system which lasted almost untouched until the present century. There were numerous water-channels which led to the medieval nickname 'The Venice of England' and it may be that the drainage effect of these channels gave Bishop Wyvil and his architect, Richard of Farleigh, the confidence to add the audacious and elegant 404foot spire in 1334. Aware that vibration is the cause of collapse, the master-builder housed the peal of bells in a separate campanile. Over 400 years later, it was left to the 18th century architect James Wyatt to add, or rather subtract, the finishing touches. He was much criticised at the time for his ruthlessness, but it is to him that we owe the parity and beauty of what, externally, is the most beautiful cathedral in the country. Wyatt demolished the campanile, cleared away the jumble of tombstones in the graveyard and laid out the great sward of mown grass that surrounds the building. He removed much of the ornate that was within, including much of the early glass; the result is the austere Gothic nobility of the original craftsmen, who dared in those far off times to construct such a great and lofty edifice on marshy grounds; their decision must have been an act of faith in it'self.

The great spire is a landmark from far and wide and every year thousands come to wonder and pay homage to those old master-builders. Glorious as the building is, with it's great cloisters, massive Purbeck pillars, lovely choir vaulting, copy of Magna Carta and ancient clock (1386 - and still ticking!), it has to be said that part of it's attraction lies in it's incomparable setting. The Close is rectangular in shape, surrounded by an intact medieval wall, with a wonderful collection of buildings, houses, some contemporary with the great church, others fine examples of Queen Anne or Georgian. Three of these are not only fine examples of the architecture of their day but also excellent museums. A 13th century house, The Wardrobe, so named because it was once used for storing clothes belonging to the Bishop and his entourage, is now home to **The Museum of the Duke of Edinburgh's Royal Regiment.** It contains a fascinating collection of the historical items relating to 250 years of military history. The King's House is a 14th-century building housing the award-winning **Salisbury and South Wiltshire Museum** with a fine collection of archaeological and historical artefacts. The classic facade of **Mompesson House**, built in 1701, conceals a fine collection of glassware and furniture together with a delightful garden.

Salisbury is altogether a beautiful city and one which rewards the interested visitor with hours of pleasure. A Cathedral city always attracts the arts and Salisbury is no exception; there is a festival in September, music in the Cathedral and the Guildhall, exhibitions in the Arts Centre and live theatre at the excellent Playhouse. There is an attractive and well patronised racecourse whilst virtually all forms of recreation and sport are catered for in and around the city.

The Avon runs south from Salisbury; passing the great estate of **Longford Castle**. The splendid mansion is a testament to one woman's ambition; she was Helena, wife of Sir Thomas Gorges, Governor of Hurst Castle during the reign of Elizabeth I. Hurst is on the Hampshire coast and during the battle of the Spanish Armada, a galleon was driven aground closeby. Lady Gorges prettily asked the Queen if she might have the wreck, omitting to inform her sovereign that the galleon was laden with silver! Consequently Sir Thomas' modest medieval manor-house was transformed into a large and imposing castle. Unusual in that it is triangular in shape with a tower at each corner; the castle is now the home of the Earl of Radnor, whose family have owned it since the 18th century.

The little town of **Amesbury** is always worth visiting for many reasons. It is one of the oldest continually-inhabited sites in the country and has a strong connection with the Arthurian legends. Legend has it that after the death of Arthur, Queen Guinevere became Abbess of Amesbury. Modern Amesbury is a friendly, bustling place, providing shopping facilities and accommodation for many of the modern military establishments that lie around it. The great expanse of Salisbury Plain to the north and west is the principal area where the weaponry and soldiers of today exercise to protect our civilisation - but surrounding Amesbury are the mysterious relics and memorials of civilisations of which we know little. The best known of these, of course is **Stonehenge**. Viewed from the main road, the stones appear insignificant against the sky-line; approach closer and they become massively impressive, the largest weighing some 50 tons. The image is so familiar to us we almost take it for granted until closer contact with it's scale and brutal bulk begin to impress on our consciousness together with an almost indefinable sense of wonder and awe. Gazing at the marvellous circle of upright stones with their huge lintels, the question that comes to mind are Who, When, Why and How? The answers range from the wildly fanciful to the reasoned and scientific, but it must be admitted that even the soundest of answers is but theory and there are still great gaps in our knowledge when it comes to a matter of actual fact.

The high ground of the Plain is divided from the richer and lower soil of Northern Wiltshire by the road that runs from **Westbury** to **Upavon**. Protected by the bulk of the downland, numerous villages, hamlets and farmsteads are spread along the road. Solidly prosperous **Westbury** made it's money from cloth-weaving, glove-making and later from foundries exploiting a seam of iron-ore that was discovered nearby. It is a nice town with an imposing Town Hall, fine Georgian houses and a nice little market place, but the chief attraction for most visitors lies on the hillside to the east of the town where a great White Horse is carved into the chalk downland. Some 160 feet high, the present shape was cut out of the turf in 1778 and overlies an earlier, somewhat oddly shaped animal of unknown origin. It is claimed that the original was made to commemorate King Alfred's victory over the Danes at the Battle of Ethandun in 878 A.D. This is by no means certain since no-one is sure where Ethandun actually is; no matter, the great horse is undoubtedly impressive and worth a visit. On the heights above is the 23 acre site of **Bratton Castle**, a massive and ancient earthwork hill-fort whose presence gives some credence to theories about that battle so long ago.

Continuing eastwards, **Edington's** past is reflected in it's great church. Edington Priory was built between 1352 and 1361 and is therefore a fine example of the style known as Perpendicular. The Priory was the scene of a brutal and scandalous murder in 1449; at the time, the county was unsettled by the peasant's revolt, known as Jack Cade's Rebellion and the Bishop of Salisbury, one William Ayscough, felt Edington to be safer than his own cathedral. Sadly he was wrong, for the mob sought him out and dragged him from High Mass. At the top of the hill he ws savagely stoned to death. These days the church is widely known for it's annual music festival.

Erlstoke has a connection with the legendary Dick Turpin for Tom Boulter, a highwayman whose exploit's were often attributed to Turpin, stole a horse - and it's name really was Black Bess!

Devizes lies not far to the north and close to the geographical heart of Wiltshire. It is a pleasant small market town. There are two attractive Norman churches and it has a thriving market. The town is an important centre for agriculture and light industry. In medieval times it was second only to Salisbury in cloth-manufacturing and was one of the principal corn-markets in the West of England. There are a great many interesting and picturesque buildings including **The Bear Hotel**, an old coaching inn where, in the 18th century, the father of Sir Thomas Lawrence, the portrait painter, was once landlord. There is also the excellent **Devizes Museum**, which makes a speciality of displaying many of the Bronze Age finds taken from the county's innumerable sites.

Every year the Devizes to Westminster canoe race takes place using much of the old Kennet and Avon Canal which once linked London to Bristol. The Trust now administers the canal and has an exhibition centre on the wharf and, to the west of the town, at Caen Hill there is an amazing example of early 19th-century civil engineering where the canal is made to 'climb' the steep gradient by means of a flight of 16 locks.

The Vale of Pewsey runs between the high ground of the Plain to the south, and the even higher ground of the Marlborough Downs to the north. The Vale is some twelve miles long by five wide and contains some of the richest farmland in the country. The settlements between the hills are quiet and peaceful, their pasts containing no great historical dramas or events. The ecclesiastical architecture is particularly fine, probably as a result of agricultural wealth, and at **Chirton** there is one of the finest Norman churches in England. Built in 1170, it has a magnificent timber roof and fine decorative work, particularly around the doorway and the font.

The little town which lends it's name to the Vale, **Pewsey**, is a friendly and cheerful place with good buildings and a fine statue of King Alfred gazing across the River Avon from the crossroads, a reminder of the time when the community was owned by Saxon Kings. The marketing and milling of corn and an iron foundry contributed to past wealth and every September there is a riotous celebration described as 'the Mother of West County carnivals'.

South of Pewsey, **Upavon** is situated at the foot of downland and overlooked by the extensive earthworks of **Casterley Camp**, a fortification dating from the first century A.D. To the east of the village is another, but more modern reminder of military activity in the area. **RAF Upavon** was one of the earliest purpose-built airfields in the country, constructed in 1912 to house the Central Flying School of the Royal Flying Corps.

The nobility who came to **Ludgershall** for sport would have looked to the preserves of the **Chute Forest** for their entertainment; the great medieval woodland spread from Hampshire through to Wiltshire and would have harboured huge herds of deer. The border between the two counties is hilly and broken and still contains large clumps of woodland. It is beautiful countryside, crossed by the **Chute Causeway**, a Roman road that is far from being perfectly straight and populated by a number of attractive little villages sheltering amongst the trees.

To the north-west, via the Causeway, is the pleasant village of **Burbage**, once totally surrounded by the **Savernake Forest**. Nearby **Wolfhall** was the home of the Seymours, hereditary wardens of another once vast forest, a favourite hunting ground for Norman kings. It was at Wolfhall tht Henry VIII met and courted Jane Seymour, his future queen who later died in childbirth. Half a mile from Burbage Wharf is the **Bruce Tunnel**, which is some 1500 feet long; horses were not used here since the boats were pulled through by hand using chains strung along the tunnel wall..

On the edge of Savernake is another of those ancient burial mounds known as **Barrows**; this particular one is believed to have been the last resting place of Maerla (in local legend, Merlin the Wizard) and the conjunction of names has been taken by the town that lies alongside, **Marlborough**. A handsome and popular town with fine, predominantly Georgian architecture lining the immensely wide main street. Where cars are parked down the middle of this street today, market stalls and livestock were tethered in the past; in fact, life in this cheerful town often seemed to be little short of one great long street party. A visitor in the 19th-century reported that there were '1333 partakers of conviviality seated at one long table from the market house to St Peter's Church, nearly half a mile'. Because of the town's past importance as a staging post on the main London to Bristol road, the modern 'partaker of conviviality' is well provided for at the many coaching inns that have survived.

The road to the west passes through small rural communities in the Downs, containing many a delight so typical of Wiltshire, sites where the historic and pre-historic sit peacefully side by side. **Fyfield** has a 13th-century church with a splendid 15th-century tower, complete with pinnacles and gargoyles. Half a mile away are the strange stones that comprise the **Devil's Den**, actually the remains of the stone-framed burial chamber that was once covered by a barrow, or mound. At first glance, **Avebury** appears little more than a picturesque downland village with an attractive grouping of part-Saxon church, the gabled Elizabethan **Avebury Manor**, thatched cottages and farmsteads - and then one notices the stones. Massive weather wrought lozenges of sandstone, many weighing more than 40 tons, stand upright in groups, around and amongst the village.

Avebury Stone Circle pre-dates Stonehenge by some two centuries and differs particularly in that the great stones are undressed; called sarsens (a local corruption of 'saracen' or foreign) they are found locally on Marlborough Downs. They surround the village, contained within the remains of a large earth ring, some 1200 feet across. Many are missing, having been broken up over the centuries for use in local houses and barns, but expert excavation has revealed their originl placement. The Stone Circle is by no means the only prehistoric site in the area and by no means the most mysterious. A 50 foot wide avenue of megaliths, nearly a mile long, once led to an older site, named the **Sanctuary**, near the village of **West Kennett**. The stones here have long vanished but, once again, patient archaeological detective work has established their positions. On the southern flank of Avebury is perhaps the strangest object of all, the vast conical earthwork of **Silbury Hill**; an earthen pyramid, 130 feet high whose base covers a staggering five and a half acres, large enough to fill Trafalgar Square and reach three quarters of the way up Nelson's Column. Described as ' the largest man-made mound in Europe' it's purpose and origins are obscure; since the 18th century, shafts have been driven into it's mighty bulk in search of burial chambers or similar but with no success. All that we know is that it was built over 4,000 years ago, that a million cubic yards of chalk were excavated and, given the simple tools of the period, would have taken 500 people ten years to build! Local legend has it that a certain King Sil or Zel, is somewhere beneath the mound buried upright on his horse and clad in a suit of golden armour.

Close by Silbuy Hill is **West Kennett Long Barrow**, a 350 foot long burial mound from around 3,500 BC while to the north is **Windmill Hill** a series of concentric earthworks which was the home of a Neolithic race of farmers who were probably responsible for the long barrow. The excellent small **Alexander Keiller Museum** has many exhibit's and finds relating to these ancient sites, and is named after the archaeologist who did so much to interpret the extraordinary works of so long ago. Nearby the splendid thatched Great Barn houses **The Museum of Wiltshire Folk Life**, with fascinating displays of rural crafts, skills, tools and equipment.

There is no doubt that it can be extremely breezy up on the downs and it has been suggested that specialised forms of miniature tornadoes or whirlwinds are responsible for a phenomona known as **Corn Circles**, strange geometric shapes that appear in the great cornfields around this area. Ineveitably, fanciful theories have been produced linking the shapes with the ancient stone circles, or even with aliens from outer space. Undoubtedly, some are the work of hoaxers but others are not so easily explained although cosmic doodling seems highly unlikely.

The highest village in the county **Baydon** stands at 750feet and is set in the heart of race-horse training country, close to the famous **Lambourne Downs**. An ancient settlement it's name may be derived from Mount Badon, the last of Arthur's twelve great battles against the invading Saxons in the 6th century. St Nicholas church has internal piers of chalk blocks, put in place some 700 years ago, which aptly illustrate the old Wiltshire dictum that chalk was an excellent building medium providing that it has 'a good hat and boots', a sound roof and foundations to keep out the damp.

The M4 motorway effectively chops off the flatter lands of the northern tip of the county and contains the great mass of **Swindon**, the largest industrial town in Wiltshire. It was the railway that brought prosperity to the town, particularly since the town became the centre of Brunel's Great Western Railway, affectionately referred to as 'God's wonderful railway'. By 1867, the town could boast that it was 'neatly and regularly built.... and is lighted by gas. The Mechanics

Institute is a noble building, having a library with upward of 3,650 volumes, and is one of the finest institutions in the kingdom; lectures, concerts and dramatic performances are frequently given in it. A free recreation ground, with a permanent pavilion, has been established for the use of cricketers, of whom there are several clubs. At the factory locomotives for the whole line are manufactured. Such is the perfection to which the building of engines has arrived here that one engine per week can be turned out. Also about 330 tons of rails per week are turned out at the rolling mill, The works cover about eighteen acres of ground.....'

Although the great locomotive works have been phased out **Swindon** remains one of the principal termini for goods and passengers and the great days of the GWR are remembered in the **Great Western Railway Museum** in Farringdon Road, which has a comprehensive display of old locomotives and railway memorabilia. Just opposite is **The Railway Village House**, a perfectly restored foreman's house from the turn of the century. Both exhibit's are situated within the area known as the Railway Village, a model community built by GWR for their workers.

The River Thames, although little more than a stream, takes a meander into the extreme north of Wiltshire, running under **Cricklade**, an ancient market town, important from Roman days onwards because it sit's on the old Roman Road of Ermine Street.

An ecclesiastical establishment of great importance was situated at **Malmesbury**, a handsome small town, built on a rocky outcrop above the waters of the Avon. The abbey and the town flourished trading in wool and exploiting the rich agricultural land that lay around. It reached it's heyday in the 14th century when riches gained from the wool trade led to the Abbey having a spire higher than that of Salisbury. However pride comes before a fall, and at the end of the next century, that is precisely what happened; the spire collapsed and the great gilt ball that adorned it's tip ' rolled unceremoniously down the High Street'. With the Dissolution the Abbey fell into the hands of an upwardly mobile clothier, one William Stumpe, who promptly filled the great building with weaving looms and cared nought for the great literary treasure house; manuscripts and parchment torn from books were put to varied uses, including making patterns for gloves,wrapping parcels, making bungs for beer-barrels and scouring guns. Stumpe went on to make a vast fortune, married his daughter off to the aristocracy, and perhaps to make amends for his earlier philistine behaviour, gave the great nave of the Abbey to the town as a parish church. What remains is lovely, with a splendid porch with fine, intricate Norman carving and a simple and elegant interior of the same period.

Malmesbury went on to establish it'self as a centre of excellence in the manufacture of silk, gloves and lace and there are some fine Cotswold stone houses from the 17th and 18th century that bear testament to the wealth of those who dealt in these trades.

South of the M4 lies a mecca for tourists to this area of the county. **Castle Combe** is almost impossibly pretty, with it's immaculate grouping of houses of golden Cotswold stone, thatch, and tile, trout-laden stream, church, old market cross, and manor house set below wooded hills, where a castle once stood. It looks like a film set, indeed it has been used as one, but it's original prosperity came from weaving.

Chippenham was once the site of a Saxon palace, which would appear to have been a comfortable and hospitable establishment since the normally alert King Alfred was caught napping by the

Danes, whilst spending Christmas here in 877 AD. Chippenham's greatest attraction to me is **Maude Heath's Causeway**. Maude was a market woman who, in the reign of Henry VII would make her way to **Chippenham** from her home in **Langley Burrell**, carrying heavy baskets full of eggs and butter. The roads in those far off days were generally appalling and the fact that most of the area was low-lying, boggy and riven with streams did not help matters. The good Maude was evidently industrious, far-sighted and charitable for, when she died, in 1474, she left all her savings to build and endow a cobbled footpath between Wick Hill and Chippenham Clift, linking the little villages of the Avon Valley with their principal market. She is commemorated not only by her Causeway, but also by a statue set high on a column on Wick Hill and by an inscription near Chippenham church which reads:

'Hither extended Maude Heath's gift,
For where you stand is Chippenham's Clift'

To the east of Chippenham is **Calne**. Once again weaving was the original basis of prosperity but when the Industrial Revolution ended that trade, it became famous for bacon-curing and the production of sausages and pies. This came about through the enterprise of a local family of butchers, the Harrises. At the time, the town was on the principal route for livestock being driven from the West to London and among the animals were large quantities of Irish pigs, having been off-loaded at Bristol. The Harris family realised that if they bought the pigs at Calne, before they became weary and lost weight on their long trot to London, then the pork would be of superior quality. From 1770 until the 1980's, their factory dealt with literally millions of those versatile beasts of whom it is said, 'everything can be used except the grunt.' Economic and regulatory factors conspired to close the factory and the only memorial to this once great business that made the name of Calne synonymous with bacon, is a bronze pig by the small shopping precinct.

Two miles to the south-west is the great estate of **Bowood**, home of the Marquesses of Lansdowne since 1754. Robert Adams spent eight years enlarging and improving Bowood House while Capability Brown was at work on the gardens and glorious parkland. The house has fine collections of sculpture, paintings and costumes. There is a Laboratory in which Dr Joseph Priestly discovered oxygen in 1774, a fine library and chapel, but undoubtedly the real glory is the setting, the wonderful park and gardens, over ninety acres of which are open to visitors.

Lacock Abbey was founded in 1232 by Ela, Countess of Salisbury, the grieving widow of William Longspee. An Augustinian order flourished there until the Dissolution, when it fell into the hands of one William Sharington, a man described as 'being of dubious character'. Fortunately, he also had excellent taste and did not go in for the usual large scale demolitions that most of the ecclesiastical property developers of that time seemed to enjoy. Indeed, such additions that he had made were very well-executed and in perfect harmony with the preserved Abbey. The Talbot family were next on the scene, but not without incident; Sir William's niece, Olivia, was being secretly courted by young John Talbot and in a scene reminiscent of Romeo and Juliet, she offered to leap from the battlements of the abbey church to join her suitor below. The young man not believeing that she would jump told her to go ahead. The young Miss Sharrington, however was no simpering ninny and happily leapt into her lover's arms, flattening him to the ground. The story goes that 'she cried out for help, and he was with difficulty brought to life again. Her father told her that since she had made such a leap she should e'en marry him.' The Talbots were fine stewards of both Abbey and the village of **Lacock** and in 1944 Miss Matilda Talbot presented both, together with 284 acres of land to the National Trust. There is no building later than the 18th-century in the winding streets of grey stone and half-timbered cottages. The perpendicular church, dedicated to St Cyriac, has an elegant interior and beautiful east window. **The George** is one of the oldest continuously licensed pubs in England while **The Sign of the Angel** dates back to the 14th century. A stone barn contains a museum dedicated to William Fox-Talbot, pioneer of photography. One cannot help but wonder what he would think of his invention now as yet another coach-load of tourists arrive with motor-driven self-focussing cameras at the ready.

Another lovely house lies some six miles to the south-west at **Great Chalfield. Great Chalfield Manor** was built about 1480 by a prosperous wool-merchant, one Thomas Tropenell. Now under the care of the National Trust, the Manor is one of the loveliest houses of it's era, lying in rich meadowlands on the edge of a moat.

Tropenell's wealth came from the same source as that of the neighbouring town of **Bradford-on-Avon** - wool. It is hard in these days of man-made fibres and multi-national fashion corporations to appreciate just how important fleece was to medieval life; suffice it to say that there were no other fibres that were so adaptable or so economical to produce and that the best wool came from the backs of English sheep raised on the chalk downlands. Until the early Middle Ages, wool was the country's principal export; later, with the development of the weaving trade, finished cloth, took that position. An indication of the little town's one time importance in this vital trade is the fact that the Yorkshire wool and textile town of Bradford was named after it.

It is a charming, picturesque town today with some wonderful buildings. The medieval Shambles is now a charming shopping area, full of antique shops and tea-rooms, light-years removed from it's original purpose as the place where the town's slaughter-men worked. Wherever you go through the twisting winding streets there is always something to interest and delight.

To understand the history of **Trowbridge**, now the administrative centre of Wiltshire, a position gained by virtue of it's old rail links, make a visit to **Trowbridge Museum** in the Civic Hall where the life and times of the community is well recorded.

Heading south and within sight of the White Horse at **Westbury**, the gentle countryside seems so peaceful and idyllic, the villages so friendly and welcoming that it is hard to imagine what life must have been like when that ancient Anglo-Saxon chronicler set down his despairing account of anarchy and misrule. Yet many of the small communities one drives through existed then and it is a tribute to the spirit and purpose of their habitants that they survived.

At **Hawkeridge**, there is a fine example of those characteristics that brought the countrymen and women of Wiltshire through the worst of times to the best of times. It is not the saga of a wealthy wool-merchant or rich clothier who became landed gentry, but a rather more modest account: in 1851, Mr Ephraim Dole and his wife Sarah invested their savings into converting three labourer's cottages into an ale-house. Nearly one hundred and fifty years later **The Royal Oak** is still going strong, complete with skittle-alley and dining room. Just goes to show that 'there ain't no flies on Wiltshire volk...'

HAMPSHIRE

Michael Drayton, a Warwickshire contemporary of Shakespeare, intended nothing derogatory in his description of one of England's finest counties. In ancient times, the thickly wooded downland of the northern part of the county must have been something of a procine paradise for the hirsute and thick-set wild boar, rootling amongst the myriad oaks in a never ending quest for acorns and other such delicacies. No true son of the county has ever objected to the sobriquet of Hampshire Hog, for the long vanished beast represented those qualities of independence, nimbleness and strength that has enabled the area to cope amd come to terms with both invasion and innovation. Romans, Danes, Saxons and Normans found the rolling countryside much to their liking, whilst in recent times, industry and urban development have stamped their mark on the landscape. Nevertheless, adjacent to the roar of the motorway and the bustle of the conurbations, there exists a seemingly timeless world rich in history and bucolic charm. The Wild Boar of Hampshire, had he been somewhat less tasty and rather more intelligent, would still find much to please him.

An apt example of this happy balance is to be found in and around the county town of **Winchester.** The M3 noisily snakes it's way past to the east of the town, cutting a giant's furrow through the chalk downs. Motorways may not be the most attractive of man's creations, but they are far from being the worst; merely the 20th century equivalent of the railway bringing life and prosperity, even in these difficult times.

Winchester was once the capital of England until it was supplanted by Westminster (London). It is the county town of Hampshire and rich in historic associations and remains with a wealth of fine old architecture but it is not somewhere in which one feels trapped in a time-warp or historical 'experience'. The city bustles and flourishes; there is room for both tourist, citizen and trader. Much of the city centre has been set aside for pedestrians and it is a real pleasure to meander amongst the thoroughfares and narrow medieval streets, enjoying the wealth of shops and buildings, yet never being far from greenery or running water, for the River Itchen, one of the finest trout rivers, flows rapidly through the city towards the water-meadows to the south.

The great grey Cathedral dominates; at 556 feet, it is the longest medieval churh in Europe. Magnificent and awe-inspiring, it was founded in 1079 and consecrated in 1093. Over the centuries it has beome a graceful melange of styles, reflecting the energy, determination and skill of those who built 'to the greater glory of God'. The broad lawns and fine buildings of the Close set off the ancient Cathedral to perfection. To my mind, one of the greatest glories of English cathedral liturgy is to be found in it's music and Winchester's choristers are trained at the Pilgrim School, with it's fine Pilgrim's Hall, worth visiting for it's magnificent hammer-beamed roof that dates back to the early 14th century. I can remember reading that Sir Andrew Lloyd-Webber used to visit the Cathedral regularly when he lived nearby and found much inspiration for his own work from the music that poured out.

Education has long been an integral part of ecclesiastical life. In 1382, Bishop William of Wykeham founded **Winchester College** which is to be found south of the Close. 600 years later, the school is still going strong and using many of the same buildings. You will find a profusion of interesting museums to visit, good restaurants, old inns and shops. Although Winchester places a strong emphasis on preservation and heritage, it's real charm comes from the fact that it possesses a past that is truly alive; clerics still tread the cloisters, scholars are still in the school-room and quadrangle, soldiers stamp the parade-ground, and traders hawk their wares in the market place.

Sport and recreation are strong in Hampshire traditions, the ethos of 'work hard, play hard' obviously appealing to the county character, yet even in play it is hard to escape a sense of the past. For example in the village of **Littleton**, to the north-east of Winchester has a recreation area which seems to accommodate an amazing range of sport including Cricket, Tennis, Bowls, Football and Croquet and closeby are some grassy mounds which are Bronze Age burial chambers dating from perhaps 1000 BC. As I watched children play, it was strange to reflect that those earthworks were created at about the same time King David ruled from Jerusalem.

Skirting the north of Winchester and heading east, I crossed the M3 and almost immediately found myself in fine countryside. Woods and coverts speckled the broad acres of rich plough and pasture through which ran the gin-clear waters of the Itchen. My first stop was at **Alresford** (pronounced Allsford), a delightful, predominantly Georgian town, whose fortunes were founded on the 14th-century wooltrade In more recent time, the inhabitants turned to the cultivation of watercress and because of the importance of the industry, the Mid-Hants Railway became known as **The Watercress Line**. A victim of Dr Beeching's now infamous cuts, the railway has been happily restored by dedicated individuals and is now one of Hampshire's most popular - and most useful - attractions. The steam railway runs via **Ropley, Medstead and Four Marks**, to the market town of **Alton**.

South of Alresford I came across another example of 'living history'. At **Tichborne**, the Tichborne Dole, in the form of a gallon of flour, bread or money has been handed out yearly to each deserving adult since the 12th century. It is said that the custom originated with the dying Lady Isabella who begged her husband Sir Roger Tichborne, to grant her enough land to care for the sick and the needy. In reply, Sir Roger, a chauvinist if ever there was one, took a flaming brand from the fire and told his sick wife that 'she could have as much land as she could crawl round before the flame was extinguished'. Astonishingly she managed to cover some 23 acres before the flame burnt out, and the land thus enclosed is known to this day as The Crawles. Tradition has it that tragedy will befall the family if Lady Isabella's request for the Dole is ever ignored, and, astonishingly, on the few rare occasions that this has happened, the consequences have been singularly unpleasant.

Close by lie the small and attractive villages of **Hinton Ampner** and **Kilmeston**. The wonderful countryside provides a fitting setting for the handsome facade and beautiful gardens of **Hinton Ampner House**. The house, it's origins going back to the Middle Ages, has been re-built several times - the last time as recently as 1960. Now in the care of the National Trust, the house is a tribute to the dedicated persistence of one man, Ralph Dutton, the last Lord Sherborne. In 1936 he lovingly restored the house and it's contents. In 1940, he relinquished the house to a girl's school, and in 1960 he saw the house destroyed by fire. Undeterred, he started again to rebuild and refurbish and the house is now immaculately maintained and has fine displays of Regency furniture, pictures and paintings.

It is difficult when writing a guide to this part of the world to avoid the over-use of the word 'attractive'. So many of the small villages and hamlets nestling in the chalk downland catch the eye and are worthy of mention; not necessarily because they are linked with historical sites or notable personages, or because they possess a fine church or noble house, but simply because of their charm and character - their very individuality attracts. Six miles east along the A272, I turned south to visit **East Meon**, a village, which to me, represents the epitome of the Hampshire downland village. Old Izaak Walton fished the trout-rich waters of the River Meon, which rises from the chalk not far from the village to run under and beside the main street. The Norman church is one of the finest buildings of it's type and set to perfection above the village in what was once a bishop's deer park.

I wandered roughly south-east from here to where the landscape is dominated by the imposing mass of **Butser Hill**. At nearly 900 feet, it is the highest point in the western end of the South Downs and is contained within **Queen Elizabeth Country Park**. Jointly administered by Hampshire County Council and the Forestry Commission, it is an admirable example of how an area can be successfully managed to incorporate a multitude of quite different interests. Recreation, forestry, conservation and education all take place within the 1,400 acres which is liberally strewn with nature trails, bridle ways and woodland walks I was fascinated by a modern reconstruction of an Iron Age farm of around 300BC, partly based on information gathered from local excavations. Crops of the period are grown here and it was intriguing to learn that the prehistoric varieties of wheat produce have nearly twice the protein content of today's. Not only that, but experiments have shown that yield per acres would have been not far off our modern figures - so much for selective breeding and generic engineering!

Petersfield is a handsome market town that has much to offer, but has suffered heavily since the introduction of the internal combustion engine; too many people pass through and never stop to investigate. In a sense, it was ever thus since the town sit's astride the main Portsmouth to London road and was an important coaching stop long before the car was invented. In the square, there is a heroic statue of William III on horseback, dressed for some odd reason as a Roman emperor.

North of the town, there is some of the finest scenery to be found in the South of England. Around **Steep**, and further north at **Selborne**, the remarkable landscape features great beech 'hangers', great clumps of mature trees hanging (hence the name) precipitously over almost sheer chalk inclines that run down to a base of greensand rock. Known as 'Little Switzerland', it is an area of great beauty and contrasts favourably with the more serene charms of the **Meon Valley**.

Selborne is, of course, the mecca for all English naturalists. It was the birthplace and home of Gilbert White (1720-93), four times curate of the church and author of that delightful classic 'The Natural History and Antiquities of Selborne'. Published in 1789, it is based on his forty years of observations of the wildlife, plants and habitat found in the immediate vicinity. The book, in the form of letters to the interested parties, has a singular freshness and charm which reflects the enthusiasm and character of the man. His old home, The Wakes, contains much relating to his studies, and also houses collections belonging to a later owner, the explorer Francis Oates, uncle of Captain Oates who perished with Scott on the expedition to the South Pole in 1912. The joint exhibitions are housed together as **Gilbert White's House and Garden and The Oates Exhibition**.

Leaving the Selborne area, where the National Trust has done so much to preserve and maintain the landscape, other literary and botanical connections are to be found a few miles further north. At **Chawton, Jane Austen's House** provides an insight into the life led by the novelist and her family from 1809 to 1817, while she wrote or revised her six great novels. The delightful garden surrounding the house contains many old fashioned varieties of flowers and visitors are welcome to picnic on the lawns.

Nearby **Alton**, a busy and good looking market town, is home to the **Curtis Museum** named after William Curtis, the founder of the Botanical Magazine. As well as exhibit's relating specifically to Curtis, the museum possesses excellent displays relating to local industry and crafts and all manner of historical exhibit's including the exquisite **Alton Buckle**, a 1500 year old item of Saxon jewellery. There are also exhibitions of children's games, toys, silver and pottery.

My next destination was amongst the big wooded downland that lies close to the border with Berkshire and to the south of Newbury. Trees fringe wide expanses of chalk soil either under cultivation or down to rich pasture. This is a county of quiet wealth and great estate, with small villages, hamlets and farms scattered across the countryside.

At **Highclere** a steep climb up **Beacon Hill** is worthwhile for the splendid view over the Downs. The summit is crowned by an Iron Age hill-fort and the grave of the fifth Earl of Caernarvon, who, with Howard Carter, led the expedition to find the tomb of Tutankhamun. The Earl's palatial home, **Highclere Castle** lies close to the foot of the hill surrounded by lovely parkland and laid out by the inimitable Capability Brown. The Castle, the largest mansion in the county, was rebuilt in the middle of the last century and is renowned for the richness and variety of it's interior decoration.

On the subject of decoration, I recommend a visit to the **Sandham Memorial Chapel** at **Burghclere**, to view the paintings by Stanley Spencer (1891-1959). They are considered to be the most important of English murals. They reflect on the futility and horror of war and were painted between 1926 and 1932 ; the chapel was built in memory of Lieutenant H.W. Sandham who died in the First World War.

The largest of the 'Cleres' is **Kingsclere**, at the foot of **Watership Down** - made famous by the author Richard Adams. His hero was a rabbit, but for many years mine was a horse, the great Derby winner Mill Reef. He was trained at Kingsclere and throughout the area, studs and racing stables breed and train in an endeavour to produce another such equine star.

The most notable of Hampshire's rivers is The Test, and seven miles south of Highclere lies the attractive ancient town of **Whitchurch**. Here the fast running alkaline waters once served both sport and industry, providing power for silk-weaving and at nearby **Laverstock**, for the manufacture of bank-note paper. Both industries have survived and **The Silk Mill** is beautifully preserved and open to the public with a shop well worth visiting; not surprisingly the banknote contract with the Bank of England dates back to 1727 and continues to this day.

The nearby town of **Andover** is representative of much of the change occurring within the County in recent times. The area has been home to man since ancient times; at **Danebury**,

338

together with some fascinating reconstructions and audio-visual displays. Andover was first recorded in 955AD and grew to become a prosperous market town and coaching centre but perhaps the most dramatic changes in the town's history occurred in the early 1960's when it became an overspill area from London. However, it must be said that Andover has not suffered quite so badly at the hands of the planners as have other such communities within Hampshire; the handsome town centre, with it's market place, guildhall of 1825, fine Victorian parish church of St Mary's and numerous coaching inns, have survived. The coaches, with post horns blowing and horses snorting, no longer rumble down the high street, but it is nonetheless a cheerful and lively place.

Thatch is common throughout the area and doubtless owes it's origins to the readily available supply of reed from along the river banks. The splendidly named Wallops, (the name means, rather disappointingly, 'valley of the stream') also have a wealth of thatched cottages. Strung along the valley of Wallop Brook, the three villages retain a wealth of character and tradition, with **Nether Wallop** being noted for it's fine Saxon wall paintings in the church, **Over Wallop** for a magnificent 15th century font, and **Middle Wallop** for it's **Museum of Army Flying**. This award winning museum houses a unique collection of flying machines, equipment and displays depicting the history of Army Aviation since the end of the last century, from balloons to kites to the latest in helicopters.

It is a truly lovely part of England with plenty of footpaths for the walker and bridleways for the rider. At **Stockbridge**, the Test flows under the London to Salisbury road and the wide main street reflects it's past as a drover's town.

Income, and not an inconsiderable one at that, is unfortunately a necessity to enable one to fish much of the Test, and on the rare occasions that private stretches of river come on the market they change hands for quite astronomical sums. Even if you are not interested in the 'gentle art of the angle', a walk along the accessible sections of the river bank will offer a clue to the extraordinary costs involved. The water is alkaline, crystal clear and the brown trout thrive growing prodigiously within the food rich waters whilst the banks, feeder streams, wiers and sluice-gates are immaculately kept and maintained; skilled work on such a scale does not come cheap. Sadly, the river, like so many of it's kind is under threat. The rapidly increasing populations of the new urban developments within the country require water for both domestic and industrial use and increased abstraction by the water companies mean a decrease in flow and greater threat of pollution.

My journey around North Hampshire ended close to where it began, just a few miles to the west of the ancient capital of Wessex. In 1201, a group of followers of St Augustinian established a priory in one of the most idyllic situations imaginable. **Mottisford Abbey** became a private house after the Dissolution and work over the centuries has resulted in the present handsome Georgian south front, perfectly complemented by the wonderful gardens that sweep down to the Test. Green lawns are shaded by great trees and the celebrated rose garden contains the National Trust's collection of old-fashioned roses. It has to be said that this is the most harmonious setting of any house in England - and one can well believe it.

The River Avon, noted for the variety of it's fishing (particularly it's fine, though sadly declining runs of salmon) runs southward, marking the eastern boundary of the county spur. The A338, from Salisbury to Bournemouth follows the river for much of it's course, passing through the attractive towns of **Fordingbridge** and **Ringwood.** Ringwood is a cheerful market town. Tourism plays an important part of the town's economy and angling is a major attraction. Many of the hotels and inns cater especially for those enthusiasts who travel from all over the country to fish the Avon and it's tributaries. It is popular too with those who love the diversity of sport to be found in the waters of the Avon. Because of it's depth, the river offers unrivalled opportunities to both the game-fisherman after trout, salmon or grayling, and the coarse angler, pursuing the like of the chub, pike, dace and barbel.

The town lies on the western edge of another great area of natural beauty within this county of contrast - **The New Forest.** It is an area of over 90,000 acres of heath and mixed woodland with an abundance of wildlife. Paradoxically, it is the oldest of the forests of England but that is simply because the word 'forest' is of Norman origin; it means an area set aside for hunting and the New Forest was the first of these preserves to be created by William the Conqueror. Savage penalties were exacted on those who broke the forest laws; at one time a person could be blinded for merely disturbing deer, whilst death was the automatic penalty for poaching. The modern day visitor might like to be reassured that the passing of the centuries have seen extensive modification of these draconian measures: apart from occasional necessary culling the deer are left in peace while the tourist can wander freely through much of the beautiful country. There are three distinctive habitats within the forest boundaries. The high heath-lands, covered with heather and gorse together with Scots pine and birch, give a somewhat barren impression - particularly to the motorists travelling along the main east/west route of the A31. However the lower slopes and better-drained land provides true forest in the modern meaning; superb traditional woodland planted with oak, beech, yew and thorn, producing in the summer great sweeping canopies of foliage. Finally there is the marsh land where the white cotton-grass conceals the bogs and where the alder and willow grow.

Amongst this vegetation can be found all manner of wildlife, from grouse on the high heath to the four varities of deer (Red, Roe, Fallow and the tiny Sika) who favour the woodland. Domestic animals, their numbers strictly controlled by the Verderers, graze amongst the trees and shrubs. These include cattle, pigs, donkeys and the celebrated New Forest ponies. Mention was first made of wild 'horses' at the time of King Canute (1017-35) while some believe them to be descendants of the Jennets, the small Spanish horses which swam ashore from the wrecks of the Spanish Armada in the 16th century. Many of them are employed in the numerous riding stables and schools to be found within the forest.

Leisure is the principal 'industry' of the New Forest and much has been done to encourage it's development. Picnic area, camping sites, trails, drives and paths are to be found throughout, and hotels and boarding houses, inns and pubs all do their very best to make the visitor welcome.

'Badger's Wood' is the meaning of **Brockenhurst**, a village that grew in popularity with the arrival of the railway in 1847. It has a fine Norman church with many memorials; one of which is of particular local interest. 'Brusher'Mills, who died in 1905, earned his nickname because he brushed the cricket pitch at Balmer Lawn between innings. Of singular appearane, with a grey beard, long coat and furry hat, he made his living by catching snakes, mainly adders, with his bare hands. It is said he was never bitten because he drank a bottle of rum a day and never washed !! Undoubtedly, he would have approved of his other memorial in the village, a pub named **The Snake Catcher** - although I doubt whether the customers would have enjoyed his company.

A couple of miles to the south of Brockenhurst lies **Boldre**, one of the best looking villages in the New Forest, where the thatched cottages spread out along the numerous country lanes. The church is a happy mixture of Norman and early English but is most celebrated for having been the living, from 1777 to 1804, of William Gilpin. Gilpin was a contemporary of Gilbert White, and like him, a writer and naturalist. He must have been something of a saint, for he recorded, on first arriving in the parish, that the village was 'utterly neglected by the former pastor, and, exposed to every temptation of pillage and robbery from their proximity to the deer, the game, and the fuel of the forest, for these poor people were little better than a herd of banditti.' Thirty years later, the 'herd of banditti' clubbed together to erect a memorial within the church to Gilpin's memory, a tribute earned by remarkably few vicars in English village history. There is also a memorial to the ship's company of the battle-cruiser HMS Hood, sunk in May 1941; the 1,406 officers and men are remembered in an annual service.

In her eighteen years in commission HMS Hood frequently sailed through the narrow patch of water that guards the western entrance to the Solent. **Hurst Castle**, built at the end of a shingle spit less than a mile from the Isle of Wight, was built by Henry VIII with a formidable armament of 70 guns. It can be reached on foot from **Milford on Sea**, a small but popular resort, or by ferry from the little harbour of **Keyhaven**.

The mud flats and marshes run eastward to **Lymington**, an attractive market town whose popularity attests to it's position by the water and close to the southern fringes of the New Forest. Now a popular yachting centre, it's elegant streets lined with nautical boutiques and smart hostelries while every inch of shore-line appears dedicated to the parking of cars or the mooring of boats, it is hard to visualise this chic little town as being the great trading port that it once was. It's origins are ancient; it has to be one of the oldest charters in England, dating back to 1150.

Although the present facade of Lymington would appear smart and leisurely, it's trading past has far from disappeared; the international reputation of it's yacht designers, boat builders, sail makers and marine electronic manufacturers contribute significantly to the national export market, albeit in a less obvious manner than when the quays and warehouses bustled with rude life. The only commercial shipping that survives comes from the operation of the Lymington-Yarmouth ferry and a handful of fishing boats.

Some five miles to the north-east, set in the Forest and at the head of a lovely stretch of river, lies **Beaulieu** (the beautiful place), founded by the Cistercian monks more than 750 years ago. Now a ruin it's remains are still singularly beautiful and well-kept. The second Lord Montagu did much to preserve it and his successors have carried on the tradition in like manner. The present Lord Montagu took over the Abbey and retained only the Great Gate House (now known as Palace House), the porter's lodge, the cloisters, the lay brother's dormitory and the refectory, which has long served as the parish church.

Beaulieu apart from it's attraction as the site of a great religious house, lovely situation and immaculate small village is also home to the splendid **National Motor Museum**, which was founded by the present Lord Montagu in memory of his father, a pioneer motorist.

Downstream from Beaulieu lies the neat little community of **Bucklers Hard**, a single wide street of Queen Anne cottages that runs down to the river. Originally created by a Montagu for the importation and refining of sugar, political events in the West Indies made the development obsolete. Instead the site became one of the most famous naval shipyards in Britain, building many of the Royal Navy's most famous ships, including Nelson's favourite command, the Agamemnon. Today, yachts moor where the ships grew upon their slipways and **The Maritime Museum** at the top of the village recounts it's past glories.

Exbury Gardens, on the opposite bank of the river, are made up of 200 acres of the most stunning displays of shrubs, trees and flowers. Particularly beautiful are the spring-time displays of the noted Rothschild collection of rhododendrons, azaleas, magnolias and camellias.

A meandering cross-country drive brings one back to the heart of the New Forest, to it's capital **Lyndhurst.** This pleasant little town is the administrative headquarters of the Forest; the Verderer's Court meets six times a year at the Queen's House which is also the headquarters of the Forestry Commission. At **The New Forest Museum and Visitor Centre**, an excellent introduction to the history, customs, traditions, flowers and fauna of the area is provided through the medium of displays and audio-visual presentations. To my mind **Minstead** is the perfect New Forest village and it is here that Arthur Conan Doyle is buried. Although best known for his Sherlock Holmes stories, he also wrote many fine historical novels. His principal character in 'The White Company' becomes the spelndidly-titled Socman of Minstead, and Doyle obviously had much affection for the place for he and his wife spent several years there.

Heading eastwards, after the peace and tranquillity of the forest glades, the heavy traffic rumbling towards **Southampton** comes as an unpleasant shock. The city, much of it modern, appears initially as an industrial sprawl, with pylons marching along the low marshy ground towards the tall cranes that indicate the presence of the docks. Further investigation of this unprepossessing facade is richly rewarding; Southampton is a city that rewards the inquisitive - it's history is ancient and it's treasures many.

Although the M27 and it's associated developments are essential to the livelihood of this area of the country, there is no doubt that the great swathe of countryside that it occupies is lost to us forever; nevertheless charming pockets of rural calm are to be found with little trouble and often lie remarkably close to the motorway. Equally, if you have small children in tow who are not enamoured of churches and museums, then there are plenty of suitable entertainments. Both forms of attractions can be found in close proximity to each other, just off Junction 2 of the M27. **Paultons Park** is 140 acres of gardens and woodland that was once part of a large estate and has now been transformed into a family leisure park with fairground rides, boating lake, aviary, pet's corner and numerous other features that appeal particularly to the young.

The River Test flows south through the town of **Romsey**, where it once provided the power for milling and water for the many breweries. The town grew around the building of **Romsey Abbey**, founded in 907AD by Edward the Elder for his daughter, Ethelflaeda. Sixty years later, it was re-founded as a Benedictine nunnery by King Edgar. The abbey church was begun in the early part of the 12th century and construction continued over the next hundred years; it is second only to Durham cathedral as the finest Norman building in England.

The North Aisle acted as the townspeople's church and they must have been more than fond of the building and it's wonderful proportions because, at the Dissolution, they raised the sum of one hundred pounds to save it. The conventual buildings were destroyed but the church was saved; a wonderful bargain which is recorded by the Bill of Sale being displayed inside.

The peaceful tranquillity of the abbey is a cheerful contrast to the bustling little market town surrounding it. Some idea of the town's history can be gained in the **King John's House**, a 13th century stone upper-hall house containing a small museum. Tudor, Georgian and Victorian domestic architecture are to be found throughout the town centre and the local Preservation Trust has done an excellent job.

Broadlands, to the south of the town, once belonged to the Abbey. The Palladian style mansion was remodelled for the Palmerston family (a statue of the third Viscount who became Prime Minister stands in Romsey market place) by Capability Brown, who also laid out the surrounding parkland. It was later the home of Earl Mountbatten until his tragic death, and the stables have been converted to an exhibition of his life and career.

From Romsey it is easy to visit the **Hillier Arboretum** at **Ampfield**, where a world renowned display of rare and beautiful plants is set in 160 acres together with a magnificent collection of trees and shrubs.

The reformer William Cobbett (1763-1835) farmed at **Botley** to the east of Southampton and described it as 'the most beautiful village in the world.' Much has changed since he penned those words but the large village still retains a rural atmosphere. An important market was held here for many years and at one time there were fourteen inns catering to the coach and carriage trade. Two of them still survive, **The Bugle** and **The Dolphin**, as does the mill, the only one in Hampshire to be listed in the Domesday Book and still working. Until the 1930's small trading vessels would come up the River Hamble to Botley to load timber and corn.

I think Cobbett would have approved of the **Upper Hamble Country Park** to the south of Botely. This is a clever blend of working farm and preserved wood and marshland: bridle paths and walkways allow almost unlimited access and the traditional farm buildings house livestock as well as displays of old farm machinery.

The lower reaches of the Hamble River must contain more yachts than any other waterway in the world. A forest of masts bristle upwards from the marinas and moorings that run the entire length of the river, from Swanwick Bridge to the rivermouth. At first sight it hardly seems possible for any of them to move, but on closer inspection a reasonably wide channel is revealed, running up the middle of the rows of moored pleasure craft. Like Lymington, the industry on and alongside the water is yachting and from the boatyards have come many notable vessels, including America's Cup yachts and record-breaking power boats. Two pubs, **The Jolly Sailors** at **Burlesden**, and **The Bugle** at **Hamble**, are ideally situated for eating and drinking and watching life on the river go by.

Both villages were once renowned for ship-building and The Elephant, Nelson's ship at the Battle of Copenhagen was built next to the Jolly Sailors; the boatyard still exists there and proudly carries the same name.

Of course, the name of Nelson will always be associated with one ship in particular, that of HMS Victory, both she and many other links with the Royal Navy are to be found less than ten miles to the east, at **Portsmouth**. 'Pompey', as it is affectionately known to both servicemen and natives alike, is situated on a peninsula that projects southwards between the two natural harbours of Portsmouth on the western side and Langstone to the east.

Like it's civilian counterpart, Southampton, Portsmouth enjoys certain natural advantages: there is deep water throughout a large part of the harbour, the Isle of Wight offers shelter from much of the Channel weather and the narrow entrance is easily defended. These assets were first recognised by the Romans who ignored the site of present day Portsmouth and sailed right up to the top of the harbour, landing at what is now **Porchester**. Here they built **Porchester Castle**, the best preserved Roman fortress in northern Europe.

Undoubtedly the best place to start a tour of the city and it's heritage is at **The Royal Dockyard** which houses three of the world's major maritime attractions as well as an excellent museum. Indisputably the most famous of the three is **HMS Victory**, Nelson's flagship at Trafalgar. Beautifully restored and maintained she still serves as Flagship to the Commander-in-Chief, Portsmouth. Once on board, it is not hard to imagine the appalling conditions in which officers and men lived and worked, fought and died. Close by are the impressive remains of the **Mary Rose**, complete with exhibit's of thousands of artefacts salvaged from the ship. The third historical ship is **HMS Warrior**, who saw no battle action, but was the world's first steam-powered iron-hulled warship and was launched in 1860.

No visitor to the Dockyard should leave without viewing the excellent **Royal Naval Museum**, which contains much of interest relating to the Navy over the centuries. Other aspects of Naval and Military life are displayed in **Fort Nelson** near **Fareham**, the splendid **Royal Marines Museum** in Eastney Barracks on the Southsea front, **The D-Day Museum** which is adjacent to **Southsea Castle**, and **The Royal Naval Submarine Museum** across the water at **Gosport** (a good excuse to get afloat and see something of the harbour it'self).

For those with young children, **Southsea**, the southern tip of the peninsula, has much to offer with it's promenade, beach and common, which includes a boating lake and attractive gardens. Pleasure cruises around the Solent depart from **South Parade Pier** which, true to it's Edwardian beginnings, offers entertainment seven nights a week. Alongside **Clarence Pier** the only hover-craft passenger service in the country runs to the Isle of Wight.

North of Portsmouth one rapidly finds oneself back in the quiet charm of rural Hampshire. One moment it is all hustle and bustle with lorries, coaches and cars shooting past, while the next moment the scenery changes to narrow lanes, rolling green fields and small rural communities. A pleasant meandering drive westwards brings one to **Hambledon**, an isolated red-brick village celebrated as the early home of cricket,and in recent times for the fine vineyards planted on the chalk slopes behind the village. Cricket actually began some two miles to the north-east, on **Broadhalfpenny Down**, where Hambledon Cricket Club was the parent of the celebrated Marylebone Cricket Club. Hambledon's finest moment came in 1777; they played All-England and beat them by an innings and 168 runs. It is interesting to note that they played for the huge sum of one thousand pounds.

It seems only fitting in this area of England so riddled with contrast to finish with;'something completely different'. A little to the west is an area of gentle downland, once the site of a great estate belonging to the brother of Henry VIII's third wife, Jane Seymour. In this quintessentially English landscape, the visitor can come face to face with one of the world's rarest animals. Such exotica as Przewalski's horse, the snow leopard, or a scimitar-horned ibex are all to be found within the confines of **Marwell Park**. The park is a charitable foundation that exists to promote breeding and conservation of rare animals that are threatened with extinction. It is both a zoo, as well as a scientific and educational trust with the administration housed in the Tudor facade of Marwell House. For the young and young-at-heart, it is a splendid place to visit and a fine example of the many and diverse attractions that South Hampshire has to offer.

WEST SUSSEX

My tour began in the cathedral city of **Chichester**, just a few miles east of the border with Hampshire. A by-pass takes the heavy road traffic to the south where a beneficial by-product of modern development exists in the form of man-made lakes, created by excavation for gravel; now home to a rich variety of wild-life. Other than the Cathedral spire, little of the city's fine heritage can be glimpsed from the outskirts by the passing traveller, who sees a flat countryside bounded to the north by the distant South Downs. This fertile land used for growing a wide variety of crops, is also home to numerous light industrial estates that seem to fringe the northern edge of the by-pass.

From the north the approach is much more promising; the foothills of the Downs lead through handsome woodland and broadfields to catch the rise of the city's outskirts with a gentle slope to the copper-clad spire rising in the centre. Chichester is no grand cathedral city. It's scale is domestic and has the air of a prosperous market town: friendly and unpretentious with nothing to intimidate. Even the lovely Cathedral seems to stand at the pavement edge without benefit of grand close or walled surround. No great avenues or parades, merely a sensible crossroads of four main streets running out in the direction of the cardinal points and the areas in between being filled with a happy warren of lanes, narrow alley-ways and delightful little squares.

The cathedral started in the time of William the Conqueror has had many alterations. Bishop Seffrid added stone vaulting to the roof and the flying buttresses to take the external thrusts. These works are the essentials of the English Romanesque building we see today, with it's elegant internal proportions and soaring beauty. The Campanile that stands beside the Cathedral was built in the 1400's and the spire added about a hundred years later. Miraculously there was no loss of life when the spire collapsed on it'self in 1861 with ' no more than the noise produced by tilting a cartload of stone into the road'. Sir Gilbert Scott rebuilt the tower and spire between 1865 and 1867 and they stand as the principal landmark on Chichester Plain.

The four main streets meet adjacent to the north-east corner, and in the centre of the junction is a fine canopied **Market Cross**, built in 1501. These crosses generally marked the trading and administrative centre of a market and it is easy to imagine the streets thronged with people and produce brought in from the surrounding countryside. It is a delightful place and well worth your attention.

Chichester is representative of much of the county in that it's prosperity comes from it's ability to adapt without losing it's essential character. Outside the city, one does not have to travel far in order to find something of interest, and it was to **Fishbourne** I went to see **The Fishbourne Roman Palace and Museum**, one of the most important Roman relics in Britain and contains much of the remains of a magnificent 1st-century villa.

Just west of Fishbourne lies one of the jewels of the Sussex shore, the small Saxon village of **Bosham** (pronounced 'Bozzum'). Lying at the top of Chichester Harbour, this is a delightful little community jumbled around the waters of Bosham Creek. It's church, Holy Trinity, a fine Saxon building, is one of the most important in Sussex. Harold prayed here before departing from the village on his visit to Normandy in 1064, in a vain attempt to pacify his cousin William, and the scene is depicted in the Bayeux Tapestry.

I worked my way northward to the very border with Hampshire to visit **Stansted Park**, near **Rowlands Castle**. Ancient woodland, once part of the Forest of Bere, sets off this most decorative Wren-style house which is full of treasures. Collections of china and porcelain, fine furniture, tapestries and paintings are all displayed in the elegant rooms. There is an extraordinary and highly-decorative chapel which owes it's appearacne to a previous owner of the house who spent most of his time trying to convert Jews to Christianity.

From here, head across country to the B2147, a splendid Downland drive, where thick woodland alternates with pasture and plough and the road steadily climbs to the crest of the chalk hills. The Mardens, West, North, Up and East are all worth a diversion to visit the small churches and to admire the way in which the little communities seem to typify the essential South Down village. If you feel like stretching your legs, the **Stoughton Down Forest Walk** can be found to the south of **East Marden**.

Uppark is a National Trust property which was partially destroyed by fire in 1989 and has now been restored. One must admire the handsome facade designed by the architect William Talm who was also responsible for Stansted Park, the gardens by Humphrey Repton and the quite breath-taking views. Uppark has had a number of owners since it was built at the end of the 17th century and the most colourful of these must have been the splendidly rakish Sir Harry Fetherstonhaugh. He was in his early twenties when he inherited the house which soon housed his then mistress, the beautiful Emma Hart. Before long she had left the rackety Sir Harry to marry the diplomat Sir William Hamilton and later achieved further notoriety by becoming Lord Nelson's mistress. Her former lover never forgot her though, and when she fell on hard times after Nelson's death in 1805, Sir Harry helped her out.

The country to the north of Chichester is both varied and well-endowed with numerous attractions, both natural and man-made. From **West Stoke** a delightful walk takes one up to the escarpment of **Kingley Vale**, now under the administration of the Nature Conservancy Council. The Vale is most notable for it's ancient yew-woods, dark, dense and silent

A cheerful and lively contrast to the mystical, perhaps Druidical, stillness of Kingley Vale can be found in the nearby village of **Lavant** where the 17th-century pub, **The Earl of March**, dispenses good food and hospitality. The pub's name is the honorary title given to the eldest sons of the Dukes of Richmond, owners of the famous estate of Goodwood. **Goodwood House**, set in lovely parkland, lies a couple of miles to the east. The house is superb and contains innumerable treasures, but to me, the real attraction of Goodwood is the magnificent setting and the fact that the 12,000 acre estate is a diverse and working entity. Agriculture, forestry and recreation go hand in hand; the small airfield is surrounded by a once famous motor racing track (now used for testing and club events), and there is a golf course and a country park. The first Duke purchased the original Tudor house as a hunting lodge and, above all, it was the passion for all things equine that the Duke and his successors made the estate world famous. Today, international dressage competitions, horse trials and the principal attraction of 'Glorious Goodwood', Goodwood Races, bring enthusiasts and competitors from all over the globe.

During the Second World War the skies over this region of sleepy Sussex reverberated to the sound of supercharged aero-engines and cannon-fire. The Battle of Britain was fought principally from the RAF airfields of Sussex and Kent; one of the most famous being just south of the A27 at **Tangmere**. Headquarters of 11 Group, RAF Fighter Command, Tangmere played a key role in the Battle and it's importance was reflected in the savage German air raids of 1940. Later in the conflict, unit's based there were instrumental in developing night-fighting techniques and also in the covert delivery and retrieval of Allied agents in France. The airfield was closed in 1970, but the small village of Saxon origin has never forgotten the tragedies and glories of those days; on the green, a simple stone monument commemorates the airfield and it's squadrons. The graveyard of the simple little Early English Church of St Andrews contains neat headstones of British, Allied and German airmen, lying amongst the older monuments to generations of Sussex folk who could never have dreamt of war in the air. There is a small Military Aviation Museum close to the old runways with an excellent display of memorabilia and, fittingly, the village pub is named after one of the most famous of all fighter pilots. **The Bader Arms** opened in 1981, is one of the nicest modern pubs I have visited and an apt way to remember 'The Few'

The flat countryside was, of course, ideal for the construction of an airfield, but for centuries it's real worth has been agricultural and horticultural. **The Selsey Peninsula** has produced grain, vegetables, fruit and flowers for generations, and it's rich soil is keenly exploited. Nevertheless, it is an attractive area with small villages and reed-fringed rivulets, popular with holiday makers and yachtsmen. On the western side it is bounded by Chichester Harbour with the yachting centre of **Dell Quay** (once the original port of Chichester), **Birdham** (with it's Marinas and ancient Mill) and **Itchenor**, neat and trim beside the water. On the westernmost tip, close to the popular sands of **East Head**, is the small resort of **West Wittering**. Sounding rather like the title of an old BBC radio comedy, the village is attractive with a welcoming pub, **The Lamb Inn**, and a church that is definitely 'organic' - in that it is a happy mixture of period and styles. Since St Wilfrid landed not far from here on his zealous mission to convert the heathen Saxons, it is reasonable to suppose that the church's origins may lie in the first century AD.

The southernmost community of the peninsula, **Selsey,** looks out over a dangerous patch of water where shoals and currents have caught many a mariner unawares and the RNLI have a lifeboat station that is well worth a visit. Old Selsey, site of St Wilfrid's cathedral, lies under the sea off **Church Norton**, a remote hamlet on the southern side of the silted waters of Pagham Harbour, where wildfowl nest amongst the tall reeds.

Across the plain, the spire of Chichester cathedral with the muted Downs behind, acts like a beacon. My next foray was back into the hills, where I stopped at **West Dean** to admire the amazing variety of crafts being taught at the former home of that eccentric patron of the arts, Edward James. James was an early collector of surrealist art which may account for the strange sight in the grounds of two ancient beech stumps, complete with fungus, that are encased in resin. **West Dean College**, built in 1804 by James Wyatt, is now an educational trust teaching everything from furniture restoration to drystone-walling.

You must take the time to visit the **Weald and Downland Open Air Museum**. This is a collection of vernacular buildings from all over the county that have been painstakingly re-erected and restored to as near their original condition as possible. Cottages, mills and farm buildings are grouped attractively, and the site is brought alive by the presence of the rural crafts of the period - wheelwrights, potters, sawyers and charcoal burners. To inspect some of these 'idyllic' rural dwellings is to receive a salutary lesson; no sanitation or glazing and the 'central heating' being literally central - merely a fire in the middle of the earth floor! Some five miles to the north is **Midhurst**, a charming and prosperous little town with good brick and half-timbered buildings from across the centuries lining the streets around the centre. It's origins as a market town since the early 13th century are reflected in names such as Sheep Lane, Wool Lane, Duck Lane, and Knockhundred Row. A curfew bell is still rung at eight o'clock every evening; a tradition that was begun when a lone traveller was lost in the mist one night and the tolling of the Midhurst bell led him to safety. In gratitude the man bequeathed a piece of land to enable the bell to be rung in perpetuity.

Cowdray is the name given to the large estate that virtually surrounds Midhurst and the great blackened ruins of **Cowdray House** can be seen to the east of the town. It was begun in 1530, at the instigation of Shakespeare's patron, the Earl of Southampton and then passed to Viscount Montague, who had received Battle Abbey from Henry VIII. Legend has it that the last monk to leave the Abbey cursed Montague, prophesying that his family would perish by fire and water. It was an effective, although somewhat slow-acting curse; the house was burnt down in 1793 and shortly afterward, the then Viscount was drowned in Switzerland and his two sons at Bognor. The remains of the house have a tragic splendour and a look around gives an indication as to why it was once compared with Hampton Court as an example of courtly Tudor splendour. The estate, however, has prospered in the hands of the present owners, the Pearson family, and the great Park, with it's immense oaks, is internationally known as a venue for polo. From Midhurst, a pleasant drive takes one north towards the gentler hills of the Surrey border, although to the east of the main road lies **Blackdown**, the highest point in Sussex at 919 feet. It was a favourite beauty spot of Tennyson's, who described the view as 'green Sussex fading into the blue, with one grey glimpse of the sea.' The character of the countryside changes; it becomes more intimate with wood and copse interspersed by streams and small fields. The soil is heathy and acid with huge banks of rhododendrons hanging over some of the small lanes.

Heading south again, the third of Sussex's great estates is centred on **Petworth**, a lovely, if cramped little town, which has the reputation of being a centre of the antiques trade. It has a number of interesting 16th and 17th century buildings set around winding narrow streets and a small market place with a simple arcaded Town Hall from the 18th century. The town's condensed effect comes from being huddled against the great east wall of **Petworth House** which, with it's 700 acre deer park, dominates both town and surrounding countryside. It is a wonderful house now looked after by the National Trust, and contains magnificent paintings, sculpture and furniture, together with much exquisite carving by Grinling Gibbons.

To the east, the A283 runs close to the pretty village of **Fittleworth**, once the home of Sir Edward Elgar. A little further along the main road, passing over the medieval bridge at **Stopham**, is the 'longest village in Sussex', **Pulborough**. Settled since Neolithic times and lying beside a flood plain of the River Arun, Pulborough was once an important Roman encampment guarding Stane Street, which ran from Chichester to London.

The South Downs Way is some 80 miles of bridle and footpath that runs along the crest, affording riders and walkers views of some of the most lovely scenery in the country. South-west of the little hamlet of **Hardham**, the Way runs close to the **Bignor Roman Villa**. Site of an enormous farmstead and house where the wonderful Roman mosaics discovered in 1811, are displayed in a covered area. The wealth and importance of Sussex in earlier times are also seen in three other major attractions that lie not far away to the east. **Amberley**. A truly lovely village seated at the foot of downland overlooking grazing marshes, was considered of such strategic importance in the 14th century that the Bishop of Chichester built a massive castle, the remains of which surround the ancient manor house. The name Amberley is reputed to mean ' fields yellow with buttercups', and the setting is exquisite.

The nearby **Amberley Chalk Pit's Museum**, contains fascinating displays of bygone Sussex industries, crafts and skills including lime-kilns, wheelwright's shop, steam engines, a timber-yard, ironmonger's shop and narrow gauge railway. Further to the east is **Parham House**. One of the loveliest Tudor mansions, set in a deer park with a church standing on the lawns - all that is left of the medieval village. Surrounded by beautiful gardens, the house contains some wonderful treasures, including needlework said to have been done by Mary, Queen of Scots, and her ladies in waiting whilst imprisoned. Returning to the south-west, the village of **Slindon**, has a most attractive setting on the southern slope of the Downs. In common with much of the area, flint and brick are the principal building materials and the National Trust looks after many of the cottages and the 3,500 acre Slindon Park Estate. Cricketing enthusiasts will know that Slindon was the birthplace in 1718 of Richard Newland, considered by many to be the father of modern cricket. **Arundel** is the home of the premier Duke and hereditary Earl Marshal of England, the Duke of Norfolk, and it undoubtedly looks the part. Narrow streets wind up from the fast-flowing River Arun towards the immense turreted mass of **Arundel Castle**, with a great grey cathedral thrusting alongside. Trees and hills provide a backdrop to a sight that has the air of a Gothic fairytale. The interior is every bit as impressive as the exterior, with it's immense Hall, baronial library and lengthy gallery. The castle's owners have nearly always been Catholics and the fourth Duke of Norfolk's son, Philip Howard was canonized in 1970; he kept the faith, although persecuted and imprisoned during the reign of Elizabeth I. His remains are interred in the Cathedral of Our Lady and St Phillip, which was designed in the 1879's by A.J. Hansom, of Hansom cab fame. It is not a particularly distinguished building, unlike the parish Church of St Nicholas, a Perpendicular construction of the 14th century which is unique in containing the Catholic Fitzalan Chapel, divided from the Protestant main body by a screen. The town it'self has a great deal of charm, with some handsome Georgian frontages and buldings of timber, flint and brick crowding the narrow, steep streets.

Naturalists will be drawn to **The Wildfowl and Wetlands Centre**, a mile north of the town, where 64 acres of marsh and watermeadows are home to a wide range of tame and wild waterfowl, ranging from the humble mallard to the rare and exotic New Zealand Blue Duck.

The Arun flows into the sea at **Littlehampton**, a cheerful little portion of 'Sussex by the Sea'; a popular family resort with all the usual attractions of an English seaside town. Originally a small fishing settlement in Saxon times, the arrival of the railway in 1863 helped develop the small port into a resort. However, medieval Littlehampton was a far cry from the cheerful and unpretentious town of today; stone from the vast quarries of Caen was landed here and some of Henry VIII's warships were constructed on the banks of the Arun.

Remains of a far more ancient industry are to be found in the downs to the east of **Findon**. A pick, made from an antler, has been carbon-dated to 4000BC, and was one of the tools used by the Neolithic flint miners of **Cissbury Ring**. It is fascinating to stand on the slopes and contemplate these vast works which are still something of an archaeological conundrum, since no-one seems quite sure who the creators of this 78 acre fortress were, nor who were their enemies. All we know is that enormous numbers must have been required to raise the 60,000 tons of chalk that went into the construction of the ramparts and that a garrison of over 4,000 would have been required to effectively man it - but to what purpose?

Not far to the north lies an even better vantage point which must be the most famous landmark in Sussex. **Chanctonbury Ring** is a great clump of beeches planted around the remains of Neolithic earthworks. Although many of the beeches were blown down in the October 1987 storm, by a freak of nature, it was principally the inner trees that suffered and not those on the perimeter. Although it is a stiffish walk, the views over the magnificent rolling hills are wonderful. The site has mystical significance: the Romans built a temple here and witches used to meet here on Midsummer's Eve.

Echoes of Belloc are to be heard in the picturesque village of **Washington** where the beer served in **The Frankland Arms** so inspired the poet that he described it as 'nectar brewed in the waxing of the moon'. The Anglo-French Belloc would still approve of the pub to-day. The ale is well kept and the price is right!

Until the River Arun silted up in the 14th-century, Steyning was a busy port, but with the loss of a navigable waterway, it turned it's attention inland to become a busy market town and has retained much of the cheerful bustling atmosphere that goes with such activities. There are a number of good buildings including the splendid **Grammar School** founded in 1614.

The vagaries of the sea which turned Steyning into a market town were to benefit **Shoreham**, a town that is a thriving port and with a history stretching back to Roman times. The modern port of Shoreham Harbour is an enclosed dock, the largest between Southampton and Dover, and handles a tonnage nearly as great as the latter. Shoreham it'self is a busy little town, quite proud of it's historical importance; somewhere that is enjoyable to explore.

West Grinstead should not be confused with it's larger, but far distant relation, East Grinstead. They lie some 17 miles apart and whereas **East Grinstead** is a town, West Grinstead is little more than a hamlet. The real attraction here is the Church of St George, tucked away at the end of a lane overlooking the river. Once again the homely exterior belies the treasures inside; there are several brasses, one to a knight who fought at Agincourt, and a number of classical-syle monuments.

Lower Beeding is separated, like the Grinsteads, from **Upper Beeding**, by several miles of countryside. Also, for some unaccountable reason, Lower Beeding is well to the north and higher than Upper! However the real reason to visit has nothing to do with the somewhat eccentric nomenclature, but to see the wonderful gardens at **Leonardslee**. The Loder family have lived here since 1889 and have created magnificent woodland gardens within a deep valley. Streams and ponds lead the visitor past magnificent trees and shrubs, including world famous displays of rhododendrons, azaleas and camellias. Although springtime is obviously the most spectacular, the gardens are a year round attraction with deer and, believe-it-or-not, wallabies living semi-wild among the trees and grassy banks.

Leonardslee takes it's name from the surrounding forest of St Leonard, where the Saint, a French hermit is reputed to have slain a dragon. The blood from St Leonard's wound dripped to the ground where lillies-of-the-valley immediately sprang up. Later the hermit, who must have been more than a touch grouchy, banned nightingales from the forest, on the grounds that they disturbed his meditations. Whatever the truth, it is a fact that lillies still grow there and the nightingale is never heard....

Horsham is not unlike Chichester, in that it has a sensible arrangement of streets in the centre based on the cardinal points. The market town stands on the edge of St Leonard's Forest, and although it has become a commuter town, modernisation has not spoiled the charm to be found around the Carfax, the old centre (the word means a cross-roads), and in particular, the Causeway, a delightful tree-lined street of mainly 17th-century houses. **Causeway House**, a lovely late Tudor building houses the fascinating **Horsham Museum**. Just south of the town is **Christ's Hospital School**, and the pupils can often be seen walking around in their distinctive uniform of dark blue coat, white neck-band and yellow stockings. The dress is based on the Tudor uniform worn by those who attended the original school established by Edward IV in 1553.

South of **Crawley**, the bland new town close to Gatwick Airport, and close to the small community of **Handcross**, are the lovely National Trust Gardens at **Nymans**. These are a whole series of quite different gardens set in 30 acres around the gaunt but romantic shell of a burnt out house. The gardens are both formal and informal yet not in the least overpowering: Nymans has been described as a domestic garden on a grand scale rather than a grand garden on a domestic scale. Without a doubt, this is a truly Sussex garden.

Moving into what I am calling 'Mid-Sussex' one finds place names which are a delight. For example **Cuckfield** derives from the Saxon word 'Cucufelda' meaning a field full of cuckoos. This is a friendly village on the western skirts of the more sophisticated **Haywards Heath**. The two communities have a common link in that their past prosperity was based on transport. Cuckfield was a major coaching centre which survived until the advent of the railway in the middle of the 19th century which effectively killed off this lucrative and colourful trade almost overnight. However by refusing to accommodate this new fangled innovation, Cuckfield lost the financial rewards but retained it's rural charm, while the nearby hamlet of Haywards Heath rapidly expanded into the commuting and shopping centre of today. The excellent little **Cuckfield Museum**, in the High Street, is well worth a visit for it's wealth of local historical information, displays and relics.

The other community to refuse the benefit's of steam was **Lindfield**, on the opposite side of Haywards Heath. Although the financial penalties must have been severe at the time, the village's loss has been Sussex's gain; this is truly picturesque, situated on a gentle slope with the village pond at the bottom and the church, with it's tall spire, at the top. The houses are nearly all a delight, ranging from Tudor through to Georgian. There is a wonderful story concerning the Church House, which was once a pub called the Tiger Inn: apparently the ale it served to the bellringers in 1588, triumphantly signalling the defeat of the Spanish Armada, was so strong that it caused them to crack a bell and break all the ropes!

Hickstead is internationally famous in the equestrian world as the home of the **All-England Show Jumping Ground**; the arena with it's grandstand and supporting facilities is set in an attractive area just to the west of the A23 and close to the pleasant little village of **Sayers Common.**

The rear escarpment of the South Downs, the last geographical obstacle before reaching the coast is breached by the **Devil's Dyke**, where the Devil is said to have tried to dig a giant ditch through the Downs in order to let the sea through. His intention was to flood the lower Weald and drown the churches, but he was foiled by a woman holding a candle. The Devil, who could only work in the dark, mistook the light for the rising sun and fled.

It is well worth a diversion to the east, to skirt the hills on their northern side and to visit **Newtimber Place.** Although busy traffic rushes by within a few hundred yards, the moated house built in 1681 is close to perfection with mellow brick and flint facade. The steep woodlands of Newtimber Hill, together with the dewponds are owned and maintained by the National Trust.

High above the village of **Pycombe**, best known as a centre of the crook-maker's craft, stands two well-loved landmarks, a pair of windmills, christened Jack and Jill. A mile or so to the east, one of the highest vantage points on the South Downs gives some wonderful views. **Ditchling Beacon** stands at 813 feet above sea-level, towering over the village of **Ditchling** that lies in the lee of the Downs. Artists such as Sir Frank Brangwyn and Eric Gill lived here and the village has some lovely buildings; the best known being **Wing's Place** said to have been given by Henry VIII to Anne of Cleves.

South of the Downs is truly 'Sussex-by-the-Sea', and it's capital **Brighton** is the best loved town in the country. Like the favourite aunt in fiction it is now settling into quiet and prosperous middle age although the fondness for eccentric dress and garish make-up hint at it's lowly beginnings and a picaresque past.

The Royal Pavilion built for the larger than life, Prince Regent, has always been the most outrageous building but much of the other contemporary development was in restrained, albeit fashionable, form. Great crescents and squares, in classical Regency style, were built to house the cognoscenti and their households, and the town expanded into the neighbouring borough of **Hove**. Craftsmen and shopkeepers, provender-merchants and the like moved in to take advantage of the expansion. The railway came in 1840's bringing the town in reach of many more people. Hotels and boarding-houses sprang up to cater for this new trade, and the three miles of seafront were provided with elegant wide promenades, splendid piers, amusements and fairgrounds. Brighton has remained popular, if at one time having a slightly sleazy reputation both for those seeking extra-marital sex and a hideaway for the more disreputable members of London's gangland. Whatever the state, whatever the time Brighton has always welcomed visitors.

Newhaven is the second of the county's two main harbours and an important cross-channel ferry and cargo terminal whilst **Seaford** once the principal port of the area found a series of events caused the mouth of the River Ouse to be diverted to Newhaven. Now it is a quiet, prosperous seaside town. From Seaford Head, where there was once a Roman cemetery, there is a fine view of the **Seven Sisters**, the dramatic vertical chalk cliffs that mark the end of the South Downs. At their far end stands the towering bulk of **Beachy Head**; on a clear day the seaward view extends to over 60 miles from the 536 foot cliff.

Close to the meandering River Cuckmere which runs into the Channel and to the north of the secluded and idyllic village of **Westdean**, is the lovely **Charleston Manor.** The house dates, in parts, back to Norman times and is reputed to have been built for William the Conqueror's cupbearer. Later additions are Tudor and Georgian with medieval dovecote. This splendid mixture is handsomely set off by a remarkable garden, created by the artist Sir Oswald Birley. The rich alluvial soil has been planted in terraces divided by low yew hedges to give an effect that is a delightful combination of English and European.

Some three miles further up the river valley and set amidst lush water-meadows is **Alfriston**, once the smuggler's headquarters. Stanton Collins, the leader of the gang lived in the Market Cross Inn, otherwise known as the **Smugglers Inn**. By a trick of fate he was eventually caught and sentenced to transportation - but for sheep-stealing, not smuggling! The village is a popular beauty spot and has a setting that delights the eye. The National Trust made it's first ever acquisition here in 1896: **The Clergy House**, a simple thatched and timbered building of about 1350 - it cost them ten pounds!

Drusillas Park, to the north of the village, has been a favourite with families for over 60 years: a winning combination of children's zoo, gardens, workshops, amusements and restaurants. Attached to this is the rather more grown up attraction of **The English Wine Centre** which has it's own vineyard and museum.

Wilmington's attraction is obvious: carved into the chalk face of the downs above the village is the outline of a giant, with a staff in either hand. No one knows the origin of **The Long Man of Wilmington**, first recorded as late as 1779; it has been variously suggested that he was a Bronze Age chieftain, or the Saxon King Harold, or even an advertisement to guide pilgrims to **Wilmington Priory**. At **West Firle, Firle Place**, a Tudor mansion extensively remodelled in the 18th century, has been the home of the Gage family for 500 years. Set amongst wooded parkland beneath the 700 foot Firle Beacon, the house contains a fine collection of paintings and furniture.

North of the main road lies another handsome house, **Glynde Place,** also a mix of Tudor and Georgian architecture. The house contains much of interest, including collections of Bronzes, needlework and a small aviary.

Glyndebourne, is world renowned for the quality of it's opera. For over 50 years, opera lovers have flocked here to listen to the music and to enjoy picnicking in full evening dress, during the long interval.

Lewes has a solid and respectable charm with the old houses clustered round the castle on the hill, and it's steep streets and alleyways. **Anne of Cleves House**, Southover, once belonged to Henry VIII's 'Flanders Mare' and is an excellent place to begin a tour of the town since it is also a museum, containing items of local and county life and history.

Simon de Montfort spent the night before the Battle of Lewes in prayerful vigil at the Church of St Mary and St Andrew, **Fletching**. The church has a number of interesting brasses and Edward Gibbon (1737-94), the historian and author of 'Decline and Fall of the Roman Empire', is buried here. A close friend of John Baker Holroyd, the first Earl of Sheffield, Gibbon spent the last months of his life staying at **Sheffield Park**. The battlemented lodge and gateway lies just across the road from the church. The Park, landscaped by both Capability Brown and Humphrey Repton and now administered by the National Trust, was at one time as renowned for it's cricket as for it's beauty; the Australians used to play their first tour game here before Arundel became the venue. James Wyatt built the lovely Gothic Revival house in the 1770's and it is perfectly complemented by the superb landscape with rare trees and shrubs arranged around five lakes, set at different levels and linked by cascades.

One of the finest steam railways in the country is **The Bluebell Railway** which has it's southern depot, headquarters and museum close to the park entrance. Named after the flowers which grow along the entire length of the line this famous railway has operated steam locomotives to Horsted Keynes for over thirty years, and it is a sheer delight to chuff gently through the wooded Sussex countryside.

Uckfield grew with the advent of the railway although originally it was a small village at the intersection of the London to Brighton turnpike road and the more ancient pilgrim's route from Winchester to Canterbury. Just north of the town and with the charming postal address of **Herons Ghyll**, is the enterprising **Barnsgate Manor Vineyard**. This is a commercial vineyard and farm with a wine museum, vineyard trail and restaurant, together with banqueting and conference facilities.

The easternmost area of Sussex stretches along the coast from Eastbourne to Rye. It is lower lying than the county to the west, a pleasant, welcoming and varied landscape where small winding lanes take the visitor past farms, hamlets and villages which possess an almost timeless air. Deer browse in the shelter of thickets and wood, while fat fleecy sheep graze in gentle rolling pasture and ancient meadows. Well-pruned orchards are laid out with military precision, and along the Kentish border, the coned towers of oast houses denote hop-growing. Although the vast majority of these buildings seem to have been converted into what an estate agent's love of abbreviation would describe as a 'des res', the hop is still grown to flavour our ale.

Eastbourne is a refined, elegant and restrained town which started life as three sepearate communities: there was the old village of Eastbourne, some two miles inland, a small hamlet nearer to the sea called Southbourne, and Seahouses, a small resort on the shore, which was developed about 1780. The three mile seafront with it's terraced parades and fountained gardens is elegant, dignified and striking. In contrast to other South Coast resorts, one is immediately struck by the absence on the front of shops and amusement arcades. At night, with the gardens and fountains floodlit, the effect can be breathtaking. After having seen the sweeping grandeur of the front, with the sea breaking gently on the shingle and sand beach, it no longer seems unusual or incongrous that Claude Debussy should have written his greatest orchestral work 'La Mer' while staying here in 1905.

Martello towers are to be seen from the shore road leading eastwards, but at **Pevensey** there are traces of an older and greater fortification. The Saxon Shore Forts were built by the Romans and at Pevensey they constructed the fortress of Anderida to repel the northern invaders. When the Romans departed, the Romano-British took the fortress over, but after a six-month siege in 491AD, the Saxons took the castle and slaughtered every inhabitant. It is said that the Saxons never inhabited Anderida because of the savage deeds done that day and that the village was thus created. They took the name of the fortress and applied it to the vast hinterland of forest - Andreadswald, the Forest of Andred, later known as The Weald.

Pevensey has had a very bloodthirsty past; William of Normandy loomed out of the Channel haze and grounded in the creeks and inlets of what was then a swampy natural harbour. This was the beginning of the Norman Conquest. Even as late as 1940, **Pevensey Castle** was armed and manned against the threat of a German invasion. The Roman curtain walls still stand along with the 11th and 13th century gatehouse and keep. For all it's past history, it is now a pleasant place where tourists, holidaymakers and weekenders have been coming for years, enjoying the sea-breezes and the walks along the foreshore and visiting the local pubs.

The Pevensey Levels is the name given to the low-lying area of marsh inland from the town, once a region of shallow dykes and creeks until silting and storms filled the watery shallows. At the head of this area stands the striking shape of **Herstmonceaux Castle** built of Flemish brick in 1440. By the time it was finished, the introduction of the cannon had made that form of medieval fortress redundant; nevertheless, it is a satisfyingly solid structure that could grace any romance involving knights in armour and damsels in distress. When it was finished it had a window for every day of the year and a chimney for every week; it was restored after decades of decay in 1913 and occupied by the Royal Observatory until recently. Herstmonceaux is the centre of a peculiarly Sussex craft - the manufacture of trugs; gardening baskets made of willow and somewhat boat-shaped in construction.

Bexhill is the next coastal town to the east. It was created almost by Lord de La Warr, who in 1885 began by building on his land that lay between the original village and the sea. It's outstanding feature today is the **De La Warr Pavilion**, a grade one listed architectural masterpiece, designed in 1933 by the German, Erich Mendelsohn. Overlooking the sea, it houses an 1,100-seat theatre, restaurants, bars and function rooms. Popular for conferences, seminars and the Annual Bridge Congress. Whilst it does not have quite the character of Eastbourne, it is nonetheless a neat and clean community with good shops and facilities. It has a large retired population and a solid core of faithful holidaymakers who return year after year.

St Leonards is another resort created in the 19th century around an ancient parish and then there is **Hastings**, who in common with other towns on this once troubled shore, has had an epic history; a past that is not easy to divine at first sight of this cheerful and easy-going seaside resort. In addition to it's well documented history, from the 14th century onwards smuggling, fishing and boat-building appear to have been the principal occupation of the inhabitants, who managed these occupations from the unprotected shingle beach. Immediately below the East Cliff is an area known as The Stade, from the Saxon meaning landing-place. To this day, boats are still drawn up the shingle by winch to lie alongside the extraordinary narrow tall net-sheds. These structures date from Tudor times and were built in this odd manner for two remarkably sensible reasons. The smallbase area meant paying less ground rent, and the tall height meant that the fishermen could work out of doorways on the mast and rigging as well as the hull. The nearby fishmarket is also of historic interest; by local custom the auctioneer starts with a high price and works down, leaving the bidder just one chance to buy. Along the quaintly named Rock-A-Nore Road there is also a Fisherman's Museum, Shipwreck Heritage Centre and an aquarium, the Sea Life Centre.

Linked closely with the story of Hastings is the little town of **Battle**, where Harold met William at what is known as the Battle of Hastings although it actually took place some six miles from the town at Semlac Hill, on October 14th 1066. The town is delightful, with a mainly Georgian High Street running up from the Abbey, with a number of arched entrances between the buildings acting as reminders of the days when coaches needed to pull into the yards of inns. The town has good inns and hotels and in Langton House is the **Battle Museum** with it's reproduction of the Bayeux Tapestry and diorama showing the disposition of William and Harold's troops. The High Street leads on to the original London Road, Mount Street, where period cottages, houses and shops line the road, has a white painted windmill at it's summit.

Talking of windmills, the A259 takes one past the oldest windmill in Sussex, dating from 1670, at **Icklesham**, and on to **Winchelsea**, sometimes described as the smallest town in England. It really is no more than a small village, although it still boasts a mayor and corporation. Peaceful and utterly charming in the late 20th century, it's past is every bit as bloodthirsty and tragic as any of the ancient towns of the Sussex Shore, having been destroyed by storm, razed by French raids and de-populated by plague.

Looking eastwards across the flats where the River Brede wanders is arguably the most beautiful small town in Britain, **Rye**. Like it's neighbour, it also suffered at the hands of the sea and the French, but survived through a combination of good fortune and the tenaciousness of it's citizens. Julius Caesar noted that they were ' fierce and hostile' and the citizens of the little town had no compunction about turning to piracy and smuggling when times were hard. The town stands on a hilltop, now two miles from it's harbour mouth. It's narrow cobbled streets probably have a greater concentration of old houses and more of the atmosphere of a 16th-century town than anywhere else in the country. G.K. Chesterton described it as ' that wonderful inland island, crowned with a town as with a citadel, like a hill in a medieval picture.' The waters of three rivers, the Tillingham, the Brede and the Rother combine to scour a channel through the marshy flats to the sea and small craft can still make their way up on the tide to lie alongside the ancient wharves under the town.

Although the town is a major tourist attraction, it is still very much a working community and there is no feeling of being 'preserved in the Aspic of Time'. Rye is a market town and still retains a fishing fleet. There are boat yards, chandlers and marine engineers alongside the more obvious attractions of the antique shops and craft galleries.

North of the town is **Rye Foreign**. There are two theories as to the origin of this odd name and both equally convincing since they are based on fact. The first is that the manor of Rye was given by King Canute to the Abbey of Fecamp in Normandy. This was fine until King John lost

Normandy in 1204; a legal and political wrangle then began which was not resolved until Henry III negotiated the town's return to crown governance. However, one small area was not returned - hence Rye Foreign. The other theory is that most of the French Protestant refugees, the Huguenots, who settled in Rye during the 17th-century, chose to live in their own community on the edge of the town - hence Rye Foreign. Take your pick!

Northiam is an interesting place with it's fine green surrounding an ancient oak. Queen Elizabeth I dined under this tree in 1573 and left her green shoes behind as a memento. These are kept in Brickwall, one of the two most notable houses in this attractive village. **Brickwall**, an elaborate timbered house of 1633 is now a school and occasionally open to the public and takes it's name from the high surrounding wall. The other house is **Great Dexter**, a 16th-century timbered half-house which was beautifully restored and enlarged by Sir Edward Lutyens, while the superb gardens were laid out and planted by Gertrude Jekyll and the house's owner, Nathaniel Lloyd.

If you have an interest in gardening - not for nothing is this area known as the 'Garden of England' - then it is well worth heading north to visit **Sissinghurst Castle**. This was once a great fortified Tudor manor house, built by a courtier of Henry VIII's known locally as 'Bloody Baker'. Sir John Baker came from neighbouring Cranbrook and his grasping and self serving ways, not to mention his persecution of Protestants, made him distinctly unpopular. After a generation or two, the family fortunes declined and the massive brick structure lay neglected, unused except as a prison for French prisoners-of-war, and later, as the Parish Poor House. Horace Walpole described it as 'a park in ruins and house in ten time greater ruins'. The main part of the building was pulled down in the early 1800's, probably rendered unsafe by the fact that the French prisoners had torn out much of the woodwork and many of the structural timbers for use as fuel. This desolate wreck was rescued by Harold Nicholson and his wife, Vita Sackville-West, in 1930. The home and garden they created from such dereliction is magnificent: a White Garden, a walk of limes, roses climbing all over the ancient brick and a medieval herb garden. The house, created from ruins, is unusual and romantic: the whole is a memorial to two writers whose creativity did not end with pen and ink.

Another writer, the historical novelist, Jeffrey Farnol, used the village and it's delightful pub, **The Bull**, in a number of his books. Obviously, there must be something inspirational in the atmosphere.

Rye is brought back to mind by the village of **Hawkhurst** - headquarters of a notorious smuggling gang.

'Five and twenty ponies
Trotting through the dark -
Brandy for the parson,
Baccy for th clerk:
Laces for a lady, letters for a spy,
And watch the wall, my darling, while
The Gentlemen go by'.

Kipling, who knew the area well, caught the atmosphere of those days in his 'Smuggler's Song' As we know the gangs terrorised the neighbourhood in much the same manner as the Mafia have behaved in Sicily. 'Watching the wall' was the only way for most ordinary folk to survive; the smugglers openly flouted the law, bribing and threatening where appropriate, and openly spending their ill-gotten gains in building large houses with large barns for storing contraband. Some of these houses were built in Hawkhurst, which was ideally positioned for the 'carriers' bringing their contraband from Rye and Romney Marsh. Although many petitions were sent to Parliament it was not until 1747 that matters came to a satisfactory conclusion - although not from the smuggler's point of view. The inhabitants of another village, **Goudhurst**, who had also suffered from the criminal activities of the 'gentlemen' and who additionally had the misfortune to be fellow-villagers of the gang's leader, one Tom Kingsmill, banded together to form a well-organised militia. Kingsmill, hearing of their activities, swore that he would ' boil four of the militiamen's hearts and eat them for supper'. In the pitched battle that ensued Kingsmill was killed by 'the discharge of a lead bullet'. In this he was fortunate, for several of his fellows were hanged and their bodies displayed in chains throughout the area. Hawkhurst is now a quiet and peaceful village-cum-town, and the only excitement in recent years was when the lovely glass in the church was blown out by a flying-bomb in 1944.

Finally on this tour I went to the village of **Lamberhurst**, known for it's vineyard and also for the wonderful garden in the care of the National Trust, **Scotney Castle**. This has to be one of the most romantic gardens in England: the moated ruins of a 14th-century castle with a 17th-century manor house attached, surrounded by an abundance of trees, rhododendrons and azaleas. Not far away is another lovely garden that of the **Owl House**. A small 16th-century timber-framed building, the house once belonged to a wool smuggler; it's treasures today are in it's grounds and gardens.

Restaurant - **CORIANDERS**

66 Devonshire Road, Bexhill-on-Sea, East Sussex TN40 1AX

Tel: 01424 220329

For the last decade Ken and Carolyn Simmons have run this very successful vegetarian restaurant in the centre of Bexhill. Imaginative and beautifully presented dishes are created by Ken Simmons for a menu that changes according to the season and the availability of fresh produce. Vegan options are always on offer. The food is 100% wholemeal which is very apparent in the wonderful array of cakes and pastries. Corianders is a warm, cosy and intimate place seating 50 people comfortably. The restaurant is strictly non-smoking and at all times it is self service. Whilst the wine list is small it does have some very interesting English wines, 50% of which are vegetarian and four are organic. Lager and ales are on sale and Kaliber is stocked for those who prefer a non-alcoholic tipple. The Simmons also have self-catering holiday flats on Bexhill Seafront. Anyone staying there will be very comfortable and have the added advantage of a 10% discount on all meals taken at Corianders.

USEFUL INFORMATION

OPEN; 9-5pm daily. Closed Christmas Easter and Bank Holidays
CREDIT CARDS; None taken
CHILDREN; Welcome
LICENSED; Yes. English wines only

ON THE MENU; 100% wholemeal. Specialises in cakes and pastries
DISABLED ACCESS; Yes + toilets
GARDEN; No
ACCOMMODATION; Not applicable

Hotel - **GRANVILLE HOTEL**

124 Kings Road, Brighton, BN1 2FA

Tel: 01273 326302 Fax: 01273 728294

The ethos of this excellent hotel on Brighton's Regency seafront is that staying in an hotel should be an adventure and a memorable experience and with this in mind the hotel has been designed with flair and style to offer something excitingly different. There are 23 individually designed bedrooms each with a sumptuous en-suite bathroom and most have sea views. The rooms have interesting names as well. The Brighton Rock Room is pink and white, the Noel Coward room has a superb Art Deco bathroom, the magnificent Balcony Room with it's large four-poster bed and balcony overlooking the sea, has a double jacuzzi in the bathroom, the Marina room boasts a water bed and for something really different The Black Rock Room is - all black! Trogs Restaurant offers gourmet cuisine in a very pretty candlelit room and you will see from the menu that the hotel prides it'self on it's outstanding vegetarian food as well as other dishes. All the dishes are prepared using organic ingredients whenever possible. In the Cafe Bar you can enjoy continental beers and organic wines as well as light snacks and other drinks. Positioned in the Town Centre Glanville's is ideal for many reasons. The visitor will find it is convenient for everything that goes on in Brighton and for the business man or conference delegate the hotel is a mere 300 yards from the Brighton Conference Centre and next door to the Metropole Hotel Conference and Exhibition Halls.

USEFUL INFORMATION

OPEN; All year
CHILDREN; Welcome over 5 years
CREDIT CARDS; All major cards
LICENSED; Yes
ACCOMMODATION; 23 ensuite rooms
PETS; Welcome

ON THE MENU; Superb gourmet food
CAFE BAR; Light snacks
VEGETARIAN; Excellent choice of dishes
DISABLED ACCESS; No special facilities
Parking available nearby

Hotel - **PASKINS HOTEL**

19 Charlotte Street, Brighton, East Sussex BN2 1AG

Tel: 01273 601203 Fax: 01273 621973

In 1783 the Royal Pavilion was built for the Prince Regent, it has wonderful onion domes which imitate Indian Palace architecture, it was extended in 1812 by John Nash, at night the floodlights transform it into an enchanting fairytale palace. Brighton is charming with graceful Georgian and late Victorian buildings, antique shops where a bargain or two could be had, history and art displays at museums and galleries, and natural history in the Booth Museum. Promenade and piers, the Volks Electric Railway and the Sea Life Centre, your days here will be filled to overflowing.

With so much going on you will need a place to stay and there is nowhere better than Paskins Hotel. Situated in Kemp Town, just off the sea front, this hotel has so much to offer, from the comfortable bedrooms to the lounge bar. The bedrooms are well appointed, most with ensuite, all with direct dial telephone, television and a tea and coffee tray, several even have the luxury of a four-poster bed. The Resident's Lounge Bar is inviting where you are able to relax, enjoy a drink and the company of your fellow guests. The food here is very special with delicious breakfasts including various fruit's, compote, juices or cereals followed by a sumptuous cooked meal. Most of the food is produced organically and bought fresh from local farms, including free range eggs, organic tomatoes and mushrooms, the difference in taste is incredible. All the meat is local. The vegetarian breakfasts are a real treat with such tempting delights as tarragon and sun dried tomato sausages and ten nut and seed sausages. Superb. Paskins Hotel is ideally situated close to all of Brighton's amenities. There are lots of restaurants to chose from all serving a variety of dishes. So come and taste the delights of Brighton and stay at this comfortable and friendly hotel.

USEFUL INFORMATION

OPEN; All year

CHILDREN; Welcome

CREDIT CARDS; Visa/ Mastercard/ Access/Eurocard/Diners

LICENSED; Wines & Real Ales

RESTAURANT; Excellent fresh organic and local produce, free range eggs

VEGETARIAN; Delicious breakfast with choices

DISABLED ACCESS; No

ACCOMMODATION; 20 rooms, ensuite and standard

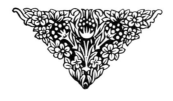

BURPHAM COUNTRY HOUSE HOTEL

Old Down, Burpham, West Sussex. Tel: 01903 882160

V/VG. Children. LIC.

Restaurant & Tearoom - **CASSANDRA'S CUP**

Winchester Road, Chawton, Nr Alton, Hampshire GU34 1SB

Tel: 01420 83144

Follow the signs to Jane Austen's house and there, immediately opposite, is Cassandra's Cup, in the picturesque village of Chawton. This is an enchanting tea room with antiques, crafts and gifts as well as offering delicious home-cooked English food which includes a number of dishes expressly for Vegetarians, although it has to be admitted that they are so tasty carnivores are frequently tempted. Most of the food is prepared and cooked on the premises but a small percentage of desserts and main courses are bought in.

Cassandra's Cup is licensed and has a small but interesting number of European wines. Everything is reasonably priced and the standard extremely high, indeed they have been awarded a certificate of excellence. It is a treat to look forward to after visiting the fascinating home of Jane Austen, one of England's favourite authors.

USEFUL INFORMATION

OPEN; 10.30-4.45pm (winter 4.30pm) **ON THE MENU;** Excellent homecooked fare
The days & hours are limited from **DISABLED ACCESS;** Yes + toilet with a little
October-March   difficulty
CREDIT CARDS; None taken

Restaurant - **CLEMENTS VEGETARIAN RESTAURANT**

Rickmans Lane, Plaistow, West Sussex RH14 0NT

Tel: 01403 871246

Unashamedly Upmarket, Clements vegetarian restaurant in Rickmans Lane, Plaistow, a small village on the Surrey/Sussex border and 12 miles from Guildford, is one of the best anywhere. Liz and Dave Clement bought an old pub in 1989 and converted it into this stylish and beautifully run establishment. Here you will find a strictly no smoking environment with an attractive decor, in which every table is laid immaculately. The napkins are crisp linen, the fine glasses sparkle and the soft candlelight enhances the atmosphere.

Listed as one of the 10 top restaurants in the 'Vegetarian Good Food Guide' and runners up in the 1993 National 'Vegetarian Restaurant of the Year' competition, one would expect the food to be outstanding and one is never disappointed. For such an outstanding establishment the prices are realistic. The menu changes regularly. All the food is freshly prepared on the premises. The 24 choices on the wine list are all organic and vegetarian from around the world. In summer there are 10 tables in the pretty garden - an additional reason for coming here. A brochure is available, if you ring the restaurant, which includes a copy of the take-away menu and price list.

USEFUL INFORMATION

OPEN; All year Lunch: Tues-Sat 12.30-2.30pm **ON THE MENU;** International dishes
(last orders 1.30pm)By reservation only everything made on premises. Outside
Eves: Tues-Sat 7-11pm catering for weddings etc
CREDIT CARDS; Access/Visa **DISABLED ACCESS;**
                                                            Yes, but no special toilets
CHILDREN; Welcome at lunchtime **GARDEN;** Delightful countryside
LICENSED; Yes. All vegetarian & organic setting
wines from around the world

Guest House - **THE FESTING GROVE GUEST HOUSE**

8 Festing Grove, Southsea PO4 9QA

Tel: 01705 735239

This comfortable, conveniently situated Guest House has been awarded the AA 3 Q's and the English Tourist Board 2 Crowns Commended but that does not really do justice to the care and consideration given to guests. For example early morning ferry travellers are catered for, and the Good Food Hygiene Standards 'Seal of Excellence' confirms how spotless the house is. Business travellers find themselves welcomed all year round and given the opportunity to relax totally after a strenuous working day. You will find Festing Grove Guest House near the seafront and the Ferry Port in a quiet residential area of Southsea and yet only 3 minutes walk from the Canoe Lake, Rose Gardens and the South Parade Pier. It is ideal for anyone wanting to visit the maritime attractions of Portsmouth and the historical sites of Hampshire.

The bedrooms are well furnished with hostess trays and colour TV. Ensuite rooms are available. In the Lounge Satellite TV is available, there is easy parking. In fact there is everything you could wish for including a first class breakfast for both Vegetarians and others. The Festing Grove is a predominantly non-smoking house.

USEFUL INFORMATION

OPEN; All year
CHILDREN; Welcome
CREDIT CARDS; None taken
ACCOMMODATION; Comfortable rooms, some ensuite

ON THE MENU; Excellent vegetarian breakfast as well as other choices
DISABLED ACCESS; No special facilities

Hotel - **SEASHELLS HOTEL**

7 Burlington Road, Swanage, Dorset BH19 1LR

Tel: 01929 422794

This very nice RAC Acclaimed Vegetarian and Non-Smoking hotel is opposite a sandy beach with glorious countryside in the Purbeck Hills. Owned and run by Brian Slater, Annie Campbell and her mother, Mary Lloyd, it is a delightfully informal establishment in which guests feel comfortable and very much at home. Open all the year there are special off season breaks available and quite frankly, Dorset is almost nicer in the autumn and winter when there are less people about and one can enjoy great bracing walks along the beach and coastline sometimes without seeing another human being. The Spring and Summer are lovely as well. Dorset is one of the most attractive of English counties and offers everything from sporting activities to stately homes, wonderful gardens, fascinating villages and splendid old towns like Sherborne and Shaftesbury.

The food at Seashells is memorable with dishes for vegetarians and vegans. The bedrooms are charmingly furnished with ensuite facilities, colour television and a well supplied tea/coffee tray. There is ample parking.

USEFUL INFORMATION

OPEN; All year
CHILDREN; Welcome
CREDIT CARDS; None taken
PETS; Not permitted

ON THE MENU: Excellent breakfast with a wide choice. Evening meal on request
LICENSED; Yes
NO SMOKING THROUGHOUT

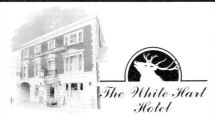

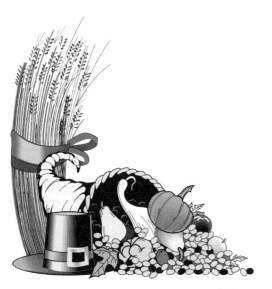

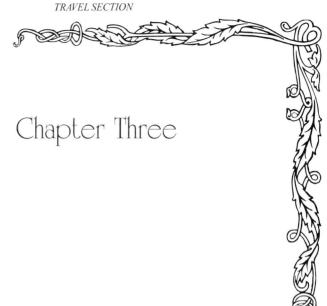

Chapter Three

The Home Counties
The Thames Valley
& Greater London

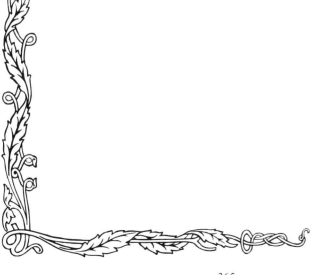

HOME COUNTIES, THE THAMES VALLEY & GREATER LONDON
GLOUCESTERSHIRE, OXFORDSHIRE, BERKSHIRE, BUCKINGHAMSHIRE
BEDFORDSHIRE, HERTFORDSHIRE & SURREY

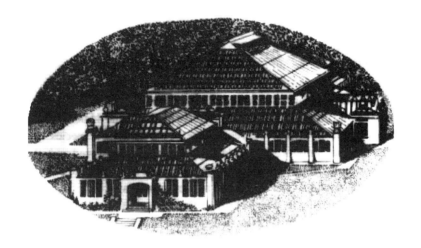

INCLUDES

The Home Counties, The Thames Valley and Greater London includes Gloucestershire, Oxfordshire, Berkshire, Buckinghamshire, Bedfordshire, Hertfordshire, Surrey and Greater London

These counties, from the upper estuary of the Severn to the broad, chalk basin of the lower Thames valley, have all been prosperous, for a variety of reasons, throughout much of this millenium, and therefore have a wealth of fine large buildings - domestic, church and state - from many periods. These are now mixed in all but the western part of the region with large new estates, and even with new towns which have been a feature of this century as the counties' populations have increased in dramatic stages. The region also contains much natural beauty, the many pretty small woods and valleys dominated by the high points of the Cotswolds, the Malvern Hills, the Chiltern escarpment and the Berkshire Downs, crossed with ancient paths and offering some quite breathtaking views, often across many counties.

Gloucestershire, the western-most and most rural of these counties offers a diversity of landscape, history and culture: from the timeless scattered stone villages of the Cotswolds, through the rivermeadows of the Severn Valley to the natural magnificence of the Royal Forest of Dean. There are several Roman relics in the county, the remains of some of the fifty luxury villas that once stood.

Rare species of flora and fauna can be found in the lush undulating tree-lined landscape of the Cotswolds and this 'Area of Outstanding Natural Beauty' also has man-made beauty - even the largest farmhouses blending into the landscape with a mellowness that stems from the local stone used.

The Cotswolds have remained open country because of the suitability of the land for sheep rearing, and the wealth earned from the wool trade as far back as the 15th century. It was the wool merchants who were responsible for the building of many wonderful Cotswold churches which often appear to be far too ostentatious for the villages they serve. It would seem the predelictions of the patrons were frequently given their due, and the superb stained glass windows of the church at **Chipping Camden** include one showing the Eternal Pit into which the damed are being pitchforked - all the damned being women!

Each year in early summer the streets of Chipping Camden are alight with a torch procession, to mark the close of the **Cotswold Olimpicks,** founded in 1612 and more recently revived. The extraordinary 'games' include 'Shin Kicking' and 'Pikes and Cudgels'! If you love gardens then **Hidcote Manor Garden** is one of the most delightful in England, famous for it's rare trees and old roses as well as it's open-air Shakespeare performances in the summer. Only a few miles away is **Kiftsgate Court,** another garden worth visiting.

Magnificent views on the edge of the Cotswolds are to be seen from **Birdlip** and from **Leckhampton** by the 'Devil's Chimney'.

In contrast to the Cotswolds, the vale of the Severn river is a flat land with **Tewkesbury** showing it's Tudor origins in the black and white timbered buildings in the centre of town. The town has one other special feature, the Norman **Tewkesbury Abbey**. Here are buried the remains of the Duke of Clarence who, it is said, drowned in a vat of Malmsey wine. If you want to learn more of this lovely old town and it's surroundings then take a look at **John Moore Countryside Museum** in the abbey precincts. The Abbey it'self is a feast for the eye and balm for the soul.

It was in the 12th century that William of Malmesbury wrote 'no county in England has so many or so good vineyards', and the tradition continues with vineyards such as the **Three Choirs Vineyards** near **Newent**, a producer with a particularly high reputation and many awards. Having started with an experimental ½ acre it now covers 65 acres with several grape varieties and a potential for 250,000 bottles annually.

From Tewkesbury the River Severn flows to the county town of **Gloucester** with it's several excellent museums including the **National Waterways Museum** at the historic **Gloucester Docks**, both of which are on the riverside walk from Tewkesbury, which then passes the extraordinary **Severn Bore**, a noisy wave from the Bristol Channel that, at high spring tide, can reach seven feet high. Near the docks is the **Museum of Advertising** and in the **Gloucester Folk Museum** a roughly carved stone figure holding an animal is said to be of Dick Whittington and his cat. Dick Whittington lived at **Pauntley** before moving to London where he became Mayor, but unlike the story he was in fact born into a wealthy family.

Along the main road from Cheltenham towards Oxford one passes through **Northleach.** This quiet old village has a magnificent church and also is home to **The Countryside Collection** on the **Fosse Way**. Once a House of Correction it now houses displays of rural life along with the 'Below Stairs' gallery and special exhibitions each season. Here too, on a smaller scale is the **World of Mechanical Music** dedicated to antique clocks, musical boxes, automata and mechanical musical instruments, a special and magical place.

Further still down the river path in the Vale of Berkeley, as the river widens into the Severn estuary, the saltmarshes at **Slimbridge** are famous as **The Widlfowl and Wetlands Trust Centre,** founded by Peter Scott. It's 73 acres protect the largest and most diverse collection of wild waterfowl in the world with, in winter, over 2,300 birds of 180 species including swans, ducks, geese and flamingoes as well as rare and exotic wildfowl, some of which can be seen from the hides, and some which will feed from your hand. The Centre even includes special facilities for not only wheelchair-bound but also the blind.

By the opposite bank of the river, close to the Welsh border, the largest holly trees in England are dotted among the oaks and the birches of **The Royal Forest of Dean**, one of the few true forests remaining. Some 2,000 miles of woodland paths pass alongside grazing land used by commoners who are referred to rather oddly as 'Ship-badgers'. Many of the hills and dales are actually tips and dips caused by coal and tin mining over the past 2,500 years as can be seen on a journey deep underground at **Clearwell Caves and Mining Museum. The Dean Heritage Centre** is a museum of forest life, it's industrial heritage and natural history, coming up to date with craft workshops. Contemporary art is also on view on the **Sculpture Trail**, a circular walk from Beechenhurst, featuring 18 sculptures among the trees.

Some of the many, especially pretty, villages and small towns in Gloucestershire include **Bourton-on-the-Hill** with the manor of **Sezincote** in Hindu-Gothic style which was the inspiration for Brighton Pavilion: **Bourton-on-the-Water** which has a number of small museums and similar attractions: **Stanton**, a single street of pretty houses: **Adlestrop** where King Alfred took refuge when Wessex fell to the Vikings in the 1st century AD: **Lechlade** where the three counties meet, a town with a suprising number of gazebos and summer houses; and **Chalford** with it's very narrow and winding lanes.

For sheer elegance little could surpass **Cheltenham's** Regency terrace and wide tree-lined avenues, an ideal location for the annual festivals of music and literature. I love it for it's shopping and most of all for probably the prettiest race course in the country. Everything stops in Cheltenham at the time of race meetings. Every hotel, guest house etc is full to the gunnels and wherever you go the conversation has an equestrian flavour.

Gloucestershire's eastern border along the Cotswolds gives onto Oxfordshire. In the north the county is gentle and undulating, running down to the Thames Valley towards the south and rising in the east towards the Chilterns with **Oxford**, 'That sweet city of dreaming spires' in the centre.

The university influences much of life in and around Oxford. The earliest Oxford colleges were founded in the 13th century, and many exceptionally fine and hugely impressive college buildings elegantly dominate the town centre. Most of the college quadrangles are occasionally open to the public as are some of the halls and chapels and other important buildings.

Oxford is a lively place, with many concerts, plays and meetings each evening, and with delightful pubs and restaurants. It can also boast what is not surprisingly, the only **Marmalade Museum**, in the world, and there is an enchanting **Museum of Doll's Houses**.

On any fine summer day punts aplenty are to be seen on the Cherwell, whilst not far away the university rowing crews practice for their many challenges, including the University Boat Race. **Henley-on-Thames**, a straight wide stretch of river is the site each July of the Henley Royal Regatta, and the town it'self is not unexceptional although it is overshadowed by the beauty of the surrounding wooded hills.

Henley is the finishing point of **The Oxfordshire Way** which takes walkers on a route linking the Cotswolds and the Chilterns, starting in Bourton-on-the-Water. A walk beside the Thames from Henley to **Goring** is said to be one of the most beautiful walks possible, just one tiny stretch of the newly opened **Thames Path** developed by the Countryside Commission, running from the source of the Thames in Gloucestershire through London to the Thames Barrier.

Oxfordshire has many attractive towns and villages: the village of **Burford** is renowned as one of the most beautiful in Britain and one where I stay whenever I get the chance to attend a Cheltenham Race meeting. Close enough to Cheltenham and peaceful enough to relax over a splendid dinner at night, hopefully paid for by ones winnings! The county also has other contenders for the title such as **Great Tew, Ewelme, East Hendred, Adderbury; Dorchester**, a cathedral city from 634 to 707AD; **Cornwell** rebuilt in the 1930's by the eccentric Clough Williams Ellis of Portmeirion fame: and **Uffington**, well described in 'Tom Brown's Schooldays'.

Abingdon, once the County Town of Berkshire, offers wonderful buildings from the medieval period onwards, and **Faringdon** too is an elegant town with fine architecture. The notable **Farringdon House** gardens are occasionally open, and here you can see the doves, their feathers stained in bright colours! The town of **Witney** bears witness to it's success in the wool trade, having long been famous for blankets. At **Hook Norton** the **Brewery** is the source of some highly regarded real ale, the Victorian building it'self being an odd mixture of all sorts of random materials.

This is Morris Dancing country, **Bampton** Morris being one of the most important traditions, their dances often now performed in other places, but the Bampton men will insist that no other can be genuine. Folk tradition is also associated with **Banbury** as reflected in the verse 'Ride-a-cock-horse to Banbury Cross'. The original cross was destroyed by the Puritans in 1602, the replacement being a Victorian monument.

A strong puff through the hole of **The Blowing Stone** - which originally stood on the Ridgeway but is now to be found at **Kingston Lisle** - produces a note which, tradition has it, Alfred the Great used to gather his chiefs in a fight against the Danes. An excellent pub which has taken the name of **The Blowing Stone** is the centre of attraction in Kingston Lisle both for the quality of it's food and the attractive accommodation. Most local people are involved with horses in some way or another and the chat in the bar is always full of lively conversations about racing and training. Alfred was born in **Wantage** and the town is worth a visit for the museum which shows much of the past history of the area.

Oxfordshire's Bronze Age stone circle, the **Rollright Stones** or King's Men is next in importance only to Stonehenge and Avebury, set in a superb situation with fine views over Warwickshire.

The Chilterns, dividing Oxfordshire and Buckinghamshire, with their centuries old beechwoods were the home at one time of hundreds of 'bodgers', wood turners making chair legs with manual lathes, and whittlers of clothes pegs. The area is one of outstanding beauty, the mainly small buildings a mixture of brick with knapped flints. Where the Chilterns meet the Berkshire Downs and the river has created the **Goring Gap** through the chalk, the ancient **Icknield Way** and **Ridgeway** come together.

The Ridgeway runs along the Berkshire Downs (now in Oxfordshire) heading towards Stonehenge and Avebury although the ancient road pre-dates the great monuments. Being away from modern roads, the Ridgeway provides for peaceful walking or horseriding with extensive open views. Towards the west of it's Oxfordshire section the Ridgeway passes by the **White Horse of Uffington**, nearly 40 feet high, cut through the turf into the chalk. If you leave a horse and a coin in the nearby **Wayland Smith's Cave**, rumour has it that by the morning the horse will have been shod. Here too is **Dragon Hill**, said to be where St George slayed the dragon.

Over the Berkshire Downs from Oxfordshire is the Royal County of Berkshire it'self, now a small county with, sadly, much of it's Iron Age and Roman history obscured by recent development. For all that it is an interesting county and the whole is really overshadowed by the majesty of **Windsor Castle**. This enormous fortress which dominates **Windsor**, is the largest inhabited castle in the world. It has been one of the principal residences of the sovereigns of England since the days of William the Conqueror, who built it. When you come to examine it closely you will see that almost every monarch since William's time has taken a hand in rebuilding. For our present Sovereign Lady, Queen Elizabeth II, the rebuilding has been forced upon her by the devastating fire just five years ago which destroyed much of value, although the works of art, furniture and books were saved by a human chain passing the priceless masterpieces gently down the line, hand to hand - hands that included the Queen, the Duke of York and many local people. The damage has now been restored and the castle is as magnificent and awe inspiring as ever. Three wards or enclosures make up Windsor Castle. The Round Tower in the Middle Ward was built by Henry II to replace the wooden Norman fortress. George IV added it's upper half in 1828-32. The Lower Ward contains St Georges Chapel and the Upper Ward has the State Apartments.

Within the Castle, parts of which are open to the public, you must not miss the 15th and 16th century St georges Chapel. It boasts some of the finest fan vaulting in the world, the helmets and banners of knights, the tombs of Henry VII and Charles I and a memorial to Prince Albert. The State Apartments also must not be missed. These magnificently furnished rooms on the preciptous north flank of the castle are still used on official occasions.

On a quite different scale is the world's most famous **Doll's House** designed by Sir Edwin Lutyens in the 1920's for Queen Mary. Everywhere in Windsor there are Royal connections. Indeed the town grew up because of the presence of the castle. It is a delightful town with a good theatre, attractive shops, fine museums and a beautiful parish church built in 1820 on the site of an erlier church. The building was supervised by Jeffrey Wyatt who later, as Sir Jeffrey Wyatville, designed the Castle's Waterloo Chamber for George IV.

Eton is always inextricably mixed with Windsor but it is a little town in it's own right. It has always had a fascination for people especially because of the world famous school, Eton College. Each year on the 4th June Eton College celebrates it's founding by Henry IV in 1440 with a firework display on the river. Also in June is Ascot Week when royalty, the gentry and celebrities as well as other racegoers, many of them in huge flamboyant hats, attend the meetings at **Ascot Racecourse**.

There are some wonderful drives along the River Thames to small towns and villages, **Maidenhead, Taplow**, amongst many. I always enjoy visiting **Cookham**, the home of the artist Sir Stanley Spencer (1891-1959). He loved his birthplace with an intensity that shows in his paintings. Cookham High Street, the parish church, the River Thames, the meadows, are all recognisable in his works. It is fitting that Cookham should be the home of the **Stanley Spencer Gallery**. It stands in the centre of Cookham in the former Wesleyan Chapel to which he was taken as a child by his mother. Pride of place is held by the immense, unfinished Christ Preaching at Cookham Regatta. There are some touching reminders of this talented man; his spectacles, easel, palettes, sunshade, and folding chair, and even a baby's push chair that he used to carry his equipment when he was off on a painting expedition.

Over the Thames from Windsor and beyond the town of **Slough**, Berkshire joins the tall narrow county of **Buckinghamshire** on it's short southern boundary. At this point Buckinghamshire is low and leafy, rising sharply further north to the Chilterns with it's thick beechwoods, then further north still becoming a land of streams and marshes.

A prehistoric boundary known as **Grim's Ditch** runs across the Chilterns near to **Great Hampden** and nearby are two crosses cut through the turf into the chalk. Not as exciting as the White Horse of Uffingham but nonetheless intriguing.

The Chilterns are renowned for the many footpaths and there are walks both short and long, but rarely strenuous, that can take advantage of the scenery, giving just occasional glimpses through the trees of distant views. The **North Bucks Way** starting near **Wendover** on the Chilterns escarpment takes walkers down to **Wolverton** in the Vale of Aylesbury. On the North Bucks Way can be found the **Quainton Railway Centre** with trains in steam on the last Sunday of each month.

The ancient trees of **Burnham Beeches** east of **Maidenhead** form a beautiful area which was bought for the people by the City of London in 1879. At one time this area was also home to Romany gypsies, now long gone.

Along the Thames, Buckinghamshire has some attractive towns such as **Marlow** which is particularly beautiful. This was the home of the poet Percy B. Shelley and Mary Shelley of 'Frankenstein' fame. The poet William Cowper spent the second half of his life in **Olney** where the **Cowper Museum** celebrates his works, including 'Amazing Grace' which was written here.

Stoke Poges church is where Thomas Gray wrote his 'Elegy written in a country Churchyard' and at **Beaconsfield** lived G.K. Chesterton and Enid Blyton who it is believed was inspired by the **Bekonscot Model Village** with tiny houses spread over a large garden. Milton lived in **Chalfont St Giles** when he fled to London to escape the plague and in addition to a small museum, his cottage is now open to visitors.

Near Beaconsfield the small town of **Jordans** was home to William Penn, the founder of Pennsylvania and he is buried at the small 17th century **Quaker Meeting House. The Mayflower Barn**, also open to the public, incorporates beams taken from the Mayflower after the Pilgrim Fathers sailed to America in 1620.

Hughenden Manor near **High Wycombe** was the home of Benjamin Disraeli and the house still contains much of his furniture and other belongings. Today's Prime Minister has a country residence southwest of **Wendover**, a Tudor house known as **Chequers**, presented to the nation for just this purpose during World War I.

From pretty, small villages such as **Hambleden** to modern towns like **Milton Keynes,** Buckinghamshire has absorbed a large increase in population in the latter part of this century, yet outside these conurbations retains it's character as a rural area.

Bedfordshire to the north east is very much more rural, a green and peaceful county where water meadows flank the River Great Ouse and the rolling downs climb towards the mighty Chilterns. John Bunyan was born in the village of **Elstow** in 1628. Later he was imprisoned for his religious views in the county town of **Bedford**. Both places have much to remind us of this great man. **Elstow Moot Hall** is a beautiful brick and timber building built about 1500. It's purpose to house the goods for the famous May Fair at Elstow. It was also used as a court house and it has been suggested that Bunyan might have had Elstow Fair in mind when he described the worldly 'Vanity Fair' in the Pilgrim's Progress. The Hall belonged to the nuns of Elstow

Abbey and after the abbey was dissolved at the Reformation, the Moot Hall continued as a court house. For centuries it was neglected until in 1951 it was restored. The upper floor has been opened up to display the superb medieval roof, with massive beams and graceful uprights.

Two miles south west of **Dunstable**, the rolling hills of **Dunstable Downs** form the northern end of the Chilterns chalk escarpment and from them there are wide views over the Vale of Aylesbury and beyond. Thousands of years ago they were a highway for prehistoric man, who trudged along the Icknield Way (now the B489) at their foot. In a 300 acre area the ground has been left untreated by chemical weedkillers or fertilisers and the result is stunning. Rare plant species flourish,including fairy flax and chalk milkwort. Little muntjac deer browse among the scrub, and whinchats and grasshopper warblers dart over the hillside.

At **Whipsnade Heath** there is a reminder of the First World War. Here is the Tree Cathedral, in a sun dappled grove, laid out to a plan of nave, transepts and chapels. It was planted in the 1930's by Edmund Kell Blyth in memory of his fallen friends. Quite moving and very beautiful.

Nearby on top of the downs, more than 2,000 animals roam over 500 acres of **Whipsnade Park Zoo**, in conditions as nearly as wild as climate and safety will permit.

If you are a narrow gauge railway enthusiast you will want to visit **Leighton Buzzard Narrow Gauge Railway.** An average speed of five and a half miles an hour might not seem much by to-day's standards but it is quite enough for the locomotives of the Leighton Buzzard Railway which was built to carry sand from the quarries north of the town to the main London and North Western Railway. Due to be scrapped at the end of the 1960's, it was saved by a band of enthusiasts who have acquired steam and diesel engines from as far away as India and the Cameroons, constructed rolling stock, and built an engine shed for maintenance.

Market gardening flourishes around the town of **Biggleswade** set amidst highly productive arable land, showing the diversity of one of the smallest counties in England. Near here you can visit **The Swiss Garden**, a beautifully restored 19th century garden with fine trees. An intricate French garden features in a park that was laid out in the 18th century and partly re-landscaped by Capability Brown around **Wrest Park House** at **Silsoe**, modelled on the French chateaux style. The history of gardening through the ages can be seen here in a setting which includes some splendid water features.

Judging by it's huge popularity, no visit to Bedfordshire would be complete without a tour around the splendid **Woburn Abbey**, home of the Dukes of Bedford, with it's stately parklands, complete with wild animals, boat trips, art galleries and shops.

Hertfordshire, along with the extinct county of Middlesex, made up the Northern Home Counties and it is here that the mix of grand country houses and new towns is in greatest contrast - or greatest harmony depending on your viewpoint. **Letchworth** was the first of the new 'Garden Cities', created as early as 1903 in a bid to bring better housing to ordinary people. It's **First Garden City Museum** tells the story of the somewhat radical social ideas which were held by those who originally created this town as well as those who lived here. **Welwyn Garden City** followed in 1920 and several other new towns, often around old town or village centres, sprung up in the post-war period of the 1950's.

I have to admit that for me Hertfordshire is principally **St Albans** with it's fine cathedral in which thousands of years of worship have continued on the site of St Alban's martyrdom. Many centuries ago Alban was the first Christian martyr in this country and his shrine has always attracted pilgrims in search of spiritual and physical healing. It is a beautiful place which emanates strength. You feel as if the Almighty is reaching out for you and endeavouring to pour into your soul the fortitude shown by St Alban, and at the same time give you hope for the present and peace eternal. The history of the cathedral is well documented and you will do no better than to purchase the beautifully presented, colourful Pitkin Guide to St Albans Cathedral which will cost you about two pounds and be a constant reminder of your visit.

Almost surrounded by motorways, St Albans is easy to reach and having done so you drive into quieter realms and begin to realise that you are going to discover in this one place, which offers the unusual combination of the dignity of a Cathedral City and the intimacy of a rural market town, the full span of British history. For a moment or two the sense of history is overwhelming. St Albans is full of museums, beautifully laid out and providing easily digested information.

A totally different atmosphere you will find at **The Mosquito Aircraft Museum** in Salisbury Hall, **London Colney**. The historic site of the moated Salisbury Hall, mentioned in the Domesday Book, was chosen by the de Havilland Aircraft Company in 1939 to develop in secret the wooden, high speed, unarmed bomber, the Mosquito; with 41 variants of the type of the most versatile aircraft of the war. This began the museum's long association with Salisbury Hall making it the oldest Aircraft Museum in the country. Visitors to the museum soon discover that it can offer more than a collection of static aircraft. Close inspection of the exhibit's provide a unique hands-on experience. Members are always on hand to assist the visitor and demonstrate the working displays. With a varied programme of regular events that include flying displays, vintage car and motor cycle rallies and model exhibitions, there is always something to appeal to all ages.

From the air to the ground. **The Royal National Rose Society** at Chiswell Green, St Albans on the outskirts of the town, invites you to enjoy the world famous 'Gardens of the Rose' at the Society's showground where there is a collection of some 30,000 roses of all types. The 12 acres of gardens are a marvellous spectacle for the casual visitor and fascinating to the rose enthusiast. The gardens are being continuously developed - in particular by associating roses with a great many other plants - to create greater interest for visitors and to stimulate ideas leading to more adventurous gardening.

The British Rose Festival is a spectacular national event held every year in July. It includes amagificent display of roses organised by the Society and the British Rose Growers Association on an excitingly new and different theme each year. The competition is for the leading national amateur rose exhibitors and floral artists. All the best of British roses can be seen at this unique show.

Of particular interest in this county for vegetarians will be **Shaw's Corner** at **Ayot St Lawrence**. **Sir George Bernard Shaw,** playwright and critic, vegetarian and humanist, lived here for the second half of his long and active life. His vegetarian ideals were based on both moral and health grounds, proclaiming that 'Animals are our fellow creatures. I feel a strong kinship with them.; The house has been kept exactly as it was at the time of his death in 1950.

The many houses on a truly grand scale include **Hatfield House** originally home to the Bishops of Ely and later to Henry VIII's children and other members of the Royal family, **Brocket Hall** which was the home of Lord Melbourne and Lady Caroline Lamb, **Moor Park,** the historic home of Cardinal Wolsey later transformed into a Palladian mansion and now a golf club. and **Basing House** home of William Penn founder of Pennsylvania.

Sadly others have fared less well, such as the Castle at **Bishop's Stortford** now just a mound, and another earthworks with just a little masonry which was the Castle at Berkhamsted, presented by William the Conqueror to his brother, later visited by Thomas a Becket, Chaucer and three of Henry VIII's wives and involuntarily visited for a long term, by King John of France. Another was Ware Park which originally housed the 'Great Bed of Ware' mentiond by Shakespeare in his plays, now in the Victoria and Albert Museum.

Near **Ware** at **Amwell** is one of the most unexpected of museums in Britain, a **Lamp-Post Museum.**

Similarly bordering on the outer suburbs of London, the county of **Surrey** has a very high population, much of it in large villages or small towns, and all of it spread out in pleasant green surroundings.

The well know geographical feature of the **Hogs Back** is a part of the North Downs and other high points such as **Leith Hill** with it's view of 13 counties, and **Box Hill** offer outstanding panoramic views. On the high point of **Chatley Heath** stands a tower which was part of the communication system, sending messages from London to Portsmouth in less than one minute in the days before telegraph.

Box Hill overlooks some of the prettiest of scenery along the River Mole. Despite it's rather unpoetic name it is probably the river most written about in poetry, by Spencer, Milton, Pope and others, and the riverside village of **Brockham** is said to have given the name of 'brock' to the badger, many of which used to live here.

The riverside meadows of **Runnymede** are famous as being the site of King John's signing of (actually fixing his seal to) the Magna Carta in 1215. The memorial buildings at Runnymede were designed by Sir Edward Lutyens.

Architecture from the early part of this century can also be seen to great effect at **Whiteley.** Built according to the will of William Whiteley who left one million pounds for the creation of this retirement village for staff of Whiteley's Department Store. Surrey contains other fine recent buildings such as the **Yvonne Arnaud Theatre** at **Guildford**, as well as **Guildford Cathedral**, started in 1936 but not consecrated until 1962 due to the intervening war. With it's position high on Stag Hill on the edge of the town it makes a magnificent spectacle.

Surrey has several special gardens, the most important of which is **Wisley Gardens**, for over 80 years the show gardens of the Royal Horticultural Society and a source of inspiration for all kinds of gardeners. There are features at their best at each time of the year; the Alpine Meadow in spring, the rhododendron-clad Battleston Hill in early summer, and for winter the Orchid House with it's naturalistic 'rainforest setting'. Wisley is full of fascinating shapes, textures, sounds and smells, and the special garden for disabled people enables all those with a handicap to take full advantage of them all. There are occasional guided walks and the RHS also runs a series of courses, some of them on aspects of gardening, others on flower arranging or botanical painting. The Information Centre is reputed to sell the most extensive range of horticultural and botanical books in the world, and the range of plants for sale, is staggering with something like 8,500 varieties, many of them far from common-or-garden.

Peppermint used to be an important crop in **Banstead**. The watercress beds at **Abinger Hammer,** fed by underground springs are one of the claims to minor fame for the village, and it's history as a centre for the iron industry is another. The iron working made use of a hammer mill (hence the name) driven by the stream.

Loseley Park between **Godalming** and **Guildford** is a splendid Elizabethan house, the home of the More-Molyneux family from the 16th century to the present day. The family farms 1,400 acres around the house, and it is here that Loseley ice-cream and yoghurt is made. All Loseley dairy products are free from artificial additives and they also grow organic crops. However the farm tour shows little of the dairy aspect and does incorporate other farm animals.

One of the most interesting of the many towns in Surrey is **Farnham**, an attractive small market town with elegant Georgian housing and with some interesting literary associations including Sir Walter Scott, Swift and William Cobbett (who described the beauty spot of **Hindhead** as 'the most villainous spot God ever made') There are several historic houses open to the public in and around the town.

Mystery surrounds **Shalford Mill**, an early 18th century water mill which was in full use until 1914 when it fell into some disrepair. It was acquired by the 'Ferguson's Gang some years later and after restoration was given to the National Trust. The 'Gang' members used code names such as 'Bill Stickers' and none of their identities has ever been known.

Ending on a happy and smiling note, **Cranleigh Church** is believed to hold the inspiration for Lewis Carroll's Cheshire Cat, a grinning cat head carved on the transept arch.

Greater London offers so much to see and do that all I can do is to skim the surface and tell you about one or two unusual places to visit. You will see in this book that there is a wide selection of vegetarian restaurants offering great food and at prices which will suit most people's pockets.

Of course, London has good vegetarian restaurants and it also has vegetarian personalities! One important figure is to be found greeting visitors in the main hallway of the **Natural History Museum**. 'Dippy', otherwise known as the Diplodocus, Britain's best loved dinosaur, is -or at least was - a vegetarian. Despite dinosaurs' fearsome reputations, this 26 metre giant was purely a herbivore.

The Museum of Mankind also has information on early vegetarians, and more evidence seems to be available to support man's early origins as at least mainly a vegetarian. London is crammed with excellent museums, most of them in **South Kensington**, and no visitor should miss the splendid **Victoria and Albert Museum**. On **Butler's Wharf** is Britain's first **Tea and Coffee**

Museum, featuring hundreds of different coffee grinders and machines, over 1,000 teapots, teabags, prints, photographs, maps and drawings documenting the history of tea and coffee drinking over the past 350 years. There are even tea bushes growing in the museum!

Visitors to **Greenwich's Fan Museum** are introduced to fans and their history through displays which also show their making and the materials used. There are some exquisite examples of 18th and 19th century fans in an elegant Georgian setting, in this, the first and only museum dedicated to the art and craft of fan making.

Just a few of the other exceptional museums around London are the **Bank of England Museum** with the history of the bank, displays of gold and banknotes: **The Design Museum** in the Docklands which has collections of well designed, mass production items along with a series of special exhibitions; **Dickens' House Museum** where the great man lived: **Florence Nightingale Museum** telling the story of her life and work, the **Freud Museum** in Sigmund Freud's last home. **The Guinness World of Records** with lifesize models and electronic displays to show the biggest, fastest etc. **Kew Bridge Steam Museum** with it's unique collection of impressive, working steam pumping engines; and the **London Diamond Centre** where you can see the diamonds being cut and polished.

An extraordinary museum, if you can call it a museum, is to be found at 18 **Folgate Street** in the heart of what was the Huguenot rag trade district of **Spitalfields**. The house is opened a few times a week by the owner who lives there as the house was when it was built in the 18th century, perfect in every detail of decor and, of course, with only candle and gas power. However those intending to visit are requested to 'telephone' for details!

The underground **Cabinet War Rooms** features a Transatlantic Telephone Room and another 20 historic rooms which were operational during the 2nd World War. Very closeby in **Horseguard's Parade**, and also underground is **Henry VIII's Wine Cellar** which can only be seen by appointment, on a Saturday afternoon.

At **Wimbledon** is what must surely be the only **Lawn Tennis Museum** in the world. It is open during the Wimbledon Tennis season to ticket holders.

Also at Wimbledon, as part of the **Polka's Children Theatre**, is a toy and puppet exhibition. In Scala Street in central London, **Pollock's Toy Museum** displays not just Pollock's card cut-out theatres but puppets, dolls' houses and teddies of the past. The **London Toy and Model Museum** covers a similar subject, in Craven Hill in **Bayswater**. Somewhat different, but on the theme of puppets, is the **Spitting Image Rubberworks** in **Covent Garden**.

Also in Covent Garden, displays of work on an environmental theme are often held at the **London Ecology Centre**, founded on World Environment Day in 1985. The Centre's focus is the Information Service for the general public, a forum for environmental organisations and a single point of contact for the channelling of enquiries. It's 'London Sustainable Development Network' collects information on examples of good environmental practice which it then publicises to those interested. The offices of the Bat Conservation Trust and the Environmental Film Festival are also within the Centre, as is a Meditation Centre.

Covent Garden is an exciting development of mainly shops, cafes and small museums, several of them quite specialised and unique, mixed with street entertainment and an electric atmosphere, in what was the old fruit and vegetable market. No longer are there flower girls to be found under the portico of St Paul's church, but although the area has changed considerably since those days it has retained it's lively spirit.

A short walk from Covent Garden via the Aldwych brings you to **Fleet Street,** another part of London now much changed. For centuries until just recently, Fleet Street was the home of all the important national newspapers, now most have moved, mainly to the **Docklands.** The other association with this area, that of the legal profession, continues. Although different, the charm of the old pubs and alleys persists, with much of it's history on view such as the **Pepys Exhibition** within the **Prince Henry's Room**, and the **Wig and Pen** where lawyers and journalists have traditionally met, but Sweeney Todd's Barber Shop and the Pie Shop on the other side of St Dunstan's Church are no longer there. In the Strand, **Twinings** tea shop is said to be the longest established shop on it's original site and also claims to be the narrowest. The names of the streets and alleys sum up something of their past history, with Wine Office Court and Old Cheshire Cheese.

An aerial view of London will show that much of it is covered in green. Not only are there large numbers of private gardens, but there are hundreds of public gardens and parks right up to the size of **Richmond Park**, which with deer roaming wild, really does seem to be a bit of the countryside within London. In **Westminster** the pretty **College Garden** with it's **Little Cloister** is only occasionally open to the public. It is said to be the oldest garden of it's type in England.

The ancient walled **Chelsea Physic Garden**, just along from the Chelsea Royal Hospital with it's red-coated pensioners, was only the second botanical garden to be opened in Britain. It is a serene and beautiful place. It was the seed of a cotton plant taken from here that resulted in America's successful cotton industry.

The most famous London garden is undoubtedly **Kew Gardens**, and indeed it is accepted as being the finest botanic garden and plant research centre in the world, aimed at creating a better future for our planet. It consists of 300 acres of magnificent tranquil gardens alongside the River Thames in West London, with 6 acres under glass from the exquisite Victorian Palm House to the stunning new Princess of Wales Conservatory. There are buildings too, including Kew Palace and **Queen Charlotte's Cottage**. One of the most unusual features is the Pagoda, completed in 1762 as a surprise for Princess Augusta, the Dowager Princess of Wales, who had founded the gardens only a few years earlier. The ten storey octagonal structure reaches a height of 50 metres, and was at the time the most accurate imitation of a Chinese building in Europe, (although to be accurate it should have had an odd number of storeys). Vistas through the garden enable the Pagoda to be seen in superb settings. The 18th century Kew Gardens was just a tiny portion of that seen today, having the Richmond estate added to it early in the 19th century, with some of the areas coming more recently into cultivation.

In addition to the nine exceptional glass houses, the dozen other buildings, the many special garden features and the wonderful parkland of the three arboreta, work goes on behind the scenes to preserve endangered plant species and to conserve habitats. The 44,000 different types of plants at Kew represent one in six of known species (it is believed that there are many plant species still undiscovered and work too continues in this direction), with 13 species extinct in the wild and 1,000 threatened. The botanists at Kew now have some 6 million preserved specimens which through their research could be found to contain important medicines, fuels or food.

Another very important although less well known garden is in **Enfield.** The National Gardening Centre at **Capel Manor** is actually not just a garden but a College for the study of landscape and garden maintenance and management, a Countryside Centre predominantly used by schools, and it incorporates 'Which? Magazine's' demonstration garden. The gardens extend over 25 acres and illustrate many different designs, styles and periods, from formal images to habitats for attracting wildlife.

In the centre of London, next to Lambeth Palace, is the **Museum of Garden History**, run by the Tradescant Trust. The Trust was founded less than 20 years ago to save the historic church of St Mary at Lambeth from demolition. There they establised the Museum of Garden History as a centre for plant displays, lectures and exhibitions. The Tradescants, father and son, were royal gardeners in the 17th century and brought back from their frequent travels many of the plants which we know, making them still today possibly the best known name in plant collecting. The plants were propagated in their famous 60 acres garden in Lambeth. Development of the garden is ongoing, with some exciting plans for the future.

Vegetarian Brasserie & Tearoom - **FROG ISLAND BRASSERIE**
Hatch Marsh, Abinger Hammer, Nr. Guildford, Surrey RH5 6SA
Tel: 01306 731463

This is an exciting vegetarian brasserie situated in between Abinger and Gonshall on the A25. It is the ideal spot for those who enjoy it's rustic, homely charm. The moment you enter this one hundred year old building you sense the warmth of it's atmosphere and acquire an awareness that this is essentially a happy establishment. The owners have the ability to produce an ever changing menu which constantly surprises. They will tell you that many of the dishes on offer are there at the suggestion or request of regular customers, of whom there are many. For this reason there are now delicious fish dishes on the menu.

One menu might offer carrot and coriander soup, spiced basmati baskets, cheesy almond croquettes or courgette and feta triangles followed by parsnip and peanut loaf, country ale pie or calzone with a creamy spinach, leek and mushroom filling. The next week there would be a total change. The desserts are always delicious and very tempting. There is a set price for two or three courses. There is a very small wine list of organic wines from France. In the summer months the small garden is used for eating out and has ten tables. It is lovely on a warm day. The service is quiet, friendly and unobtrusively efficient.

USEFUL INFORMATION

OPEN; Mon-Sat:12-2pm
Dinner: Mon-Sat 7pm-11pm
Sundays: 12-3pm
CREDIT CARDS; None taken
CHILDREN; Welcome
LICENSED; Yes

ON THE MENU; Wide range of delicious Vegetarian dishes. Vegan options + Chicken dishes also available
DISABLED ACCESS; Yes + toilets
GARDEN; Small with tables in summer

Inn & Restaurant - **THE KNIFE AND CLEAVER**
Houghton Conquest, Bedford, Bedfordshire MK45 3LA
Tel: 01234 740387 Fax: 01234 740900

Situated 5 miles south of Bedford about 1 mile from the A6 turn off this 500 year old hostelry is an atmospheric, brick-built inn which has been sympathetically extended by the erection of a Victorian-style conservatory restaurant. This leads on to a flowery terrace where you can eat al-fresco on sunny days by the fountain. The award-winning restaurant, which specialises in fresh fish and shellfish, serves affordably priced vegetarian dishes using highest quality fresh ingredients. The unusual and innovative menu changes on the first of every month but always includes home-made vegetable soups and other vegetarian starters as well as two vegetarian main courses. The dark Jacobean panelling in the bar is said to come from Houghton House, 'House Beautiful' in Bunyans 'Pilgrims Progress. More informal meals are served in the adjoining Trellis Room accompanied by hand pumped real ales or a choice from over 20 wines by the glass. There are nine ensuite bedrooms in the quiet orchard garden.

USEFUL INFORMATION

OPEN; 12-2.30pm & 7-10pm Closed Sunday nights
CREDIT CARDS; Visa/Amex/ Mastercard/Diners

ON THE MENU; Interesting dishes with vegetarian fare across the board
DISABLED ACCESS;Yes + suitable toilets

Hotel - **THE OLD MANSE**

Victoria Street, Bourton-on-the-Water, Gloucestershire GL54 2BX

Telephone 01451 820082 Fax: 01451 810381

Built in 1748 in a period of wealth for all the settlements of the Cotswold hills, the family owned and run Old Manse in Bourton-on-the-Water is now a delightful hotel with 12 well furnished en-suite bedrooms. Bourton is one of the most famous of the Cotswold villages and is frequently called 'Little Venice' because of the many picturesque low bridges spanning the wide and shallow River Windrush which flows past only a few feet from the porch of The Old Manse on it's leisurely way to the Thames. The whole village has houses which are solidly built and honeyed with the famous limestone.

The Old Manse was the home of the Reverend Benjamin Beddome, the village's Baptist pastor. He was renowned for his biblical knowledge and as a prolific hymn writer. In recent years a modern wing has been added to the hotel. It too is built in traditional Cotswold stone and sit's in harmony with it's older parts.

The spacious 50 seater restaurant is elegantly decorated and furnished and offers excellent food, using fresh local produce wherever possible. Any special dish of your personal choice will always gladly be prepared by the chef so that even if you prefer something other than the many super vegetarian dishes on the menu, a meal to your taste is readily available. The menu changes daily in the restaurant and in the bar there are specials each day. The delicious home-made soups are almost always vegetable based and with fresh granary bread become a meal in their own right.

USEFUL INFORMATION

OPEN; Bar, Mon-Sat: 10am-11pm
Sun: 12-10.30pm
Restaurant: Mon-Sat: 6.30-9.30pm
Sun: 12-2.30pm & 6.30-9.30pm
CREDIT CARDS; Access/Visa/Amex
Diners

ON THE MENU; High percentage of vegetarian dishes across the board
DISBALED ACCESS; Yes+ suitable toilet
LICENSED; Yes
GARDEN; Small garden
CHILDREN; Welcome

ACCOMMODATION; 9 dbl, 3 twin. 1Bedroom has a king size four poster

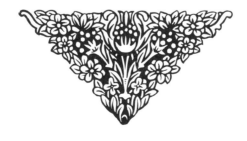

NATURAL THERAPY CENTRE

10 New Street, Chipping Norton, Oxfordshire OX7 5LJ

Tel: 01608 641995

The Natural Therapy Centre, at Chipping Norton in the heart of The Cotswolds, revitalises the natural way with successful therapies enjoyed for thousands of years. A days treatment can be designed especially for you giving you he opportunity to experience everything from Floatation Therapy to Thalassotherapy Seaweed treatments, or an Indian Summer Treat which includes Aromatherapy Indian Head Massage Solarium (whilst oils penetrate) and Hydro/steam seaweed treatment.

A full Day Treat offers a Rebound session - a great way to exercise - Hydro'spa seaweed treatment. Full relaxation therapy massage. Healthy lunch and relax. Delux Floatation therapy, Solarium, Hydro/steam seaweed treatment. Optional hair treatments are also available in the salon. Wholesome food and drinks are served all day in the reception lounge where you are welcome to call in for coffee and a chat or stay all day.

Wine Bar and Bistro - **SEVENS**

7 The Borough, Farnham, Surrey GU9 7NA

Tel: 01252 715345 Fax: 01252 737849

Sevens wine bar and bistro is one of the great meeting places for local people and for visitors who come to Farnham either on business or for pleasure. An attractive place in a black and white beamed building. This is an establishment which is run with easy informality and the service is friendly yet unobtrusive. In the summer the pretty walled courtyard provides a Barbecue at lunchtimes in a colourful floral setting. Inside the benefit of an efficient air conditioning system keeps the air fresh. Sevens is somewhere in which you can spend a relaxed evening or be in and out quickly if the demands of the day dictates it. The food is all home-cooked with a selection of traditional and speciality dishes. It is excellent value for money and for vegetarians offers the opportunity to enjoy some excellent vegetarian dishes right across the board. The menu is changed every month. The wines are superb in quality, come from around the world and are sensibly priced. A bottle of the very good house wine costs approximately £8.20.

USEFUL INFORMATION

OPEN; Mon-Fri: 9.30-11pm
Sat: 9.30-3pm & 6.30-11pm
Closed Sundays & Bank Holidays
CREDIT CARDS; Mastercard/Visa
GARDEN; Walled garden
CHILDREN; Welcome to eat

ON THE MENU; Home-cooked,
traditional Good selection for
Vegetarians at every course.
DISABLED ACCESS; Yes but not -
suitable toilets

Restaurant - **RIVERSIDE VEGETARIA**

64,High Street, Kingston-upon-Thames, Surrey

Tel: 0181 546 7992/0181 546 0609

This award winning restaurant together with it's take-away service specialises in International Vegetarian and Vegan cuisine, prepared and cooked to a very high standard. The menu is vast and whether it is a starter, a main meal or a dessert, the prices are sensible. The most expensive main course will cost you under six pounds. It is a fun place to be, always busy, and with a cheerful staff. Licensed, it has quite a range of wines primarily Italian including organic wines of English and French origin.

Outside catering is a comparatively new venture for the Riverside Vegetaria but the food and the service is excellent and it has become highly successful in a very short space of time. The restaurant opens every day of the week, even Christmas Day.

USEFUL INFORMATION

OPEN; Mon-Fri: Lunch 12-2.30pm
Dinner 5.30-11pm. Sat 12-11pm
Sun 12-10.30pm

CHILDREN; Welcome

ON THE MENU; Wide range
Vegetarian and Vegan cuisine
DISABLED ACCESS; Not really
CREDIT CARDS;All major cards

Restaurant - **GREENHOUSE VEGETARIAN RESTAURANT**

16 Chenies Street, London WC1E 7EX

Tel: 0171 637 8038

The Greenhouse Vegetarian Restaurant has been flying the flag for good vegetarian eating for some time. You will find it just off Tottenham Court Road - the nearest tube is Goodge Street, two minutes away. This popular venue is in the basement of an old drill hall and very popular it is! At lunchtime it is a busy, bustling restaurant coping with people who come from far and wide to sample the hundreds of different dishes from around the world that appear on the ever changing menu. At night it takes on a totally different personality and becomes quietly relaxed allowing one to take in the contemporary art exhibit's on dislay and the gentle unobtrusive music mainly classical and jazz. The Greenhouse is strictly non-smoking and does not have a licence.

The chef has a superb range of recipes and enjoys trying them out on willing customers. His secret lies not only in presentation but in the imaginative use of the ingredients with which he concocts dishes. It is not just a job to him but an art form. Here you can have a snack, a light meal or a full meal and if time is the essence there is a take-away service. The only food bought in is the bread which comes from a local bakery. You will find the menu contains several options that are suitable for vegans.

USEFUL INFORMATION

OPEN; Mon:10-6pm Women only 6-8.30pm
Tues-Fri: 10-8.30pm Sat: 11-8pm Sun: 12-6pm
Closed Xmas,New Year & Easter weekend
CREDIT CARDS; None taken
LICENSED; No

ON THE MENU; Ever changing menu
Featuring hundreds of different
vegetarian dishes
DISABLED ACCESS; Not for wheelchairs
CHILDREN; Welcome

Indian Vegetarian Restaurant - **MANDEER**

21 Hanway Place, off Tottenham Court Road, London W1P 9DG

Tel: 0171 323 0660

Mandeer is the oldest of London's Indian vegetarian restaurants. It has been suitably showered with accolades, the most recent being Vegetarian Living's 'Ethnic Restaurant of the Year 1993'. You will find it two minutes from Tottenham Court Road tube station, just behind the Virgin Megastore. You go downstairs to a basement area into a place of enchantment, reminiscent of an Indian temple. It is low lit and very atmospheric. Classical Indian music playing in the background heightens the sense of the Orient. Occasionally the music is live with classical concert.

The menu is made up of Gujarati, Punjabi and South Indian dishes, all created on the premises by the talented chefs under the watchful eyes of Mr and Mrs Patel, the proprietors. Every ingredient is traditional and no compromises are made. Each dish is freshly cooked and comes to the table with all the artistry of true Indian cuisine. The smiling attentive staff make you feel that their whole reason for being there is to ensure your pleasure. In addition to the many vegetarian dishes on the menu, there are a number of vegan options and Mandeer caters for those on a Jain diet - in other words no onion or garlic.

Wine complements any meal and with the emphasis on wines from France and Germany at sensible prices, there is an excellent organic chateau des hautes combes house wine. Indian and organic beers are available as well as the usual run of spirit's, sherry, liquers and exotic fruit juices. Mandeer is a wonderful culinary experience.

USEFUL INFORMATION

OPEN; Lunch: 12-3pm Dinner 5.30-10pm   **ON THE MENU;** Exclusively vegetarian
CREDIT CARDS; All major cards   Gujurati, Punjabi, & South Indian
CHILDREN; Welcome   **DISABLED ACCESS;** No. Restaurant in
LICENSED; Yes   Basement

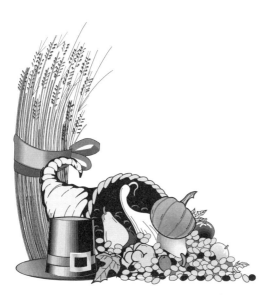

Restaurant - **NUTHOUSE**,

26 Kingly Street, Oxford Circus, London W1R 5LB

Tel: 0171 437 9471 Fax: 0181 691 9366

In a capital city renowned for the variety and excellence of it's restaurants it has to be somewhere very special to stand out. This is the reason that the Nuthouse Vegetarian Health Food Restaurant has become so popular over the years. It has been established since 1969 and in the same skilled, creative hands since 1979. You will find it in Kingly Street just two minutes from Oxford Circus tube station or three minutes from Piccadilly. There are two rooms devoted to the first class cuisine, it is self-service and partly no smoking. People come here knowing that they will enjoy the food, find the prices sensible and, if needs be, the service speedy.

One cannot pin down the range of dishes to any one culture or region. There is a large selection of vegetarian food with vegan options. It is definitely imaginative and many of the dishes on offer are unique to the Nuthouse. People come here expecting to find their time-honoured favourites on the menu and they are not disappointed.

Wine is always enjoyable with a meal. No one could call the wine list here vast but the limited choice comes from England, Italy and France and is extremely reasonable. Less than five pounds a bottle on the whole. For non-drinkers there are some unusual and refreshing drinks. The Nuthouse is a relaxed, informal place in which to eat and will please carnivores as well as vegetarians when they realise how tasty and exciting the menu is.

USEFUL INFORMATION

OPEN; Mon-Fri 10.30-7pm Sat 11.30-6.30pm **ON THE MENU;** Imaginative unique dishes
CREDIT CARDS; None taken   For vegetarians and vegans
CHILDREN; Welcome   **DISABLED ACCESS;** No
LICENSED; Yes   **GARDEN;**No

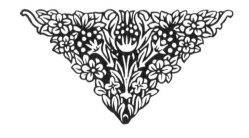

Hotel with Brasserie and Public House
ROYAL TRAFALGAR THISTLE HOTEL
Whitcomb Street, London WC2H 7HG

Tel: 0171 930 4477 Fax: 0171 925 2149

This busy hotel which stands between Trafalgar Square and Leicester Square behind the National Gallery is a modern building with excellent, well-appointed bedrooms, the Battle of Trafalgar pub and a Brasserie designed in the style of 19th century Paris. It is all charming, friendly and well worth seeking out.

Come to the Royal Trafalgar Thistle to stay and you will find yourself in the heart of London. Every room is en-suite and has satellite television, direct dial telephone, trouser press, hair dryer and that blessing to travellers, tea and coffee making facilities. For anyone wanting to enjoy a weekend break in the capital, there is a special rate.

The Brasserie is busy every day but it is restful and the service excellent. The menu is full of exciting dishes and many of them suitable for vegetarians. For example you could start with Avocado Mediterranean with Mozarella, Black Olives and Pine Kernels, followed by Mushroom Korma served in a filo pastry basket with seasonal vegetables and rice. Every day additional dishes are featured on the blackboard and many are suitable for vegetarians.

The wine list, although not specifically vegetarian, has some interesting choices from around the world. The extensive cocktail list offers both alcoholic and non-alcoholic exotic drinks.

USEFUL INFORMATION

OPEN; 7am-11.30pm. (Sunday 10pm) Closed at Christmas
CREDIT CARDS; All major cards
CHILDREN; Welcome
LICENSED; Full licence

ON THE MENU; Brasserie type food with wide vegetarian choice
DISABLED ACCESS; Yes
GARDEN; Terrace dining area
ACCOMMODATION; 24 dbl 36 sgl 48twin all en-suite

Bed & Breakfast

WINFORTON COURT

Winforton, Herefordshire HR3 6EA
Tel: 01544 328498

Mrs Jackie Kingdon, in her charming 16th century home, Winforton Court, offers a warm welcome and country hospitality at it's best. The house is set in old world gardens close to the Black Mountains. Owned by the Earl of March - Roger de Mortimer - until 1523, Winforton Court abounds in period features, oak beams, early 17th century stencilling and fine oak staircase. There is evidence of the 20th century but only where ones creature comforts are concerned! Furnished with antiques, collections of old china, samplers and bygones, the house has three delightful bedrooms - one with four-poster bed and private bathroom. Fresh fruit and flowers are always placed in each bedroom. There is a spacious lounge, open fires and good books. Breakfast is a sumptuous feast whether it is traditional or vegetarian. Bed and Breakfast is from £18 per person per night. Reductions for five or more nights. Also available, Kilverts Cottage, an attractive, comfortable, detached self catering cottage sleeping four persons. Special diets catered for.

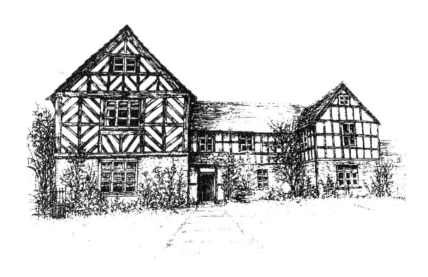

Country House - **COOMBE LODGE**
Wotton-under-Edge, Gloucestershire GL12 7NB
Tel: 01453 845057

One mile from the town centre of Wotton-under-Edge is Coombe Lodge a Grade II Listed house built around the 1800's. Set in an acre of lawned gardens surrounded by mature trees and overlooking the Coombe Valley. This delightful non-smoking Georgian Country House is owned and excellently run by Chris and Sylvia Mayo who extend a warm and friendly welcome to all their guests. The spacious, comfortable bedrooms are tastefully decorated and well appointed with central heating, wash bain, TV and tea and coffee making facilities. The elegant Victorian dining room is where Sylvia will serve a delicious breakfast, you can choose from fruit juices, grapefruit, cereals, yoghurts, choice of cooked breakfast, wholemeal toast, marmalade, honey and a selection of teas and coffees. The guest's sitting room is full of local guide books and maps ready for you to plan your day's outing, you can watch television or just sit and chat with the other guests. If you really want to pamper yourselves, why not relax in the Sauna available on request Coombe Lodge is ideally situated for touring the surrounding area with many attractions to suit the whole family, Slimbridge Wildfowl and Wetlands Trust, Berkeley Castle, Prinknash Abbey, Potteries and Bird Park to name a few. Stroud and Tetbury are two nearby towns well worth visiting, further afield are Bath, Cheltenham, Cirencester and Gloucester. However long you stay you are sure to enjoy this English Tourist Board '1 Crown Highly Commended' Country House.

USEFUL INFORMATION

OPEN; All year except Xmas & New Year

DINING ROOM; Good home-cooking

CHILDREN; Welcome over 3 years
CREDIT CARDS; None taken
ACCOMMODATION; Comfortable rooms

VEGETARIAN; Excellent selection
DISABLED ACCESS; No
GARDEN; Yes, delightful

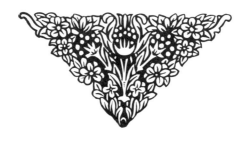

GILBERT'S

Gilbert's Lane, Brookthorpe GL4 0UH Tel: 01452 812364 Fax: 01452 812364
V/VG/Trad. WH. ORG NS. Children welcome. ETB 2 Crown Highly Commended
RAC Highly Acclaimed. Which Good B & B Guide. Welcome Host.

HALLERY HOUSE HOTEL

48 Shurdington Road, Cheltenham GL53 0JE Tel: 01242 578450.
Family run hotel with a welcoming relaxed and comfortable atmosphere. Much
used by business people who appreciate the elegance and comfort after a busy
working day. It is equally equipped to please the visitor who comes to visit the
Cotswolds or simply enjoy the charm of Cheltenham. Excellent food with plentiful
choice for vegetarians.

SOPRANO RESTAURANT

1-5 Broad Street, Oxford OX1 3AH Tel: 01865 240973
Open all year. Mon-Sat 11am-11pm No smoking area. Vegetarian & Traditional.
LIC. Children welcome.

Chapter Four

The South East

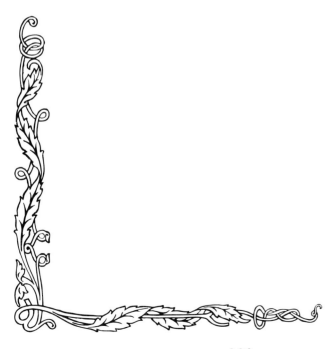

KENT, ESSEX, SUFFOLK, NORFOLK & CAMBRIDGESHIRE

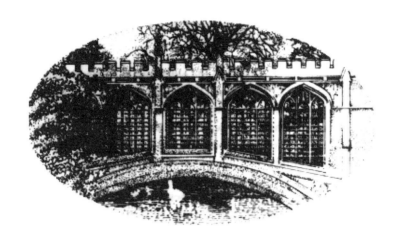

INCLUDES

Chapter 4

The South East
Kent, Essex, Suffolk, Norfolk & Cambridgeshire

𝕴f one wanted to choose somewhere that spelt out beauty, history, heritage and national pride, then **Canterbury** in Kent, the Garden of England, would probably top the poll. You have only to stand back and watch the expression on the face of visitors as they see Canterbury Cathedral, a building of incalculable beauty to underline what I have just said. Canterbury was welcoming pilgrims 900 years ago and even then it was an ancient city. Three hundred years later Chaucer brought attention to it with his Canterbury Tales. The Cathedral dominates the city and is the spiritual centre for Christians who belong to the Church of England in many countries but the non-believers in the tenets of the Anglican Church are as much addicted to it's beauty as anyone else.

Canterbury's beginnings go back to the Iron Age and oddly enough the damage caused by German bombs in World War II which destroyed almost a third of it's buildings, assisted archaeologists. The craters disclosed foundations more than a thousand years old and enabled them to trace it's history from the time man first settled there long before Christ.

Over the years I have found it beneficial to stay in Canterbury and to alternate my days there by taking a full day in the Cathedral and the following day going out to the Kent countryside and exploring there. Too much Cathedral, beautiful and inspiring as it is, becomes a recipe for mental indigestion and almost being sated with loveliness, making one unable really to appreciate all that one sees. When it is time to leave at the end of a day my feet are aching and my head bursting with the overwhelming beauty. In my nostrils linger the very special smell of the Cathedral.

There is so much to see in Canterbury. The High Street is an unending source of delight. For example at No 37 there is a 12th century crypt and across the road is The Beaney Institue where archaelogical items such as Roman glass, silver and Saxon finds from local excavations are exhibited. In a former church in St Margaret's Street is 'The Pilgrims Way', a fascinating exhibition portraying both the Canterbury Tales and medieval life generally. Just past the Yeomanry War memorial is Queen Elizabeth's Guest Chamber which began as a 15th century inn and was modernised in restoration times. And so the delight goes on. You will need many days and many walks if you are to uncover all Canterbury's treasures. On each of them you will discover many new delights and reminders of past ages. Nothing is farther than twenty minutes from the heart of the city when you take a walk round the city walls which enclosed the original Roman town.

Beyond Canterbury is **Hernhill** where you will find **Mount Ephraim Gardens** at the heart of an 800 acre estate, comprising the house and gardens, a progressive fruit farm, woodland and grazing, which acts like a magnet to those who enjoy the glory of a garden in a superb setting. The house rebuilt in 1870 but the home of the Dawe family for over 300 years, commands magnificent view over the woodland park, orchards and the Swale and Thames Estuary. Then there is **Forwich on Stour** which was once the port for Canterbury. **Hackington** near the University was once a village in it's own right. **Harbledown** appears in the Canterbury Tales as the last village before the destination of the pilgrims and it was here they would get their first glimpse of the Cathedral. To the east of Canterbury is the attractive village of **Wingham** home to the famous **Tanner of Wingham**.

Supposing one were to decide on a longish tour that took one around the coast of Kent which is possible from Canterbury, then within fifteen minutes to the north you would come to **Whit'stable**, long renowned for it's oysters but it has more than that to offer. There is good fishing, bathing from a shingle beach and excellent yachting facilities. A spit of land known as 'The Street' juts about a mile and a half into the sea and provides a pleasant promenade.

To the east the seaside resorts of **Westgate on Sea** and **Margate** have been popular for generations. The former is less boisterous than the latter but both have their adherents who would not go anywhere else. I cannot say that it is a holiday that would appeal to me but the countryside and the sea are both beautiful and you see a lot of happy smiling faces, so who am I to judge?

Broadstairs just round the North Foreland is a different kettle of fish. Here is a Regency resort which has not changed much since the society of those times put their stamp on it. It has miles of sheltered and sandy bays and to the north stand the chalk cliffs and lighthouses of the North Foreland. Dickens lived here and there is a Dickensian festival every year.

Down past **Ramsgate, Sandwich** and **Deal**, one comes to the beautiful **St Margaret's Bay** part of the Foreland Heritage Coast. Here at **West Cliff** is the stunning **Wallets Court Hotel** with the tiny church of St Peters opposite. It is a fascinaing hotel in it's own right but add that to the history of the building which first gets it's mention in the Domesday Book and you cannot help being enthralled. The White Cliffs and St Margaret's Bay have provided great inspiration for many writers, poets and artists over the years. The quintessential Englishman, Noel Coward and also the man who created James Bond, Ian Fleming, both lived in the Bay at one time. The spectacular cliff tops are famous for their rare wild flowers and birds. One can lie there in the long grass for hours listening to the skylarks and watching the traffic in the Channel. On a clear day you can even see the French coastline which lies just over 20 miles away.

Dover at the end of the North Downs is famous for it's White Cliffs but it is also of great historical importance. Apart from being an ancient port linking Britain and the Continent it was once the walled Roman town of Dubris, and the beginning of the Roman road, Watling Street. One of the best vantage points from which to view Dover is from Langdon Cliffs belonging to the National Trust, where you will have a bird's eye view of the bustling Eastern Docks and miles of waymarked footpaths across the flower rich cliff tops. Nowhere else will give you such a panoramic view over the Strait's of Dover.

'The Garden Coast' encompasses **Folkestone, Hythe & Romney Marsh** which offers me endless pleasure both in the beautiful countryside, the sea and the history of the area together with the monaticism of the Romney Marshes. You will see in the list of attractions in the back of this book that there is so much to see and so varied that it must please everyone whatever age.

Royal Tunbridge Wells is beyond **Sissinghurst** and a town that must delight the eye. A distinguished spa at one time especially among persons of fashion in the 18th century, though the waters can still be drunk. Samuel Pepys and John Evelyn both visited and Beau Nash left

Bath to become the master of Tunbridge Wells ceremonies in 1735. However it was Lord North who made the waters popular a hundred years earlier. The town is blessed with many parks and gardens and a fine common with outcrops of weathered sandstone rocks. From Royal Tunbridge Wells you can take a leisurely cruise around **Bewl Water**, Southern Water's beautiful reservoir at **Lamberhurst**. This is the largest area of inland water in south east England and set in the most attractive countryside. Also at Lamberhurst is **Scotney Castle Garden**, one of England's most romantic gardens surrounding the ruins of a 14th century moated castle. Rhododendrons, azaleas, waterlilies and wisteria flower in profusion.

Groombridge Place Gardens and **Enchanted Forest** provide another stunning day out. Surrounded by breathtaking parkland this mystical medieval site includes the famous Grade I Listed 17th century walled garden set against the backdrop of the classical moated mansion and Enchanted Forest, which have inspired writers, artists and connoisseurs of beauty for hundreds of years.

To the north of Tunbridge Wells is **Tonbridge** a prosperous market town at the navigable extremity of the River Medway, where it diverges into formidable streams. The River Walk along the Medway, through willow-lined meadows gives a fine view of **Tonbridge Castle**. It's Norman to 13th century ruins on a site defended since 1088, are substantial: the shell of the keep, curtain walls, round-towered gatehouse. Some of Tonbridge's 18th century houses are built of castle stone. It is an exciting place to visit and you are invited to travel back over 700 years to join the Lords of Tonbridge Castle and experience a vivid recreation of the sights, sounds and excitement of 13th century castle life.

Penshurst Place and Gardens near Tonbridge must be visited. The beautiful medieval stately home of Viscount de L'Isle, with it's magnificent Barons Hall dates from 1341. The splendid gardens were first laid out in the 16th century. Two of the loveliest castles in Kent and some say in the world, are **Leeds Castle** 4 miles east of Maidstone and **Hever Castle** near Edenbridge, the childhood home of Anne Boleyn.

The Medway towns must not be forgotten. Made up of **Strood, Gillingham, Chatham** and **Rochester**, they are steeped in history and none more so than the ancient cathedral city of **Rochester** on the lower reaches of the River Medway. The city is closely associated with the novelist Charles Dickens, and features more often in his books than any other place apart from London, although Portsmouth, where he was born, has The Charles Dickens Birthplace Museum. Rochester's Norman legacy cannot be missed. The great square keep of **The Castle** towers above the River Medway, a daunting reminder of the history of the city. It was on this site that the Romans originally built the first fort to guard the bridge which connected the Imperial Route of Watling Street, leading from London to Dover. The Cathedral is the second oldest in England and is a regular place of pilgrimage for historians and worshippers alike. It has many visitors from all over the world who delight in the majesty even though it is much altered and reconstructed, with a spire dating only from the early years of this century.

Chatham has had a long and distinguished history and until recent years been inextricably involved in the life of Her Majesty's Navy. Those days are gone but a visit to **The Historic Dockyard** will give you at least five hours of absorbing interest. There are no less than 47 Scheduled Ancient Monuments, forming the most completely preserved Georgian dockyard in the world, dry docks and covered slips, timber mast houses and seasoning sheds, huge storehouses and the quarter mile long working ropery stand beside the elegant Commissioner's house and garden, officers' terrace and dockyard church. Now a living working museum this tells of the lives of the dockyard craftsmen whose skills- from carpentry and caulking to rigging and forging - made the British fleet the finest in the world. No one can fail to be fascinated by what they see. With seven main attractions plus skills and crafts in action, it is not surprising visitors stay an average of 5 hours.

I lived in Suffolk for a while on the Shotley Peninsula looking over the River Stour to **Harwich.** This allowed me to become happily familiar with the corner of Essex that includes the old Roman town of **Colchester**, and the glorious **Dedham Vale**, as well as many of the smaller villages including **Wix**, between Harwich and Colchester, bypassed by the A120 which is a direct route to London. It is a place surrounded by local beauty spots like **Mistley** where one of Great Britain's largest population of mute swans live and the twin 'Mistley Towers' stand as the only remains of Robert Adams' ecclesiastical work in England.

Colchester is Britain's oldest recorded town and has 2000 years of fascinating history and heritage to discover. It is a history involving the Romans, the Saxons and the Normans which has been interpreted and displayed using the most up to date methods in the town's museum.

Colchester Oysters were famous in Roman days and are still so today, but as a fishing and trading port, the town is no longer significant. The town however is significant for the 1000 acres of public gardens and parks. You should not fail to walk in the glorious surroundings of the Castle which was built by William the Conqueror in 1076.

The Vale of Dedham is something very special and immortalised by John Constable. This north-east corner of Essex is where the River Stour forms the boundary with Suffolk and is an area of outstanding scenic beauty. It is still possible to stroll through the meadows and along the river banks with their abundance of flora and fauna, or explore the delightful villages with their impressive medieval churches and old pubs. It is constantly changing scenery.

From **Bures** to **Harwich** the river loses it's quiet willow-lined banks enclosing the gently flowing water, home to colourful ducks, elegant swans, and moorhens and becomes tidal flats beyond Manningtree and the dominant east coast. From here it is easy to reach the enchanting wool towns and villages like **Lavenham, Hadleigh, Kersey** and **East Bergholt,** just over the Suffolk border and of course **Dedham** it'self.

The three counties which make up the region of **East Anglia** share a common topography, all basically being flat lands. In addition all have excellent soil for agriculture, and all have many areas that are important for our native plant, animal and bird life. Even today the region is sparsely populated, and almost completely without motorways as it is not actually on the way to anywhere!

Cambridgeshire is a county of two extremes: in the south are the chalk downs with their gentle hills and crops of corn, barley and rye, topped with beech and majestic elms; but to the north the countryside could hardly be more different, the treeless prairie of endless fens and the dark lonely landscape with it's cutting winds and endless horizons. Much of it was at one time no more than a continuation of the Wash, but over the many years of dedicated work by the inhabitants more than 2,000 square miles have been reclaimed. Today it has some of the richest, yet bleakest terrain in England.

In the centre of Cambridgeshire fens **Ely** was at one time an island, and is still referred to as the Isle of Ely. It's Norman Cathedral is exceptionally beautiful, dominating the flat landscape for miles around. The last of the old fens, still undrained is **Wicken Fen**, a truly natural environment of dense reed-beds, sallow-bushes and sedge jungles, a habitat that is home to many rare butterflies and moths. It is fortunate indeed that nearly all of Wicken Fen is now owned by the National Trust, meaning that not only is this eerie landscape in secure hands for future generations, but also that there is still a place for the indigenous wildlife to breed and prosper.

Cambridge is somewhere that has no need of explanation - it speaks for it'self with it's truly splendid college buildings and lively atmosphere that university life engenders. **The Fitzwilliam Museum** is one of the principal collections of fine and applied arts in Britain, and also for art lovers is **Kettle's Yard** off Castle Hill and the **Botanic Gardens** with it's Chronological Bed showing the diversity of plants introduced over the centuries, and there is much more of interest in this pleasant city which although quite large is on a small market town scale.

I listened to Jeffrey Archer talking about Cambridge, a city he loves, and one in which he almost lives at **Granchester**, made famous by Rupert Brooke, only two miles away. He gave some good advice to people wanting to visit the city. 'Do not allow the academics and students to make you feel you have no right to be there. Cambridge is as much your city as theirs'. Good advice, for this famous seat of learning can be a bit intimidating.

There are all sorts of things you need to know about Cambridge. For example during the year there is constant activity and one thing is for certain one visit will not suffice. No matter when you come it is lovely and very special but if you remember that accommodation is difficult during the major events such as May Week, Degree Days and the Festival, that may influence your decision. If you have thoughts of going to Evensong in Kings College Chapel for example, the service only takes place during the University terms. Lastly during the University examination period, May to June, many of the colleges are closed to the public..

Beyond Cambridge the county has many delightful places. A little way west on the A45 is **Stow-cum-Quy** and **Anglesey Abbey**, a place of great beauty bequeathed to the National Trust in 1966 by Lord Fairhaven whose nephew the third Lord Fairhaven now lives there. It's history has been chequered with several owners since the 16th century one of whom was a carter from Cambridge by the name of Hobson and from whom we have derived the expression 'Hobson's Choice'. Of the original Augustinian priory only the chapter house and vaulted monks' parlour survive. It is a wondrous place to visit and the gardens are nothing short of superb.

Waterbeach is a pleasant village with the River Cam flowing nearby. The church is 500 years old and well worth a visit. If you went further west and then drove northwards up the A1, the Great North Road, you would come to the historic village of **Buckden**. In 1533 King Henry VIII imprisoned his wife, Catherine of Aragon in Buckden Towers following the annulment of their marriage, allowing him to marry Anne Boleyn.

Swaston lies to the south of Cambridge. This small town has a bustling High Street and abounds with delightful eating places in which to refuel and stoke up the energy for a visit to the mighty **Imperial War Museum** at **Duxford** two miles away. **Melbourn** was an important place in the Middle Ages. It still has moated houses and a medieval church as well as many attractive cottages and is an ideal place to stop and relax after visiting the museum. Here one can sit and watch the world go by in pastoral surroundings.

2 miles from the Duxford Museum and only 4 miles from the historic **Audley Hall**, is **Hinxton**. It sit's just one mile inside the Cambridgeshire border, 6 miles from Saffron Walden. It has no shops, just one street and it's biggest disturbance is the River Cam flowing nearby. The tiny spire of the old church rises from a dome set in the battlement of a 650 year old tower. The church is mainly 14th and 15th century and has old benches in the chancel and old beams in the roof. A wonderful inspiring house of God.

Now for **Huntingdon**, a county within the county of Cambridgeshire and famous as the home and constituency of Prime Minister, John Major. There are many picturesque villages to visit which are a shining example of rural life. Inns with a story to tell abound, waiting to welcome the weary, thirsty and hungry traveller. Enjoy Huntingdon which is rich in history and has attractive countryside. It is a land of wide skies and church spires, pretty riverside villages, historic market towns and tranquil waters.

Norfolk has an atmosphere entirely of it's own and is both exciting and quietly rewarding with it's splendid towns and villages. **Norwich** the county town, should be explored on foot. For example at the Back of Inns is the Royal Arcade which has a tesselated pavement, laid by imported Italian workmen and over the delightful Victorian/Edwardian shops, the walls and glass roof can only be described as Art Nouveau. In Theatre Street is the Assembly House, set back behind wrought iron gates and well manicured lawns. It is the venue for thousands of people every year who flock here to enjoy concerts, exhibitions and meetings.

Norwich has more pre-Reformation churches than London, York and Bristol put together. One of them is **St Stephens** in Theatre Street. It was the last of a great series of Norwich churches to be built. It is eye catching. The tower is superbly decorative in contrasting flint and stone in roundels, diamonds and window outlines. The 16 clerestory windows have some notable glass and the sun shining through them throws immense light on the glorious hammerbeam roof. I have only touched on some of Norwich's gems and there are many more including **Elm Hill** which looks almost like a film setting.

A visit to the Castle and the Cathedral are musts. The battlements of the castle provide a vantage point to look down on many of the sights and streets you will have already seen. It really does dominate the city and all the streets go round it. In contrast the cathedral does not dominate the skyline. It is quite low lying and surrounded by buildings which make it's spire, one of the tallest in the country, hiding it's beauty for privileged eyes. What a wondrous place it is. Before you enter you will find yourself embraced by the arms of Cathedral Close. It's effect is immediately to make you feel withdrawn from the modern world. You can choose to enter this enchanted world through Bishop's Gate in Palace Street, the Erpingham Gate or St Ethelbert's Gate in Tombland. Any of them reveal the stunning beauty of Upper Close or Lower Close as well as Green Yard and Almery Green. The grander houses are in Upper Close with delightful cottages in Hook's Walk. At every corner there is another vista on which to feast your eyes. Lovingly tended gardens are an offering to the Lord, and when the sun shimmers on the mullioned windows you know you are in a magical land.

The Cathedral was begun in1096 by Bishop Herbert de Losigna on the orders of the Pope, as a penance for the sin of simony. The penance could not have been performed better. I have my own special favourite spots in the cathedral, one of which is going in through the south transept door, passing through the transept and then turning left into the nave south aisle until I reach the end of the nave. From here I have a view of the full length of the building which takes my breath away every time.

It is almost a relief to leave so much beauty and if your departure happens to be at eventide when The Close is at it's best, I suggest you walk slowly through to Pull's Ferry from which you can turn back and see the cathedral from the river, an unforgettable and glorious sight.

Norfolk is so full of great places that I am forced through the limitations of space to tell you only of a very few.

Billingford just west of Diss, has a handsome five storeyed windmill which is open to the public. **Blickling**, one mile north of Aylsham, has **Blickling Hall**, owned by the National Trust and undoubtedly Norfolk's most wonderful Jacobean house. **Burnham Market** is one of seven pretty vllages in a group. All the villages seem to be in sight of the sea and you reach them through a network of high hedged narrow lanes.

Coltishall is a village you must find time for. It is at the head of navigation on the River Bure and a favourite place for boating people. It has pleasant, mellow brick Georgian houses with many of the gardens running down to the river bank. Roman urns have been unearthed and Roman tiles frame two of the Saxon windows in the hilltop church. **Cromer** is a fishing village that was developed into a seaside resort by the coming of the railways at the end of the 19th century and has been bustling ever since. It has great charm especially round the centre which highlights the old flint buildings of the fishing village it once was.

Fakenham has all you might expect of a market town. Go there on Thursday and you will find it transformed into an open market full of bustling shoppers and friendly chatter. It is a splendid centre for antique auctions too. There is a racecourse with regular meetings, and on the outskirts of the town is the village of **Thursford** which is the home of **The Thursford Collection**. I was there a few years ago when this exciting place played host to Songs of Praise; it was magical.

Fritton is a straggling village scattered around a vast marshy common. It's glory is the church of St Catherine reached up a grassy track. It is a thatched building with a little round tower. Nearby is **Fritton Lake Country Park** part of the **Somerleyton Estate**, which offers hours of interest and activity to the visitor. The lake is two and a quarter miles long and probably one of the most beautiful expanses of water in East Anglia. A house filled with love is how I would describe **Somerleyton Hall**, family home of Lord and Lady Somerleyton and their five children. It is a perfect example of a house built to show off the wealth of new Victorian aristocracy. Sir Morton Peto made a vast fortune from the railways, and promptly spent a large part of it taking what was a comparatively small 17th-century manor at Somerleyton and creating around it an extravagant concoction of red brick and white stone. Inside he made it nothing less than lavish. He went too far and subsequently went bankrupt, selling his beloved house to Sir Francis Crossley, whose great-grandson is the present Lord Somerleyton.

Horning is one of the best loved Broadland boating centres. It is a charming place with one long street containing a happy mixture of inns, shops, cottages and boatyards. Many of the buildings have reed thatch and most of them are built with brick that has mellowed with age. The pretty half-timbered houses have moorings and thatched boathouses alongside.

King's Lynn you will either love or hate and you will learn to refer to it as 'Lynn'. There is so much that is beautiful here and so much that has been spoilt in careless development because of the need for new industry which became obvious immediately after World War II. Lynn's most famous building is **The Guildhall**. It is fabulous, with it's handsome facade of chequered flint and stone. Built in 1421, it was originally the hall of the Trinity Guild, a wealthy merchant guild, existing before King John gave the town it's charter.

Mundesley has one of the nicest sandy beaches on the Norfolk coast. It is unspoilt, a place for families and for those who just enjoy a walk across an uncrowded beach watching for the 'lowies' at low tide. This is the odd name locals use for the small rock pools.

North Walsham's quaint Market Cross with three tiers of bell-like roofs each lessening in size, built by the Bishop of Norwich in 1550 is still the focal point of this prosperous market town which caters for Mundesley, Bacton, Happisburgh and the northern part of The Broads. The Paston Grammar School taught Horatio Nelson for three years before he went to sea.

Sale pronounced Saul, has the marvellous church of St Peter and St Paul which rises high above the land. The foundations were laid in the 15th-century and it was built to last, as it has done and been saved the fate of restoration by the sometimes over zealous Victorians. The noble families included the Boleyns, and there are many brasses to the family but none to the sad Anne, Henry VIII's second Queen. It has been said though that she is secretly buried here and not in the Tower of London.

Sandringham - 'Dear old Sandringham, the place I love better than anywhere in the world' wrote King George VI about this most private and beloved Royal home. It is an enormous estate of 20,000 acres taking in several villages. The grounds are open to the public from April to September when the family are not in residence.

Sheringham on the North Coast is designated an area of outstanding natural beauty. The small, attractive town has one of the finest seaside golf links to be found anywhere.

Swaffham is an elegant small town with some lovely buildings situated around a triangular market place. The Butter Cross which is not a cross at all, immediately demands attention. It is a circular pavilion built by Lord Oxford in 1738 and at it's apex sit's a life size figure of Ceres. East of the Market Place is the church of St Peter and St Paul in which the north aisle was built by a wealthy man, John Chapman, known as the Pedlar of Swaffham. Legend has it that he discovered two pots of gold in his garden.

Wells-next-the-Sea has a name that enchants. It manages to combine a working port with tourism successfully. Wandering the narrow yards (lanes to us) is a delight.

Wroxham which considers it'self to b the unofficial capital of The Broads, is linked to **Hoveton** by a hump back bridge over the River Bure. The banks of the river are alive with boatyards and the waterway is so busy that traffic lights would not come amiss. The marina is the place to go if you would like to take a boat trip by paddleboat or motor launch through the adjacent broads.

Going back to happy stomping grounds can produce feelings of dismay because what was once treasured has disappeared to be replaced by foreign objects or simply erased to make way for a new road. My return to **Suffolk** in the 1990's has given me nothing but pleasure. Of course things have changed but in most cases it has been for the good.

Ipswich, the county town offers a choice of many things to see and do. For starters there are no less than 12 medieval churches. The loveliest of these is St Margaret's. Flanking the north side of St Margaret's Plain, it is almost as beautiful as Norwich's St Peter's Mancroft., with a spectacular 15th-century roof, painted in the time of William III. Five of these churches are floodlit at night and most are open in daylight hours.

The Tudor **Christchurch Mansion**, which was built in 1548 is furnished as a country house and contains the finest collection of Constable and Gainsborough paintings outside London. **The Worsley Art Gallery** is another must on a visitor's list remembering that Cardinal Wolsey was one of Ipswich's most famous sons. My favourite building is **The Ancient House** in the Butterwalk. Once a hiding place of Charles II, it is the finest example of pargetting in the country and is now a used bookshop. One must not forget that Ipswich is still a busy port but much of the marine activity on the waterfront today is for leisure with yachts large and small berthing there.

Aldeburgh has always been a gentle backwatr and only came to prominence with the advent of the composer Benjamin Britten who, together with his friend, Peter Pears, the opera singer, lived here for many years. **The Moot Hall** is one of Aldeburgh's treasures. It is a herringbone brickwork building of the 15th century and is still used as the Town Hall.

Bramford close to Ipswich is a village of picturesque houses and a beautiful church, St Mary the Virgin. It has a handsome 14th-century tower with an 18th-century lead spire. Look closely and you will see panelled stone parapets and carved figures, including a monkey wearing a monk's cowl and hurling stones. The extraordinary presence of boulders round about it are thought to indicate a pagan sacred site.

Bury St Edmunds is one of the most pleasing and splendid Suffolk towns. It is full of treasures and has managed to remain almost untouched by large scale modern developments. Almost 1,000 of it's buildings have preservation orders on them.

Clare named after the long line of the Earls of Clare from William the Conqueror. Gilbert, the 7th earl was one of the most powerful men in the land during King John's reign and his son founded the famous Priory of Clare. The town is beautiful with handsome houses, several of which are pargetted - intricately patterned plasterwork.

East Bergholt was the birthplace of John Constable in 1776 who wrote 'I even love every stile and stump and lane in the village'. He painted innumerable pictures of the village of which 21 are now in the Victoria and Albert Museum in London.

Felixstowe gained popularity as a south facing Edwardian seaside resort, round a wide shingle bay with totally safe bathing. It lost it's Pier at the end of World War II but it is still a favourite place for Ipswich people to come at weekends.

Kersey is designated as the prettiest village in Suffolk and has to be seen to be appreciated like **Lavenham**. Quaint streets will lead you into enchanting medieval prospects, including those of the Guildhall, the Old Wool Hall, Tudor Shop and Woolstaplers in Prentice Street, a house that is 14th century at the back and 16th century at the front. Set at the end of this miraculously intact timber-framed Tudor wool town is the incomparable church of St Peter and St Paul, built by rich clothiers to celebrate the end of the War of the Roses in 1485.

Newmarket is where horseracing started 2000 years ago whilst **Saxmundham** is an unsophisticated small town dating back to Norman times and before that to the Danish Conquest. **Saxtead** is a little village close to Framlingham which has **The Saxtead Green Windmill**. This gem is preserved in beautiful order. It is an 18th-century post mill with a three storey roundhouse. There are four patent sails, two pairs of stone and a fantail.

Snape is the home of the Aldeburgh festival. Set right on the banks of the River Alde, it is a trustee of a wonderful collection of 19th-century buildings which includes the Snape Maltings Concert Hall.

Southwold with Blythburgh and Walberswick, cradle the River Blyth in their beautiful arms. The tower of Holy Trinity Church soars out of the reed beds. The beach is famous for it's coloured pebbles and the old Edwardian pastel painted beach huts. You will not find fast food shops, arcades or souvenir shops. St Edmunds Church rises proud and tall, a monument to light and airiness. 'Southwold Jack' stands by the tower at the rear of the chuch. It is he who strikes the bidding bell to mark the beginning of a service. He has been doing this since the War of the Roses.

Finally **Woodbridge** does not have an ugly building to my mind. Once a busy commercial port it is now a haven for those who love to sail. St Marys Church is a must for you to visit. The 15th-century tower and north porch are magnificently decorated.

Restaurant - **BRAMLEYS RESTAURANT**
16, Market Place,
Aylsham, Norfolk
Tel: 01263 732103

This interesting restaurant is housed in a 16th century building, in the far corner of the Market Place, at the main access to the church. It is part of this historic market town which is still busy every Monday with it's Market day. Because of the number of aged and preserved buildings it has been nominated as a National Trust Conservation area. In the restaurant you will find that all the original oak beams are still there which, added to the low ceilings, gives the place a feeling of intimacy. This is endorsed by the friendly Childerhouse family who have run the business the last 25 years. Today it is Mother and Daughter who are in charge and they have a particular concern for senior citizens who make up quite a percentage of their regular clientele. The Childerhouse's main aim is to provide good food using local produce wherever possible, and to offer the customer good service with the personal touch. They succeed admirably both in the restaurant and in the Coffee House at the rear. Every morning, except Sundays, home-made quiches, pies and cakes, which are made fresh daily, can be bought from the restaurant. Before 11am you may enjoy an excellent set breakfast or coffee and cakes. For those wanting a light snack there is a special menu called 'Just a Bite' which includes simple dishes such as Vegetarian pancakes, Cheese Omelettes, Deep fried Scampi. On the main menu there are a number of starters followed by a whole range of grills and a dessert list which will please anyone with a sweet tooth. The price range is within everybody's pocket and it is good value for money.

USEFUL INFORMATION

OPEN; 9-2pm. Eves reservations only
CHILDREN; In Coffee House only
CREDIT CARDS; All major cars
LICENSED; Most wines & spirit's

RESTAURANT; Good traditional food
BAR FOOD; Light snacks in Coffee House
VEGETARIAN; Menu is 20% vegetarian
DISABLED ACCESS; Small entrance step
GARDEN; Small seating area at rear

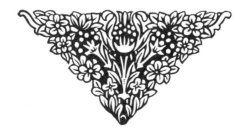

Public House & Restaurant - **DUKE OF YORK**

Southend Road, South Green, Billericay, Essex CM11 2PR

Tel: 01277 651403

For almost 12 years the White family have made the Duke of York one of the most welcoming and popular venues in Billericay. You will find it on the A129 Billericay to Wickford Road about one mile from Billericay High Street. Built at the turn of the 19th century, one of the nicest things about the pub is it's total lack of gaming machines and juke boxes. It is a place where soft music plays in the background encouraging the art of conversation. The whole of the Duke of York is furnished in a comfortable, olde worlde style, especially the Tudor style restaurant. The wide ranging menu is mainly French and English in it's cuisine. It includes a selection of 10 starters and 10 main courses especially for Vegetarians. Vegans can be catered for on request. Where possible everything is home-made and fresh produce is used. For those not wanting to eat in the restaurant, bar meals and snacks at reasonable prices are available. Awarded Les Routiers Corps d'Elite for outstanding wines, there are some 120 wines from around the world on the list and approximately 100 malt whiskies. The range of liquers and brandies are frequently topics for discussion.

USEFUL INFORMATION

OPEN; Restaurant: Mon-Fri 12-2pm & 7-10pm. Sat 7-10pm Bar food similar times except Sat 12-2pm & Sun 12-2.30pm

CREDIT CARDS; Access/Visa/Diners

CHILDREN; Welcome

ON THE MENU; Good range of vegetarian dishes. Vegan on request

DISABLED ACCESS; Yes but no special toilets

Restaurant - **ARUNDEL HOUSE HOTEL**

53 Chesterton Road, Cambridge, Cambridgeshire CB4 3AN

Tel: 01223 367701 Fax: 01223 367721

The Arundel House Hotel occupies one of the finest sites in the city of Cambridge overlooking the River Cam and Jesus Green. This elegant, privately owned, 105 bedroom hotel is only a short walk from the city centre and the wealth of fascinating architecture for which Cambridge is famous.

The hotel is well known for the friendly, welcoming atmosphere of it's bar and restaurant and has achieved a reputation for providing some of the best food in the area, all freshly prepared in it's scrupulously clean, award winning kitchens. The comparatively recent refurbishment of the restaurant makes it one of the most attractive places to eat in Cambridge and yet it is not expensive. For vegetarians, it is not only a delightful place to stay but it offers a superb range of delicious and imaginative, mouth watering dishes on a specially created vegetarian menu.

The hotel has excellent facilities for conferences, seminars and weddings, with it's friendly, efficient staff and ample car parking it forms a perfect base for your visit to Cambridge.

USEFUL INFORMATION

OPEN; All year except Xmas & Boxing Day

Rest: 12.15-1.45pm & 6-9.30pm (last orders)

CREDIT CARDS; All major cards

ACCOMMODATION; 105 bedrooms

ON THE MENU;
Wide choice for vegetarians at all meals

DISABLED ACCESS; Bar & restaurant Designed for wheelchair access. Bedrooms not Ideally suited

Restaurant - **PASTA GALORE**
5 Jordan's Yard,
Cambridge CV2 1UA
Tel: 01223 324351

Just off Bridge street and opposite St John's College you will find the delightful and unusual Pasta Galore in Jordan's Yard, a pedestrian walkway to the car park. Run by two talented ladies, Jessica Johnston and Celia Honer, this busy place has brought the charm of Italy to Cambridge. It stands on the site of three cottages one of which was damaged in World War II and subsequently demolished leaving room to create this pretty 2 storey building. It will seat 60-65 people on the two floors and in typical Italian fashion welcomes children and also party bookings. Before Jessica and her sister Celia started their two restaurants - the other is in Bath - they took several trips to Italy and to America, the homes of purely pasta restaurants, to ensure that they got the formula correct. They did, and the result is there for you to enjoy. Tantalising smells greet you as you walk through the door. They serve many traditional sauces and starters. The pasta, which contrary to popular belief is not fattening and is extremely healthy, is made on the premises daily as are all their sauces. For the vegetarian there is an excellent selection. The menu has a range of non-pasta Italian dishes and, like the starters, they are all tempting. Every day there are specials and a fine array of cakes, desserts, sorbets and dairy ice creams. Finish your meal with an Italian cheese and you will have had a feast. The wines naturally are Italian complementing the food beautifully. Pasta Galore is a great experience.

USEFUL INFORMATION

OPEN; 10am-10.30pm
   (11pm Fri & Sat)
   Sun: 6-10.30pm
CREDIT CARDS; Access/Visa
CHILDREN; Welcome
LICENSED; Italian wines, lager etc. liquers, Spirit's

RESTAURANT; First class Italian
BAR FOOD; Not applicable
VEGETARIAN; 1/3 of menu is vegetarian
DISABLED ACCESS; No
GARDEN; None

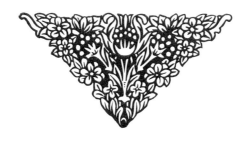

Hotel - **THE SOUTH LODGE HOTEL,**

196 New London Road, Chelmsford, Essex CM2 0AR

Tel: 01245 264564 Fax: 01245 492827

This comfortable hotel is known in Chelmsford for the excellence of it's food and it's efficiency. Not strictly vegetarian but it does offer dishes every day that are suitable and it is worth eating here for the quality of the dishes. The Garden Restaurant is used at lunchtime beacuse of the speed with which people are served and for the special Business Lunch prices. For example three courses are ten pounds, two courses eight pounds and one course seven pounds. The menu is available in the Restaurant, the Bar and in warmer weather, the garden. There is also a very good a la carte menu if you would prefer it and of course simpler bar snacks for those who do not want a meal. Dinner is also popular with a wide ranging menu, a good wine list and special dishes for vegetarians.

The ensuite bedrooms are comfortable and for those who want to use the hotel for business there are a number of rooms available for small conferences. Four rooms are available for one to one interviews, but may also be used for small boardroom meetings of up to six people.

USEFUL INFORMATION

OPEN; All year	**RESTAURANT;** Good menu
CHILDREN; Welcome	**BAR MEALS;** Wide range
CREDIT CARDS; All major cards	**VEGETARIAN;** Several dishes daily
ACCOMMODATION; En suite rooms.	**DISABLED ACCESS;** No special
GARDEN; Yes	facilities Conference facilities

Guest House - **SPRINGFIELDS**

Ely Road, Little Thetford, Ely, Cambridgeshire

Tel: 01353 663637

Springfields is a lovely large home set in an acre of beautiful landscaped gardens and orchard where guests are invited to wander and sit awhile to enjoy the tranquillity of the setting and (in summer) to smell the roses!

Guests stay in a separate wing which is absolutely charming. There are three pretty double rooms which have each been tastefully furnished and appointed with many delightful touches, and everything you could wish to make your stay a happy and memorable one. Breakfast is served in a pleasant dining room in which guests sit around a large table to enjoy together the delicious, freshly prepared food. Springfields richly deserves it's classification as 'English Tourist Board De-Luxe'.

Springfields is set in a very quiet location yet is only two miles from historic Ely with it's famous cathedral and is a perfect base from which to explore the changeless beauty of the Fens!

USEFUL INFORMATION

OPEN; All year except December	**ON THE MENU;** Delicious, freshly cooked
CHILDREN; Not under 12 years	food
CREDIT CARDS; None taken	**VEGETARIAN;** Catered for
LICENSED; No	**PARKING;** Private (Off road)
ACCOMMODATION; 2 twin 1 double	

Restaurant with Rooms - **THE ARK**

The Street, Erpingham, Norfolk NR11 7QB

Tel: 01263 761535

Vegetarians are extremely well catered for at The Ark, a small restaurant of national renown in the Norfolk village of Erpingham. The food is exquisite, cooked and prepared by Sheila Kidd and her daughter Becky. Sheila together with her husband Mike owns this enchanting place. Some people have an inborn ability to cook superbly without any need of formal training and this is so with Sheila who is self-taught and very individual in her cooking styles. She is quite happy to admit that she has been much influenced by Elizabeth David. This is apparent when you study the menu which changes daily. Imagine starting your meal with local Asparagus accompanied by a Maltaise sauce and following that with a Walnut and Chestnut Pate en croute with a Wild Mushroom Sauce. The desserts are equally superb and irresistible.Chefs Sheila and Becky use their organic garden, which produces the freshest vegetables and herbs. The dining room is small, serving a maximum of 36 covers, so ensuring a personal touch to all the dishes which emerge from the kitchen. Mike Kidd is the front of house man and it is he who selects wines from around the world for the excellent list. It is no wonder that newspapers and magazines are constantly writing about The Ark. It is a culinary experience - and there's more! You can stay here. The three bedrooms are full of character and delightfully appointed. Breakfast is totally flexible - there is no menu you simply ask for what you want. The countryside is superb so to really enjoy The Ark and all it has to offer, book in and relish the comfort, the food and the friendliness of the Kidds.

USEFUL INFORMATION

OPEN; All year	**ON THE MENU;** Wonderful, innovative food
CHILDREN; Welcome	**VEGETARIAN;** Always dishes available
CREDIT CARDS; None	**DISABLED ACCESS;** No special facilities
LICENSED; Yes	**GARDEN;** Yes

Restaurant **- SPINNING WHEEL RESTAURANT**

117-119 High Street,

Hadleigh, Ipswich, Suffolk IP7 5EJ

Tel: 01473 822175

This heavily beamed 15th century restaurant has been owned by Dominic Fazzone for 22 years and boasts approximately 60 covers. It is conveniently situated between Ipswich and Sudbury with easy access available to Colchester and the A12.

Both the blackboard and the A La Carte menus offer a wide range of vegetarian meals including Mozzerella Caprese, Chilled Melon with Sorbet, Vegetable Risotto and a variety of pasta dishes. Dominic is always pleased to offer vegetarian alternatives to the main menu.

With comfortable surroundings and friendly staff, the Spinning Wheel at Hadleigh is a popular choice for vegetarian diners. There is a non-smoking dining area.

USEFUL INFORMATION

OPEN;6 ½ days for Morning Coffee	**RESTAURANT;** Wide range vegetarian food
Afternoon Tea,Lunch, Evening Meals	**DISABLED ACCESS;** No special facilities
Sunday Lunch. Sunday evenings bookings only	
CHILDREN; Welcome	**CREDIT CARDS;** All major cards

Restaurant - **ROCOCO RESTAURANT**

11, Saturday Market Place, King's Lynn, Norfolk

Tel: 01553 771483

Situated right next to King's Lynn Guildhall, which is probably the town's biggest attraction, is The Rococo Restaurant. The building is a 300 year old Grade II listed building, sympathetically renovated in the Rococo style, and is one of the nicest restaurants in the whole of Norfolk. It has panache. The owners, Anne and Nick Anderson, are true professionals with good pedigrees in the restaurant business. Nick is a chef of many years experience who has been featured both in the Good Food Guide and the Michelin Guide. They demand a high standard in everything they do. The food is always of the finest quality. The wines have been carefully chosen to give a good selection of European and New World wines. In addition to the set menu light lunches are also available. At night there can be no better place to enjoy a pre-dinner drink whilst you await what will assuredly be a gastronomic delight. Food is always of a very high standard and most creative. Vegetarians are very well catered for with several excellent dishes. There are also simpler light lunches. The Rococo would be an ideal place for a special occasion. For a function it can hold 40 people.

USEFUL INFORMATION

OPEN; Mon: Dinner 7pm
Tues-Sat 12-2pm. Dinner 7pm
CHILDREN; Yes. No pets
CREDIT CARDS; Mastercard/Visa
GARDEN; No

RESTAURANT; Quality fresh food
BAR FOOD; Not applicable
VEGETARIAN; Yes, several dishes, the menu
is 20% vegetarian
DISABLED ACCESS; Yes + toilets

Restaurant - **THE MOORINGS**

6 Freeman Street,Wells-next-the-Sea,Norfolk NR23 1BA

Tel: 01328 710949

Bernard and Carla Phillips have owned this very nice restaurant since 1986 and whilst it is not strictly vegetarian, they have always made a point of having interesting vegetarian dishes and they also try to use organic produce whenever possible. Tucked away in Freeman Street, in summer it has a profusion of hanging baskets and flower boxes which highlight the old building. Inside it is warm and attractive with nice furniture and table settings. You will find the service efficient and friendly, the wine list well thought out. In fact you will be hard to please if you do not enjoy eating at The Moorings.

Wells-next-the-Sea has many delightful hidden places and a great beach complete with fishing boats, nets and that nose twitching smell that comes from a combination of fresh sea air and fish. Walking along the beach after lunch or in the quiet of the evening after enjoying a good dinner is very therapeutic and thoroughly enjoyable.

USEFUL INFORMATION

OPEN; Fri-Mon inc for lunch Thurs-Mon inc for Supper
CHILDREN; Welcome

CREDIT CARDS; None taken
LICENSED; Yes

RESTAURANT; Superb food
With interesting vegetarian
dishes
DISABLED ACCESS; Yes
PETS; No

LES AMANDINES
Norfolk House Yard, Diss IP22 3LB Tel: 01379 640449
Established in 1987 this non-smoking cafe/restaurant with it's glass covered courtyard, is out of the ordinary. Daily newspapers and magazines are for your edification whilst you drink Cappuccino and sample the delicious cakes which are served all day. Lunch is served from 12-4.30pm. Service is always fast and friendly, especially in the lunch hour. It is wise to book for evening meals. Specialises in Mediterrannean cuisine and unusual desserts. Many Vegan choices. Italian Pasta, biscuit's, home-made jams etc for sale. OPEN: Mon-Sat 9.30-5.30pm. Fri & Sat evenings 6-10pm(last orders).LIC. Children welcome.
LIC.

OSTRICH INN
Stocks Greeb, Castle Acre, Kings Lynn PE32 2AE Tel: 01760 755398

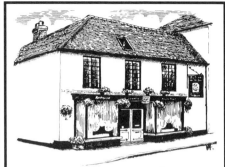
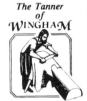
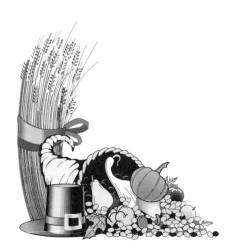

Chapter Five

Wales

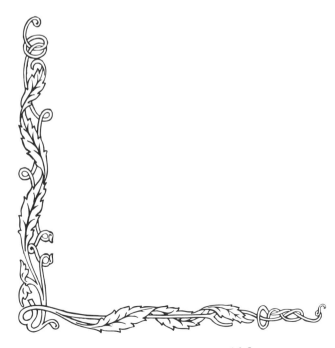

WALES

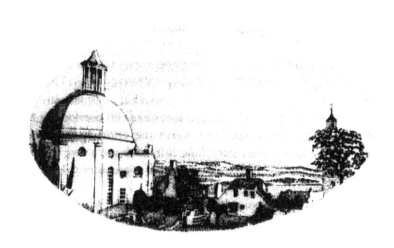

INCLUDES

Wales

℃ rossing from England into Wales, in a very short time you notice a country of different speech and different historical and cultural traditions; this is a Principality with deep-rooted national pride, which is vigorously defended. In this small chapter I can only hope to give you a taste of the excitement, wonder and delight you will find almost everywhere. The scenery is spectacular whether it is the majesty of Snowdonia, the glory of the Brecon Beacons or the magnificent stretches of golden sands.

Possibly one of the best examples of Welsh tradition is the Eisteddfod, the celebration of song and poetry in the Welsh language, which dates back to the Middle Ages and has remained an annual event. Welsh people from all over the world attend, from as far afield as the Welsh colony around Trelew in Patagonia. There is no one centre for the Eisteddfod and the venue is changed each year.

The southern corner overlooking the Bristol Channel, around **Swansea, Cardiff**, and **Newport**, is densely populated, with much heavy industry, but throughout the rest of Wales there are no very large towns and very little commercialism. What there is in abundance, is scenic natural beauty: three large National Parks, four important 'Areas of Outstanding Natural Beauty', rare flora and fauna, impressive mountains and pretty valleys, lakes, exquisite river scenery and some quite wonderful coastline, much of which is designated Heritage Coast.

The Snowdonia National Park is the largest National Park in Wales, with a landscape of deep valleys and rugged mountains formed by the glaciers of the Ice Age, giving lakes, rivers and splendid waterfalls which are legendary. The main feature is **Snowdon** it'self, the highest mountain in England and Wales at 3,560feet. The long sloping ridges to the peak and the steep drops between them give the climber great scope. Many of the wood and forests reach down the sharp valleys and add a much needed softness to the area.

As always in an area of such diverse terrain, there is a great variety of plants and wildlife. The coastal areas are a particular treat with wide sandy bays and sweeping dunes, and the estuaries are teeming with wading birds of all kinds.

There are Neolithic stone circles above **Penmaenmawr** and Bronze Age burial chambers at **Capel Garmon**. The old Roman road Sarn Helen can be traced running through the Park, and medieval Wales is brought dramatically to life with the castles at **Dolwyddelan** and **Castell-y-Bere**; The Edwardian **Harlech Castle** gives access to the wild, western mountain area. From the not too distant past you can see the remains and marks that the slate industry has left on the Park, not all bad; the narrow gauge railways are always popular with tourists. The Park covers an area of 827 square miles and the whole region is a stronghold of Welsh language and tradition.

The Brecon Beacons National Park is an area covering some 522 square miles, with the wild **Black Mountains** in the west and the old Norman hunting grounds of **Fforest Fawr.** The broad

Usk Valley in the north separates the Brecons from the Black Mountains, and in the south the different landscape of millstone grit and limestone has spectacular waterfalls and caves.

The Brecon Beacons contain many remains of castles and hillforts such as **Garn Gogh** at **Bethlehem**. Come to Bethlehem in December and you will find it probably has the busiest post office in the United Kingdom. Everyone wants to send their cards from Bethlehem. In the winter months this area can be a foreboding and desolate place with the terrain stretching on for as far as the eye can see. At these times of the year walkers should be prepared for extremes of weather.

The Pembrokeshire Coast National Park has over 100 miles of rugged coastline with broad bays and numerous islands, and is very popular with the sailing fraternity. Further inland are the tree-lined creeks and open moorland of the **Preseli Mountins.** The mild climate means that wild flowers flourish in abundance here and the area is famous for it's seal and bird colonies. At **Brynberian** the **Pentre Ifan Cromlech**, just north of the village, is the most impressive prehistoric monument in Wales, four vertical tapering stones hold a capstone. There are other ancient monuments as well as the reconstructed Iron Age hillfort at **Castel Henllys**, and early Christian relics are to be found throughout the Park.

Situated halfway between the Pembrokeshire National Park and the Brecon Beacons and on the far south coast, the 73 square miles of the **Gower Peninsula** in West Glamorgan was, in 1965, the very first area in Britain to be designated an 'Area of Outstanding Natural Beauty', chosen not only because of it's classic coastline and outstanding natural environment but also as a last outpost of unspoilt beauty in this otherwise industrial heartland.

Gower's scenery is rich and varied, ranging from saltmarshes and fragile dunes to the rocky drama of one of Britian's finest limestone coasts. The commons that lie inland dominate the landscape eventually merging into wooded valleys and traditional small fields.

The wild **Llyn Peninsula** in Gwynedd, most of it an 'Area of Outstanding Natural Beauty', is edged around it's 60 square miles on the north and west coast by rocky coves and sheer cliffs and on the southeast by picture-postcard bays. Next to the bay of **Porth Neigwl** or 'Hell's Mouth' so called because of it's treacherous tides, the sheer black cliffs of **Mynydd Mawr**, described as the'Land's End of Wales', overlooks the holy **Bardsey Island**. Inland the volcanic peaks of Yr Eifl abruptly give way to neat countryside with narrow lanes and hedged fields.

At the top of the Llyn Peninsula lies Anglesey, an island but linked to the mainland near **Bangor** by the Menai Bridge. Anglesey is wonderful. It has a tremendous sense of freedom. Gone are the immensity of the mountain ranges, so much part of this journey and instead there are gently rolling hills, low white cottages, and skies which seem endless. The whole of the island is criss-crossed with enticing small roads although there are two or three excellent A roads. Around the dunes of **Aberffraw Bay** and the high **Holyhead Mountain**, bird and plant life is plentiful. Further east **Great Orme's Head,** with the town of **Llandudno** the largest resort in Wales, rises spectacularly, with exposed fossils from the tropical sea that this area once was. From here are superb views of the mountains of Snowdonia.

Everywhere there is much to commend Wales to the visitor. **The Wildfowl and Wetlands Centre,** 2 miles east of **Llanelli** just above the Gower, is Wales' premier estuary for wildfowl and waders;

it has a visitor centre and many observation points. In 1993 it received Wales' 'Green Award' from the Tourist Board.

Castle Narrowboats at **Gilwern** in Gwent is another Green Award winner, it's canal boat hire business located on the original wharf from where the **Monmouth and Brecon Canal** was started 200 years ago. The canal is within the **Brecon Beacons National Park** passing through some of it's most beautiful and environmentally sensitive areas. In 1982 the first Monmouth and Brecon electric narrowboat was introduced, there are now four of them, one a 40 seater passenger boat. These boats have proved very popular due to their environmentally friendly characteristics - with no exhaust fumes and very little noise, the canal and surrounding environment is hardly disturbed and the recharging stations have been very carefully sited. Companies intending to operate boats within 'Sites of Special Scientific Interest' are being very much encouraged to use only electric boats, a clear signal as to future trends and legislation.

Nestling among historic remains at **Averdulais Falls** near **Neath** in West Glamorgan is a unique hydro-electric scheme, which is open to the public. The new **Turbine House** provides access to the top of the falls and visitors are able to see Britain's largest electricity generating water wheel.

The Stackpole Walled Garden Sense Centre in **Stackpole** near Pembroke, was opened in 1979 to provide unparalleled accommodation and facilities for the disabled visitor. The object of the sensory garden is to create a place where the primary senses can be stimulated in a therapeutic manner: through sound, based on the concept of outdoor musical instruments; sight, using optical illusions; scent in the form of a raised garden for the blind; and through all of them the sense of touch. It is believed that such a centre on this scale is unique in the UK.

Of great importance to those with a concern for the environment is the **Centre for Alternative Technology** at **Machynlleth** in Powys. It is unique in Europe. The Centre was started in 1974 on an abandoned slate quarry and after many years of hard and dedicated work there is now a seven acre display circuit (on a 40 acre site) open to the public. They have been experimenting with and demonstrating ways in which individuals, families and small communities can have a sustainable, whole and ecologically sound way of life. It has only been in the last few years that governments and consumers have started to look seriously for more environmentally friendly ways of producing the power needed for sustaining our modern day way of life. The number of visitors who find their way to **CAT** is continually on the increase, and with over 100,000 visitors each year there is no doubt the message is getting through.

The Centre is proving that a comfortable, varied, but in many ways rather ordinary lifestyle can be carried on with a fraction of the resources normally considered necessary, and in general with much lower environmental impact. Obviously this is not achieved without care, organisation and above all efficiency in the matching of resources to their uses.

At the Centre you can spend a very interesting and enlightening day. On arrival you can choose either to walk to the upper station by the main 250m track or by the woodland walk, or better still you can get to the upper station by a unique piece of environmental engineering, the centre's water-powered cliff railway, one of the steepest such railways in Britain, which operates on the principle of 'water-balancing'; with the two carriages connected via a winding drum at the top, water is run into a tank beneath the upper carriage until it is just heavier than the lower carriage plus it's passengers, then the parking brakes are released and gravity does the rest.

At the upper station, displays are arranged in a more-or-less circular route, and range from organic gardening through hydro and solar power onto composting and recycling and much more. The centre also holds courses on subjects as diverse as birdwatching, alternative sewage systems, wind power, and vegetarian cookery.

The area all around **Machynlleth** along the Dyfi Valley has much to offer the visitor. There are nature reserves, forest trails and a heritage trail, a pony-trekking centre, enigmatic stone circles, magnificent water falls and lakes, an organic vegetable garden, a wind farm, a craft centre and a railway museum. There is also the steam, narrow gauge **Tal-y-Llyn Railway** running from near **Abergynolwyn** through Snowdonia National Park to the coast at **Tywyn**.

Not far from here is **Craig-yr-Aderyn**, otherwise known as 'Bird Rock', created when the sea receded with the silting up of the Dysynni, leaving the rock stranded four miles inland. It is a strange oddity with it's craggy cliffs soaring over 700 feet above the fertile meadows of the Dysynni Valley. Cormorants still nest here, not seeming to care about the extra distance to go for lunch!

North from this valley rises the **Cader Idris** mountain range beyond which is Snowdonia. As Snowdonia joins the Llyn Peninsula around **Porthmadog** is the small town of **Tremadog**. In 1888 T.E. Lawrence, better known as Lawrence of Arabia, was born here as shown on a plaque on the house which is on the south side of the town, now the Centre for Christian Mountineering which opens it's doors to all faiths who wish to participate in it's environmental, climbing and adventure courses. The town also has connections with the poet Shelley who incurred the anger of the locals by his belief that sheep were in general unhappy and ill, which led him to put them out of their misery without first making sure they were not incurable.

Very close by is **Portmeirion**, by any standard a 'different place' and one that never fails to delight me. Often referred to as 'Little Italy', it was built between 1920 and 1972 by Sir Clough Williams-Ellis who moved to Dyfed to reproduce his dream, supposedly using Portofino as a template. With it's peculiar architecural style Portmeirion has succeeded in creating a place of lightness and beauty with an air of tranquillity. Critics who prefer a more serious architectural style would say that the diversity of buildings and the air of unreality make this place too much like fairyland, but Portmeirion is one man's attempt at capturing a certain ambience and culture, built with love and with no intention of creating a theme park.

I love the place for it's beauty and it's escapism. To stay here either in self-catering accommodation in one of the villas or houses or to enjoy the superb hotel, is a never forgotten experience. It is equally pleasureable for day visitors to wander round the village, have a meal in one of the restaurants, sit a while on the Piazza and dream dreams.

Those of us old enough to remember the television series 'The Prisoner' will recognise Portmeirion as the place where the programmes were made. Noel Coward is said to have stayed here while he was writing 'Blithe Spirit'. Portmeirion is unique, probably best described as a surreal village, a bold statement. You may love it or hate it, but you could not dispute it was worth a visit.

More conventional buildings are to be found at the **Welsh Folk Museum** at **St Fagan** near Cardiff. Over 20 buildings from all over Wales have been brought together on a 20 acre site to form an open air museum. There are various types of farmhouses and agricultural buildings, a Unitarian chapel, woollen mill, smithy and toll houses. These are important collections of Welsh social history, supplemented by displays of costumes, material culture, agriculture and vehicles to work the land, some in the reconstructed houses others in a special museum.

St Fagan also gives the visitor a good idea of the social and cultural life in Wales, over the past couple of hundred years through regular demonstrations by craftsmen, such as smithying and wood turning, dyeing and weaving. The museum also sells traditional Welsh bedspreads. To find out what it was like to be a successful merchant in the 15th century visitors can walk around the **Tudor Merchant's House** in **Tenby**. To find out, on the other hand, what it was like to be a gold miner in the 1930's, visitors can now explore the **Dolaucothi Gold Mines** near **Lampeter** which were first exploited by the Romans some 2,000 years ago. Welsh gold has been used for many important items for the Royal Family for centuries.

Three and a half miles east of **Llangollen** stands **Pontcysllte Aqueduct**, the longest aqueduct in Britain at 1007 feet long and 127 feet high, built by Thomas Telford and completed in 1805. The stupendous structure has 19 sets of arches, and is still in use, although more now by holiday cruisers than by the commercial barges for which it was built. In a former warehouse is an exhibition on the subject of the part canals have played in Britain's history.

Halfway between Llandeilo and Ammanford and well off the main road near the hamlet of **Trapp** is **Careg Cennen Castle**. The medieval masonry may be unkempt and ruinous but it sit's defiantly and breathakingly on top of a sheer-sided limestone cliff overlooking the forbidding Black Mountains. Well worth the effort is the walled passageway, hewn out of the side of the cliff leading to a cave beneath the castle it'self, unarthed here were a number of prehistoric skeletons.

Llantrisant in Mid Glamorgan was the home of Dr William Price, a preacher who in his time was considered something of a revolutionary with strong views on subjects such as vegetarianism, politics, nudism and sex, and he was not averse to preaching about them. In the 1800's even thinking about these issues could make you extremely unpopular. A statue of this unusual character with his fox-skin head-dress stands, appropriately, in Llantrisant's **Bull Ring.**

Knighton is the only town that stands on top of Offa's Dyke. King Offa of Mercia in the 18th century had the earthworks constructed as the first official border between England and Wales. The **Offa's Dyke Centre** is able to give information on the 170 mile footpath which follows as nearly as possible the line of the Dyke, running close to the border with England.

Guest House - **GRAIANFRYN**

Penisarwaun, Caernarfon, Gwynedd LL55 3NH

Tel: 01286 871007

Graianfryn, set in spectacular countryside on the edge of Snowdonia with it's wonderful walks is also close to Anglesey's sandy beaches making it an ideal centre for touring North Wales or for a walking, climbing, or beach holiday. It is just three miles from Llanberis at the foot of Snowdon with it's lake and mountain railway.

Amongst the many tourist attractions within close proximity to Graianfryn are the castles of Caernarfon, Beaumaris and Conwy, narrow-gauge railways (including Ffestiniog railway), Portmeirion and Bodnant Gardens. Road communications to North Wales have been greatly improved making it easily accessible from England and there is a railway station at Bangor.

The early Victorian ex-farmhouse is beautifully furnished throughout with beams, original fireplaces, log-burning stove, antique furniture etc and offers luxurious accommodation. Catering is to a high standard and is exclusively vegetarian and wholefood. The dishes are imaginative and created on the premises using healthy and fresh ingredients (organic and from the garden where possible). Specialities include home-made bread, ice-creams and tempting desserts and cakes.

The evening meal is served by candlelight in the romantic setting of the pretty and intimate dining room. Vegans and special diets are well catered for. The house is strictly non smoking. A brochure is available from Christine Slater at the above address. As all meals are freshly prepared please telephone in advance.

USEFUL INFORMATION

OPEN; All year, please give advance notice of arrival

CHILDREN; Welcome to share parent's room

CREDIT CARDS; None taken.

LICENSED; No. Please bring your own wine.

ACCOMMODATION; For 6 adults. Ensuite rooms available.

ON THE MENU; All wholefood vegetarian. Vegans & special diets with advance notice.

DISABLED ACCESS: No

GARDEN; Patio with picnic benches. Herb fruit and vegetable garden. Views across open countryside and to the mountains.

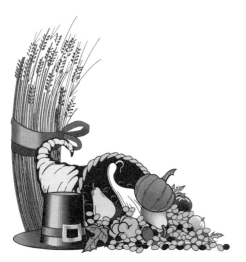

Hotel - **TREGYNON COUNTRY FARMHOUSE HOTEL**

Gwaun Valley, Nr. Fishguard, Pembrokeshire SA65 9TU

Tel: 01238 820531 Fax: 01239 820808

If you have a love of good, imaginative food, fine wines, a wonderful atmosphere and want to marry that with somewhere that seems to be out of this world, then Tregynon must be the place for you. For starters the hotel stands overlooked by Carn Garli, Mountain of Angels, and perched on the edge of the spectacular, and almost forgotten Gwaun Valley with it's banks carpeted with ancient oaken forests. This 16th-century farmhouse is full of character, has a wealth of old beams, fascinating nooks and crannies and in addition to the comfortable, centrally heated, ensuite bedrooms in the main house there are charming cottages adjacent which have been converted to provide Tregynon's finest bedrooms. Peter and Jane Heard are your hosts. Jane is an inspired cook who has won many awards for Tregynon. It is not only that she cooks well that makes the food so good, it is the fact that she constantly brings imaginative thinking to existing traditional recipes and the result is what makes Tregynon special. One of the specialities of Tregynon is wholefood and vegetarian dishes but the menu spans across many choices. Dining in a low, beamed ceilinged room with walls of rough stone which may well be similar to the stone used at Stonehenge, produces an atmosphere that is conducive to relaxed and enjoyable dining and without young children for whom a meal is produced at 6pm leaving their elders and betters to relax and enjoy both the food, the wine and the company.

USEFUL INFORMATION

OPEN; All year
CREDIT CARDS; All major cards
LICENSED; Yes
ACCOMMODATION; Ensuite centrally heated rooms

DINING ROOM; Award winning food specialising in wholefood and vegetarian dishes
DISABLED ACCESS; Yes

Exclusively Vegetarian Country Hotel - **TREMEIFION**

Talsarnau, Nr Harlech, Gwynedd LL47 6UH

Tel: 01766 770491

Tremeifion is a wonderful base for exploring the many attractions in the area and the owners' aim is to make their guests' stay a relaxing and enjoyable experience. Enjoy unrivalled and spectacular views from the sun lounge and 3 acres of private garden. Browse through a wide range of books and magazines in the comfort of the spacious lounge. Breakfast on the special 'Tremeifion Muesli', fresh and dried fruit's, home-made breads and full cooked breakfast. relax in the evening with a candlelit dinner of three courses, with a choice for each course, followed by coffee/tea and mints. A selection of vegetarian organic wineis available. There are five individual bedrooms, all with tea/coffee making facilities, hair dryers and radio clocks. No smoking throughout the hotel.

USEFUL INFORMATION

OPEN; All year. Bargain weekend breaks Oct-Jun inclusive

CREDIT CARDS; None taken
CHILDREN; Welcome - special rates
PETS; Welcome - by arrangement
LICENSED; Full on Licence
ACCOMMODATION; 3 dbl ensuite, 1 tw, 1 fmly. H & C throughout. CH.
No smoking within hotel.

ON THE MENU; Wide range of exclusively Vegetarian meals.
Open to non-residents.
Booking essential
DISABLED ACCESS; No wheelchair
GARDEN; 3 acres garden with seating

Hotel - **THE OLD RECTORY**

Maentwrog, Gwynedd, North Wales LL41 4HN

Tel: 01766 590305

If you want to stay somewhere which will allow you to explore Portmeirion Italianate Village-the film location for the TV series 'The Prisoner', the beaches of Harlech, Porthmadog and Shell Island, take a ride in the Ffestiniog Railway, visit wonderful gardens, explore castles, climb Snowdon, go horse-riding, play watersports or golf or go for some superb walks. then you should stay at The Old Rectory at Maentwrog which is within easy reach of all these delights. Built around 1845 as the dower house for local landed gentry, becoming a rectory in 1890, the hotel is constructed of handsome Welsh stone and features an unusual chimney construction known as flying buttresses. The three acre garden is bordered by the river Dwyryd, and surrounded by fields. The ensuite accommodation in the house overlooking the gardens, is spacious and well furnished with king size beds and TV's. The budget annex, originally the stables, has double, twin or family rooms all en-suite. Dogs are accepted in the annex rooms for a nominal charge. You will be extremely well-fed whether you are Vegetarian, Vegan, non Vegetarian or on any other diet. It is a friendly, happy house - a good place to stay.

USEFUL INFORMATION

OPEN; All year

CHILDREN; Welcome

CREDIT CARDS;All major cards

ACCOMMODATION; En suite rooms and in budget annex house

ON THE MENU; Excellent food for Vegetarians, Vegans & non-Vegetarians

DISABLED ACCESS; No special facilities

GARDEN; Lovely grounds border in in house

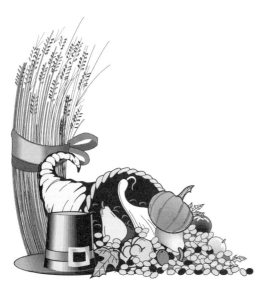

Restaurant - **PEPPERS RESTAURANT**
Puzzle Square,Welshpool, Powys SY21 7LE
Tel: 01938 555146

PEPPERS has grown in stature as a restaurant which provides as much good food for vegetarians as it does for meat eaters. The philosophy behind the running of this attractive, light, airy, establishment was accentuated by Wendy Waldron and Judith Ward who became the energetic and perceptive owners some five years ago. They took stock of Peppers which had been in being for about six years and decided it had much they liked but even more that they could improve upon. The regular clientele, who have discovered this quiet oasis, in a secluded square to be found off many of the alleys that lead from the main street of Welshpool, will tell you that they come here as much for the ambience as the excellent food. Peppers is not large, it has 32 covers added to in the summer months when you can sit outside and enjoy a meal in the sure knowledge that your children and animals are safe in a traffic free area. The criteria for any good eaterie has to be home-cooked food using as much as possible of both local produce and ingredients. This is very much so here. You will find that everything is made on the premises and covers a wide range from snacks, which are 75% vegetarian to light meals where 50% of the starters are vegetarian and both the main courses and desserts on offer are 50% vegetarian. There is a wide range of pies and quiches, also jacket potatotes with numerous fillings and hot dishes of the day. The cheese, onion and potato pie is a by-word for many a mile. There are few people who do not rave about the excellence of the home-made scones and cakes. Whilst there is a very limited wine list, there are a number of delicious and unusual specialist teas including many herbal varieties.

USEFUL INFORMATION

OPEN; Mon-Sat 8am-5pm,
Sun: 10-5pm Closed Autumn/Winter
Sundays & Christmas and New Year.
CHILDREN; Welcome
CREDIT CARDS; None taken
GARDEN; No, but secluded square.
ACCOMMODATION; Not applicable.

ON THE MENU; A mixture of
vegetarian and meat dishes
All home-cooked
DISABLED ACCESS; Yes, but no
special toilets.
LICENSED; Restaurant. Limited
list

OLD STATION COFFEE SHOP

Dinas Mawddwy SY20 9LS Tel: 01650 531338 Situated on A470, 1 mile north of Mallwyd.
Built as a railway station in 1868, the coffee shop has been in the capable hands of Eileen Minter for 22years. 75% of her dishes are suitable for vegetarians. OPEN; March-early Nov 7 days. Licensed.
No smoking inside. Garden. D/Acc.

BICYCLE BEANO

Cycling Holidays, Erwood, Builth Wells, Mid Wales LD2 3PQ UK.
Tel: 01982 560471.
E-mail: bicycleabeano.kc3Ltd.co.uk.
Internet: http://www.kc3Ltd.co.uk/local/beano/. NS V/VG Lic. Children ESR

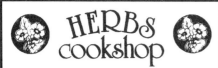
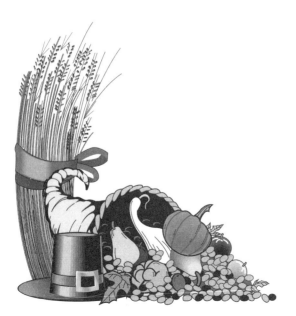

Chapter Six

Central England

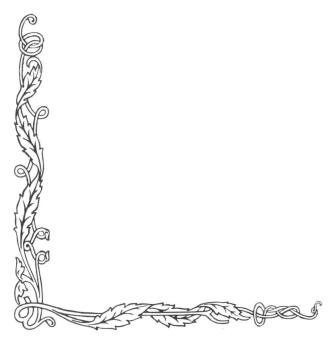

CENTRAL ENGLAND, HEREFORD, WORCESTERSHIRE, SHROPSHIRE, WEST MIDLANDS, WARWICKSHIRE, DERBYSHIRE, LEICESTERSHIRE, NORTHANTS, LINCOLN & SOUTH HUMBERSIDE

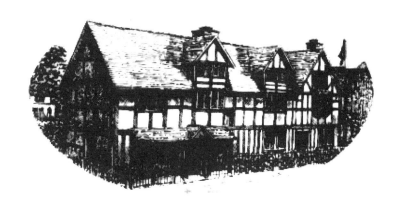

INCLUDES

Chapter 6

Central England

Hereford & Worcester, Shropshire, Staffordshire, West Midlands, Warwickshire,
Derbyshire, Leicestershire, Northamptonshire, Nottingham,
Lincolnshire & South Humberside

*A*ctually further south than north, and right over to the west of England bordering Wales, this region has become known as the 'Heart of England'. Right in the centre the county of West Midlands is very much an industrial one, and industry has thrived around this core, particularly to the north in Staffordshire, but there are too, particularly good farming lands and some, on the whole, very pretty countryside.

Hereford has an indefinable air of well being. In the far south west of the region close to the county town, the red soil, is rich and well farmed. It derived from old red sandstone and when the fields are ploughed the contrasting colours of the soil and the green of the trees will leave most people lost for words. This is a stunning district, it's numerous rivers and oak woods, it's wild daffodils and it's superb black and white timbered buildings, giving the impression of a managed landscape. They may not actually farm to beautify the countryside here, but that is what they achieve.

Various small towns and villages appeal to me in this lovely county. **Ross-on-Wye**, a delightful market town built on a steep rocky outcrop, has been a favourite with visitors since the early Victorian era when, as now, the attractions of the surrounding countryside and the excellent salmon fishing brought people back year after year. South of Ross, there are a multitude of attractions to be found as the Wye loops it's way round to enter the precipitous gorge known as **Symonds Yat**, one of the most beautiful and spectacular views in England.

Apple trees, some of them of unknown age, proliferate throughout Hereford and Worcester and cider has always been an important industry here, from the large scale to the various farmhouses advertising their wares with signs by the road. At **Much Marcle,** an attractive village, blessed with a fine church of 13th-century origin, **Putley** and **Lyne Down**, the old fashioned cider farms are opened to visitors and there are several organised cider events each year. Recently grapes have become almost as commonplace as apples, and there are now many vineyards in this region. **Ledbury** is a lovely, ancient market town set by the old cross roads to Tewkesbury, Hereford and Gloucester.

The **River Teme** wriggles through the three counties of Herefordshire, Worcestershire and Shropshire in the area around **Tenbury Wells**. A borough since 1248, Tenbury has remained an attractive small market town surrounded by hopyards and apple orchards.

Leominster (pronounced 'Lemster) lies nine miles to the south-west and is Herefordshire's second largest town, set amongst a gentle landscape of fields, hills and meadows where stream and brook wander. The town's fortunes were based on the fine quality of the wool from the local breed of sheep, the Ryeland, an animal that thrives on the poorer grazing to be found on the neighbouring hills and the less fertile outcrops of sandy soil from which the name is derived.

Hereford the county town, which one approaches along a road dotted with cider orchards, hint at one of the city's major industries. **Bulmer's** have been making cider in Hereford for well over a century and their premises in Plough Lane are open for tours and samplings. The Cathedral, begun in the 7th century, is wonderfully handsome but quite small compared to most cathedrals. It is full of many unique treasures, chief amongst these is the Mappa Mundi, a map of the world drawn around 1290 and of great importance because it shows us how the scholars of that time saw their world, both in spiritual, as well as geographical, terms. The choral traditions of the cathedral are long and the origins of the magnificent Three Choirs Festival can be traced back to an 18th-century chancellor, Thomas Bisse. To listen to soaring music in such surroundings is surely close to the 'rudiments of Paradise'.

Fine half-timbered buildings are to be found at **Weobley** (pronounced 'Webley) where the first tough Hereford strain of cattle, dark red with white faces, bellies and hocks, were first bred on the Garnstone Estate. **Eardisland**, a picture postcard village, on the banks of the River Arrow continues the half-timbered black and white theme and almost next door is the beautiful and unspoilt village of **Pembridge** with a wealth of 13th and 14th century buildings.

The venerable Cathedral City of **Worcester** is capital to the region and reflects much of the contrasts to be found within the region as a whole with historical associations, architectural contrast and industrial, as opposed to agricultural wealth; yet even it's industry has a bucolic air to it, for the black smoke and noisome forges of the industrial revolution have little place in the manufacture of gloves, Royal Worcester porcelain, or that secret blend of 'brown vinegar, walnut ketchup, anchovy essence, soy sauce, cayenne and shallots' known world-wide as Worcestershire Sauce. The Cathedral, a place of beauty, harmony and full of interest, stands on a rise overlooking the River Severn and the **Worcestershire Cricket Ground**, giving the ground a splendidly English backdrop, ideally suited to our summer game.

The Vale of Evesham with it's dark fertile soil, produces the finest of fruit and vegetables while farmers throughout the region happily indulge in the old-fashioned concept of mixed farming with seeming success. The River Avon almost entirely encircles **Evesham**, an attractive market town and where **The Almonry Museum** chronicles much of Evesham's fascinating history.

The area between Evesham and Pershore has a number of most attractive villages and on the other side of the A44 and on the B4080 is **Eckington**, a quiet village on the edge of the Cotswolds. **Pershore** is the second town in the Vale and was once the 'third town' of the county after Worcester and Droitwich. A handsome town with a predominance of seemingly Georgian architecture (many are facades built onto older buildings) it lies to the north of Bredon Hill amongst water-meadows beside the Avon's meanderings. To the south-west lies another small town of considerable appeal whose fortunes have also been linked to a river: **Upton upon Severn**. It is a charming place with an abundance of good pubs and hotels.

Worcestershire's greatest natural glories are to be found to the west of the Severn. **The Malverns** are perhaps the originators of that well-known phrase ' as old as the hills' for this ridge of pre-Cambrian rock is more than 500 million years old. The name means 'the bare hills' and they rise gently from fertile soils and woodlands to stand guardian against the prevailing winds. Although of no great height (the highest point is only 1394 feet) their appearance is impressive in contrast to the lowlands from which they spring, and the infinite permutations of light and shade sweeping over their bracket strewn slopes and barren summit's have inspired musicians, poets and artists over the centuries.

If **Warwickshire** can be described as the heartland of England then the Avon must be the principal artery in that it's waters have provided means of irrigation, transport and power. **Stratford-Upon-Avon** is without doubt the central tourist attraction of the county- perhaps of the entire country. Shakespeare may be synonymous with Stratford, but the town was of importance long before his birth (reputedly on St George's Day, 23rd April 1564) and had it's beginnings as a Roman camp, and a Saxon monastic settlement. Quite rightly, Stratford-Upon-Avon is home to the **Royal Shakespeare Theatre.** Originally known as the memorial theatre, it was designed by Miss Elizabeth Scott, a niece of the great Victorian architect Sir Gilbert Scott, and was opened by Edward, Prince of Wales in 1932. Considered controversial and innovative when first built, it stands massively beside the river and is a wonderful place to spend an evening being entertained by one of the greatest companies in the world. In the **Bancroft Gardens**, adjacent to the theatre is the impressive Shakespeare Monument, cast from sixty-five tons of bronze which shows the dramatist seated on a plinth surrounded by four of his principal characters (Hamlet, Lady Macbeth, Falstaff and Prince Hal). Also in close proximity to the Theatre are the **Other Place**, a small intimate theatre which presents a wide range of drama, and the **Black Swan Inn,** a favourite theatrical haunt that is better known as the Dirty Duck.

West Warwickshire is often referred to as Shakespeare country, providing numerous literary and historical connections, some true and some apocryphal, but one does not have to travel far from the centre of Stratford to find one of the most famous sites associated with the Bard of Avon. His wife, Anne, came from the picturesque little village of **Shottery**, now part of the modern borough of Stratford, and her family home, once called Hewland's Farm and now known as **Anne Hathaway's Cottage,** still exists.

Shakespeare's mother came from a well-to-do farming family who lived at **Wilmcote**, three miles north-west of Stratford, and, to my mind, **Mary Arden's House** is the most fascinating of the properties managed by the Birthplace Trust

Kenilworth will always haunt me because of the extraordinary and impressive sight of tall windows rising beside a massive fireplace in the ruins of the 14th-century Great Hall of Kenilworth Castle. You will see the red-sandstone castle keep standing foursquare on a grassyslope, aloof from the bustling market town below, serene in it's own world. Though it's towers are crumbling and it's windows as blank as sightless eyes, it still retains the imposing strength and grandeur that made it one of England's chief strongholds in Norman times.

Shipston-on-Stour dating from Saxon times has the flavour of other days. The streets are lined with houses and inns of the Georgian period built when the woollen industry made Shipston a more prosperous place than now. It is charming with weathered roofs of Cotswold tiles, quaint little dormers and handsome doorways with brass knockers.

The Grand Union Canal and the River Avon make their way through **Royal Leamington Spa**, whose tree-lined avenues, river-side walks and wealth of handsomely proportioned architecture are laid out in a grid pattern. Although the town has expanded further since the 19th century, much of the architectural interest has been retained around the centre and the original source of prosperity, the spring water, can still be sampled at the **Royal Pump Room and Baths.** This elegant building designed in the classical style with a colonnade, was first opened in 1814. It is a town blessed with many parks and gardens, perhaps the best known being **The Jephson Gardens** whose entrance lodge faces the Pump Room.

Industrialisation is the word that springs automatically to mind when thinking about the **West Midlands,** but the county does have rural areas mixed in with it's two great cities, it's three cathedrals, three universities and many old schools. It is said that Queen Victoria ordered the blinds of the royal train to be lowered so that she could not see the belching chimneys and furnace fires as she passed through the area. Thankfully the area has changed a great deal since her time, and there is now a dignity, both in the Georgian and Victorian buildings and the many modern constructions, be they artistic or utilitarian, along with parks and other amenities built for the enjoyment of the people.

Birmingham is certainly a city which has seen an improvement in it's standard of living in recent years, and is now an important centre for the arts. It has quite a lot worth seeing, all well documented in other publications, as are the attractions of **Wolverhampton** and **Coventry.** Due to the many businesses and activities taking place in these conurbations their inhabitants have come from all over the world, giving a great diversity of culture to this area.

The county of **Staffordshire** has probably some of the dullest and most depressing industrial areas in the land, but within a short drive the visitor can get right into the countryside. In the east of the county around **Uttoxeter** there is some of the best dairying countryside in England, and the scenery around **Dovedale** is wild and rugged and has a presence of foreboding, even more so when the black clouds cling to the snarling peaks and ring out their thunder which echoes and groans in the valleys for miles around.

In the north, Staffordshire shares the **Peak District** with Derbyshire and this area is a National Park to be explored again and again. There is a tendency to think of the Peak district as belonging exclusively to Derbyshire, but natural physical features have a distressing habit of ignoring man-made boundaries, and there is more than a little truth in the local boast that 'the best parts of Derbyshire are in Staffordshire'. This is fascinating countryside, almost cosy in scale one minute, then possessed of a wild grandeur, the next. North east of **Oakmoor,** through the hills and dales lies one of the most beautiful valleys in the region, **The Manifold Valley.**

The village of **Ilam,** standing at the southern end, makes a good starting point for exploring the area. The valley is relatively flat at this point but becomes increasingly deep and narrow as one journeys northwards. The River Manifold has a disconcerting habit of disappearing underground and at **Ilam Hall,** now a Youth Hostel, it re-emerges from it's subterranean journey from **Darfur Crags.** In the south is **Cannock Chase,** a 16 square mile area which attracts hoards of local people and visitors. Half this area is afforested with incongruous foreign conifers, but the other half is beautiful, open moorland with natural woods of oak and silver birch. Visitors should be warned that Cannock Chase is immensely popular and it is necessary to walk quite a way to avoid the crowds and to be rewarded with a sight of the wild deer and grouse.

The county town of **Stafford** is a city constructed on the site of a hermitage built by St Pertelin some 1200 years ago. Commercial development has left the town surprisingly untouched - apart from the jutting intrusion of a few tower blocks. It still wears the bubolic air of a country town even though it has been an important manufacturing centre for centuries. Here you have **Stafford Castle** built in 1070, an impressive example of an early Norman fortress. **Chetwynd House**, a handsome Georgian building is now the Post Office but it was here the ebullient playwright, theatre manager and MP for Stafford, Richard Brinsley Sheridan, would stay on his visit's to his constituency.

Due west of Stafford on the very tip of Cannock Chase, is **Shugborough**, ancestral home of the camera-wielding Earl of Lichfield. A beautiful mansion, dating back to 1693, and set within a magnificent 900 acre estate, Shugborough contains fine collections of 18th-century ceramics, silver, paintings and French furniture. **The Staffordshire County Museum** is housed in the old servants quarters and there are splendid recreations of life 'behind the green baize door'. Shugborough Park Farm is a working agricultural museum where rare breeds are kept, horse drawn machinery is used and an old mill grinds corn.

Longnor is a tiny market town in the farthermost corner of north-eastern Staffordshire on the same road which once used to carry the intrepid Greyhound as it rattled it's way across the rutted pot-holes over the moors. The road may have improved, but Longnor is little altered with it's stone lined streets and alleyways, houses with 18th-century facades and a small Market Hall dated 1873. Wandering westwards one comes across the highest village in England, set close by the high road from Leek to Buxton. The oddly named **Flash** claims this title at 1,158 feet above sea-level. A Nepalese would doubtless fall off his mountain with laughter, but it is a respectable height for our 'sceptr'd isle' and probably just as cold in winter as the Himalayas.

Leek is a neat mill town standing in magnificent countryside. Like so many of it's kind Leek has a cheerful and generous nature and welcomes visitors especially on Wednesdays when the old cobbled market square is thronged with stalls and the air filled with cheerful banter. There are a surprising number of antique shops and many of the mills have their own shops.

The great canal builder, Brindley, started his working life as a mill-wright and the **Brindley Mill** in Mill Street, tells the sory of his life and graphically demonstrates the many facets of this once important craft. One of his later works was the **Caldon Canal** which runs with the River Churnet in the valley alongside the hillside village of **Cheddleton**. The canal's successor, the railway, is commemorated at the **Cheddleton Railway Centre,** with displays, mementoes, engines and other paraphernalia set in and around the attractive Victorian station.

The two different forms of transport were obviously of major importance to the development of the industries of the north-western sector of the county. **Newcastle-under-Lyme** and **Stoke-on-Trent** lie side by side, geographically close yet separate in terms of history and character.

Coming from the east, the first is Stoke-on-Trent, a combination of the six communities of **Tunstall, Burslem, Hanley, Longton, Stoke** and **Fenton** - known the world over as **The Potteries**. The companies based here, both large and small, have a world-wide market for their products and their heritage dates back many centuries. Wherever fine china-ware is used and appreciated, names such as Spode, Copeland, Minton, Coalport, Royal Doulton and Wedgwood are revered and respected.

The Potteries have the flavour of a rural area; a feeling of continuity and a sense of tradition. The same family names crop up time and time again, and even in these difficult times, there is a pride in the past and enormous efforts have been made to clean up the detritus of yesteryear and make Stoke an attractive place in which to live and work. **Trentham Gardens** cover 800 acres of parklands, gardens and lakes with numerous sporting facilities. **Festival Park**, is an amazing 23 acre complex which includes a sub-tropical aquatic playground with flumes, water slides and rapids.

Newcastle-under-Lyme is the oldest of the two cities, dating back to it's incorporation as a borough in 1180, at a time when the neighbouring Potteries were hamlets or villages. Although Stoke-on-Trent and Newcastle have grown into each other, they still retain their separate identities; the delicate craft of the potteries being complemented by the ruder skills of the iron workers and colliers of their older neighbour. Modern Newcastle is an attractive town with much good architecture and is host to **Keele University**. Markets and a fair date from medieval times.

The surrounding countryside is immensely attractive with villages containing much good domestic architecture and a number of beautiful gardens, such as the **Dorothy Clive Gardens** at **Willoughbridge** and country parks like **Bathpool Park, Kidsgrove**.

Shropshire is such a wonderful mixture of countryside, architecture, agriculture and industry. It has wonderful places to visit, history which is fascinating and at times awe inspiring, stately homes, gardens and all manner of other attractions.

Telford is a new town that is light years ahead and well worth visiting. Nearby **Lilleshall** has six fully equipped sports and leisure centres of it's own. The Telford Ice Rink is one of the finest in the Midlands, and the home of one of the country's top ice hockey teams.

Cosford Aerospace Museum close to **Shifnal**, is one of the world's most spectacular collections of civil and military aircraft, with more than 70 aircraft, missiles and engines on display. It is outstanding and for anyone with a feel for aircraft, Cosford has to be seen. Allow plenty of time, one afternoon is hardly sufficient.

Market days are good fun in **Shifnal**. They are held on Wednesdays and one can just imagine walking with Dickens, who mentioned it in the Old Curiosity Shop, between houses in narrow streets, their timbered eaves and gables burdened with age.

Newport is only eight miles to the north-east of Telford but it is as different as chalk from cheese. Here I found a pleasant, unspoilt market town, centred around the broad, elegant High Street, a street just asking to be explored.

Just 3 miles north of Junction 3 on the M54 is **Weston Park** on the A5 at **Weston-under-Lizard**. The classic 17th century stately house is the historic home of the Earls of Bradford. The interior has been superbly restored, there is one of the country's finest collection of paintings, superb tapestries and letters from Disraeli which provide a fascinating commentary on Victorian history.

From Weston Park it is only a short distance to **Boscobel House**, in which Charles Stuart sought refuge after his defeat at Worcester. The Giffords of Chillington owned Boscobel and as staunch catholics they had honeycombed the house with hiding places for priests. If you see the house today many of them still exist. One will be pointed out to you as the kings, which is reached by a short flight of stairs leading to the cheese room.

You must visit **Tong**. It is only a small village but the magnificent 14th-century church of St Bartholomew would not be out of place in a city. It is frequently referred to as 'the cathedral of the West Midlands'. Just north of the village, off the A41, you can see a peculiar pyramid-shaped building set back a few hundred yards from the road. It's called the **Egyptian Aviary**, and it is a bizarre hen-house designed by a celebrated local eccentric, George Durant in the early 19th century.

The whole of **Ironbridge Gorge** is one big real-life museum that tells you every chapter of the fascinating story, on the spot, where it happened. There is no other place like it anywhere in the world. Make sure you allow yourself plenty of time to enjoy it. The Severn flows through this deep gorge and the houses cling to the hillsides, looking as though a puff of wind would blow them into the swirling river, but they have been there for hundreds of years and are as much a part of this incredible place as the Museums. The chief distinction is, of course, the bridge, believed to be the first iron bridge ever built. It was built by Abraham Darby of Coalbrookdale in 1777. It is 196ft long with one span of 100feet and two smaller ones, the total weight of iron being about 380tons.

Much Wenlock cries out to be visited; it is a lovely old market town full of history. Arthur Mee described it as somewhere that 'sleeps in the hills, dreaming of all that has been, stirring with the memory of warrior kings and the ancient strife of the Border Valleys, and inspired by the natural spectacle of Wenlock Edge'.

The steep wood escarpment known as **Wenlock Edge**, runs for 16 miles and provides a series of spectacular viewpoints across to the Stretton Hills and the Long Mynd. It is essentially a geological phenomenon; the rock, Wenlock limestone, was formed more than 400 million years ago in a tropical sea. It developed as a barrier reef built up largely from the skeletons and shells of sea creatures.

Three miles north-east of Much Wenlock on the B4378 you will come to **Buildwas Abbey**. Standing in a beautiful situation on the banks of the River Severn quite close to Ironbridge Gorge, it is a wonderful place to visit. It must be one of the country's finest ruined abbeys. Dating back over 800 years to Norman times it is surprising that so much is still standing today.

When you are in Telford, Wellington, Ironbridge or Much Wenlock you should make the effort to reach the summit of **The Wrekin**. It is a curiosity and one of the most distinctive landmarks in the Shropshire Hills. It is the site of an ancient Iron Age hill fort and it has been the focus of local legends and superstitions for hundreds of years.

Bridgnorth is two towns in one perched dramatically on a steep cliff above the River Severn. It is naturally beautiful and quite unlike anywhere else in England. The picturesque market town has High Town and Low Town linked by the famous Cliff Railway, which climbs up a hair raising incline. The only other I know like it, is the Cliff Railway which joins Lynton and Lynmouth in Devon.

There is something reminiscent of old Italian towns as you climb the Stoneway Steps cut sheer through the rocks, or wander about the maze of old half-timbered buildings and elegant 18th-century houses. One of these is the curious 17th-century Town Hall. This timber-framed building is built on an arched sandstone base partly across the roadway in the middle of the High Street. **Bridgnorth Castle** is famous for it's leaning tower which is 17 degrees out of straight. The leaning tower of Pisa is only 5 degrees!

I would think that almost everyone would be enchanted by the long established **Midland Motor Museum**, the only one of it's kind in Europe. Added to the collection of some of the world's fastest cars and motorcycles are the more laborious, but equally absorbing relics of the steam era. The exhibition covers a 25 acre site in the converted stable area of **Stanmore Hall,** an historic house on the outskirts of Bridgnorth.

To the east of Bridgnorth is **Claverley**, a pretty village with black and white houses and a fine Norman church. There is a nice story told about a friend of this village who left eight shillings a year for a man to be employed to drive dogs out of the church and wake up sleeping people. The man was given a long rod with a knob on the end and a fox's brush at the other. He would tap the heads of sleeping men with the knob and touch the faces of the women with the tail.

There are few better ways of seeing the Shropshire countryside with it's wooded valleys and changeable moods than from the **Severn Valley Steam Railway** which runs from Shrewsbury to Hartlebury, north of Worceser. It is designed to capture the atmosphere of railway history to the last detail with enchanting, evocative little stations like Highley, Hampton Loade and Arley, signal boxes and railway inns. Some two hundred thousand people, many of whom come from overseas, travel on the Railway each year, making it one of the most popular tourist attractions in the Midlands. It has become the home of the largest collection of working steam locomotives and restored railway coaches and wagons in Britain.

Ludlow is probably my favourite place in Shropshire. Here is a town that has few equals. It's river rings it like a moat and to walk about it's castle and streets is quite thrilling. We are lucky to claim it as part of England because it is almost on the Welsh border. It became a fortress from which Wales' unruly and mutinous tribes were eventually knocked into submission. The church of St Lawrence soars upwards and vies with the castle for supremacy. It is an outstandingly beautiful Perpendicular church with an earlier foundation, twice restored in the 19th century. The church is open in summer from 9-5pm and in winter until 4pm.

There are some beautiful places to visit between Ludlow and Shrewsbury. One of my favourite haunts is **Stokesay Castle**. It stands just off the Ludlow-Shrewsbury Road half a mile south of **Craven Arms**. There is a car park up the signposted lane and past the church, only a few yards from this romantic ruin.

The A49 going towards Shrewsbury will take you to **Little Stretton** which must be one of the most beautiful villages in Shropshire complete with a little thatched church and a village inn, **The Green Dragon** which is 250 years old. The pub is a popular haunt of walkers on the **Long Mynd Hills** and **Ashers Hollow**. Little Stretton's big neighbour, **Church Stretton**, is somewhere else you should visit. Houses dot the valley and climb the slopes. To the west is the great moorland ridge of Long Mynd rising nearly 1700 feet, with the beautiful Cardingmill Valley below and the prehistoric Portway running along the top. To the east are the rugged Caradoc Hills with Watling Street at the foot, and the banks and trenches of Caer Caradoc's stronghold 1500 feet up.

Bishops Castle to the west and surrounded by the beauty of the South Shropshire hills was plundered by Royalists during the Civil War in 1645. Here you are on the edge of the **Clun Forest**, a delightful place and if you have ever read A.E. Housman's 'A Shropshire Lad' you will know his description of the Cluns, he thought it a quiet area:

> *Clunton and Clunbury*
> *Cluganford and Clun,*
> *Are the quietest places*
> *Under the sun.'*

And so to **Shrewsbury** where once again A.E. Housman says it all:

> *High the vanes of Shrewsbury gleam*
> *Islanded in the Severn stream;*
> *The bridges from the steepled crest*
> *Cross the water east to west'*

It is almost an island with it's castle standing in a narrow strait and more than half-a-dozen bridges crossing to and fro. It has old black and white houses, half-timbered, of the Elizabethan era, fine brick buildings of the 17th century and wonderfully elegant Queen Anne and Georgian town houses, narrowstreets and alleyways with strange names - Grope Lane, Shoplatch, Dogpole, Wyle Cop and Pride Hill. Everywhere oozes history and clamours for your attention.

There are people who may tell you that North Shropshire is dull. That is absolutely untrue: it may be flatter than the south but within it you will discover it has miles of gentle green countryside, reed fringed meres, the excitement of the Shropshire Union and Llangollen Canals, red sandstone hills, a wealth of small villages and five historic market towns, Oswestry, Ellesmere, Whitchurch, Wem and Market Drayton.

Powys Castle you will find south of **Weshpool** on the A483. Not in Shropshire of course, but as you are so near the Welsh border it would be a pity to miss it out. What an atmposhere it has, that has been steadily increasing since it was built around 1200AD by Welsh Princes. The Castle contains the finest country house collection in Wales.

The 17th-century terraced gardens are wonderful and both historically and horticulturally important. So much history has gone into the centuries since the Castle was built and it has so many associations. It houses the **Clive of India Museum**.

Oswestry is back on the Shropshire side of the border. It is a delightful market town and cries out to be explored. It is equally splendid to wander the hilly, sparsely populated border country. This is a town that has so much to see and do that you could well stay here for a month and still not have seen everything.

Canals are very important to the way of life in this part of Shropshire and provide so much more than just water transport. Following the canal or the 'cut' is a wonderful way of exploring this area whether you have a boat or not. The towpath is a splendid, traffic free footpath on the level for miles albeit in some places it is distinctly rough going and very muddy. You are rewarded though by the wildlife that abounds on the water, in the bankside vegetation, and along the hedges. You can learn so much for the canal tells it's own story of our industrial and architectural heritage.

At **Whittington** you will meet with the **Llangollen Canal**, which wends it's way across the country right up into Cheshire where it joins the main Shropshire Union Canal close to **Nantwich**. Whittington is a very large village in the centre of which is the remains of Whittington Castle. All that you can see today of this important border castle is the magnificent gatehouse and the moat. It is a delightful place to visit, with a children's play area, ducks to feed and a tearoom in which to relax. The village is reputed to have been the birthplace of Dick Whittington, the famous Lord Mayor of London and cat owner!

From here I went north a little until I came to **Chirk** where it is the only way to cruise from England into Wales over the aqueduct on the Llangollen Canal, one of the seven wonders of Wales. This is quite a place with lots of history, right on the borders of Shropshire and Clwyd; it has withstood the slings and arrows of outrageous fortune. **Chirk Castle** which belongs to the National Trust, is a place you must visit and you should make sure you get to **Llanrhaedr Falls,** another of the seven wonders of Wales. They are stunning.

The Shropshire Union Canal, a popular waterway for pleasure craft, has played a great part in the history of **Ellesmere**, and the **Old Wharf** with it's warehouse and crane is a reminder of a prosperous period of development of the town when nearly 200 years ago it was the centre of plans for a link to the River Mersey, at what was to become **Ellesmere Port.**

Another place to join the canal is by the junction of the Whitchurch to Shrewsbury road east of Ellesmere. The junction stands above one of the earliest tunnels to carry a towpath through it. To the east is **Blakemere,** a lake left by glaciers some 12,000 years ago. In Autumn the trees on the opposite bank attract innumerable artists trying to capture their elusive beauty.

Ellesmere is not blessed with any major historical buildings but it is known as the capital of Shropshire's Lake Country because it stands on the biggest of ten wonderful meres. The most important are **Blake Mere, Kettle Mere, Newton Mere, Cole Mere, White Mere, Crose Mere,** and the biggest of all, called simply, **The Mere**. The very nature of the lakes makes them unique in Britain and indeed a rarity in global terms.

Naturalists have long been interested in these meres because of the phenomenon, which occurs occasionaly after a period of warm, calm weather; millions of tiny water plants, that we call algae, suddenly appear on the surface so that the mere becomes like thick soup. This indicates the abundance and importance of this tiny plant life as the basis of food chains supporting the wildlife of the mere.

Fringed by trees and rushes, **The Mere** covers 116 acres. It is home to swans and abundant wildlife, a place of beauty and of peace. It offers boating and fishing and is an ideal place for bird watching, most especially in the Winter Migration season when many rare birds are seen. On the shores of the Mere are the **Cremorne Gardens**, given by Lord Brownlow for the use of the people of Ellesmere. This lovely waterside park is a place beloved by the people of the town. It is a sheer delight to walk amongst it's well kept lawns and avenues of trees always with The Mere and it's wildlife in sight.

Wem is a town that still manages to preserve more of the old market town atmposphere than most others. It dates back before the Conquest in 1066 and can boast that it is the only town mentioned in the Domesday Book which can trace descendants from before and after the Conquest.

Whitchurch is the most ancient of the market towns dating from 60AD when it was founded as a garrison for the Roman legions marching between Chester and Wroxeter. Many Roman artefacts and buildings have been found in the town centre, notably in 1967 and 1977, and Pepper Street, High Street and Bluegates occupy the same situation as the Roman streets.

Market Drayton is a market in name and by nature. Ideally you should come here on a Wednesday and join the bustling bargain hunting tradition that has been going on for over 750 years. Since the Norman Conquest this seemingly sleepy and isolated town has been the scene of revolt, riot, murder, adventure and trade; it's links have extended worldwide. Clive of India was born here and will never be forgotten for many reasons and not the least because of **The Clive and Coffyne**, a splendid old inn in which the landlord makes Clive Pies from a recipe that Clive gave in 1768 to the French town of Pezanas... If you are worried about the second part of the pub's name, don't be - a coffyne is the local name for a pie crust. You will find much to enjoy in Market Drayton, including the celebrated product of the local bakers' shops - Gingerbread Men, which come in a range of novelty shapes and packages, all faithful recipes over 200 years old. A true taste of history!

You must find time to travel 6 miles down the A53 to **Hodnet** where the **Hodnet Hall Gardens** covering 60 acres are unrivalled for their beauty and natural valley setting. The magnificent trees, lawns and lakes provide background to an ever changing seasonal colour and interest. Between April and July the rhododendrons are fantastic.

From the high peaks of the Pennines in the northwest to the flat flower fields in the east and the undulating farm lands in the south **The Midshires** is one of mixed terrain. It has always been crossed by major roads, from truly ancient tracks to Roman roads, trunk roads and more recently motorways, resulting in an area rich in history. It is also crossed by hundreds of miles of canal linking the area to important centres of trade, mostly further to the west.

Northamptonshire is often given no more consideration than being somewhere it is necessary to travel through to reach an intended destination. This is the county of 'Spires and Squires'; it's Saxon churches and it's grand country houses, being very fine, although it's domestic architecture is generally less impressive. Many of the large country houses are still privately owned and many of them not open to the public or only by appointment.

Northampton it'self is the busiest place in the county, famous for it's boots and shoes since King John bought a pair of shoes here for ninepence in the early 13th century. It is a thriving market town and a wonderfully convenient place to use as a base for seeking out the beauty of the county. The Norman church of **St Peter** in **Marefair** is beautiful with no structured separation between the nave and the chancel. **The Central Museum and Art Gallery** in Guildhall Road not surprisingly has a strong collection of boots and shoes, the largest in the world. **The Leathercraft Museum** in Bridge Street contains leatherwork from Ancient Egypt, Roman Britain, the early Middle Ages, gloves, Spanish leather, saddlery and the work of leathersellers. It is an amazing collection and very well displayed.

One of the most famous stately homes in all England is **Althorp**. The home of the Spencer family since 1508, it is known throughout the world now as the birthplace of Diana, Princess of Wales. It lies only a few miles to the west of Northampton off the A428. Althorp has been altered over the centuries but in one sense it has changed little, the site is the same and the basic structure is Elizabethan. The setting of the house, between formal gardens and in the middle of the park, is essentially a picture of Northamptonshire at it's very best.

Another masterpiece of English architecture is **Castle Ashby** which lies on the outskirts of the village of the same name and a mere seven miles from Northampton. The building was started in 1674 by Henry, 1st Lord Compton. The original plan of the building was in the shape of an 'E' in honour of Queen Elizabeth I, and about sixty years later the courtyard was enclosed by a screen designed by Inigo Jones. The most interesting feature of Castle Ashby is the lettering around the house and terraces. The inscriptions when translated read 'the Lord guard your coming in' and ' the Lord guard your going out'. The Compton family are still there today so I think the prayer has been answered, don't you?

Turner's Musical Merry-Go-Round to be found near the village of **Wootton** off the A508 has the most unusual collection of mechanical instruments. If you enjoy gardens you will be well advised to visit **Holdenby,** six miles north west of Northampton off the A50. It is a tiny place but it contains one of the jewels of Northamptonshire. **Holdenby House** was the home of Queen Elizabeth's Chancellor, Sir Christopher Hatton who became her favourite Lord Chancellor. Hatton Garden, home of the diamond dealers in London is named after him. The original house is no longer there but it's successor is a building of great beauty and dignity with fine transformed windows, seven picturesque dormers in the roof and some arresting chimney stacks. The grounds are particularly interesting with one of the finest Elizabethan gardens in Englnd. As you wander around the fragrance of the silver borders assails your nostrils. It is quite lovely.

Coton Manor Garden off the A50, 10 miles north east of Northampton, is another gem. It forms the framework for a charming 17th-century stone manor house. You can wander around the gardens to your hearts content watching the activity of the water gardens, admiring the herbaceous borders, revelling in the glorious colour and scent of the roses. It is beautifully kept and home to a collection of waterfowl, cranes and flamingoes.

Racing on the pretty course at **Towcester** is a very pleasant outing but even if there is no racing it is still a delightful place to visit and historically the oldest town in Britain. **Silverstone Motor Racing Circuit** is only four miles away.

Stoke Bruerne is just to the east of Towcester, It is a pretty place in it's own right with it's thatched cottages climbing the hill, but most people come here to see the canal winding slowly by until it's waters are raised by seven locks and vanish into a tunnel. **The Stoke Bruerne Canal**

Museum will keep you interested for hours and give you a deep insight into 200 years of history and tradition on the canals and waterways.

The land now given to farming covering much of Northamptonshire was at one time the ancient **Rockingham Forest**, with just a few small areas remaining. On a hill overlooking the thatched and slate village of **Rockingham** is the magnificent castle which dates from Elizabethan times. William the Conqueror gave orders for the keep to be built and King John used it as his hunting lodge. The castle was host to Charles Dickens on many occasions and it was to the then owners, the Watsons, that he dedicated David Copperfield.

Between **Grafton Underwood** and the village of **Geddington** is another wonderful stately home, **Boughton House**, the Northamptonshire home of the Duke of Buccleuch. The beauty of Boughton lies in the wonderful light from the 366 windows. It has been described as a vision of Louis XIV's Versailles transported to England. You will find it full of beautiful things. It should be remembered that Boughton House is an integral part of a thriving and progressive rural estate of some 11,000 acres. The 350 acre Park has broad avenues with 200 year old trees, with river and lake walks, nature trails and an Adventure Woodland Play area

Where the A6 joins the A6116 is the little village of **Islip** separated from it's bigger neighbour, **Thrapston** by the fine old bridge that spans the River Nene with many arches. Both places are like magnets for our American visitors. At Islip it is the elegant medieval church they come to see with it's great east window. It is as fine inside as out and high on the south wall of the sanctuary is a monument to Mary Washington, whose husband was John Washington of Thrapston, uncle of Laurence Washington who sailed to America in 1657, becoming the great-grandfather of the President.

In the west of the county **Daventry** will always be thought of for it's association with radio communications but it goes back to the Prehistoric Age when it was a fortified camp and the stronghold for men of the Stone Age. It lies on Borough Hill and is part of the ride which forms the Water Divide of the Midlands. From it's highest point the line of the ancient Watling Street may be followed. When the day is clear you can see into seven counties.

It is in **Oundle** in the north of the county that I leave you. This is a treasure of the county with it's fine houses, ancient pubs and St Peters Church with it's glorious Decorated tower and spire. If all this were not enough Oundle has one of the country's oldest and most famous public schools. The streets are wide and the gentle waters of the River Nene embrace it on three sides. Oundle illustrates all that is best and beautiful about this lovely county, the 'Rose of the Shires'.

The Grand Unon Canal continues through **Leicestershire** via **Foxton Locks**, an incredible flight of ten locks which raises the water by 75 feet. This county is a stronghold of fox hunting. It dates from the days when the area was heavily forested, and although now mostly farm land the hunting continues, with some of the most important hunts in the country. It is even said that the modern landscape 'has been moulded for the needs of fox hunting'. Leicestershire is said to be the least visited of all counties in England. Some people might say this is because of fox hunting but I think that would be unfair. I equally think it is a pity that it is not popular for it has much to offer.

Leicester is where people have lived and worked since before the Roman Conquest. The Romans recognised it's position as worthy because of it's many trade routes. Today it still has an enviable central position within two and a half hours drive of many of Britain's largest centres of population. Leicester is Britain's first Environment City and it shows in it's surroundings and green spaces - those used to more built up cities will be impressed by the parks and the gardens, green hedges, foot and cycle paths and wildlife sanctuaries in the city centre it'self.

The town has some fourteen museums and a host of other places to see and you will see a list of them in the Visitor Attractions section in the back of this book.

Ashby de la Zouch whose unusual name comes from the La Zouch family who acquired Ashby Manor in 1160, is a charming place which, in the 19th century, was quite a fashionable spa town. It is a place of mellow half-timbered buildings, impressive churches, delightful green parks and the ruins of an old castle which underlines it's historic past.

Coalville, as it's name suggests, is an industrial town originally centred round coal mining. I mention it because it is pleasantly situated on the fringe of **Charnwood Forest** and within walking distance of **Bardon Hill**, the highest point in Leicester.

Castle Donington is another nice small town. The Norman castle built to command the River Trent crossing was demolished by King John to punish the owner for supporting Magna Carta. It was rebuilt in 1278 and no less than four of it's subsequent owners were executed. The 13-14th century church has a spire that reaches for the heavens, the timber-framed houses are delightful and the shops will tempt you to spend money.

At **Donington Park**, where the vast Hall of 1793 was built in the 'Strawberry Hill' Gothic style, is the famous motor racing circuit, racing car collection and a new exhibition centre.

Between Ashby and Castle Donington is **Breedon-on-the-Hill** from which nothing blocks quite the most stunning and panoramic views in Leicestershire. It's Norman and 13th-century church stands with The Bulwarks, remains of an Iron Age fort, on one side and to the east a limestone quarry drops precipitously down creating an unbelievably beautiful setting.

Market Bosworth found fame nearly five centuries ago when the Wars of the Roses ended on the stricken Field of Bosworth two miles away. It has slumbered ever since, almost as if it was happy to step back into obscurity. It attracts visitors of course. **The Bosworth Battlefield Visitor Centre and Country Park** is signposted from the town off the A5, A44, A447 and B585.

Lutterworth just off the M1 and on the border of Warwickshire must be one of the loveliest places in the county, where the High Street climbs steeply from the bridge across the shallow River Swift and leads the way to it's famous church, with a tower stretching upwards as if to reach the heavens.

Market Harborough is a pleasing old market town and deep into hunting country - in this case the Fernie Hunt. The town was the creation of Henry II. Here in three days in 1645 the balance between King and Commonwealth swung. It was the eve of the Battle of Naseby and the streets and square were filled with Royalist soldiers. At the end of three days the church of St Dionysius was filled with Royalist prisoners. The first part of the dramatic turn of events took place when Charles I, sleeping at nearby **Lubenham** was roused at two in the morning with the news that Fairfax had marched from Northampton to Naseby. Charles came riding down the street in the darkness to meet his Generals at a Council of War. He allowed the rashness of the Cavalier, Prince Rupert, to prevail and the Royalist Army marched from it's entrenched positions to give battle to the New Model Army. At Midday the fight began and by nightfall the King was a fugitive, his army destroyed and his throne lost.

Finally in Leicestershire a visit to **Melton Mowbray** famous since Roman days and still famous now for it's pies, Stilton cheese, Melton Hunt Cake and hunting. You will want to stay in and around Melton for a while both to savour the town it'self with it's quaint customs, attractive buildings and a parish church that Leicestershire men acclaim as the most beautiful in England. Wherever you go in Leicestershire you will find warm-hearted people. Leicester has become a renaissance city with so much to offer. Yes, I do not rate the Cathedral compared to the might of Canterbury and the beauty of Wells but it is still a joy to see and the regeneration of the city makes it a place that should come high on any visitor's itinerary.

Rutland, the smallest of all counties is a gem, but in reality and officially it does not exist in it's own right but merely as an appendage to Leicestershire, although as I write, there is a move to restore it's independence. Those who live here will claim it as Rutland and not Leicestershire. It would take 300 Rutlands to make up England and 40 to cover Yorkshire but that does not phase this little brother of the shires. I started my journey in **Uppingham**, a small town which is home to one of England's finest schools known throughout the world. The great school with it's splendid halls and courtyards appears to stand sentinel over the quiet town with it's attractive bow fronted shops, peaceful streets and sombre ironstone houses.

Wing has one of the oddest survivals of any English village. The ancient turf maze is forty feet across and still preserved, a wonderful example of the mazes that were once commonplace in England. Here the maze is made up of little turf banks about a foot high winding round and round. Tradition has it that it's was devised by the Church as a means of penance, the wrongdoer was put in and left to find his own way out

Tinwell, a small village with a green and a good hostelry is very close to the magnificent **Burghley House**, home of the Cecil family. Burghley is one of the finest examples of late Elizabethan design in England. Entering it is like walking into an Aladdin's cave, full with every imaginable treasure. If the interior beauty was not enough, you have the additional thrill of walking in a 300 acre Deer Park landscaped by the inimitable Capability Brown under the direction of the 9th Earl. From Tingwell you are only moments away from the man made masterpiece, **Rutland Water**. Spanning 3,100 acres, it is the largest man-made lake in Western Europe. It is surrounded by delightful villages, offers all sorts of sporting facilities as well as charming walks.

My journey around Rutland Water finished at the capital of this small county **Oakham**. It is in the very heart of Rutland and quite lovely. The wide streets have delightful houses and flower filled gardens. Glimpses of hills and wooded lanes can be seen from the ancient cobbled market square. All that is good has been preserved including the ancient stocks and buttercross. It is all quaint and it would not evoke much surprise if one saw a prisoner in the five hole stocks.

Oakham is famous for it's magnificent church, it's old school and what is left of the castle. If you look upwards you will see high above All Saints, Cock Peter, a weather vane which must be the oldest in England. It is said to have shown the way of the wind to men on their way to the Battle of Agincourt.

Nottinghamshire is a delight, redolent with history, landscape and culture, yet intensely alive, taking advantage of it's very centrality to attract business and visitors from all over the world. The land is fairly flat with the highest country being in the western region - perhaps the only off putting fact about the county is that it's name is derived from the Saxon for 'the followers of Snot!'

More famous than anything happening today in Nottinghamshire, and more famous than any positively documented history, is the legend of Robin Hood and his exploit's in and around **Sherwood Forest**. There are some known facts which tie into the legend, and much of what is only recorded in the form of a story is likely to be true, but Robin Hood nevertheless remains something of a mysterious character, and perhaps it is best this way. Sherwood Forest once covered a huge area, and although what remains is still reasonably large by today's standards it is not on the large and daunting scale of past centuries. Possibly the best known tree anywhere is the **Major Oak**, a hollow tree several hundred years old. In the same area, **Edwinstowe** is an interesting forest visitor centre. **Nottingham Castle** has been rebuilt a couple of times and now houses a **Robin Hood Exhibition.**

In addition to the restored and converted castle, **Nottingham** has everything, with good theatre, concert hall, museums, pubs and hotels. Trent Bridge caters for cricket fans at county and Test level, whilst soccer enthusiasts can choose between the oldest football league club in the world, Notts County, or Nottingham Forest. Particularly impressive is the **National Watersports Centre** at Holme Pierrepoint, a 250 acre country park complete with 2,000 metre Olympic rowing course and white water slalom canoeing course - all this just four miles from the city centre. Under the city is a honeycomb of ancient caves, some linked by passages, used as dwellings until quite recently. There is even a pub here, carved out of the rock, the 'Trip to Jerusalem' which dates from the Crusades.

Eastwood is known as the birthplace of D.H. Lawrence and the family house in Victoria Street is now a museum to him, although he did not live there in adult life. He did however use the town and surrounding area with lightly disguised names in many of his novels, and the local library has a **Lawrence Study Room.**

At **Kirkby-in-Ashfield** is **Newstead Abbey**, ancestral home of one of England's greatest poets, Lord Byron, although he and his mother were too poor to move into it when they first inherited the vast place, and it was sold a few years later. Byron sold it to an old friend who spent a quarter of a million pounds on remodelling the house into it's present style incorporating the ruins of the priory. It is a site worthy of a romantic such as Byron, and the surrounding parkland with it's lakes and waterfalls and gardens provide the appropriate backdrop. Thanks to another two great benefactors the house and the land were presented to the City of Nottingham, whilst a third bequeathed a unique collection of Byronic relics.

Newark is almost a guide book cliche - an ancient market town with a strong sense of it's own importance in the history of our country. Situated where the ancient Fosse Way crossed the

Great North road and by the banks of the River Trent, where the wool was once shipped to Calais via the Lincolnshire port of Boston, it was an important geo-political centre from earliest times and it was considered the Key to the North in the turbulent days of the first King of All England. The town's buildings reflect it's importance in historical terms, particularly around the large cobbled market square with an enchanting blend of architecture, predominantly medieval and Georgian inlet with narrow streets and alleys.

The tall and well proportioned spire of the parish church of St Mary Magdalene rises to well over 200ft from behind the square and the building is mainly 14th century, although there has been a church here since Saxon times. However, to my mind, the town's greatest glory is to be found in the forbidding and noble ruins of **Newark Castle**, which stands guard over the entrance to the old town from the north. It is a wonderfully impressive structure and I think best viewed from one of the cruise boats that sail past it's ancient walls.

Before leaving Nottinghamshire I went, once again, to what has been described as 'England's least known Cathedral', the beautiful Mother Church of Nottinghamshire, **Southwell Minster**. If you admired the carvings in St Mary Magdalene, Newark, then you will be staggered by the work to be found in the 12th century Minster with it's octagonal chapter-house and twin spires.

Southwell it'self is an attractive small town and was once described by the late Sir John Betjeman as 'unspoilt', a description that is true today. The heavily beamed Saracens Head Hotel, an old coaching inn, was where Charles I spent his last night of freedom whilst **Burgage Manor** was the residence of Lord Byron and it was friends in the town who first encouraged him to publish his poems.

Just in **Derbyshire** on the Leicestershire border **Chalke Abbey** is one of the fairly new introductions to the list of National Trust properties to be opened. The huge house in an immense park was hidden from everyone for more than a century, the reclusive family keeping totally to it'self, not even allowing any motor vehicles within the grounds.

Another abbey of note is **Dale Abbey**, the largest surviving remnants of a dissolved abbey in Britain. Here too is the smallest church, a part of which is actually a house, and closeby is a cave occupied in the 12th century by a pious baker.

A large corner of Derbyshire is taken up by the **Peak District National Park**, for the most part a wild, desolate moorland. The outside edge is the Dark Peak of peat, the centre a landscape of undulating limestone with caves, criss-crossed by dry stone walls and deep wooded valleys with delightful unspoilt villages. One such is **Castleton** with spectacular panoramic views over the Peaks and perching high above it is **Peveril Castle**. The area abounds with spectacular caves and caverns, the show caves at Castleton being some of the best. At **Eldon Holt** it is an apparently 'Bottomless Pit'.

The elegance of the Peak District town of **Buxton** owes it's existence first of all to it's spa water and later to the lime industry and to copper. There is an important, international but also low budget opera season here each year. The town is the centre for exploration of the Peak District and has several museums including **A Natural World Exhibition**.

Matlock is another spa town, home to the **Peak District Mining Museum** and many other interesting places worth visiting.

The county has many Neolithic stone circles as well as a wealth of medieval castles and 18th century grand houses including **Chatsworth**, the seat of the Dukes of Devonshire. The 'Stonehenge of Derbyshire' more generally known as **Arbor Low Stone Circle** with it's giant stones around a sundial and beside it the slightly later round **Gib Hill Barrow,** are important Neolithic and Bronze Age monuments. Nearby are similar monuments at High Low, Lean Low and Carder Low. Other early monuments include the **Nine Ladies Stone Circle** and to the north **Eyam Moor Tumulus and Stone Circle.**

Eyam is also known for being the 'plague village' which in 1666 created it's own quarantine to prevent the plague from spreading. It is a tragic story and something no one in Eyam ever forgets. The tradition of 'Well Dressing' has associations throughout this region with the plague, the people who were not affected being grateful for the untainted water that their wells supplied. It is believed however that the tradition has even earlier roots. The small town of **Tissington** dresses five wells with flower pictures on Ascension Day each year.

One of the impressive grand houses of the area was the project of the then 71 year old Bess of Hardwick, widow of four husbands. The Elizabethan **Hardwick Hall** not far from **Chesterfield** was built to replace an even older house, the ruins of which are still to be seen, and now under the ownership of the National Trust, it is one of the country's most popular historic houses. In **Crich** visitors can travel back in time at the **Tram Museum**, with over 40 steam, horse-drawn and electric trams making it one of the finest transport museums anywhere.

Derby is an important industrial town: home to **Royal Crown Derby** porcelain, which has it's own museum; birthplace of the Rolls Royce and with various associations with railway engineering, as can be seen in the **Industrial Museum.** My first stop and my first love in **Lincolnshire** is the wonderful town of **Stamford**. It took me quite a while to get to know this fascinating county. Until I did I had always thought of it's as nothing else but fens and tulips with the occasional sausage and pork pie thrown in for good measure. It is no such thing and it burst forth upon me with a matchless and unique beauty of it's own. I suppose today I should refer to it's as the County of Lincolnshire and South Humberside which is it's official title.

This time I was determined to spend more time in and around **Stamford.** What an elegant town it is, probably the finest in the county standing at it's southern gateway, where Lincolnshire, Northamptonshire and Rutland meet and where the bustling River Welland makes a last dash down from hilly country to enter the Fenland plan. It was one of the five towns, Lincoln, Stamford, Leicester, Derby and Nottingham from which the Danes ruled Lincolnshire and the Midlands. For nearly a thousand years it has been a market town. It's beautiful buildings range mostly from medieval times to the Georgian era, and despite the centuries that separate them, the harmony is superb. No intrusion from the 19th century, the age of the Industrial Revolution, or one of our own 20th century have been allowed to spoil Stamford.

You will have much to explore when you stay here including perhaps a visit to **The Steam Brewery Museum** in All Saints Street, where you can watch the brewing process from start to finish. In All Saints Place is a church of that name, one of the five medieval churches in the town. I visited three of them and found All Saints the most beautiful, with an exterior distinguished by the 13th-century blank arcading and it's fine Perpendicular steeple. It is a church that makes a statement about the wealth of the rich merchants who endowed the church and to whom there are splendid brasses.

A little to the east of Stamford along the A16 is **Market Deeping** where the market is still a busy place and the rest of it's name (with the other Deepings) reminds us that once it's deep meadows were flooded every year by the River Welland from time immemorial. There are records that will tell you that the land was so fertile, gardens of great beauty were made out of it's pit's and bogs. The lands are still fertile, the floodings gone and the little town is a thriving place. The Old Market Place is where the A15 and A16 converge as well as several minor roads.

It would be a pity not to take a look at **Woodhall Spa** which you will find on the B1292 off the A153 between **Sleaford** and **Horncastle**. No longer operative as a spa town, the unique spa town atmosphere is still very much in evidence.   By the Golf Hotel and situated next door to the famous Woodhall Spa Championship Golf Course, there is a little **Cottage Museum** which will tell you how the town started and became a spa. You will then understand the enterprising John Parkinson, who set out with three aims in the early 19th century; 1. Build a town. 2. Plant a forest. 3. Sink a coalmine. The town sadly was not built in Woodhall but a street of fine town houses lies in the nearby village of **New Bolingbroke**. The forest was planted near Woodhall. As for the coalmine, John Parkinson chose a spot in Woodhall. When the shaft reached a depth of 540feet, there was an inrush of clear salty water. So the Spa began. The Museum is open daily from Easter to October.

Throughout the year the woodlands in and around Woodhall Spa provide a cavalcade of colour. There are picturesque walks. The Viking Way, a long distance footpath from the Humber to Rutland Water, goes through the village.

Going further towards the east coast, I made for **South Thoresby**, at the foot of the **Lincolnshire Wolds**, with it's open high landscape and peaceful villages, tucked in green valleys. An area of Oustanding Natural Beauty and beloved by Alfred, Lord Tennyson. The Wolds are crossed on their southern crest by the **Bluestone Heath Road**, a prehistoric ridgeway, passing nature reserves and some superb viewpoints, plus the deserted medieval villages of **Calceby** and **Calcethorpe**.

You will find South Thoresby one mile off the A16 and nine miles south of Louth. An ideal place for anyone to stay if they want to take a look at this coastline. An invitation to a race meeting at **Market Rasen** took me up the A16 to **Louth** and then on the A631 to this bustling town. Here is a delightful course, just east of the town and is acknowledged as one of the finest small tracks in the country, the town it'self is charming.

Twenty five years ago or thereabouts the area to the south of the Humber was part of Lincolnshire, now joined with the area north of the river which was previously the East Riding of Yorkshire to form the county of Humberside. In South Humberside evidence of our forebears abounds, place names mapping the successive invasions of the Romans, Saxons and Danes. Deserted medieval villages can be found, such as **Gainsthorpe** which was comparatively recently discovered from the air.

The now ruined Augustinian **Thornton Abbey** to the south of the Humber has a magnificent 3-storey gatehouse with a facade ornamented with finely-carved detail.

Alkborough could be described as an amazing place. There are several mazes to be found here, the largest and original is **Julian's Bower Maze** standing on a high escarpment overlooking the confluence of the Trent and the Humber, a turf maze some 44 feet in diameter, probably cut by monks in the early 13th century. In the church is a replica of it in the floor of the porch. There is also one in a stained glass window and one on a tombstone.

Restaurant - **VAL VERDE**

Diamond Court, Water Street,
Bakewell, Derbyshire
Tel:01629 814404

Whilst Val Verde is not a vegetarian restaurant, it does serve some wonderful pasta dishes and pizzas that conform to the needs of the non-meat-eater. It is a delightful place tucked away in the midst of Bakewell's intriguing alleyways in Diamond Court surrounded by a profusion of roses, ivy and clematis. It is not so long ago that the restaurant was known as the Green Apple but with it's new owners it has taken on, not only a new name, but a new lease of life and is fast earning a name for it'self not only in Bakewell but way out into deepest Derbyshire. It is a deserved reputation. You have only to look round at the happy diners to know how successful it is. Your table will be candlelit, attractively laid and you will await your starter with eager anticipation. That might well be a Greek salad or asparagus with gorgonzola, mascarpone and parmesan cheese sauce or perhaps home pickled mushrooms, roast peppers, anchovy sauce, leeks and prawns in oil and herbs. Follow that with a pizza baked to order with fresh pizza dough. Pizza con Funghi - tomatoes, fresh and wild mushrooms and pecorino cheese or Pizza Val Verde with tomatoes, goat's cheese, thyme and walnut oil will leave you wondering if you could possibly manage a bowl of Italian style ice-cream - do try it is unmissable.

USEFUL INFORMATION

OPEN;Daily from 10am for coffee, lunch & afternoon tea.
Dinner Mon-Sun 7pm-10pm
(10.30pm on Fridays & Saturdays)
CHILDREN; Welcome

RESTAURANT; Excellent range of dishes for
Vegetarians and other
DISABLED ACCESS;No special facilities
CREDIT CARDS; All major cards

Hotel - **THE FALCON HOTEL**

St. Johns street, Lowtown,
Bridgnorth, Shropshire WV15 6AG
Tel: 01746 763134 Fax: 01746 765401

The town of Bridgnorth is interesting in that it is split in two by the River Severn, the Lowtown on the banks and the Hightown on the 200ft cliff opposite. It is in the Lowtown, with it's lovely shops, preserved buildings, pubs and restaurants you will find The Falcon Hotel, a 17th century Coaching Inn. The Falcon has been providing hospitality for the traveller for many years. It is ideally situated as a base for the business person, the motorway network being only 15 minutes away, or a delightful family holiday in a county well-known for it's beautiful countryside. The high quality accommodation including 15 bedrooms all with the luxury of private bathrooms, direct dial telephone, television and a beverages tray. The Falcon offers excellent fresh wholesome fare with Daily Specials and interesting vegetarian dishes, all served in the comfortable oak beamed bar/restaurant. There is a fine wine list with a selection of quality European and New World labels. A warm and friendly atmosphere pervades this hotel, a delightful place to stay.

USEFUL INFORMATION

OPEN; All year
CHILDREN; Welcome
CREDIT CARDS; Amex/ Visa/
    Mastercard
LICENSED; Full

RESTAURANT; Excellent fresh wholesome fare
VEGETARIAN; Catered for
DISABLED ACCESS; Yes
PARKING; Private car parking
ACCOMMODATION; 15 ensuite rooms

Inn - **THE NAGS HEAD**

Hilltop, Castle Donington, Derbyshire DE74 2PR

Tel: 01332 850652

This lively, friendly inn is an excellent stopping place. Close to the M1 Junction 24 on th B6540 through Castle Donington towards Donington Park and there it is at the top of the hill, on the left. It has been a hostelry for over a hundred years and inside you will see what a welcoming place it is with it's low beamed ceiling and open coal fires which send out a great warmth in winter. It is the sort of inn where locals gather and at the same time has become the haunt of many visitors who have found great enjoyment in the bar or the dining room, over the years. The garden is well used in summer and many a good game of Petangue has been played on the Boules Pitch. Ian Davison and his partner Jennie Ison are the owners. Ian is also the chef and it is his enthusiasm for vegetarian dishes that has ensured an entry in this guide. All the food is cooked and prepared on the premises and mainly to order. Fresh produce is used at all times including vegetables and potatoes. You will never find chips on the menu! Twenty five per cent of the menu is strictly vegetarian and other diets can be catered for with notice. If one had to describe the type or style of cooking it would be difficult. Ian is imaginative and has the sort of rapport with herbs and spices that will always make the food at The Nags Head just a bit different. For those who have a sweet tooth the puddings will appeal particularly.

USEFUL INFORMATION

OPEN; Mon-Sat: 12-2.30pm & 5.30-11pm
Sun: 12-3pm & 7-10.30pm
CREDIT CARDS; Access/Visa/Switch/Amex
CHILDREN; Not in bar. Well behaved
in restaurant
LICENSED; Full Licence

ON THE MENU; Dishes for
vegetarians at every course
DISABLED ACCESS; Yes but
no special toilets
GARDEN; Yes,Boules pitch
ACCOMMODATION; Not applicable

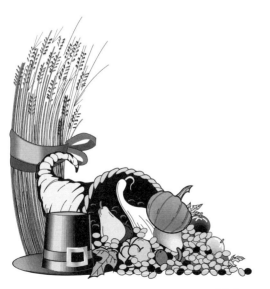

Inn - **HIGH CROSS HOUSE,**

High Cross, Claybrooke,

Lutterworth, Leicestershire LE17 5AT

Tel/Fax: 01455 220840

The fascinating history of High Cross House, once a 16th century coaching inn, would be one good reason for staying here. It is a unique historic site with the remains of the Earl of Denbigh's monument, built in 1712 to commemorate the end of the 100 Years War between England and France, still to be seen in the grounds. Many artefacts of interest have been discovered dating from the early Roman settlement known as Venonae. The Romans were the significant architects of England's road network, and they sited the main cross road of Watling Street and Fosse Way at Highcross, which is only one mile from the modern day junction of the M69 and the A5.

Whilst the delicious, imaginative menus at High Cross are not purely vegetarian, they do contain many dishes without meat. The house is renowned for it's cuisine and can cater for all occasions, from the quiet romantic dinner for two to business functions or family celebrations. The accommodation is of a very high standard with most rooms having ensuite facilities, direct dial telephones, colour television and a courtesy tray. Honeymooners are especially welcome, where you can spend your first special night in the privacy and intimacy of the luxurious Honeymoon Suite, complete with original stately antique four poster bed and en suite facilities, including large double jacuzzi.

USEFUL INFORMATION

OPEN; All year

CHILDREN; Welcome

CREDIT CARDS; None taken

LICENSED; Yes

PETS; With blind or disabled people only

RESTAURANT; Imaginative food

VEGETARIAN; Many dishes

DISABLED ACCESS; No special facilities

GARDEN; Yes

ACCOMMODATION; Mainly ensuite

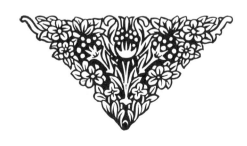

Farm Guest House - **BODKIN LODGE**
Grange Farm,Torrington Lane,
East Barkwith, Market Rasen,Lincolnshire LN8 3RY
Tel: 01673 858249

Whilst Anne and Richard Stamp have 'flitted' as they describe it, to Bodkin Lodge, they still farm the 330 acre Grange Farm, winner of the Cynamid (UK) Arable Farm Conservation Competition originated in 1985, together with the younger generation who now live in their old family home. They welcome guests to Bodkin Lodge extended in order to provide the maximum comfort for their visitors. There are two bedrooms, both ensuite, one of which is a double and the other a twin. Part of the luxury is the walk in shower in the bathroom as well as the bath. Each room has television, radios and tea trays. Wood fires, central heating and even a baby grand piano, all on ground level, just add to the welcoming atmosphere.

Food is all important to Anne. She gets Richard to cook the excellent breakfasts and then uses him as a kitchen hand whilst she prepares and cooks memorable three and four course dinners with sherry and coffee. All the Stamp family are keen on conservation and this is obvious in the produce and ingredients used in the menu. One of the favourite starters is Avocado pear pate followed by Chestnut & Walnut pate en croute. The recipes are original and exciting. Dining here is such a delicious relaxed affair - something to look forward to after a days exploration of the fascinating countryside. The award winning farm trail runs from the door. No Smoking.

USEFUL INFORMATION

OPEN; All year except Xmas & New Year
CHILDREN;Welcome over 8
CREDIT CARDS;None taken
DINING ROOM;Memorable meals
VEGETARIAN; Yes
DISABLED ACCESS; Yes

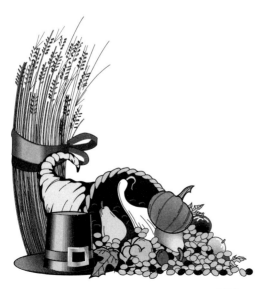

Guest House - **DERWENT HOUSE**

Knowleston Place,Matlock,Derbyshire DE4 3BU

Tel: 01629 584681

Beside the beautiful wooded Derwent gorge is the tourist resort of Matlock with it's wonderful scenery, the Rare Animal Wildlife Park in the grounds of the 19th century Riber Castle, where you are able to see animals such as the Lynx, the Mining Museum chronicles local mining going back to the Romans. A few minutes level walk from the town centre is Derwent House a delightful property built in 1620, it is very warm and welcoming. Owned by Jan Rodgers, who looks after her guests in a very friendly, efficient and professional manner, your needs are well taken care of, and the atmosphere is a happy one. The rooms are delightful and comfortably furnished. The bedrooms all have a wash hand basin, television and tea and coffee making facilities. Derwent House is renowned for it's full English and Vegetarian cooked breakfast, there is no better way to start the day. Special diets are catered for on request. Once breakfast is over and you are suitably sated, it is time to get out and about, why not take a cable car to see the magnificent views from Heights of Abraham some 750ft up, there is such a lot to do in this area. Derwent House is situated close to a well maintained park with boating lake, paddling pool, tennis courts, putting and bowling greens and a children's playground with swings and slides. You will certainly enjoy your stay at this very amiable and family run guest house.

USEFUL INFORMATION

OPEN; All year except Christmas and New Year

CHILDREN; Welcome, under 3 free 3-12 years half price if sharing 2 adults

ACCOMMODATION; 5 rooms, 1 double ensuite, 1 family/twin, 2 singles

NO SMOKING

DINING ROOM; Renowned for English and Vegetarian cooked breakfast

VEGETARIAN; Well catered for. With Special diets available on request

DISABLED ACCESS; No

PETS; Yes

Hotel & Restaurant - **THE LAKE ISLE HOTEL & RESTAURANT**

16 High East, Uppingham, Leicestershire LE15 9PZ

Tel:01572 822951

Uppingham is a pretty market town with a lot going for it as well as the famous Uppingham Public School which tends to play a leading role in the lives of the community. Uppingham is close to Rutland Water which will provide the visitor with hours of enjoyment from walking alongside this man made reservoir, to wind surfing, fishing and bird watching, even to taking a boat trip. Lots of small but interesting villages surround the water. Rutland's county town, Oakham is also a fascinating place to explore. The Lake Isle Hotel is small and personally run which makes it a particularly pleasant place in which to stay. It is in the centre of the town and the entrance is reached via a quiet yard hung with flowering baskets. The bedrooms are each named after a wine growing region in France and guests will find fresh fruit, home-made biscuit's and a decanter of sherry for their enjoyment. Excellent meals are served in the intimate restaurant with a choice for vegetarians. All meals are prepared from fresh produce. There is an extensive wine list of 300 items, including half bottles, and special wine meetings are held 8 times a year.

USEFUL INFORMATION

OPEN; All year

CHILDREN; Welcome

CREDIT CARDS; All major cards

PETS; Welcome

ACCOMMODATION; All bedrooms ensuite

ON THE MENU;Delicious food vegetarian choice

DISABLED ACCESS; No special facilities

THE OLD POST OFFICE

Llanigon, Hay-on-Wye HR3 5QA Tel: 01497 820008.
Grade II Listed building set in outstandingly beautiful countryside & only two miles from the famous Book town. Wonderful Vegetarian Breakfast. A distinctly different place to stay. Open: From Mid-Feb-December. No Smoking. Dogs by arrangement. Car Park.Prices 1997 £16-£21 per person based on 2 people sharing.

KIRTON LODGE HOTEL & RESTAURANT

Dunstan Hill, Kirton in Lindsey, Gainsborough,Lincolnshire DN21 4DU
Tel: 01652 648994
A unique,small hotel and restaurant converted from a 300 year old barn. Cosy restaurant offers a wide choice of vegetarian dishes. En suite rooms.

PENRHOS COURT HOTEL

Penrhos Court, Kington HR5 3LH Tel: 01544 230720

BRIEF ENCOUNTER

- at Great Malvern Station, Imperial Road, Malvern, Worcs WR143AT
Tel: 01684 893033.
Fascinating establishment which won a Hertiage Award in 1989. Specialises in international vegetarian food utilising the fine fresh fare availabe from this prime rural area. NS. V/VG, LIC, Children, D/Acc.

TUPPENNY RICE WHOLEFOODS

1& 2 Castle Street, Stamford, PE92RA
Tel: 01780 62739.
Cafe established for 5 years, is within well-stocked shop.Wide range delicious food prepared on premises. Mon-Fri from 8am for Veggie breakfasts.
Saturday evenings a set 3-course menu is served with live music. Bring your own wine.V/VG.NS. Children welcome. D/Acc.

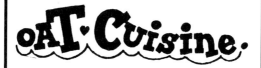
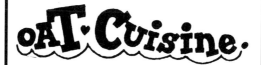

Chapter Seven

The North West Counties

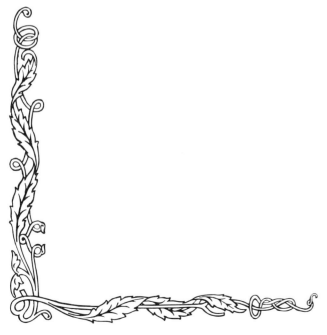

NORTH WEST COUNTIES
Cheshire, Greater Manchester, Merseyside, Lancashire, Cumbria & The Isle of Man

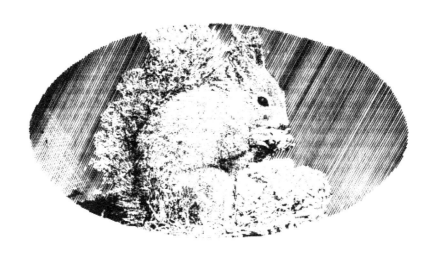

INCLUDES

Chapter 7

The North West Counties
Cheshire, Greater Manchester, Merseyside, Lancashire & Cumbria

This thin band of counties stretches from a border with Wales to a border with Scotland, and includes within it's bounds two very important cities, several elegant towns, famous seaside resorts, picturesque villages, the magical Lake District and the fiercely independent, Isle of Man.

Surrounding the mainly urban counties of Merseyside and Greater Manchester, parts of Cheshire to the south and Lancashire to the north have to some extent become commuter belts for Liverpool and Manchester. For centuries these areas have benefitted from wealth generated in both cities and from cotton growing and processing as well as dairy farming, a wealth which can be seen in the quality of much of the domestic building. The intricate black and white designs which abound in Cheshire, decorate some of what are surely the most attractive buildings to be found anywhere.

Chester appears to have been founded by the Romans, using it's strategic position at the mouth of the Dee. It may well have seen it's first fort in AD59. The Romans called it Deva, their camp, and no one can come here without their minds turning back to those far off days. There is no walled city in these islands to surpass it in completeness. From it's famous walls one looks down on a spectacle that would be hard to match anywhere. Chester stands on a rocky sandstone spur at the head of the River Dee, set in the middle of rural countryside about which still hangs the air of medievalism that I have never felt anywhere else in England

Chester is a city of steps. There are flights of them everywhere, to the houses, to the Rows, to the gates in the walls. These famous walls of red sandstone are nearly two miles round, making a raised walk from which many of Chester's interesting things can be seen. Wandering around the city is rewarding at every turn especially when you come to the unique and world famous 'Rows'. Among the interesting buildings are the 17th century **Bishop Lloyd's House.** Nearby is **God's Providence House,** the only building untouched by the Black Death during the city's 17th century plague years. Two fine museums in Bridge Street are both worthy of a visit: **The Chester Heritage Centre** and **The Toy Museum**. The magnificent cathedral is superb and should not be missed. It has both a sense of majesty and humility and is totally beautiful.

The centre and far south of Cheshire are rich in farming lands, in part overlaying bands of salt. Unstable, the salt has caused landslips and where it has been mined not far from the surface the land has sometimes collapsed into the void, both features leaving their mark on the landscape, often in the form of meres, and occasionally on buildings which can be found at strange angles. The story of the salt mining from Roman times is told in the **Salt Museum** at **Northwich.** Northwich has the unique **Anderton Lift**, water-filled tanks used to lift and lower boats from the **Trent Canal** to the **Mersey Canal** and vice versa.

Nantwich is always a delight to visit. This was once the most important town in the shire after Chester, and certainly the most famous of the three 'wiches'.

Another of the 'wiches' is **Middlewich** which goes back according to the records, to the 13th century. Here we have a pleasant little salt town with timber and brick houses. The church is mainly 14th century Perpendicular with a square 15th century tower. The gravestones amused me. One said:

> *Here lies Ann Barker*
> *Some have children, some have none*
> *But here lies the mother of twenty one.*

There is an old font in the graveyard and stocks as well. You will see the tower is marked by cannon shot which is said to have been acquired in the Civil War during the battles of Middlewich when the town stood for church and King.

From Middlewich to **Congleton** is no distance along the A54. For a long time it's prosperity was linked with gloves, lace and ribbons. It has fine houses and from the streets, hill climbers can recognise in the distance their favourite Mow Cop. I had been told of an intersting hostelry, a canal pub, **The Wharf Inn**, on the Macclesfield Canal. It stands side by side with Tudor and Georgian buildings and harmonious modern developments. A short walk along the canal will introduce you to 'The Macc' which is renowned for the beautifully designed stone bridges crossing the canal. Within easy reach of the Wharf Inn are places such as **Gawsworth Hall, Biddulph Grange Garden, Little Morton Hall** and the fascinating **Congleton Antique Market and Fayre.** Canals are very much part of the life of Cheshire and close to the M6 Crewe and Middlewich road is **Wheelock**, a pretty village through which runs the Trent and Mersey Canal.

Just off the A523 from Macclesfield is the cotton town of **Bollington**, which always seems to be quietly bustling, if that is not a misnomer, with a railway viaduct of 20 arches over the River Dean. Climb up the hill to **White Nancy**, a round stone tower, 920ft above sea level and you will see wide views all around which allow you to look over Cheshire into industrial Lancashire, and as far as the hills of the Derbyshire Peak.

For me Merseyside is inextricably a mixture of **Liverpool, Anfield, Goodison Park** and **The Grand National at Aintree**. There is something very exciting about this great city which has seen so many swings of fortune. The roar from the Kop End at Anfield when Liverpool Football Club are playing at home is my strongest memory of this unwieldy city. It is the spirit of the club that highlights all that is good about Liverpool, the sporting spirit, the ability to climb back after disaster, the solidarity in the time of greatest need. It is not only at Anfield this shows but also at adjacent Goodison Park where Everton have their base, and in the other spirited Merseyside team, Tranmere Rovers. **Liverpool Football Club Visitors Centre Museum** at Anfield captures the history and success of the club from the beginning right up to the present. Tours operate Monday to Friday except on mid-week match days, at 2pm and 3pm. Advance booking is essential.

Liverpool also boasts the most spectacular and thrillng horse race in the world, The Grand National run on the Aintree Course and attended annually by thousands of excited spectators waiting for the thrills and spills. This is a city that has provided a plethora of talent from John, Paul, George and Ringo - The Beatles - to the inimitable Ken Dodd, the fun loving comedian, Jimmy Tarbuck, the Nazi hater, funny man Stan Boardman, Les Dennis and the much loved Cilla Black of 'Blind Date' fame. Liverpool has been the seat of successful politicians - Harold

Wilson, our Prime Minister for so many years, to name but one. It is also the home of the Liverpool Philharmonic Orchestra which gives almost 100 concerts in it's Philharmonic Hall each year.

No one would call Liverpool architecurally beautiful, at least I would not. I have none the less found it a city of such wide interests and tastes that one could never be bored. It has the remarkable and probably unique achievement of having built two cathedrals in this century. The Roman Catholic Metropolitan consecrated in 1967 is unusual. Designed in contemporary style by Sir Frederick Gibberd, it is capped with a stained glass lantern tower, and is sometimes referred to as a 'wigwam wearing a lantern crown'.

The Anglican Cathedral was commenced as an act of faith in 1904 and continued to be built even through the traumatic days of World War II when the Germans were trying their hardest to destroy Liverpool because of it's strategic importance. The aftermath of the bombing and it's industrial decline has left Liverpool with many problems but the act of building a cathedral, eventually to be completed in 1978 when many dreams remained unfulfilled, is the essence of a city which has had sufficient faith in it'self to see this, and so much more achieved against a background of adversity. The site chosen could not have been better. It commands on one side the whole city and riverside, and on the other, a deep ravine enclosing an old churchyard. The sheer scale of the building is stunning, the Gothic arches the largest ever built. You stand there in awe of this vast expanse and yet wrapt around by the great love of God - His presence is real here unlike many cathedrals I have visited.

Liverpool has so much to show you as you will discover in The Albert Dock. There are Museums galore, wonderful Art Galleries, The Beatles Story in the Britannia Vaults. You can have a day out on the famous Mersey Ferries and much, much more.

Manchester is somewhere that I lived for a short time in 1961 when I thought it rather a dirty place - anyone who lives by the sea, as I do in Plymouth, does not appreciate vast cities anyway. Since those days Manchester has improved out of all recognition. Here is a bustling, prosperous city busy with commercial life, it's Universities, it's theatres and concerthalls. Life is rich, the shops are good, there are eateries of every nationality and superb hotels. It is an exciting city and justly proud of it's achievements.

In **Lancashire**, the world famous **Blackpool** with it's piers, it's holiday attractions is probably the best known place. Lord Leverhulme was responsible for the restoration of the 14th century **Hall I' the' Wood** near **Bolton**, the birthplace of Samuel Compton who invented the spinning mule in 1779, which is now a fine museum. Also at Bolton is a **Textile Machinery Museum** and the **Bolton Steam Museum**, both with displays of engineering important to the industry of the area.

There is also a **Textile Museum** at **Blackburn**, the home of James Hargreaves, inventor of the 'spinning jenny'. **Preston** was the birthplace of Sir Richard Arkwright, inventor of the spinning frame and other devices which sped up the production of the all important cotton cloth.

Blackburn has a small, but interesting cathedral, once the parish church. **Preston** has the privilege of being Lancashire's administrative capital, although **Lancaster,** with it's University is still the county town.

The high peak of **Rivington Pike** is a splendid viewing point close by the 400 acre **Lever Park** presented to the public by the 1st Lord Leverhulme. From **Pendle Hill** by **Clitheroe**, is a superb view of the Ribble Valley. This part of Lancashire countryside has long been associated with tales of witchcraft.

Oddly enough however it was to **Oldham** I went to seek out a good Vegetarian venue in the conservation Pennine village of **Delph**. Here Woody's Vegetarian Restaurant will delight anyone who enjoys good food whether or not they are vegetarians.

In the county of **Cumbria**, which makes up almost half of this north west region, exceptional views are the norm and not a rarity. **The Lake District** has been shaped by the elements, in particular during the Ice Age to produce sculptured lakes in wondrous valleys surrounded by dramatic hills and mountains. The huge variations in level can be seen to particularly great effect around **Wasdale Head** where Britain's deepest lake, **Wastwater**, is set immediately at the foot of England's highest mountain, **Scafell Pike** at 3,210 feet.

The weather still has it's part to play in the atmosphere of this area, with the highest average annual rainfall in Britain, and with sometimes fearsome skies that make the human race seem insignificant against such huge forces.

The Lake District can be appreciated fairly well from a car, but is naturally best seen on foot and well away from the few areas that are well populated with holidaymakers. The more remote areas are home to some rare flora and fauna. **Kendal** is at the southern gateway to the Lakes, where many visitors start their tours, making a visit first to **Levens Hall**, an Elizabethan house with an exceptionally fine topiary garden.

Ambleside is another of the excellent centres from which to base a walking holiday, close to **Lake Windermere,** England's largest lake with steam boats in operation, and to **Wansfell Pike** and **Loughrigg Fell**. The village of **Buttermere** is pleasantly situated between the lakes of **Buttermere** and **Crummock Water.** **Ullswater** is a truly grand lake, bordered by **Gowbarrow Park** with it's daffodils depicted in Wordsworth's most famous poem. **Coniston Water** was made famous by Donald Campbell's water speed records. **Derwentwater** is situated close to the particularly pretty and much visited valley of **Borrowdale** with it's ancient fort, **Castle Crag**, and within easy access from another of the centres for a walking holiday, **Keswick**. Near Keswick there is an enigmatic ring of 48 standing stones, known as the **Castlerigg Circle**, measuring 100 feet in diameter. Larger still is the stone circle **Long Meg and her Daughters** near **Little Salkeld.**

Eskdale is one of the few lakeless valleys, noted for it's magnificent waterfalls and it's cliff railway and for the spectacular views from the Roman fort at **Hardknott Pass.**

Many poets have been associated with the Lake District undoubtedly the most famous being William Wordsworth. Born at **Cockermouth**, he later lived at **Grasmere** and **Rydal,** and is much in evidence around the area, but generally in an informative rather than tacky manner. John Ruskin is another famous name, having lived at **Brantwood** near **Coniston** for 30 years. The museum here is now dedicated to him and includes many of his artefacts. Beatrix Potter's 17th century **Hilltop Farm** at **Sawrey** attracts huge numbers of visitors each year. One could go on forever extolling the delights of the Lake District but I would beg you not to omit **Keswick** or **Kirkby Stephen**. Then there is **Appleby in Westmoreland** another charming spot.

Today's Cumbria consists of areas which from time to time have belonged to Scotland, and both Runic and Celtic names show that the ancestry of the area is closely linked with it's northern neighbours. In addition to **Hadrian's Wall** there is significant evidence of Roman occupation here. **Penrith's** ruined castle can testify to some of the later border skirmishes, as can that at **Carlisle**. However before one gets to Carlisle do try and get to **Wigton** which is almost on the west coast of Cumbria and there you will find nearby the pretty village of **Caldbeck** which has a well established Vegetarian Restaurant, **The Watermill**, which as you may gather from it's name is housed in an old watermill. The rooms are delightful and full of atmosphere.

But not all Cumbria is either the Lake District or the northern lands, and along the flat coast are some lovely towns and villages, with much more pleasant weather, and a great contrast to the drama that is just a short way inland.

Way out into the Irish Sea the 227 square miles of the **Isle of Man** is a law unto it'self, literally, an idependent kingdom with it's own taxation system and currency and it's own government. Today the Isle of Man is known primarily as the venue for TT races and as a holiday destination, and indeed has plenty to interest the visitor, with a lot of history and with sunny beaches. From the top of the highest mountain, **Snaefell**, there is a view not only of the whole of the island but also on a clear day, of England, Scotland and Wales.

Inn & Restaurant - **THE ROYAL OAK INN**

Bongate, Appleby-in-Westmorland, Cumbria, CA16 6UN

Tel: 017683 51463 Fax: 017683 52300

Very old buildings have a special aura and sometimes age does not lend enchantment but this cannot be said of The Royal Oak at Bongate which has gradually been extended since 1200. The newest part is of the 17th century. It's years have given it a special atmosphere and the skill of the owners, Colin and Hilary Cheyne, has ensured that any refurbishment has merely enhanced and not taken character away. This is particularly noticeable in the charming ensuite bedrooms. The inn has a friendly tap room and a snug as well as a lounge and restaurant, a private sitting room for residents and a non-smoking dining room. Hilary Cheyne and Stuart are talented chefs and they have spent a great deal of time making sure that suitable vegetarian dishes, across the board, are available daily. All the food at the Royal Oak is 'organic' wherever possible. Good house wines, organic wine, country wines and a fine selection of malt whiskies are on offer, as well as a wide range of Real Ales. The Royal Oak Inn was awarded an AA Rosette for food in 1996 and an RAC Merit Award for it's restaurant in the same year - richly deserved.

USEFUL INFORMATION

OPEN; Food: 12-2pm & 6.30-9pm

ON THE MENU; Modern British.
Not exclusively vegetarian

CREDIT CARDS; Amex/Diners

CHILDREN; Welcome

DISABLED ACCESS; Yes. No special WC
Assistance available

LICENSED; Yes

ACCOMMODATION; 4dbl, 2tw, 1fam
All en suite.2sgls with private facilities

GARDEN; Terrace at front of hotel

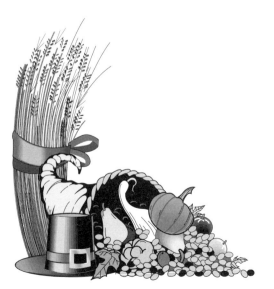

Inn with Rooms - **THE DRUNKEN DUCK**

Barngates, Ambleside, Cumbria, LA22 0NG

You may not find the Drunken Duck Inn easy to find so before we go any further let us address that minor problem, for this is somewhere you must not miss. There are dozens of delightful ways to approach the 'Duck'. We will concern ourselves with one of the most direct: Leave the M6 at Exit36. You are now well within an hours pleasureable drive. Follow the road signs to Windemere and then to Ambleside. Just before reaching Ambleside, the road forks at the Waterhead Hotel. Bear left (A593) the lake cruiser pier on your left, past Galava Roman Fort. Left over the Rothay Bridge. In half a mile, at Clappersgate, turn left. A mile through heavily wooded country then take the first obvious, right fork. Less than a mile and you have arrived. For 400 years The Drunken Duck has cared for travellers - that's a lot of practice. It is a mellow place and the good news is that it is as keen to care for vegetarians as it is for those who prefer other foods - the latter are rapidly growing to love some of the delicious vegetarian options available, resulting in The Drunken Duck being named Vegetarian Food Pub of Great Britain 1996 by the Good Pub Guide. There is a blackboard menu which has vegetarian options offering dishes that have been perfected over the last 10 years. There are three starters, 15 main courses and eight desserts on offer on this extensive menu. Try the celery, stilton and walnut pasta or the fennel, orange and butterbean bake and you will realise what a treat The Drunken Duck is for vegetarians - or for anybody else for that matter. Stay in the inn where you will be accommodated in one of their well appointed, en-suite rooms and spoilt with a splendid breakfast each morning.

USEFUL INFORMATION

OPEN; 11.30-3pm & 6-11pm

CREDIT CARDS; Visa/Access/Master/Switch

CHILDREN; Welcome

LICENSED; Full Licence

ACCOMMODATION; 10 en-suite rooms
2 day stay Nov-March, Sun-Thurs only

ON THE MENU; Wide choice especially for vegetarians

DISABLED ACCESS; Yes

GARDEN; 60 acres. Walking land, own fishing tarn

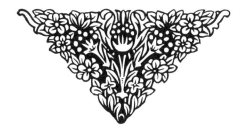

Guest House - **BEECH TREE GUEST HOUSE**
Yewdale Road, Coniston, Cumbria, LA21 8DB
Tel: 015394 41717

This totally vegetarian household is also a 'smoke-free zone' but the interesting thing is that half of the guests are non-vegetarian who, apart from coming to enjoy the amenities of the house and the countryside, want to experience the high standard of vegetarian cooking, often with a view to extending their own repertoire at home. The meals are delicious, freshly prepared and cooked every day. Wholefood, additive free ingredients are used in all the cooking and the dishes are well chosen to excite the palate and provide the energy to climb the surrounding hills! Breakfast is memorable and the delectable evening meals are optional. Vegan and other diets are catered for.

Beech Tree House is full of character, set in it's own grounds, it stands at the foot of the Old Man of Coniston. The House was formerly the Vicarage of the Parish of Coniston. It is a charming building with lots of Victorian features. The rooms are individually decorated, well furnished, warm and very comfortable. All the bedrooms have tea and coffee making facilities and there is a guest television lounge and dining room. The village of Coniston is an excellent centre for many and varied activities. Nearby is some of the most beautiful scenery in the Lake District as well as many famous houses and countryside attractions.

USEFUL INFORMATION

OPEN; All year except Christmas and January. Open New Year

ON THE MENU; Some of the best Vegetarian Food in the country

CHILDREN; Welcome over 6 years

CREDIT CARDS; None taken

DISABLED ACCESS; No special facilities

ACCOMMODATION; Ensuite & standard rooms

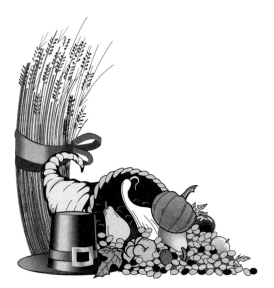

Hotel & Restaurant

LANCRIGG VEGETARIAN COUNTRY HOUSE HOTEL

Easedale,Grasmere,Cumbria, LA22 9QN
Tel: 015394 35317 Fax: 015394 35058

This house which is about 150 years old has had admirers since the first stone was laid. It is a house of timeless charm in the serenity of Easedale. There is a total absence of traffic and the peace is broken only by the sound of the waterfalls and the birdsong. There are acres of private, rare woodland, with paths and streams. It is no wonder that Wordsworth, Tennyson and Coleridge were frequent visitors. It was in Lancrigg Woods that Wordsworth wrote 'The Prelude' and other poems. The famous explorer Sir John Booth-Richardson also lived there. For the last 10 years Lancrigg has gained a reputation as probably the finest vegetarian country house hotel for hundreds of miles, if not in the British Isles. Individual descriptions are really necessary to describe the bedrooms as no two rooms are the same. Because of the rambling and unusual character of the house which blends a cottage style with that of a country house, some rooms lend themselves to luxurious en-suite accommodation with four poster beds, whirlpool baths and antique furniture. There are three luxury Country House ground floor rooms. They tend to be the most spacious and peaceful rooms and have individual characteristics and all are named. All rooms are ensuite and have colour television and tea making facilities. They have a wonderfully cosy feel enhanced by their individual decor.

The fare is the best of wholefood home-cooking using a wide range of the best fresh and natural ingredients, organic where possible and always free of artificial additives. The cheeses are vegetarian. The evening menu changes daily. All the bread, croissants and cakes are made from organic, stone-ground flour, milled by waterpower. The extensive organic wine cellar is accompanied by unusual beers, aperitifs, brandies and fruit liquors, all organic. Meals are served in the elegant chandelier lit dining room which has superb views across the valley. Lancrigg is a sheer delight.

USEFUL INFORMATION

OPEN; All year, 24 hours
CREDIT CARDS; All major cards
CHILDREN; Welcome
LICENSED; Yes
ACCOMMODATION;11 dbl,1sgl,2twn, 2 fmly, ensuite. 2dbl, 1 sgl.

ON THE MENU; The best vegetarian wholefood home-cooking
DISABLED ACCESS; Yes. No special toilets
GARDEN; Acres of beautiful woodland paths and streams

Bistro - **THE MOON**

129 Highgate, Kendal, Cumbria LA9 4EN

Tel: 01539 729254

It would be very trite to say that people are 'Over the Moon' when they have eaten at this charming, informal bistro, but it is a very fair description. Val Macconnell, the chef proprietor, has that intangible something that makes both herself and The Moon special.

The blackboard menu makes good reading with individual, imaginative and original bistro dishes on offer. The vegetarian side of the menu is most creative and is always changing. Imagine fennel, rice, mozarella and sweetcorn cabbage dolmas served on lemon and raisin couscous with tomato, garlic and allspice sauce. Everything is made by Val and nothing is bought in. The Moon's wine list is small but well chosen. Val Macconnell has published two successful cook books and has a monthly 'pudding club' with a great following. The Moon is one of Britain's top ten in the Vegetarian Good Food Guide. It deserves it's accolades.

USEFUL INFORMATION

OPEN; Every eve, Sun-Fri 6.30-10pm Sat 6-10pm. Summer open half and hour later. Closed last two weeks in January
CREDIT CARDS; Visa/Access/Switch

ON THE MENU; Imaginative, high standard
DISABLED ACCESS; Yes.
No Special toilets

Restaurant - **WOODY'S VEGETARIAN RESTAURANT**

5 King Street, Delph, Oldham, Lancashire OL3 5DL

Tel: 01457 871197 Fax: 0161 6788389 (Menus only)

When a restaurant has the accolade of being a 'Vegetarian Restaurant of the Year' finalist every year, it has reached an enviable standard and not only for it's food but for the ambience and the hospitality. Woody's has style, it's tables are beautifully appointed in the classical manner including shimmering glasses. Here you can be assured of a wonderful meal in a restaurant which is set in Delph, a conservation area Pennine village.

Music of the right sort always aids the digestion whilst every evening the gentle sound of classical music pervades a backdrop. The imaginative menu offers a choice of starters, main courses and 7 or 8 desserts. It would be virtually impossible not to find a dish to relish. The wine list includes wines from around the world all of which are organic and most vegetarian. Mike and Liz Wood are your talented hosts.

USEFUL INFORMATION

OPEN; Thurs/Fri/Sat 7.30-11pm (last bookings 9.30pm)
CREDIT CARDS; Master/Visa

ON THE MENU; First class choice of imaginative dishes at all courses
DISABLED ACCESS; Yes, but no special toilets

Restaurant **- THE WATERMILL RESTAURANT**
Priests Mill, Caldbeck, Wigton, Cumbria CA7 8DR
Tel: 016974 78267

This attractive Vegetarian restaurant is a converted Watermill in the pretty village of Caldbeck which nestles amongst the Northern fells of the Lake District. The atmosphere is warm and friendly enhanced by the original eighteenth century oak beams and wooden floor, with a cosy log stove burning during the winter months. The restaurant has been established for 11 years and Nikki and Joe are now in their successful fourth season. Nikki has been a Vegetarian for many years and is an experienced and imaginative cook making use of local and organic produce, including free range eggs and quality ingredients. Some typical favourites to try at the restaurant include Vegetable and Coconut curry, Herby carrot and Pinenut pie, Sticky Toffee Pudding, delicious scones and cakes. There is a selection of produce for sale including homemade jams and chutneys. Some tables overlook the river, or you may sit outside on the grassy terrace next to the village cricket pitch. There are monthly evening dinner parties with special menus. The restaurant is not licensed but customers are welcome to bring their own wine. Booking for evening meals is essential.

USEFUL INFORMATION

OPEN; 1st March-6th January.
March-September Every Day
Oct-Jan. Every Day except Mondays
10-5pm 11-4pm on Mondays.
Closed Christmas Day& Boxing Day.
Open New Years Day

ON THE MENU; Delicious, imaginative Vegetarian Fayre
DISABLED ACCESS; Yes
LICENSED; No. Please
Bring your own
CREDIT CARDS; All major cards

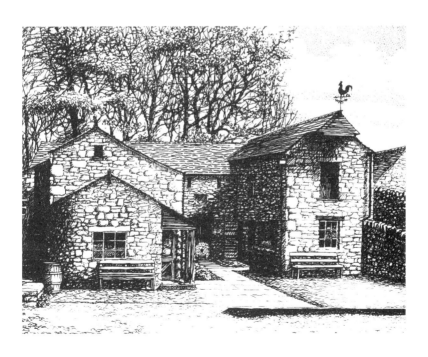

ELLERCLOSE HOUSE

Grasmere, Cumbria LA22 9RW Tel:015394 35786

Open all year.

V/VG. ESR. HT. Situated in the heart of the Lake District.

Charming Victorian Vegetarian Guest House set in delightful secluded gardens with mature trees and mountain stream. Wonderful views from every room, ensuite, centrally heated with colour TV and tea and coffee making facilities. Delicious cooked breakfasts. Nick and Pauline Greathead welcome guests to share the peace and tranquillity that this house has to offer. Self-catering also available.

Non smoking throughout.

THE GREAT LITTLE TEA SHOP

Lake Road, Keswick CA12 5DQ Tel: 017687 73545

GREENSIDE

48 Saint John Street, Keswick-on-Derwentwater CA12 5AG Tel: 017687 74491

All rooms en-suite with television and snack making facilities. £16.50 Bed and Breakfast. Private Parking. Ring 017687 74491 for Brochure.

CHESTNUT HOUSE

Crosby Garrett, Kirkby Stephen CA17 4PR Tel: 017683 71230

Off the beaten track, in Cumbria's delightful Eden Valley, and part of a beautifully peaceful village, this small, cottage guesthouse is informal and has a wonderful atmosphere. Stephanie and John Dewhurst serve exclusively vegetarian and vegan food, which the comments in their Visitors Book suggest is rather special. Two bedrooms with H & C, log fires, books, pretty garden, no smoking.

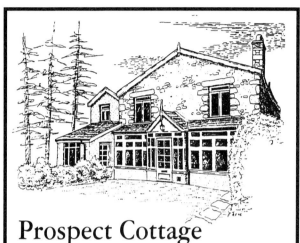

Chapter Eight

The North East Counties

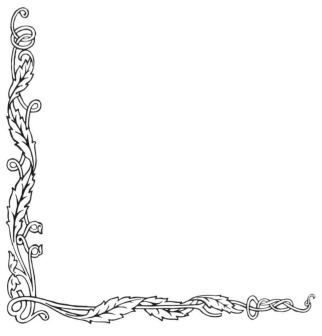

NORTH EAST COUNTIES
Yorkshire, Cleaveland, North Humberside, Tyne & Wear, Durham & Northumberland

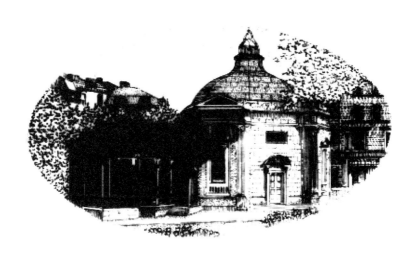

INCLUDES

Chapter 8

The North East Counties
Yorkshire, Cleveland, North Humberside, Durham, Tyne & Wear and Northumberland

From the high, sometimes desolate ground of the moorlands to the wide sweeps of the west coast, from the mellow cottages clustered in small villages to the heavy industry in densely populated conurbations, this region is one of great diversity. The newer industrial areas cannot be described as being in any way attractive and some of the areas are blighted by coalfield scars, yet many of the earlier mill sitings have a unique picturesque quality. A large portion of the region is designated either as a National Park or as an "Area of Outstanding Natural Beauty". The area's beauty is a very powerful one.

Some of the roughest of the landscape is to be found high on the **Pennine Chain**, the backbone of England, consisting of hard dark rock that can give a bleakness all of it's own.

The 256 mile **Pennine Way**, which for much of it's distance more or less marks the western boundary of the region, is a favourite with walkers. So much so that it has suffered much from erosion. From the **Cheviot Hill**, and the **Northumberland National Park** the Way crosses the **North Pennines** to the **Yorkshire Dales** with their seemingly never-ending stretches of bracken and rough long grass only interspersed in autumn with beautiful purple heather, through the **Calder Valley** where it joins the 50 mile cirular **Calderdale Way** around Bronte country near **Hardcastle Crags Valley** with it's many splendid walks to the **Peak District National Park**.

Whatever you want from a holiday, you will find it in **Yorkshire**, a county with a unique mixture of history, beautiful countryside and coastline, lovely cities and a host of different activities.

For glorious countryside the scenery of the Yorkshire Dales is difficult to beat. Miles upon miles of National Park with a stunning landscape which includes high peaks and sleepy valleys, pretty villages and bustling market towns, as well as great castles, like **Middleham** and **Castle Bolton**. More unspoilt beauty can be found in the forests, hills and vales of the **North York Moors National Park**, with heather covered moorland stretching from the Vale of York to the sea. The region has 120 miles of stunning coastline to discover. Full of character and individuality, it has a very special charm of it's own. Cliffs, coves and sandy beaches overlook quiet fishing villages like **Robin Hood's Bay** and tiny **Staithes**, and each of the main coastal towns of **Scarborough, Whitby, Filey, Cleethorpes** and **Bridlington** has it's own atmosphere.

The towns and cities of South and West Yorkshire make interesting destinations, their powerful industrial heritage combines with a new spirit of renovation and renewal. **Bradford** is a testimony to this, with the **National Museum of Photography, Film and Television**. Nearby is the Bronte village of **Haworth**, high on the Pennine Moors. Due to the abundant iron ore, to coal for power, and to water, the area in the south of this region gained importance in the steel industry, which also gave rise, more than 600 years ago, to **Sheffield's** pre-eminence as a manufacturer of cutlery, as shown in the town's **Industrial Museum**.

When the industrial revolution came, textile operatives took to the streets in revolt, there were riots and even murders, some of the 'Luddites' being tried and hung at **York Castle** having been betrayed by one of their own. Close to **Huddersfield** is the **Tolston Memorial Museum** at **Ravensknowle Hall** which has an exhibition of looms as well as relics from the Luddite riots.

In Yorkshire you will never be bored, whichever time of the year you visit. There are many historic houses and abbeys to explore, like **Harewood House**, near **Leeds**, and **Fountains Abbey** near **Ripon**, and more than 100 museums and art galleries, ranging from small folk museums to the award winning **Jorvik Viking Centre** in **York**.

This is only a taste of what is on offer in Yorkshire. I have chosen little pockets of this stunning county in order to whet your appetite, but if you want more information then do send for one of the very competent and instructive brochures issued by the Yorkshire and Humberside Tourist Board at 312 Tadcaster Road, York YO2 2HF. Tel: 01904 707070.

Naturally I have chosen to include **York**. I lived here for a while and revelled in the sheer beauty of the city dominated by the majestic and magnificent York Minster. This glorious building has three times been brought to it's knees by fire. The first in 1829 was started by a fanatic, Jonathon Martin, who believed he was acting on divine instructions; the second in 1840 was started simply by a careless workman who left a candle burning and the third in 1984 was witnessed around the world.

The South transept roof was destroyed and the precious Rose Window badly damaged. The task of restoration was put in the hands of master craftsmen once more, and now, thankfully, is complete. In a delightful gesture, children were invited to suggest designs for some of the new wooden roof bosses, and a competition was run by the BBC's Blue Peter programme. The winning entries are in place and the children of the 20th century have made their contribution to the Minster's history.

There is a well documented walk around the walls of York, but it isn't unreasonable to suggest it may once have been a well documented stagger! In 1870 Walmgate for example contained 28 pubs and every other house was a brothel. There is now only one pub and that is the **Spread Eagle**. Needless to say, but for the sensibilities of the residents the other 'business' establishments have gone too!

There is no better way to appreciate the marvels of York than by viewing it from the medieval walls. The distance of this walk is about two and a half miles, but you would be well advised to allow an afternoon to stroll at your leisure; there are too many points of interest to rush. The walls are now maintained but during the 19th century they were falling into a neglected state of disrepair. Fortunately they were saved by the endeavour of local citizens led by York painter, William Etty. York attracts millions of visitors and perhaps for that reason it is best explored out of season when you can take the time to stand and stare without being hustled by the crowds.

If you enjoy ecclesiastical splendour take the short journey from York to **Selby** where the glorious abbey is stunning - even after seeing the majesty of York Minster. **Harrogate** has always been the Eastbourne of the north to me but in reality this busy, dignified town has a much more demanding role. It has retained it's gorgeous flower beds, it's discreet ambience, but it has opened it's doors to become one of the leading Conference venues in the whole of the country. The Spa town is known as a 'floral resort' and is beautiful.

You will obviously want to visit **The Royal Pump Room Museum**, the site of the original sulphur well. Here you can sample the waters as the earliests visitors did - although in much more comfortable surroundings. There are 200 acres of land given to the people of Harrogate under an award of 1778 known as **The Stray**. It was here that Tewit Well was discovered in 1571. **The Valley Gardens** are utterly lovely. Acres of floral displays lead into beautiful pinewoods with rhododendron bushes. There is a boating lake, a paddling pool, playground, tennis courts, pitch and run and a mini golf course. On Sunday afternoons in summer the band strikes up and you can sit enjoying a concert which will cost you nothing.

Knaresborough was well established centuries before it's neighbour Harrogate even came into existence. Stand in the grounds of the ruined Norman and Platagenet Castle and you will be rewarded with the most dramatic views of this fascinating town. On one side trees clothe the steep bank to enhance the prospect from the north-east slope where Knaresborough's red-roofed houses climb one above the other. There are attractive Georgian buildings to be seen everywhere. The cobbled market square is a visitor's paradise and has the 'Oldest Chemyst Shoppe' in England dating from 1720.

Beside Knaresborough Castle, which you must see, is **Mother Shipton's Cave** and **The Petrifying Well**, probably England's oldest tourist attraction. Mother Shipton is England's most famous Prophetess. She lived some 500 years ago in the times of King Henry VIII and Queen Elizabeth I. She was born in a cave beside Knaresborough's Petrifying Well, delivered as lightning crackled and burned in a violent storm.

The Cave and Well lie at the heart of Mother Shipton estate - a relic of the Ancient Forest of Knaresborough. The beautiful riverside walks and carriage drive were classically landscaped with beech trees in the 18th century. Sir Henry Slingsby's Long Walk leads you to the Cave and Well. There is an excellent children's adventure playground, picnic area and plenty of car parking.

You might take a drive along the little B6165 frequently in sight of the River Nidd until you come to **Pateley Bridge**. This popular Nidderdale centre for walkers and bird watchers is an attractive small town with plenty going on. **The Nidderdale Museum** houses a fascinating collection in what was the Victorian Workhouse. It leaves you under no illusion how difficult life was for the dale folk. **Stump Cross Caverns** on **Greenhow Hill** is an experience not to be missed. 500,000 years ago Stump Cross area was a wilderness over which bison, reindeer, fox, wolf and wolverine roamed, preying on one another. Sealed off in the last Ice Age, the caves were not discovered until the mid 19th century. From then on exploration has yielded a richness of animal remains, the untold wonders of stalactite and stalagmite, and fossils between 30,000 and 200,000 years old. The cave is skilfully lit to enhance the underground wonders and easily reached via steps and gravel paths.

I was also impressed by what is known as 'Yorkshire's Little Switzerland'. Correctly it should be called **How Stean Gorge** where the caves are just waiting to be explored. To allow children to work off some surplus energy there is a good play area.

Within easy reach of Harrogate I visited three places. The first is **Otley** whose most famous son is Thomas Chippendale and although born in London, the artist Turner became a son of Otley by adoption. **Farnley Hall** contains probably the largest private collection of Turner paintings in the world.

Otley does not need to hang on the coat tails of the famous. It is an attraction in it's own right. Standing near the southern end of the beautiful Washburn Valley and on the River Wharfe, it is full of interesting buildings and an old Victorian Maypole at Cross Green, or more correctly one should say a replacement for the Victorian Maypole which was struck by lightning and replaced in 1962. None the less it carries on a tradition as old as the town it'self. Otley shelters below The Chevin, an 841ft escarpment with a viewpoint at the summit. For keen 'Soap' addicts it is the 'Hotton' of Emmerdale. The Chevin is much more than a backdrop for this historic market town. It is worthy of a Turner landscape and provides a wonderful area in which to wander. The rambler will find it a mini paradise, the kite flyer somewhere in which there is total freedom to enjoy this ever more popular sport. Horseriding, climbing, walking the dog, all is possible. **The White House** is the visitor centre from which you can find out all sorts of information. If you are fit, a well signed path leads from the town centre to The Chevin. It is far too steep for me and I found it easier to take my car around the back and park close to what is known as 'Surprise View' from where the outlook is stunning. You look right out over Wharfedale beyond the valley to Almscliffe crag and the thickly wooded Norwood Edge.

The medieval street patterns make exploring Otley a pleasure. The town has held a market since Saxon times but the recorded history dates are Fridays and Saturdays with the addition of Tuesdays in the summer. In December Otley holds it's annual Victorian Fayre when traders dress up in Victorian costumes and you can hear the sounds of a massive steam organ and children's choirs singing traditional carols. It is a wonderful occasion.

From Otley and Bolton Bridge there is a road on either side of the river. It is one on the east bank that I made for because it is so pretty. Much narrower than the other side but equally much quieter. I was told to turn beyond the bridge into Weston Lane and a mile on I would see the gates of **Weston Hall**. They, in themselves, are impressively ornamental but it was the footpath I wanted, in order to be able to cut across a corner of the park and so get an excellent view of the Hall with it's Tudor wings. The middle is 18th century - fire having destroyed the building earlier. What I was looking for was a sight of the unique glass turret which surmounts the 18th century Banqueting Hall. It certainly is extraordinary and well worth the detour.

My second town was **Ilkley**. Famous to most people because of the old song 'On Ilkley Moor Bar' tat' but this does not conjure up at all what one does see in this superbly set town. There it lies in the arms of a narrow section of the valley between the great curves of heather moorland, grit'stone outcrops and thickly wooded hillside. It is somewhere that has attracted visitors since before the Iron Age.

A quiet, pleasant place to live, it was happy to be in the backwater and leave the hustle and bustle to it's sister towns of Otley and Skipton, until in the 18th century someone discovered a healing moorland spring in White Wells. The local squire who lived across the river, saw the benefit of exploiting it and built a small bath-house to which were brought elderly patients who benefitted from total immersion in the stone bath, built for that purpose. The development from this simple beginning was amazing, hotels and boarding houses sprang up, and by early Victorian times, the previously quiet Ilkley was a fully fledged spa town.

The advent of the railway changed the scene once more. It became fashionable for the wool manufacturers and their senior management to live in what would now be called a commuter town. They built fine residences which can still be seen today. The incoming wealth brought other advantages. A splendid Town Hall was built and so was the Library, the Winter Gardens and Kings Hall. The Grove became the place to be seen and even today there is a sense of elegance with good dress shops, antiques and the famous **Betty's Coffeeshop.** Behind the Grove are pedestrian areas around the small market square, beyond which is a well preserved Victorian read complete with potted palms.

Ilkley is a place in which you want to abandon your car and just walk, the riverside parkland is charming. From Grove Road you can stroll gently to **Heber's Ghyll**, a natural wooded ravine with a stream which tumbles down from the moors, and man has built a series of footbridges. It is enchanting. Nearby Heber's Ghyll is the site of the **Swastika Stone**, a unique carved relic believed to have been instrumental in ritual fire worship.

Pickering is the third town. It is almost older than time it'self and has records that show it was firmly established by 270BC. Today it is a lively market town with steep narrow streets climbing the hillside. Standing watching over the town above the market place is the parish church, the walls of it's nave decorated with a series of remarkably vivid wall paintings, depicting the legends of the saints. It is believed to date from the 15th century.

Pickering Castle stands high above the town but it is in ruins. It has a fine motte-and-bailey with shell keep founded by William the Conqueror.

I always enjoy the quiet charm of **Settle** with it's air of well being and I can cheerfully recommend it well worth while making the fifteen miles or so journey along the A65 westwards from **Skipton** to see it for yourselves. It is a gem set in Ribblesdale on the edge of the Yorkshire Dales. If you want somewhere to stay while you take a look then the **Sansbury Place Vegetarian Guest House** is ideal.

Whitby is the stuff that fairy tales are made of. The quaint character of the town is a result of it's long maritime tradition. The people built their homes as close to the harbour as possible, covering the steep valley sides on both banks of the River Esk at it's mouth. The lofty ruins of **Whitby Abbey** stand guard over the narrow streets, compact houses and red rooftops nestling below. Visitors love this fascinating little town with a setting that has inspired many writers. At the bottom of the 199 steps, in a very dramatic, picturesque harbourside position, with a small sandy beach in front and an old Abbey on the cliff top immediately above, **The Duke of York** is a splendid pub. This is where Bram Stoker spent a great deal of time when he was writing 'Dracula', indeed he featured the sandy beach in his story.

To get to the pub you have to walk the length of a narrow cobbled street in Old Whitby and you can just imagine the surreptitious way in which smugglers would have crept along with their illgotten gains. Whitby was the centre of much smuggling in times past and most of the small town seems to have had some involvement with the trade; certainly fooling and outwitting the Excise Men was one of the great pastimes.

You should go to **Egton Bridge** close to Whitby. Here the pretty, creeper covered **Postgate Inn,** is named after Father Postgate who was hung, drawn and quartered for practising Catholocism in the village. The inn is popular with television companies, one of whom uses it for the popular 'Heartbeat'series. The first Tuesday in August is very special to the village when the famous 'Gooseberry Show' is held here.

Goathland my next stop has also acquired fame because in this case, it is the village at the centre of the 'Heartbeat' television series. Sturdy grey stone houses surround the large sheep-grazed greens of the scattered village which is a popular starting point for walks on the North York Moors. The charming **Mallyan Spout Hotel**, gets it's name from the cascading waterfall which is immediately behind it. Moorland streams cascade over rocks in spectacular waterfalls, the best known is the high Mallyan Spout.

Way across to the East at the edge of the Yorkshire Dales, I went to see **Leyburn** and **Middleham**. Taking the latter first I found myself in the smallest town in the country and one of the most beautiful, which clings to the rocky hillside with true Yorkshire grit. The river runs beneath, and above it all lies **Middleham Castle**, the childhood home of Richard III. A magnifcent fortress, it lies on the edge of the enchanting scenery of the Dales with a sort of brooding acceptance of the beauty it perceives. If you climb to the top of the massive keep you will enjoy marvelous views over Coverdale and Wensleydale. Middleham Castle is one of the largest ever built in England. The great tower contained all the main living rooms, while crowded around are later buildings - a chapel, gatehouse and chambers, built to supplement it.

Five main roads meet at **Leyburn** and it lies on a shelf on the northern side of the valley some distance from the river. Visiting Leyburn on Friday is good fun. It is market day, full of bustle, and very colourful. It takes place in the Broad Market which received it's Charter from Charles II. What it does lack is the old market cross, the bull ring and the stocks which were removed many moons ago.

For unrivalled views you will do no better than go to **The Shawl**, along a natural terrace running parallel with the valley. Somewhere along here at a place known as **Queen's Gap**, history tells us that Mary Queen of Scots was recaptured after an abortive attempt to escape from imprisonment in Bolton Castle. It is thought that The Shawl had much to do with the Ancient Britons, and implements used by prehistoric man have been discovered here.

Bolton Castle is just off the A684, four miles west of Leyburn. Seen from the valley below it looks almost intact. It's massive square towers, though crumbling away at the top, stand over 100 feet high. Many of the rooms remain roofed and you can catch glimpses of the windows glittering in the sunlight. It was built in the late 14th century as the fortress home of Richard le Scrope, Chancellor of England during the reign of Richard II.

I found it saddened me when I looked at a room in the south west tower which is known as Mary's room, and is supposed to be where the tragic Queen of Scots was imprisoned. In reality she would have been given the State Apartments in the north-west tower and certainly a far greater degree of comfort than the prisoners in the dungeon of the north turret - a grim chamber with only one entry - a square trap through which the victims were dropped! The five storeys of the tower are now without floors and roofless.

Further west on the same road, you would come to a sign post that said **Askrigg-in-Wensleydale**, a charming village which will be familiar to anyone who watched the television series of James Heriot's 'All Creatures Great and Small'. Askrigg is the Darowby of the story and the village pub, the splendid and atmospheric **Kings Arms Hotel**, was 'The Drovers'.

Finally I came to **Doncaster** for the sole reason of attending the races. Horse racing is a great love of mine and there are few more exciting courses than Doncaster especially for the St Leger.

Humberside, which takes in the old East Ridings of Yorkshire, has large and imposing industries in and around Hull and the Humber estuary, surrounded by flat pastures. Most of the county is underlayed by a chalk belt, the **Yorkshire Wolds** rising to over 800 feet, a dry upland with a thin covering of soil and swept by strong winds. It has over the years been reclaimed by the local people and now between August and September, field after field of swaying corn stretches into the distance as far as the eye can see.

As the chalk belt reaches the coast it can give spectacular effects, the chalk eroded by the sea into caves, chalk pillars standing defiantly alone against the elements, white cliffed bays and pebble beaches; a visual extravaganza of the forces of nature in action. **Flamborough Head,** a magnificent place for bird watching, is the only place you will find gannets nesting on the mainland.

Further south at **Holderness** the chalk is much lower and covered with alluvial soil left by the ice age. This is now some of the richest land in Britain, the boulder clay of the cliffs hold little sway against the ravages of the sea, and are worn away at an alarming rate of up to 30yards a year, ending up at **Spurn Head**, a spit of sandstone some three miles long. This area of the country is likely to change beyond recognition in the coming years, due to the Government's new thinking on erosion; whether they are right or not, whether we should fortify our coastline against the sea or allow the sea to reclaim some areas, feelings are running strong. People's views could of course be tempered by how close they live to the problem.

Northumberland, Durham, Tyne & Wear and **Cleveland** are the four counties which covered the old Anglo Saxon Northumbria, the Kingdom of Eric Bloodaxe. In the wide Dales sheep are the main inhabitants, but elsewhere the coal inudustry has left it's mark. **The Woodhorn Colliery Museum** at **Ashington** reflects the mining communities' way of life through displays of original colliery buildings and artefacts along with vivid portrayals by the Ashington Group of Artists. Shipping too has been an important industry and the historic **Jacksons Dock** incorporates **Hartlepools Historic Ships** along with a history of the ships and the docks.

As large industries creep inevitably inland, most of the coast remains a haven for birdlife and a delight to the soul. The old priory on the Holy Island of **Lindisfarne**, the beginning of Celtic Christianity, is well worth a visit, if you remember it is impossible to cross to the island from two hours before and three and a half hours after high tide. **The Castle** was converted into a private house in 1903 by Sir Edward Lutyens.

Just to the south, the **Farne Islands,** a small group of islands off the coast at **Bamburgh,** are home during the summer months to over 17 species of sea birds; puffins, kittiwakes, eider ducks, guillemots, terns and fulmars just to name a few.

Bamburgh is a seaside village unspoilt by time, clinging beneath a red sandstone fortress jutting out 150 feet above the water. From here you can get a splendid view of the **Farne Islands** and the National Trust bird sanctuary.

South of **South Shields**, around **Souter Lighthouse**, is a spectacular coastline, an area to walk the open grassland of **The Leas** and look at the famous bird colonies. **Marsden** offers the visitor a descent (by lift) into the bar of an inn excavated from the cliffs, where you can hear and see the congested colonies on **Marsden Rock**. At the lighthouse you can see the Engine Room, Battery Room, the Light Tower and Fog Signal Station, which were the summit of lighthouse technology in 1871 when it was built.

Inland down the Tyne near **Stocksfield**, wood engraver and naturalist Thomas Bewick, Northumbria's greatest artist, was born at **Cherryburn** which now houses a small exhibition on his life and work. There are occasional demonstrations of wood engraving and printing.

Durham is dominated by it's castle and cathedral, the **Castle** is a university and the buildings are a good example of 12th century construction, the best view is from the 18th century **Prebend's Bridge**. To get a good view of the **Cathedral** , the best vantage point is from the gardens of St Aidan's College. The cathedral is considered splendid due to the fact that the nave, chancel and transept were built in a single period between the years 1093 to 1140. The two principal additions were Bishop Pudsey's Galilee Chapel in 1170 and in 1230 the Chapel of the Nine Altars. The Monks Dormitory which is attached to the cathedral has some fine Anglo Saxon carvings.

Escomb in Durham has a nearly perfect Anglo Saxon church and the porch with a sundial over it is reputed to be the oldest in the country. At **Finchale**, on the bed on the River Wear, lies a 13th century priory considered to be the most important remains in the county.

Barnard Castle, near **Bowes** in Durham is a ruin overlooking the River Tees. In the castle is the **Bowes Museum**, a must for art lovers with it's fine collection of decorative arts with paintings, furniture, ceramics and textiles from Britain and western Europe.

Charles Dicken's 'Dotheboys Hall' in 'Nicholas Nickleby' was said to be modelled on the local school at Bowes. Unsurprisingly it closed soon after the book was published!

In the south Durham town of **Darlington** the **Tees Cottage Pumping Station** has a good range of motive power machines, and for the railway enthusiast there is a real treat because at **Darlington Railway Centre and Museum** Stephenson's 'Locomotion No 1' and 'The Derwent' are on display. 'Railway mania' hit the north east in the mid 19th century and the area is now very well served with railway museums. At **Wylam** near **Bywell** in Northumberland there is a **Railway Museum** as well as **George Stephenson's Cottage** which the National Trust opens to the public.

Hydraulic and hydroelectric machinery is on view at the **Armstrong Energy Centre** which has many of such inventions by Lord Armstrong who owned **Cragside House** (the first house in the world to be lit by hydroelectricity) and grounds at **Rothbury** in Northumberland, which were only recently first opened to the public. It is a high and formal Victorian house in grounds which extend to over 1,000 acres, the millions of rhododendrons being of special interest as are the orchard house, Italian garden, terraces, rose loggia and fernery with man-made lakes.

Kielder Water high on the Northumberland National Park is the largst man-made lake in Europe, 7 miles long with over 27 miles of shoreline, and said to be 170 feet deep in places. A place of great popularity for walking and water sports.

At **Chollerford** in Northumberland there have been extensive excavations, exposing a **Roman Bath House,** with hot, cold and steam baths and changing rooms in a five acre site, as documented in an excellent museum.

Hadrian's Wall, most of which is in what is now Northumberland, was built around the year 122 AD and must have been a mammoth undertaking. Built of stone it was ten feet broad and too high to be scaled by one man standing on another's shoulders, and protected by a ditch. The wall had gateways, a Roman mile apart, called milecastles, and there were watchtowers and 17 fortresses. From one in particular of them, Housteads, one can get a truly glorious view along the Wall.

The **Roman Fort** of Arabia at **SouthShields** features reconstructions along with excavations, marking it's importance in the construction and garrisoning of Hadrian's Wall.

Northumbria's history is displayed in a great many excellent museums in the area, possibly none finer than the **North of England Open Air Museum** at **Beamish** south of Gateshead.

Guest House - **SANSBURY PLACE VEGETARIAN GUEST HOUSE**
Duke Street, Settle,
North Yorkshire BD24 9AS
Tel: 01729 823840

Settle is a gem set in Ribblesdale on the western edge of the limestone and grit'stone country of the Yorkshire Dales. A traditional unspoilt Dales market town, Settle has interesting shops, many fine old buildings and a bustling street market every Tuesday. Settle is served by bus and train and the railway station is only a few minutes walk away. You can have a day out on the magnificent Settle-Carlisle Railway visiting places like Dent and Appleby. Sue and David Stark love living here in their Victorian house and they hope that when you stay you will love it too. Sue has extensive experience of running wholefood shops, teaching vegetarian cookery and catering for people on special diets. The house is spacious with splendid views of the surrounding hills and guests are welcome to enjoy the private sunny garden with it's wildlife pond. All rooms are centrally heated and you can relax in front of an open fire in the guest sitting room. There are two guest bathrooms, one with a Victorian bath. All food is vegetarian and carefully prepared with a wide variety of fresh wholefood ingredients (organic where possible). Guests are welcomed with a pot of tea and home-baking. For breakfast there is home-made bread and a choice between something hot like herby tomatoes or something fruity like Bircher-Benner muesli. Evening meals are delicious and include dishes like mushroom and walnut pate, spinach and almond pancakes and hot sticky prune cake with fromage frais. They are not licensed but you are welcome to bring your own drinks to have with your meal. Tea, coffee and herbal teas are always available. How comforting to know that after a hectic day exploring you will be returning to this peaceful and homely guest house.

USEFUL INFORMATION

OPEN; All year
DINING ROOM; Delicious fare using fresh produce organic if possible
CHILDREN; Welcome over 5 years
CREDIT CARDS; None taken
VEGETARIAN; Completely
ACCOMMODATION; 3 rooms, 2 double, 1 single
GARDEN; Secluded

NON SMOKING GUEST HOUSE

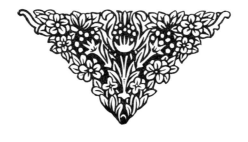

Guesthouse - **DAIRY GUESTHOUSE**

3 Scarcroft Road, York YO2 1ND

Tel: 01904 639367

The Dairy is a lovingly restored and upgraded Victorian house, retaining it's character and original features, such as stained and etched glass windows, pitch pine doors and staircase, cast iron fire grates, and wonderfully ornate ceiling roses and cornices. The Dairy is set around a flower filled courtyard with pretty cottage styled rooms which offer warmth and welcome. Each individually styled room has colour television, hot drink facilities, hairdryer and alarm clock. In addition the personal touches include toiletries, maps, books, games and information folders. Your somewhat elusive host, Keith Jackman, is an ex-accountant and was a professional drummer in Australia, many moons ago! He still performs playing hand-drums, didgeridoo and blues harmonica. The Dairy offers a friendly welcome and delicious breakfasts from continental to traditional British or vegetarian. Apart from the courtyard where one can enjoy a quiet smoke, the rest of the house is a smoke-free zone. Situated in central York, The Dairy is just 200 yards south of the medieval city walls and an easy stroll to York's many attractions and museums.

USEFUL INFORMATION

OPEN; All year
CHILDREN; Welcome
CREDIT CARDS; None taken
ACCOMMODATION; Beautiful en suite rooms

ON THE MENU; Traditional, continental or Vegetarian breakfasts
DISABLED ACCESS; 1 ground floor room available

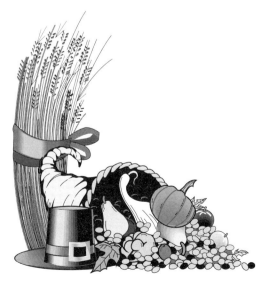

THE BAY HORSE INN

Terrington, York, North Yorkshire YO6 4PP
Tel: 01653 648416

The village of Terrington can be found from the A64 by taking the turn off to Castle Howard. If you are approaching from York then you can follow the signs to Strensall and Sheriff Hutton. Five years ago you would have found The Bay Horse Inn boarded up, yet for 150 years it had served the village well as a watering hole for locals and a welcome stopping place for travellers. The Snowdons saw the pub, liked what they saw and having purchased it, set about restoring it to what a good village inn should be. They have made it a warm, friendly and comfortable hostelry and patiently collected farming and countryside tools, harnesses etc which are attractive and add to the pleasing atmosphere.

In addition to the three bars and the dining room there is a conservatory which not only adds to the space but provides a very pleasant place in which to sit and eat.

Great thought has been put into the planning of the dishes on the varied menu. Many traditional pub favourites are there but mainly it consists of true country dishes using local and seasonal foods. Talk to Mrs Snowdon and you will discover she is very interested in researching old Yorkshire recipes in amongst which are many devised for vegetarians. In fact there are six snacks, six starters and six main courses as well as several desserts which conform to vegetarian requirements. An excellent Sunday lunch is served at an exclusive price. Wine with your meal is as well chosen as the menu. It is a list full of interest from Europe, South Africa and Australia and offered at reasonable prices; the average for a bottle is £7.

USEFUL INFORMATION

OPEN; Weekdays 12-3pm & 6.30-11pm
   Sun: 12-3pm & 7-10.30pm
CREDIT CARDS; None taken (Cheques Full on only)
CHILDREN; Welcome
LICENSED; Full

ON THE MENU; Interesting farmhouse recipes. Good range for vegetarians.
DISABLED ACCESS; Yes + toilets
GARDEN; Yes
ACCOMMODATION; Not applicable

IVY GUEST HOUSE
3 Melbourne Place, Bradford BD5 0HZ
Tel: 01274 727060 Fax: 01274 306347/411428 E-Mail:101524,3725acompuserve.com

AMADEUS VEGETARIAN HOTEL
115 Franklin Road, Harrogate, HG15EN Tel/Fax: 01423 505151
No smoking and totally vegetarian hotel. Children welcome. Licensed.
Open all year except Christmas. No Disabled Access

WENTWORTH HOUSE
27 Hudson Street, Whitby YO21 3ED Tel: 01947 602433
Guest House.

PRIORS
7 The Bank, Barnard Castle DL12 8PH
Tel: 01833 638141 Fax: 01833 638141
Non-smoking, V/VG & Gluten & Sugar Free diets. Children wlecome. LIC. D/Acc with assistance.
Open all year.

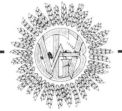

Gillygate Wholefood Bakery Ltd

CAFE, SHOP & BAKERY

- *Delicious vegetarian meals and snacks in a peaceful, friendly environment*
- *We cater for a large range of special diets*
- *We also cater for special occasions, birthdays, weddings etc*
- *All our food is made using the finest NATURAL ingredients*

There's nowhere else like us in town, so come and see for yourself.

We are located behind the Minster on Gillygate in a secluded courtyard opposite Vickers Hi-Fi shop

Millers Yard, Gillygate, York YO3 7EB

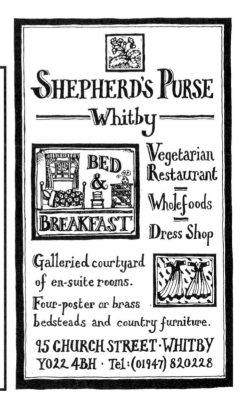

SHEPHERD'S PURSE
Whitby

BED & BREAKFAST

Vegetarian Restaurant
Wholefoods
Dress Shop

Galleried courtyard of en-suite rooms.
Four-poster or brass bedsteads and country furniture.

95 CHURCH STREET · WHITBY
YO22 4BH · Tel:(01947) 820228

Chapter Nine

Scotland

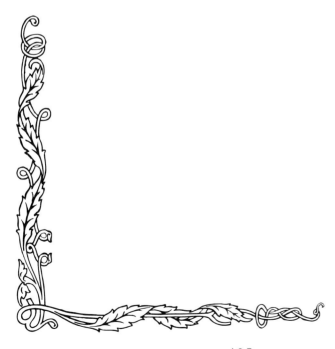

CHAPTER 9

SCOTLAND

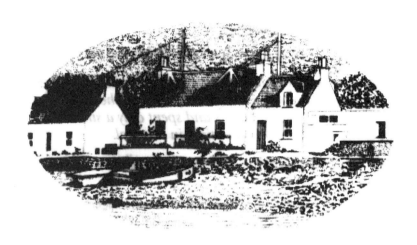

INCLUDES

Chapter 9

SCOTLAND
Dumfries & Galloway, Borders, Lothian, Strathclyde,
Central, Fife, Tayside, Grampian, Highlands & Islands

cotland covers an area of approximately 30,000 square miles, surrounded on three sides by water, which strongly influences the climate of the country and has contributed to determining the character of the people.

The culture of Scotland has been formed by successive waves of settlers and invaders throughout the 8,000 or more years that the country has been inhabited. The name Scotland was derived from the Scoti, a Celtic tribe who arrived in Scotland around the 5th century from Ireland and settled in Argyll. Other Celts arrived from northwest Europe and a strong Celtic influence has remained ever since.

When the Romans later invaded they called these early inhabitants Britons, and the peoples of the northern lands were named Picts. The Roman influence was minimal, and gradually these groups came together, a Scottish'Pictish Kingdom being formed late in the 1st century.

Since that time Scotland seems to have had more than it's fair share of wars and uprisings, the border with England in frequent dispute, and it was not until the 1328 Treaty of Northampton that England accepted Scotland's independence, but this was then short lived as the death of King Robert I in 1329 led to another crisis of succession, a theme which is repeatedly found in Scotland's history.

Despite many aspects of it having at one time been banned, Gaelic culture remains very strong, and the Highlands still have their most potent symbols, the tartan and the bagpipes, not forgetting the famous Highland Games. The rest of Scotland including the Lowland where the majority of the population live, has likewise retained it's own vigorous personality.

Scotland is divided into three geographical areas, roughly in line with the diagonal border it'self. The Highlands, about half the land area, lie north of a line known as the Highland Boundary Fault from **Helensburgh** in the west to **Stonehaven** in the east. This broad definition includes low-lying ground around the **Moray Firth**. The Lowlands or 'Central Belt', with the highest population density, lie below the Highlands, the southern boundary being another line defined by geology, running from **Girvan** in the west to **Dunbar** in the east, and below this is the Southern Uplands, running to the Border.

The fact that Scotland is on the same latitude as Moscow accounts for the sometimes Arctic weather conditions, but it is also warmed by the North Atlantic Drift, part of the Gulf Stream.

Because of the latitude, northern Scotland benefit's from the 'Aurora Borealis', the scientific name for the night sky phenomenon otherwise known as the 'Northern Lights' and sometimes called the 'Merry Dancers' by local folk. The aurora occurs as a result of solar flares sending charged particles into space, affecting the upper layers of atmosphere. Though this is most noticeable in the winter it occurs all year round, seen most clearly in country areas because street lights can make the night sky difficult to see. A good display usually starts with a greenish light observed low down in the northern sky after sunset has faded, and is well worth the wait.

A straight line placed north to south on the west coast covering just 260 miles, stretches with the indented coastline to over 2,000 miles, which gives a good guide to the kind of coast to be found. The many islands have resulted from jagged areas of coastline cut off from land by the forces of nature.

The most promising island groupings in the west are those off the Clyde estuary, **Arran** and **Bute**, the **Inner Hebrides**, where **Mull, Islay** and **Skye** are to be found and the **Outer Hebrides** with the **Isle of Lewis,** also known as the Western Isles. The **Orkney Island** are to the north, and further north still are the **Shetlands**.

As you travel through Scotland, look out for the prominent **National Tourist Route** signs (white lettering on a brown background). There are now ten separate routes and if you follow these signs you will discover areas of interest and beauty which could easily be overlooked travelling on the main motorways or trunk routes.

Single track roads are still to be found in some parts of Scotland, especially in the north west and on the many islands. Care and consideration are the order of the day and the passing places should never be used as parking spots or picnic areas. Many of these roads are not fenced so look out for straying sheep and deer.

For cycling holidays there is a network of rural roads and designated **Cyclist Routes,** in many places making use of former railway tracks and Forestry Commission access roads. The **Glasgow-Killin Cycleway** is one of the most popular. Scotland is one of the last areas of Britain where you can pitch a tent away from recognised camp sites, although it is still necessary to obtain permission from the land owner.

Scotland's history lends it'self to **Themed Trails** and you can follow a car trail in **Speyside** which takes in eight malt whisky distilleries. The Gordon district has so many castles that they are now linked in a castle trail. You can follow a trail through the gardens of Argull, or discover the Christian heritage of the Solway, or the wool trade of the Borders, and we must not forget Scotland's national poet, Robert Burns who lived in Ayrshire and Dumfries; you can follow his story from humble beginnings to his town house, to places which he made famous by association.

Much of Scotland's land mass being in the Highlands makes this a paradise for hill walkers and sightseers alike. Footpaths or rights of way are defined in Scotland as routes between 'Places of Public Resort', fortunately the difficulty that may arise in defining a 'Place of Public Resort' is avoided as most landowners show tolerance to walkers on their land.

At certain times of the year, mainly May to August on humid evenings, the midges abound, particularly where there are damp masses and marshy places, around lochs burns and woodlands in the Highlands. They seem to prefer people in dark clothing! Spending the day being pursued and bitten by these natives enables one to understand something of what it feels like to be hunted and eaten alive.

On the subject of hunting, much of the country follows the philosophy of 'if it moves shoot it'. The stalking and shooting season is around August to October. It is very important when walking in the Highlands at this time of the year to check with local estates or farmers about your intended route, for your safety as well as theirs. The 170 Tourist Information Centres throughout Scotland are of great help on this subject.

There are several **Long Distance Footpaths**, all well signposted but it should be remembered that the weather can change extremely quickly, particularly along the west coast in the path of the fast-moving weather systems off the Atlantic Ocean, turning what was a pleasant afternoon stroll into a much more serious undertaking requiring a high degree of skill, endurance and map reading ability.

Not for the faint of heart is the **Southern Upland Way** which runs from **Portpatrick** in Galloway in the west to **Cockburn** on the Scottish borders in the east. It crosses high ground in places and walkers should be well equipped for it is a 212 serious miles long.

Also not for the inexperienced walker is the 95 mile long **West Highland Way** which starts on the outskirts of **Glasgow** and runs to **Fort William** via **Loch Lomond** and part of **Glencoe**. Some parts of the Way are remote and rough going.

A somewhat easier walk is the **Speyside Walk**, 30 miles long, following the river Spey from **Tugnet** at the mouth of the river to **Ballindalloch**.

For the experienced climber 'Munro collecting' is a popular pastime. There are 279 peaks over 3,000 feet, called **Munro's** after the mountaineer who first classified them. Only seven exceed 4,000 feet, with **Ben Nevis** near **Fort William** at 4,406 feet being Britain's highest mountain. Most of these Munros and the larger hills are quite accessible and within a reasonable distance from a public road and car park. The visiting climber can in a short holiday experience the character of many mountains in several parts of the country.

Scotland is possibly more famous for it's lochs than for it's mountains. The largest Loch in capacity is **Loch Ness**, the greatest surface area is **Loch Lomond**, the deepest is **Loch Morar** and the longest is **Loch Awe**.

The longest river in Scotland is the **River Tay** stretching for 118 miles, and the highest waterfall is the **East Coulaulin** at 658 feet.

The **Caledonian Canal** is 60 miles long from coast to coast, and connects **Lochs Lochy, Oich** and **Ness** with 22 miles of canal, altogether the longest short-cut in Britain. The area around the 9 mile **Crinan Canal** is a truly beautiful sight, and it was constructed in 1801 to shorten the sea journey round the **Mull of Kintyre.**

Water sports abound in Scotland. On the **Caledonian Canal** and many areas around the west coast, boats and yachts can be chartered, and there are a good many areas of water for windsurfing, water skiing, jet-skiing and canoeing, in particular at **Loch Earn, Loch Morlich** and **Strathclyde Park.**

Diving is a well established sport in the **Orkneys** where there are many wrecks to be investigated, and the area around **St Abbs** in the Borders is especially popular bcause of the clarity of the water and diversity of underwater species to be seen.

There are five ski-resorts in Scotland, **Nevis Range** and **Glencoe** in the west, **Cairngorm** on Speyside, **Glenshee** and **The Lecht** further east in the Grampian mountains. The Lecht is particularly good for beginners, but all five cater for all abilities right up to Black runs. Cross country skiing is available at **Glenmore Forest, Glenisla** and **Glenmulliach**. Skiing is usually possible for January until April or even May.

Golf, for those who like a little exercise with their walking, is well provided for with over 400 golf courses: **Muirfield, Royal Troon, Carnoustie, Turnberry, St Andrews** and **Gleneagles**, to name just a few. There are more golf courses per head of population in Scotland than anywhere else in the world.

Another favourite occupation of visitors to Scotland is bird watching. Inland, golden eagles and ospreys are to be found in good numbers, whilst the coastal areas and islands throng with the clammer of sea birds. Of the 790 islands off the west and north coasts, only 130 are inhabited by man, many being simply too small and too wild, but they present ideal conditions for many birds, many of the islands being home to millions.

Copinsay, one of the Orkney Islands is administered as a bird sanctuary by the RSPB having been bought by the WWF as a memorial to a naturalist.

There are 70 islands in the **Orkneys**, but now fewer than 20 populated, and that number is diminishing despite the fact that the closest is only eight miles from the mainland. Most of them are low-lying, the exception being **Hoy** with some of the most spectacular cliffs anywhere, soaring to over 1,000 feet above sea level alongside the 'Old Man of Hoy' a splendid isolated stack of red sandstone. The islands have a wealth of prehistoric sites; at **Quoynes**, on **Sanday** chambered tombs date back to 2,900BC and at the unique site of **Skara Brae**, preserved beneath the sand for 4,000 years, is a real picture of neolithic life; at **Stenness** the **Ring of Brodgar** is a stone circle to equal Stonehenge. The vast harbour of **Scapa Flow** between the islands was a strategic naval base during both the World Wars. The capital **Kirkwall** is famous for the **St Magnus Cathedral**,and for the Orkney Festival under the auspices of the Orcadian composer Sir Peter Maxwell Davies.

On the **Shetland Islands,** at **Lerwick**, at the end of January each year they celebrate the ceremony of 'Up-Helly-A' when a Viking boat is burned. Many of the islands, and in particular **Jarlshof**, have many remarkable remnants of the Viking era. The island of **Fair Isle** is world famous for it's unique knitwear and traditions here can be traced back for many centuries, although discovery of oil in the North Sea has vastly changed the islands. Shetland is home to the contemporary poet George Mackay Brown.

On the mainland, the region of **The Highlands**, which covers the new administrative districts of the Western Isles, Highland, Grampian, most of Tayside and parts of **Central and Strathclyde,** has much to commend to it's visitors.

The Findhorn Foundation on the **Moray Firth** is a remarkable working community which welcomes visitors. It was started in 1962, it's aim to foster a common vision and help create a better world through spiritual growth. Workshops are open to guests from all over the world. The 'Ecological Village' at Findhorn is aimed as a technical guide to building greener houses, using natural materials and saving as many of the earth's resources as possible, in an effort to assist those wishing to help stop global warming and heal the world.

To the west is **Inverness** the rapidly growing Highland capital and home, at **Balnain House**, to a traditional music museum in the town, which is regarded as the capital of the bagpipe. Nearby at **Moniack** the **Moniack Winery** has an exhibition of country wines and jams.

Up the river from Inverness, is **Loch Ness**, created by a geological fault and so deep that a monster could well dwell there almost without detection. Loch Ness is not unique in it's monster legends as there have been many other sightings in Scotland over the past centuries. **Drumnadrochit** is the sightseeing centre for the monster, with an exhibition on this intriguing subject.

To the north, the former county of Sutherland was the 'southern land' of the Norsemen who came in the 9th century and were dominant in the 11th to 13th centuries. It has the best mountain scenery in Scotland. To the north again, in former **Caithness** pre-historic man left his mark with a wealth of brochs (round towers), cairns, forts and standing stones, as well as early Christian chapels. By the small village of **Lybster** the **Hill O' Many Stanes** comprises some 200 stones set in precise rows, an extraordinary ancient site.

On the north coast here many ships have been wrecked. **The Pentland Skerries** off **John O' Groats** are particularly dangerous due to the many vicious whirlpools with innocuous names like 'Merry Men of May'. Many of the inhabitants in these far north lands are still crofters although the land was much changed by the 'Clearances' in the 19th century.

South of the exceptionally beautiful **Spey Valley** with some of the finest Scottish castles alongside the wooded river banks, is the recreation centre of **Aviemore** in the **Cairngorm Mountains**, now home to imported reindeer. In the valley of **Kingussie**, the **Highland Folk Museum** gives a lot of information on how life was lived and is lived in this region.

On the far side of the Cairngorms is **Balmoral Castle**, the Royal Family's Scottish home.

Aberdeen is one of the richest cities in Scotland, thanks to the North Sea Oil industry, although not every aspect of this association is a positive one and many locals resent the intrusion.

Aberdeen's **Hazelhead Park** has an unusually large and complicated maze for a municipal park and the village of **Udny Green** east of **Oldmeldrum** contains a circular stone buildings called a Mort House, used to keep bodies safe from the resurrectionists!

On the opposite coast, the famous **Inverewe Gardens** stand at the head of Loch Ewe. Their superb collection of sub-tropical plants are a wonder to behold in this spectacular landscape. The area around **Glen Torridon** in Wester Ross is a must for walker, climbers and naturalists. Here is a 16,100 acre estate with some of the finest mountain scenery in Scotland.

A little to the south, by the village of **Dornie**, inland from the **Kyle of Lochalsh** at the junction of the three lochs, stands the **Eilean Donan Castle**, once a Chieftan's castle and a Jacobite stronghold, and still a magnificent sight, as are the nearby **Falls of Glomach** with a 370feet drop over spectacular black cliffs.

From the Kyle of Lochalsh the trip to **Skye**, one of the Inner Hebrides, is a short one. The island more than anywhere else shows the dramatic contrast of moors and mountains, with working crofts and ancient castle ruins, and the phenomenal rock formations of the **Old Man of Storr**, and the ragged lava pinnacles of **Kilt** and **Quirang**.

The awesome size and the blue hue of the **Cullin Hills** literally fill the sky, as best appreciated from **Glen Brittle** or **Elgol**.

Legend has it that the extraordinary **Callanish Stone Circle** on **Lewis** in the Outer Hebrides was at one time giants who were turned to stone when they refused to be baptised, although there are other legends which add further to the mystery of this atmospheric place.

The island of **Iona** off Mull has early Druid associations and has remained a sacred and magical place. The even smaller island of **Staffa** is St Columba's 'sacred isle', where, in calm weather, you can explore the basalt rocks which match those of Antrim's 'Giant's Causeway'. The cliffs on the south and west of the island are splendidly perpendicular and **Fingal's Cave** is truly impressive with it's grotesque formations which inspired Mendelssohn's 'The Hebrides' overture.

The small island of **Gigha**, west of Kintrye has very fertile soil, and is especially known for it's gardens and valuable plants. At **Achamore House** there is a fine collection of rhododendron hybrids.

The **Auchindrain Museum of Country Life** near **Inverary**, Strathclyde, is a preserved crofting settlement in situ, with more than 20 buildings in various stages of restoration, some of them furnished, showing the way of life of a communal tenancy settlement.

The Treasures of the Earth exhibition at Corpach, **Fort William** includes a mineral and fossil exhibition, and just to the south is **Glencoe**, certainly one of Scotland's most beautiful glens, the magnificent scenery with it's history and wildlife makes every step you take worth the effort.

The Central Lowlands, which include the busy cities of **Edinburgh** and **Glasgow**, as well as other important towns such as **Dundee, Perth, Stirling** and **Kilmarnock**, is made up of the regions of Lothian, Fife and parts of Tayside, Central and Strathclyde.

Th 'Fair Maid of Perth' was immortalised by Sir Walter Scott and has given readers a knowledge of this lovely area. **Perth** has many museums and parks. One such, the **Branklyn Garden** is a truly outstanding collection of alpines, rhododendrons, herbaceous and peat garden plants, gathered from all over the world.

The Doocot at **Finavon** north of Perth is the largest dovecot in Scotland and now houses an exhibition on similar buildings in **Angus**, a better occupation for the buildings than it's intended one - which was to breed doves for the table. At **East Linton**, west of Dunbar, the **Phantassie**

Doocot is a part of the centre at **Preston Mill** with one of the oldest mechanically working water driven meal mills in Scotland.

In **Airth** at **Dunmore Park** is a building in the shape of a pineapple, which started out as a two storey summerhouse, built by the Earl of Dunmore in 1761 when the pineapple was an exotic novelty. It is now owned by the Landmark Trust.

In Fife, **Anstruther** is worth a visit for those who like their houses decorated in shells.

Colinsburgh Balcarres Craig in Fife has a splendid castellated folly to the north of the town, and in **Edinburgh**, probably the most famous of all canine momuments is the one to **Greyfriars Bobby**.

In Edinburgh **The Salisbury Centre** is a residential community based in a large Georgian house with an organic garden near Arthur's Seat. This centre organises classes for meditation, massage, self-healing, yoga and shiatsu, and welcomes anyone who wishes to meet for meditation or discussion.

Robert Burns and friends formed their debating club at the **Batchelor's Club** at **Tarbolton**, near Ayr, a thatched house built in the 17th century.

The cities of Edinburgh and Glasgow are generally well documented, and include a vast array of important sites and worthwhile places to visit. Much of the interest is historical, but comparatively recently years have seen some exciting developments in the arts, **Glasgow** having been home to the art nouveau designer and architect Charles Rennie Mackintosh whose fine **School of Art** built at the turn of the century is a true masterpiece. Glasgow is home to the very special **Burrell Collection**. **Edinburgh** is famous throughout the world for it's **Edinburgh International Festival** as well as the Fringe Festival.

The Southern Uplands cover the regions of Borders and Dumfries and Galloway along with some of the far southern fringes of Strathclyde. This is a region not of mountains but of gentle hills rising from ground that is for the most part already well above sea level. The land is well suited to sheep grazing which led to the successful woollen cloth industry which took it's name from the river Tweed, around the town of Berwick-upon-Tweed, actually in England. The Border Collie was used here to help in the sheep farming.

The east coast above Berwick is a ragged one, **St Abb's Head** with it's small sandy harbour nestled beneath 300 feet cliffs, is surrounded by caves at one time used for smuggling. The fine views of the rocky coast take in the ruins of **Fast Castle**, the 'Wolf's Crag' of Scott's 'Bride of Lammermoor'. It is a most spectacular promontory described as ' the most important locality for cliff-breeding sea birds in south east Scotland'. The four abbeys all dating from the early 12th century, which lie in a line east of **Selkirk**, have been much painted and written about in prose and poetry. They are all in ruins, following many border skirmishes. **Melrose Abbey** is the most substantial of the ruins with some fine detail remaining, but **Jedburgh Abbey** and **Kelso Abbey** are in a less complete state. The idyllic setting of **Dryburgh Abbey** is where Sir Walter Scott chose to be buried.

The magnificent **Abbotsford House** was built by Sir Walter Scott in the early 19th century and he lived here until his death in 1832. It now acts as a museum to his life with artefacts still much as he left them.

The little toll house at **Gretna Green**, and later the town's Smithy were the first places in Scotland where elopers from England could make use of the Scottish marriage laws, but the law was changed in 1940 and running away to Gretna Green is no longer possible. This does not prevent thousands of visitors coming here very year to see the Smithy and the Toll House, enjoy the romantic atmosphere and perhaps catch sight of one of the legal weddings which still take place.

The red sandstone ruins of **Sweetheart Abbey** stand on the banks of the Solway Firth with views to the Lake District.

Famous for it's 13th century moated castle, **Caerlaverock**, Dumfries can also boast a very important nature reserve. **The Caerlaverock Nature Reserve** on the north shore of the Solway Firth consists of some 13,000 acres of saltmarsh, visited every winter by something like 10,000 barnacle geese. It is the most northerly area for the natterjack toad, a species so protected that it is even an offence to pick one up.

The Devil's Beef Tub, by the main route north near the spa town of **Moffat** is not a corrupted place name but it is actually associated with beef, cattle raiders hiding their animals in the deep dell.

Ten years ago Scotland was a relative wasteland for vegetarians, but things have very much improved; there are now quite a number of solely vegetarian places to eat and stay, and even though the vast majority of places in Scotland still have no leaning towards vegetarianism, there is an increasing understanding of what is required.

Brasserie - **OWLIES BRASSERIE**

Little John Street, Aberdeen, Scotland AB1 1FF

Tel: 01224 649267 Fax: 01224 626558

Built in the mid 1920's, Owlies was part of the Department of Engineering at Aberdeen University and is really a warehouse complete with chain pulleys, girders and a glass roof. The decor and the atmosphere are excitingly out of the ordinary. Secondhand wooden chairs and tables stand on a brilliantly painted cement floor.

There is absolutely nothing that matches but with candles in bottles, plenty of greenery from the plants, and walls covered with artwork, which is for sale, the whole ambience is special and great fun. Here you will be offered French country cooking to a very high standard and with a good choice of vegetarian dishes. You will be hard to please if you do not enjoy the delicious creations placed before you. Nothing is bought in and everything is freshly prepared. Owlies is somewhere that contends happily with a variety of tastes, diets and budget requirements. The brasserie is licensed.

USEFUL INFORMATION

OPEN; Monday: 5.30-10pm Tues-Thurs; 11.30-10pm, Fri-Sat; 11.30-10.30pm. Closed Dec 24-Jan 6.
CREDIT CARDS;Access/Visa/Switch.

ON THE MENU; Delicious French country cooking. Vegetarian choices
DISABLED ACCESS; Not for wheelchairs, but disabled toilets.

Restaurant - **HENDERSONS SALAD TABLE**

94 Hanover Street, Edinburgh

Tel: 0131 225 2131

This is Scotland's original Vegetarian/Wholefood restaurant and as such has maintained a high standard of food and service throughout it's career. Inside it is almost as if the world and his wife were visiting! Totally cosmopolitan, you may well find yourself surrounded by foreign tongues - and I do not mean Gaelic!. It is an attractive venue with live music at night. The menu is imaginative and innovative although it holds fast to some traditional dishes. One thing one can be sure of is value for money. Licensed, it serves a range of organic wines as well as beers and spirit's. You will find it is open from Monday to Saturday from 0800-2245 and also on Sundays during the Edinburgh Festival.

USEFUL INFORMATION

OPEN; Mon-Sat 0800-2245 Sundays during Festival
CHILDREN; Welome
CREDIT CARDS; All major cards
LICENSED; Yes. Organic wines

RESTAURANT; Wide range of vegetarian and wholefoods
DISABLED ACCESS; No basement steps

Bed and Breakfast - **CAFE BEAG**

Glen Nevis, Fort William, Inverness-shire PH33 6SY

Tel: 01397 703601

Cafe Beag is three miles from Fort William town centre in Glen Nevis it'self, and right next door to the Youth Hostel at the foot of Ben Nevis. It is a friendly cafe in a timber building that fit's well into it's beautiful surroundings on the banks of the River Nevis with Ben Nevis across the river. It is a relaxed place with an eating area, a general sitting room and games room. It is strictly non-smoking, unpretentious and inexpensive. Cafe Beag is open every day from 8am-9pm from the beginning of March until the end of October. The food is excellent, traditional home-cooking which one might describe as International in flavour with a Scottish bias. A large percentage of the dishes are suitable for vegetarians. Cafe Beag is licensed.

Walking boots, rucksacks and child carriers are available for hire, and the shop on site sells maps, socks, laces and films.

USEFUL INFORMATION

OPEN; 8am-9pm 7 days Closed end February
CREDIT CARDS; Visa/Mastercard
LICENSED; Yes

ON THE MENU; Traditional of October until end home-cooked. Many dishes vegetarians
DISABLED ACCESS; Yes + toilets

Bed & Breakfast - **NEVIS VIEW**

14, Farrow Drive, Corpach, Fort William,

Inverness-shire PH33 7JW

Tel: 01397 772447

If you appreciate wonderful views you will enjoy Nevis View with it's south facing living rooms and bedrooms which soak up all the available sunlight. However that is just one ingredient of this interesting establishment. Built 35 years ago it was architect designed and is fascinating. Everyone who stays here is intrigued. Barbara Grieve runs this strictly non-smoking house and looks after a husband and children at the same time. Her lively personality and her love and knowledge for this exciting part of Scotland, make her the ideal person with whom to discuss the places to visit.

For those who enjoy lazing about, the garden is inviting, and for everyone the beautifully cooked breakfast is something to look forward to when you wake in the morning after a good night's sleep in a comfortable bedroom. Evening meals are available on request but need to be ordered in advance. With a husband who is a vegetarian Barbara is well versed in catering for your needs. Nevis View is not licensed but you are invited to bring your own wine.

USEFUL INFORMATION

OPEN; All year
CREDIT CARDS; Access/Visa
CHILDREN; Welcome

ON THE MENU; Well chosen dishes for vegetarians, vegans & meat eaters
DISABLED ACCESS; No. The path is too steep.

Guest House

TAIGH-NA-MARA VEGETARIAN GUEST HOUSE

An Cladach, Ardindrean, Lochbroom,
Scottish Highlands IV23 2SE

Tel/Fax: 01854 655282

This remarkable guest house is quite unique by virtue of it's easy acceptance of guests who, apart from being asked to observe the no-smoking rule, are free of restrictions. The owners, Tony and Jackie like to think of you as their friends, breakfast is when you want it - treat the place as your own - and they mean it. They invite you to come, christen your wellies and find the true meaning of idyllic, secluded contentment. Children and dogs are welcome as long as children under 10 are in bed before 8pm and dogs confined to either the boatshed or scullery. Apart from the breadth of the welcome why is Taigh-Na-Mara out of the ordinary? Because in 1989 the remains of the old seashore shop were transformed into a special guesthouse for special people. It is now a 30ft (but cosy) lounge/dining room with wood burning stove, a spiral stair up to two romantic bedrooms, wood panelled bathroom and breathtaking views.

The honeymoon suite in the boat shed has a corner bath, king size bed and a huge picture window revealing the loch and mountains beyond. Lying about the place you'll find a hotchpotch of bikes, a windsurfer, a dodgy dinghy and some of the best all year round hill walking right on the doorstep. You don't have to be active to stay here but there is a 200yd descent walking down through a steep muddy, slippy croft to contend with. It is worth it though; you could sit down to a huge breakfast and watch seals, porpoises or even an otter swimming past the window. If it rains and you can't face the brae, then select one of the great selection of books to read, a musical instrument or game to play, or spend the day in bed - nobody minds! The speciality is Scottish Highland Gourmet Vegetarian/Vegan farmhouse cooking. Dinner is four courses finishing with a selection of Scottish vegetarian goat, cow, ewe and even soya milk cheeses! You are asked to bring your wine or alchohol, as Taigh Na Mara does not have a licence - nor an illicit distillery - just a free wee dram when you arrive as a reward for braving the walk down.

USEFUL INFORMATION

OPEN; All year

CHILDREN; Welcome. Children under 10 requested to be in bed by 8pm

CREDIT CARDS; Mastercard/Visa/Delta/Switch

DINING ROOM; Scottish Highland Gourmet Vegetarian/Vegan Farmhouse cooking.

DISABLED ACCESS; Not easy

Guest House   - **INVERDEEN HOUSE**

Bridge Square, Ballater, Royal Deeside, Scotland AB35 5QJ

Tel: 01339 755759

Beneath the summit of Lochnagar is the spa town of Ballater founded in the 18th century, it is surrounded by rolling hills and wonderful scenery. The Craigendarroch - 'The Hill of Oaks' - rises to 700ft, there is a well beaten path to the top and once there the view of the Dee Valley is stunning. Down in the town is Inverdeen House one of the original buildings in Ballater, the Listed building was built around 1820. The house it'self is very comfortable with a warm and friendly atmosphere, and is furnished w.ith antiques from the Victorian and William IV eras. The 3 bedrooms, 2 double and 1 family, are charming with central heating, wash basin, colour television and a tray with tea, coffee, hot chocolate and biscuit's. The period bathroom and modern showerroom are conveniently located. After a very restful night in the more than comfortable beds, you make your way to the period dining room, where seated at the large farmhouse table you are served the most superb breakfast. Your tastebuds are treated to fresh fruit, muesli, organically grown prunes, Canadian pancakes and maple syrup, muffins and jam both home-made. There is a fine selection of teas, coffees and herbal teas.Vegans and guests requiring special dietary attention are invited to consult about their requirements at the time of booking. Special needs are honoured with care and respect For the non-vegetarian there is a wonderful breakfast including venison sausages and home-cured bacon. Inverdeen House is a totally non-smoking establishment. The area is an absolute paradise for the outdoor person with hillwalking, climbing, golf, fishing, riding, gliding, and skiing. There are Whisky and Castle trails, a Sweet Factory where you can watch sweets being made, Mountain bike hire and 4 x 4 off road driving. Inverdeen House is an excellent choice, as the Visitor's Book will confirm.

USEFUL INFORMATION

OPEN; All year
CHILDREN; Welcome
CREDIT CARDS; None taken
ACCOMMODATION; 3 rooms
2 double, 1 family

DINING ROOM; Superb choice of breakfasts
VEGETARIAN; Excellent selection, Vegan
meals or other special diets by arrangement
DISABLED ACCESS; No
GARDEN; Yes
POSITIVELY NO SMOKING

DUNNET HEAD TEA ROOM

Brough KW14 8YE Tel: 01847 851774

Good vegetarian menu.

SUNFLOWERS

39 Whytescause Way, Kirkcaldy PY1 1XY Tel: 01592 646266

This is a colourful, relaxing restaurant where the food has that essential mmm...factor! There is an extensive menu catering for such favourites as shepherdess pie and vegetable chilli and for the more indulgent, Chocolate Amaretto cheescake, toffee apple cake and pecan pie. To supplement this there are specials each day. In order to promote healthy vegetarian eating there is also Sunflowers Lighter Option range. OPEN; Mon-Sat 8.30am-4.30pm. V. VG. NS. D/Acc.

THE BAY TREE
403 Great Western Road, Glasgow G4 9HY   Tel: 0141 224 5898 - Cafe - V.VG.NS.CHILDREN C.

SONNHALDE
East Terrace, Kingussie PH21 1JS Tel/Fax: 01540 661266
This Victorian villa built at the turn of the century has been modernised and centrally heated to ensure a comfortable holiday all the year round. There are seven guests' bedrooms, some with en-suite facilities, including family rooms, all with electric blankets, duvets and wash-hand basins. The Guests' Lounge has a log fire, TV and Tea/Coffee making facilities. There are two public bathrooms with shower and w.c. Ample parking and a ski store. Evening Meals are available with advance notice as all food is purchased daily. Vegetarian and Special Diets catered for. Reduced rates for children.

WOODWICK HOUSE
Evie, Orkney KW17 2PQ Tel: 01856 751330 & 0171538 5633.
'Good food, Peace and Seclusion, set in 12 acres of woodland with burn and bay. Close to Ancient Sites and R.S.P.B Reserves.

GLENRANNOCH HOUSE
Kinloch, Rannoch PH16 5QN Tel: 01882 632307 Guest House
One of those 'Off the beaten track' places. Comfortable and friendly. Peaceful, remote and unspoilt.

BURRASTOW HOUSE
Walls, Shetland ZE29PD. Tel: 01595 809307 Fax: 01595 809213
A delightful house offering ensuite accommodation in well appointed rooms. There is a no-smoking rule which applies to the bedrooms and the dining room. Children are welcome. Burrastow House has a table licence. There are facilities for the disabled. Open all year except January and February.

SEAGREEN
Plockton Road, Kyle of Lockalsh, Wester Ross IV40 8DA Tel: 01599 534388
This Restaurant and Bookshop specialises in local seafood and wholefood dishes. All the food is cooked on the premises. All day licenced cafe. Garden. Wholefood shop. Outside terrace. Exhibition space. Traditional music. Local interest literature. Open every day, all year (except mid January to end March)

GREEN INN - Restaurant with Rooms
9 Victoria Road, Ballater, Aberdeenshire AB35 5RP
Tel: 013397 55701
Don't be foled by the unprepossessing exerior. Excellent food - every dish though through. elaxed but generally smartish. Proprietor Jeff Purves delights in the challenge of vegetarian cooking. Open: All year 7-9pm except last week in Nov., first eek in Dec. 12.30-1.45pm Sunday only Mar-Oct

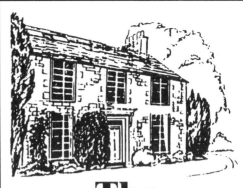
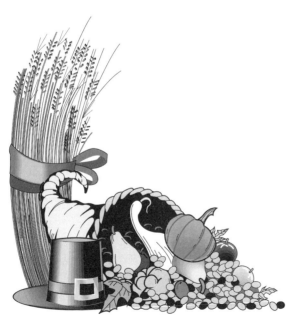

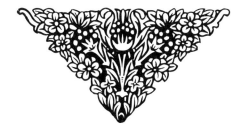

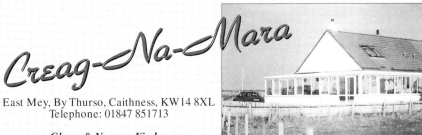

East Mey, By Thurso, Caithness, KW14 8XL
Telephone: 01847 851713

Glenys & Norman Kimber

Glenys and Norman invite you to their fully licensed restaurant with accomodation which is open to non-residents and also caters for special diets.

Our conservatory restaurant is beautifully situated with views of The Orkneys and Dunnet Head and close to the Castle of Mey. Shooting and fishing are available in season.

We cater for vegetarians and special diets & have many facilities for the disabled. Prices for accomodation & breakfast range from £16 to £17.50 per person. Dinner, bed & breakfast can be had from £23.50 per person. There is no surcharge for lone travellers who are most welcome as are children and pets. Two of our lovely rooms are en-suite and 2 have shared facilities, TV & hospitality tray in all rooms. Hairdryers & trouser press available.

Visitor Attractions

VISITOR ATTRACTIONS

BEDFORDSHIRE

BEDFORD DISCOVER THE BEDFORDSHIRE COUNTRYSIDE
Tel: 01234 228671
Discover the wonderful landscape and varied heritage by taking a family day out to visit one of the many country parks and cyclewalks that Bedfordshire has to offer. Throughout the year there is plenty to do. Visitor Centres and Country Parks are open all the year round.

BEDFORD MUSEUM
Tel: 01234 353232
This lively museum is set in attractive surroundings close to the River Great Ouse. Excellent displays interpret the human and natural history of the region. Open Tues-Sat 11-5pm Sun & Bank Holidays 2-5pm. Closed Mondays. Admission free.

BROMHAM MILL
Tel: 01234 824330.
Built in 1695, Bromham Mill is an attracive stone building set by the River Great Ouse. Now restored to its former working glory, the enormous revolving water wheel is the focal point .

DUNSTABLE WHIPSNADE ANIMAL PARK Tel: 01582 872171 Location: 20 miles from
the M25 junction 21 following elephant signs from Dunstable. Europe's largest conservation centres offering 2,500 rare and endangered species in 600 acres of beautiful parkland, including all the family favourites - elephants, tigers, penguins, bears, rhinos and many more. Free daily demonstrations of Elephant Encounters, Californian Sea Lions and free flying Birds of the World will keep all the family entertained. Open daily 10-6pm.

LEIGHTON BUZZARD RAILWAY
Page's Park Station, Billington Road (A4146) Tel: 01525 373888
This is one of England's foremost narrow gauge preservation sites; home to over fifty engines. It provides a great day out. Page's Park Station is situated alongside a large public recreational area offering grassy open space, children's play equipment and sports facilities. The station has a souvenir shop and buffet serving hot and cold snacks and refreshments at most times when trains are running. There is a picnic area, free car parking and space for coaches. The five and a half mile return journey by historic steam train takes just over an hour. A museum project display is open to visitors and much of the railway's historic locomotive and wagon fleet is based here. Steam locomotive viewing, a working quarry display and the demonstration sand trains are planned throughout the year. Industry Train Displays are live demonstrations of authentic locomotives and wagons which represent the major industries served by narrow gauge railways. Another form of heritage transport can be enjoyed on your day out to the railway. Cruises on the 19th century Grand Union Canal can be combined with your historic steam train ride. Ring or write for details. Although the trains mainly operate on Sundays from April-October, there are Festive Specials in December complete with Father Christmas, mince pies etc.

LEIGHTON BUZZARD GREBE CANAL CRUISES

Pitstone Wharf, Pitstone, Nr Leighton Buzzard LU79AD   Tel: 01296 661920.

Rod and Margaret Saunders founded this business some 20 years ago and operate passenger vessels on the Grand Union Canal on a most beautiful length of the Canal where it climbs up the Chiltern escarpment from the Vale of Aylesbury into the Chilterns themselves. Built 200 years ago, the passage of time has seen the canal mellow into the beautiful countryside, it's quaint hump-back bridges and locks complimenting the scene.

The fleet of passenger vessels operate from the purpose built base, Pitstone wharf, near to the village of Cheddington (of 'great train robbery fame') and there is a regular service of one and a half hour trips run during the peak summer months via the Chiltern Summit level of the canal at Tring, the highest point of the waterway, 396 feet above sea level. Passengers have the opportunity to leave the boat in the lock flight and view Marsworth reservoirs and nature reserve and to picnic ashore if they wish.

The boats are mainly wide-beam, offer all weather protection, and provide considerable comfort for the passengers. There are bars on all the boats and for pre-booked parties meals can be served while cruising - try the very popular afternoon cream teas.

At Pitstone Wharf the Saunders have developed a boat yard which is open to everyone, where the non-boat owner can come and enjoy the canal and if so wished, can hire a self-steer boat, from a single day hire to a week or fortnight's holiday. Tuition is available for the beginner. Superbly run, with efficient professional crews, you can relax aboard and enjoy Grebe Canal Cruises.

LUTON   WOODSIDE FARM & WILD FOWL PARK

Tel: 01582 841044.

At Woodside Farm Shop and Wild Fowl Park, there are over 160 different breeds of animals and birds to see and feed with special feed from the Farm Shop.

Large picnic areas, pony rides, tarzan trails, birds of prey displays and daily tractor and trailer rides are available. Open all year round Mon-Sat 8- 5.30pm. Closed Sunday.

THE WERNHER COLLECTION

Tel: 01582 22955

The works of the Russian Court Jeweller, Carl Faberge are part of the finest private art collection in Great Britain. There are many paintings, costumes and other personal possessions of the Russian Imperial Family Romanov.

Treasures include old master paintings, magnificent tapestries, English and French porcelain, sculpture, bronzes and renaissance jewellery. Open to the public 29th Mar-16th October Fri-Sun 1.30-5pm.

SILSOE WREST PARK HOUSE AND GARDENS

Tel: 01525 860152

The history of English gardening from 1700-1850 is set out in acres of stunning delights at Wrest Park. In the Great Garden, water catches the eye in every direction, while intersecting alleys provide splendid vistas of the many garden buildings and ornaments.

Wrest Park House was inspired by an 18th century French chateaux. the delightful intricate French Garden, with statues and fountains, enhances any view of the house from The Great Garden. Open 1st April-30th Sept weekends & Bank Holidays only 10-6pm.

WOBURN

Tel: 01525 290666

Home of the Dukes of Bedford for over 350 years, Woburn Abbey is now lived in by the Duke's heir, the Marquess of Tavistock and his family. The house contains one of the most important collections and works of art in the world and is surrounded by a 3,000 acre deer park with nine species of deer. Open 1st Jan-26 Mar weekends only 27th Mar-30th October everyday.

WOBURN SAFARI PARK

Tel: 01525 290407.

Britain's largest drive through safari park with lions, tigers, rhinos, wolves, bears, hippos, monkeys and many more are all part of the attractions which make the safari park a great family attraction. New attractions include: The Adventure Ark, Penguin World and Great Woburn Railway. Open 5 Mar-30 October everyday.

BUCKINGHAMSHIRE

AYLESBURY   AYLESBURY BREWERY COMPANY

Tel: 01296 395000

The company has been part of Buckinghamshire since 1895. It has some 200 Public houses most of them in the county, but you can see the ABC sign in parts of neighbouring Bedfordshire and Oxfordshire too. In addition to its own wide range of beers and lagers, you'll find a number of outstanding products from several other breweries. Visit Aylesbury and sample for yourself.

THE CHILTERN BREWERY

Tel: 01296 613647

Location: A413 Aylesbury.

The ancient and revered art of the English Brewer can still be discovered flourishing in the beautiful countryside of Buckinghamshire. Completely independent and family run since it's inception in 1980, this unique small brewery specialises in the production of high quality, traditionally brewed English beers with a real local flavour. Included in the large selection of home brewed ales is a 300 year old ale available in imperial pint bottles. Open Mon-Sat 9-5pm.

BUCKS RAILWAY CENTRE

Tel 01296 75440

Home to the private collection of steam locomotives. The centre boasts vintage carriages, signal box, station and gift shop. Throughout the year the centre holds special events and steaming days including regular visits by Thomas the Tank Engine, steam train rides and the extremely popular Victorian afternoon cream teas.

BUCKINGHAMSHIRE RAILWAY CENTRE

Tel 01296 75720

The centre's 25 acre site is at Quainton Road station and exchange sidings, the last remaining Metropolitan Railway county station. On display is one of the country's largest collection of historic steam and diesel locomotives as well as a comprehensive collection of coaching and freight rolling stock. Open 11-6pm daily.

BEACONSFIELD BEKONSCOT MODEL VILLAGE

Tel: 01494 672919

The oldest model village in the world is a charming minature covering over one and a half acres. Included in the many things to see are beautifully landscaped gardens, miniature houses, castles, churches, shops and railway stations, through which runs the finest outdoor model railway (Gauge One) open to the public in the United Kingdom. The 'country' of Bekonscot is planted with 8,000 conifers, 2,000 minature shrubs, and 200 tonnes of stone used for the rockeries alone.There are no less than one hundred and sixty buildings including churches, hotels, shops and private houses constituting Bekonscot and the outlying villages. Souvenir Shop. Refreshment Kiosks, 2 Picnic Areas, Childrens Playground, Miniature Tramway and many other scenes. It is a paradise for photographers, a fascination for model-makers, an admiration for gardeners, 'Heaven' for small children. In fact a must for the whole family. OPEN; Every day from 10am-5pm from 17th February to 3rd November.

CAMBRIDGESHIRE

CAMBRIDGE   OLIVER CROMWELL HOUSE

Tel: 01353 662062.

Standing almost in the shadows of Ely Cathedral this was the home of Oliver Cromwell and his family for some ten years. Several rooms have been refurbished in Cromwellian style to show features of the house which Cromwell would have known in his time. Displays tell the story of the house's history, for although Cromwell was still the most famous occupant, the house itself has medieval origins and a fascinating past. Built in the early 14th century for the collection of tithes, it was used as a brewery and inn during the 19th century. Open 1st Apr-30th Sept 10-6pm daily including Sat, Sun and Bank Holidays 1st October-30th April 10-5.15pm.

DUXFORD AEROPLANE MUSEUM

Tel: 01223 833376

Location: Duxford is next to junction 10 off the M11 motorway, 48 miles from London.

A day at Duxford is a day you'll never forget. You'll find Europe's biggest collection of historic aircraft, over 130, displayed in the giant exhibition hangers. Flimsy biplanes that fought over the trenches of the First World War through to Gulf Jets are on show at this preserved wartime airfield. See the legendary Spitfire, Lancaster and B-17 Flying Fortress. Marvel at the U-2 Spyplane that flew on the edge of space and climb aboard Concorde. Look at the only F-111 supersonic swing-wing bomber on show in Europe and be amazed by the Harrier jump-jet. Open everyday except 24,25 & 26 December. Summer 26-Mar-16 October 10-6pm. Winter 10-4pm.

ELY CATHEDRAL

Tel: 01353 667735.

Location: A10 from Cambridge.

In 673 St Ethelreda, Queen of Northumbria, founded a monastery in the centre of the Fens on the Isle of Ely where she was Abbess until her death in 679. Some 400 years later in 1081, work on the present building was begun, under the guidance of Abbot Simeon. It was completed in 1189 and the cathedral now stands as a remarkable example of Romanesque architecture. Undoubtedly, the most outstanding feature of the cathedral is the octagon, built to replace the Norman tower which collapsed in 1322. The regular free guided tours will help you appreciate all that is special about the cathedral. The Cathedral Shop in the High street offers an imaginative selection of beautiful greetings cards, pottery, glassware, and jewellery. Open daily all year round. Summer 7-7pm and in the winter 7.30-6.30pm. Sun 5pm.

LINTON ZOO

Tel 01223 891308

location: Ten miles east of Cambridge on the B1052 just off the A460.

All set in 16 acres of beautifully landscaped gardens. Find time to visit the zoo and you will find lots to interest the whole family from Sumatran Tigers, African Lions, Snow Leopards, Lynx, Wallabies and Toucans and many exciting and unusual wildlife to be found at Cambridgeshire's Wildlife Breeding Centre. The zoo is continually expanding as more of the world's threatened species are taken on board.

Open all year round every day including Bank Holidays.

CORBY KIRKBY HALL

Tel: 01536 203230

Location: Off A43, four miles North East of Corby.

Begun in 1570 and completed by Sir Christopher Hatton, an Elizabethan courtier who built on a scale matching his ambition to entertain the Queen. The ruins of this marvellous country house show the dawning influence of the renaissance on more traditional Tudor forms.

Impressive in its sheer grandeur, the house is still partially roofed and glazed with many rooms to explore, and a wealth of richly carved stonework to discover. Kirby's Great Garden is the scene possibly of the most important formal garden restoration project in England.

Open daily 10-6pm 1st April-31st October 10-4pm.

LYDDINGTON BEDE HOUSE

Tel: 01572 822438

Location: 6 miles north of Corby.

Amidst the picturesque golden stone of the Leicestershire village of Lyddington, next to the handsome medieval parish church, stands Bede House. For more than 300 years, since 1602, the building was used as an almshouse, but its beginnings were less humble.

It was once part of the rural palace of the Bishop's of Lincoln. Many fine details from beautiful 16th century wooden ceilings, 15th century painted glass and a grand fireplace remain to remind us of the original purpose.

Open daily 10-6pm 1st April-30th Septenber.

HINCHINGBROOKE COUNTRY PARK

Tel: 01480 451568.

At Hinchingbrooke Country Park you can wander freely through beautiful, unspoilt Cambridgeshire countryside, through woodland glades and meadows or along river banks and lakesides. Set in 156 acres of woodland, there is a natural habitat home to a suprising variety of wildlife. Here you can see herons, woodpeckers, snipe, foxes and even deer, especially on a peaceful early morning walk. Terns and dragonflies hunt over the lakes in the summer and butterflies drift effortlessly over the meadows. As dusk falls bats emerge and you may even hear a nightingale sing.

Open all the year round.

THE OLD HUNTINGDON CAR TRAIL

Tel 01480 425831

This wonderful car trail has been designed to allow motorists or cyclists to join at any point, journeying around until you return to your starting point. Travelling through all parts of Cambridgeshire taking in all the major sights and attractions, the trail is a great way to travel. Open throughout the year Mon-Fri 9.30-5.30pm Sat 9-5pm. Closed Bank Holiday Mondays.

CORNWALL

BODMIN AND WENFORD RAILWAY.

Bodmin Station just south of town centre on B3268 to Lostwithiel. Tel: 01208 73666.

Bodmin General Station is a typical Great Western Railway terminus connected by three and a half miles of line to Bodmin Parkway. (British Rail main-line) The railway passes through lovely Cornish countryside and gives access to walks and other attractions. Most trains are steam hauled. For timetables ring or write. Open April-1st week in November plus Christmas and New Year.

LANHYDROCK,

National Trust.

Two and a half miles south east of Bodmin-Liskeard or B3268 Bodmin-Lostwithiel roads.

Tel: 01208 73320.

The finest house in Cornwall, superbly set in wooded parkland of 450 acres and encircled by a garden of rare shrubs and trees, lovely in all seasons. Allow time to view the 42 rooms. Through the crenellated gatehouse (1641) an idyllic walk on to the River Fowey and back through the woods should not be missed. Open 30th March-31st October daily except Monday when the house only is closed, garden, shop and restaurant remain open.

Open Bank Holiday Mondays 11-5.30pm, 5pm in October.

JAMAICA INN

just off A30 at Bolventor. Tel: 01566 86250.

Made famous by Daphne du Mauriers novel of the same name. For 400 years it has stood high on Bodmin Moor welcoming smugglers, highwaymen and travellers of all descriptions. It is an experience and in addition to the bars, restaurant and accommodation there is MR POTTERS MUSEUM OF CURIOSITY - showing the remarkable work of Walter Potter the famous Victorian Taxidermist who created the most imaginative animal scenes with loving care. Jamaica Inn is open all year and so too is Mr Potter's Museum except January.

DOBWALLS FAMILY ADVENTURE PARK

Tel: 01579 20578 Look for signs at Dobwalls on the A38.

Wonderful day out for the whole family with one admission fee allowing you to travel on the Rio Grand Miniature Railroad and The Union Pacific Miniature Railroad. Access to Locomotive sheds with their 6 steam and 4 diesel locomotives including the famous 'Big Boy'. Unlimited use of Adventureland. Mr Thorburn's Edwardian Countryside. Beautiful picnic areas and Woodland Walks. Open 30th March-30th September 10-6pm. October weekends only but daily durning Devon and Cornwall Half Term holidays.

TREBAH GARDEN
Mawnwn Smith, Nr Falmouth Tel: 01326 250448.

This magical old Cornish garden is listed by the Good Gardens Guide as being one of the eighty finest gardens in the world. The twenty five acre, steeply wooded ravine garden falls 200 feet from the 18th century house down to a private beach on the Helford River. It is truly wonderful. The garden is undergoing a major replanting and the beach, which is open to visitors to the gardens, is a secluded haven with superb views. Visitors are welcome to use the beach for swimming and picnics. Open every day of the year 10.30-5pm.

MARAZION ST MICHAEL'S MOUNT
Marazion, Penzance. National Trust. Tel: 01736 710265.

This magical island is the jewel in Cornwall's crown, a national treasure which is a must for every visitor to the far west. The great granite crag which rises from the waters of Mount's Bay is surmounted by an embattled 14th century castle, home of the St Aubyn family for over 300 years. On the water's edge there is a harbourside community, an ancient trading place for tin and other Cornish goods which today features shops and restaurants. Open: 30th March-31st October Mon-Fri (shop and restaurant open daily) 10.30-5.30pm November - 29th March. Guided tours as tide, weather and circumstances permit.

NEWLYN ART GALLERY.
Approaching Newlyn, the gallery is the first building on the sea-side of the coast road from Penzance.

Tel: 01736 63715.

Presents an exciting and varied programme of contemporary art and related events throughout the year. The Gallery is a dynamic artistic activity. One of the most important visual arts resources in the South West. Open: Mon-Sat 10-5pm Admission free.

NEWQUAY TRERICE
National Trust. Tel: 01637 875404.

An architectural gem - a small Elizabethan manor house, built before the Armada in 1571. The summer-flowering garden is unusual in content and layout and there is an orchard planted with old varieties of fruit trees. A small museum traces the history of the lawn mower. Open: 30th Mar-31st October daily except Tuesday 11-5.30pm Closes 5pm in October.

SPRINGFIELDS PONY CENTRE AND FUN PARK
St Columb Major.

Well signposted from the St Columb Major roundabout. Tel: 01637 881224. All weather attraction. Friendly Shetland ponies, pony rides. Pets Corner. Enjoy feeding lambs, calves and goats and hand feed the ducks fish and Sika deer. Springfields is a paradise for children. Burger Bar. Lake View restaurant. Dogs not allowed. Open: 31st March-30th October, 7 days a week 9.30-5.30pm October 10-4.30pm.

NEWQUAY SEA LIFE CENTRE
Towan Promenade. Tel: 01326 22361.

Experience the thrill of a deep sea dive without getting wet as you journey through a wondrous watery world with a surprise around every corner. Fascinating and extraordinary experience. Open: All year except Christmas Day 10am.

PENZANCE AND DISTRICT MUSEUM AND ART GALLERY.

Off Morrah rd. Tel: 01736 63625.

New Interactive Multimedia computer technology which has been istalled in the new Archaeology gallery. Discover the shops of the 1890's and 1930's and use the new computer image data- bank to discover what the area looked like in times past. The Art Galleries contain the largest collection of Newlyn School paintings in public ownership. Open: Mon-Fri 10.30-4.30pm Sat: 10.30-12.30pm.

TRINITY HOUSE NATIONAL LIGHTHOUSE CENTRE

The Old Buoy Store, Wharf Road. Tel: 01736 60077.

One of the few national museums outside London, it houses the finest collection of lighthouse equipment in the world. Audio-visual. Open: Daily April-October.

TRENGWAINTON GARDENS

Nr. Penzance.

In the far west, the uncommonly mild climate encourages the most tender and exotic shrubs and trees to flourish. A unique feature is the complex of walled gardens with west-facing raised beds, built c1820 for the growing of early vegetables. Open: 1st March-31st October, Wed,Thurs, Fri, Sat and Bank Holiday Mondays 10.30-5.30pm (5pm in March and October) National Trust.

PORTHCURNO THE MINACK THEATRE

Tel: 01841 540147.

The theatre is on the south coast about 3 miles from Land's End and 9 miles from Penzance. At the seaward end of the Porthcurno valley go up the winding hill. The Theatre is on your left. Wonderful open air theatre.

Audience are admitted one and a half hours before 'curtain up'. The earlier you arrive the closer you will be to the stage. The sun can be very hot at matinees and it is advisable to wear warm clothes in the evening. The seats are very hard but they do hire cushions! If you are disabled, please bring at least one able bodied person with you and try to let the management know in advance. Parking is free. Sandwiches and confectionery, hot and cold drinks are available pre-show and during the interval. There is an Exhibition Centre. Hours 10-5.30pm daily from 1st April-31st October (closing at 4.30pm in Oct). On days when there is a matinee, the Centre will be closed from 12-2.30pm, and viewing of the Theatre will be restricted durning the performance. A fabulous experience and unlike any other theatre in the world.

SALTASH COTEHELE.

National Trust. On the west bank of the Tamar 1 mile west of Calstock by footpath, 8 miles south west of Tavistock, 14 miles from Plymouth via Saltash Bridge. Tel: 01579 50434.

Recorded Information 01579 51222. Enchantingly remote, perched high above the wooded banks of the Tamar. For nearly six centuries the home of the Edgcumbe family. The manor house gives the impression of having been woven through time. It retains a medieval atmosphere. Cotehele today is a romantically unique estate - the terraced garden with its pools and dovecote, a working watermill and adjoining ciderpress, the Quay with its evocation of Victorian bustle. Now the home berth of the Shamrock, one of the last surviving Tamar sailing barges. Worth spending a day here. Open: 30th Mar-31st Oct. House, restaurant and mill daily except Friday (open Good Friday) House 12-5.30pm. Tearoom on Quay, shop and garden daily 11-5pm. Quay gallery daily 12-5pm.

ST AUSTELL   WHEAL MARTYN CHINA CLAY HERITAGE CENTRE.

Follow the signs to Carthew on the B3274, 2 miles north of St Austell. Tel/Fax: 01726 85362. Historic trail - discover the history of this important Cornish industry. Open air historic clay workings, indoor exhibitions, displays and audio-visual show, 1899 locomotive working water wheels and 1916 Peerless lorry. Nature Trail - mile long walk through the beautiful wooded site and spectacular views of a modern day working clay pit. Childrens Adventure Trail - picnic area, mineral displays, gift and pottery shop. Open: daily April to October 10-6pm.

LOST GARDENS OF HELIGAN

Pentewan, St Austell. Tel: 01726 844157/843566.

Award winning gardens, asleep for more than seventy years, are the scene of the largest garden restoration project in Europe. Most exciting, must be seen. Open: every day of the year 10-4.30pm.

KIDS KINGDOM

Albert Road, St Austell. Tel: 01726 77377.

Indoor Adventure Play Centre for the under 12's who must be accompanied by a responsible adult. Great fun, plenty to do. Open: 7 days a week Easter-end September 10-9pm. October-Easter 10-6pm.

ST IVES SOCIETY OF ARTISTS

Old Mariners Church, Norway Square adjacent to Sloop car park.

Exhibits representational work. Gallery overlooks harbour that was the inspiration for so much of their work. Open: March-early November Mon-Sat. 10-12.30 & 2-4.30pm Mid-December-Mid January same hours. Closed Christmas Day and Boxing Day. Tel: 01736 795582.

BARBARA HEPWORTH MUSEUM

Barnoon Hill,. Tel: 01736 796226.

Sculptures in wood, stone and bronze can be seen in the late Barbara Hepworth's house, studio and sub-tropical garden where she lived and worked form 1949-75.

TATE GALLERY

Porthmeor Beach. Tel: 01736 796226.

Presents changing displays of 20th century modern art in the context of Cornwall. Displays are drawn from the Tate Gallery collection. Open: all year. Closed 24,25,26 Dec and 1st Jan.

ST KEW   THE CORNWALL DONKEY & PONY SANCTUARY

Lower Maidenland. Tel: 01208 84710.

Plenty to do. Help groom the donkeys and ponies. Play area. Adventure Swamp. Cart rides for children. Picnic by the stream. Under cover: The Eeyore Club for younger children. Bouncy Castle. Meet the baby animals. Coffee Shop and Tea Garden. Just off the A39 Wadebridge to Camelford road, 3 miles form Wadebridge. Open: daily one week before Easter-October 10-5pm. Telephone for winter opening hours.

TRESCO ABBEY GARDENS

Isles of Scilly. Tel: 01720 422849.

The garden flourishes on this small island only two miles long. Nowhere else in the British Isles does such an exotic and exciting collection of plants grow in the open. Within its 14 acres, palms shoot skywards; stately echiums resemble burning rockets. Quite wonderful to see. From its early days Tresco has welcomed visitors; the effect is so stunning that even the non-gardener annot fail to be impressed. Open: everyday of the year. 10-4pm.

TRURO ROYAL CORNWALL MUSEUM
River Street. Tel: 01872 72205.
Superb collections of Cornish history and archaeology, paintings, ceramics, silver and gold. Examine a genuine Egyptian mummy of the world famous collection of Cornish minerals. Shop and cafe. Open: Mon-Sat 10-5pm except Bank Holidays.

TREWITHEN GARDENS
Grampound Rd, Nr Truro. Tel: 01726 882763/4.
Adjoining Probus Gardens on A390. Covering some 30 acres and created in the early years of this century, the gardens are outstanding and internationally famous. Renowned for the magnificent collection of camellias, rhododendrons, magnolias and many rare trees and shrubs. Extensive woodland gardens surrounded by traditional landscaped parkland. Teas and light refreshments. Plants and shrubs for sale. The house goes back to the 17th century and has been cared for and lived in by the same family since 1715. Open: Gardens: 1st Mar-30th Sept Mon-Sat 10-4.30pm Nursery: All year Mon-Fri 9-4.3-pm House: Apr-Jul Mon and Tues only and August Bank Holiday Monday 2-4pm.

PROBUS GARDENS
Probus. Tel: 01726 882597.
A garden with a difference; a true centre of excellence. Here you can enjoy literally thousands of specimen plants and shrubs growing in superb settings - and find new ways to get more out of your garden. Whether you live in Cornwall or are visiting, a real enthusiast or an enthusiastic amateur you'll find something here to inspire you. Open: every day 1st April-30th Sept 10-5pm and Mon-Fri in the winter from 10-4pm

THE ORIGINAL CORNISH SCRUMPY CALLESTOCK CIDER FARM
Penhallow. Tel: 01872 573356.
Traditional Cider farm with a Jam Kitchen. Shire Horses and other friendly farm animals. Free samples of all their products. Signposted off the A3075 Newquay road at Penhallow. Designated as being of outstanding natural beauty and listed as being of special historical interest. Open: Easter-Dec Mon-Fri 9-6pm and Saturdays form Easter-end Oct. July/August Mon-Fri until 8pm. Sundays: shop only 12-3pm.

ZENNOR THE WAYSIDE MUSEUM
B3306 St Ives to St Just coast road. Tel: 01736 796945.
A unique private museum, founded in 1935, covering every aspect of life in Zennor from 3,000 BC to 1930s. Waterwheels, Millhouse, Wheelwrights, Blacksmiths, a Miller's cottage with kitchen and parlour etc. nearby is the famous Mermaid Chair in the village church. Open: Easter to October 31st daily from 10am plus evenings in high season.

DEVON

ASHBURTON THE RIVER DART COUNTRY PARK

Holne Park. Tel: 01364 652511.

Country fun for everyone. Adventure Playgrounds, Bathing, Piccnics, Woodland Walks, Pony Riding, Ananconda Run and more. Suitable for any age. Open: Easter to September.

ASHBURTON MUSEUM

1 West Street. Tel: 01364 63278.

Attractive small town museum displaying local artifacts and items of local history, geology and social customs. The home of the Paul Endacott North America Indian Collection. Open: Tues, Thurs, Fri & Sat. 2.30-5pm, mid-May to end of September.

BABBACOMBE THE MODEL VILLAGE

Tel: 01803 328669.

Unique reproduction of the English countryside often featured on TV. A Masterpiece of miniature landscaping. Press Button information in English and French. Illuminated every evening from dusk (Easter to October). Buses direct form Brixham, Paignton, Torquay, Teignmouth, Dawlish and Exeter. Open: every day except Christmas Day. Easter to September 9am-10pm. October 9am-9pm. November 9am to dusk.

BARNSTAPLE ARLINGTON COURT.

N.T. Tel: 01271 850296.

Houses one of the country's finest collection of carriages in the stables. Walk through peaceful woods, a haven for birdlife. See Shetland ponies and Jacob sheep in the park. The Regency House has fascinating Victorian collections of model ships, animals, exotic shells, pewter and snuff boxes, and the history of a 600 year old Devon family. Open: Mar 30th-Oct 30th daily except Sat 11-5.30pm. Dogs in park only on short leads. Refreshments and Shop.

MARWOOD HILL GARDENS

4 miles north of Barnstaple, signed from the A361 (Barnstaple-Braunton road).

Beautiful gardens with many RHS Awards for plants.

GREEN LANES SHOPPING CENTRE

- BARNSTAPLE - at the heart of the town. Excellent shopping centre. Every Wednesday afternoon there is the sound of live music. Throughout the week, the Centre plays host to a wealth of displays and exhibitions. So whether shopping, dining, or just enjoying the experience - make a day of it in Green Lane.

BIDEFORD THE BIG SHEEP

Tel: 01237 477916. 2 miles west of Bideford on the A39 North Devon link road.

Look for the big flag!

A working farm turned wacky tourist attraction. Combining traditional rural crafts, such as cheesmaking and shearing, with hilarious novelties such as sheep racing and duck trialling. An amusing programme of events throughout the day. Hours of entertainment for all ages whatever the weather. The main programmes start at 10.30am and 2pm. Phone for details. Shop and restaurant. Open: daily 10-6pm all year.

BLACKAWTON WOODLANDS LEISURE PARK

Tel: 01803 712598.

60 acres of indoor and outdoor fun for a full day of variety for the whole family. Experience 12 challenging Play-Zones for every age and ability plus great Entertainment Days. Go walk-about round the seven acre Animal park then linger by the exotic Waterfowl Collection. Take time to relax by a woodland pool; enjoy that cream tea on the Rose Terrace or a delicious meal in the cafe.Browse round the Gift Shop for that souvenir of a fantastic day out. Discount Ticket for 2 adults and 2 children. Open daily March until the beginning of November 9.30am until dusk. Winter opening at weekends and School Holidays except December 24,25 & 26.

BOVEY TRACEY THE DEVON GUILD OF CRAFTSMEN

Riverside Mill. Tel: 01626 832223.

Constantly changing series of exhibitions of the finest craftsmanship in Britain today. There is a shop where members of the Guild sell a wide range of top quality goods, and an attractive Granary Coffee Shop serving light meals including imaginative vegetarian dishes throughout the day. Open 10am-5.30pm seven days a week all year.

PARKE RARE BREEDS FARM.

N.T. Haytor Rd. Tel: 01626 832093.

Over 200 acres of parkland in the wooded valley of the River Bovey, forming a beautiful approach to Dartmoor. Lovely walks through woodlands, beside the river and along the route of the old railway track. National Trust and Dartmoor Park information centre and National Park headquarters. A private collection of rare farm animals. An interpretation centre and farm trail helps people to discover yesterday's farm and bring it to life. National Trust members must pay the admission charge. Open: parkland all year. Rare Breeds Farm, April to October daily 10-5pm.

HOUSE OF MARBLES

The Old Pottery, Pottery Rd. Tel: 01626 835358.

At the House of Marbles they have been manufacturing their unusual range of games, toys, marbles and glassware for many years. Visitors are welcome to view the old pottery buildings with their listed kilns. Watch the glass blowing work in progress and browse in the factory showroom/seconds shop. Coffee Shop/Restaurant. Museum area. Open: Shop. Mon-Sat 9-5pm. Sundays (easter-September). Glassmaking can be viewed Mon-Fri 9-5pm. Sundays and Bank Holidays 10-3pm (Easter-Sept).

BRENTOR ROWDEN GARDENS

Nr Tavistock. Tel: 01822 810275.

Rare, unsual and aquatic plant specialists. Open: 1st Apr-30th Sept. Sat, Sun and Bank Holidays 10-5pm.

BUCKFAST ABBEY

Tel: 01364 43723.

The Abbey is a living Benedictine monastery and the only fully restored medieval monastery in Britain. The church contains many internationally known works of art. Shops, refreshments, ample car park and caravan park. An audio-visual exhibition tells you about the Abbey from its foundation in AD 1018 to the present day. Church open daily. Exhibition: Easter to end October.

BUCKFAST BUTTERFLY FARM
Buckfastleigh Steam & Leisure Park. Tel: 01364 42916.

Wander through the tropical landscape garden with its ponds, waterfalls and bridges and see exotic butterflies and moths from many parts of the world - live - flying around you. An all weather educational attraction for all the family. Free parking for cars and coaches. Gift Shop. Picnic area. Open: daily Apr-1st Nov from 10-6pm.

DARTMOUTH CASTLE
Tel: 018043 3588.

Guarding the narrow entrance to the Dart estuary - one of the loveliest in England - the Castle was one of the first to be built for artillery. Dates from 15th century. It says much for the foresight of the burgesses of Dartmouth that the site of the fortress has not been bettered. Guns were mounted there in the Second World War. Open: all year round except for Dec 24/25/26 and Jan 1st. Car park. Toilets. Refreshment facilities nearby.

EXETER MARITIME MUSEUM
Tel: 01392 58075.

The World's biggest and best collection of World's Boats. This is a 'Please Touch' Museum where you go where you like, when you like. There are boats of every kind from Canoes to Coracles, Row Boats to Steamers. Super place. Free parking. Tea room. Summer Boat Hire. Open daily all year except Christmas and Boxing Day 10-5pm (6pm in summer).

GUILDHALL
High Street. Tel: 01392 265500.

Earliest reference contained in a deed of 1160. One of the oldest municipal buildings in the United Kingdom still regularly used for council meetings and civic functions. The City Silver and Regalia, and an interesting portrait of Princess Henrietta, sister to Charles II is on display. Open Tues-Sat subject to Civic requirements. Ring first.

THE CATHEDRAL
Open daily. Cathedral shop. Licensed refectory. Somewhere that deserves your time.

KINGSBRIDGE MINIATURE RAILWAY
- gives a half-mile return ride for the length of the quay alongside the estuary. The track guage is only 1 1/4 inches, yet the train is robust enough to take the whole family. The miniature railway is right by the quay car park, ideally placed for rides to keep the children amused while shopping in Kingsbridge or on the way to and from the beaches. Trains run at Easter, then daily mid-May to mid-Sept. 11-5pm weather permitting.

KINGSBRIDGE TO SALCOMBE RIVER CRUISES.
Tel: 01548 3607 or 3525.

Weekday scheduled Kingsbridge to Salcombe Ferry service, evening cruises, Sunday estuary and coastal cruises. The ferry operates from its boatyard and the quay, Kingsbridge and from Ferry pier, Salcombe. It takes about half an hour each way. The scenic beauty and maritime activity provide estuary and land views of unrivalled magnificence. Boats run daily from May to end of Sept. For details ring.

PLYMOUTH DOME.
On the Hoe overlooking Plymouth Sound. Tel: 01752 600608. Since the days of Drake, Cook and Darwin, Plymouth has been associated with adventure and discovery. Today, visitors can embark on their own adventures and discover the rich heritage and fascinating history of this great seafaring City in the award-winning Plymouth Dome. Atmospheric reconstructions and high-tech equipment take you on an extraordinary journey through time, through the sights and smell of Elizabethan Plymouth; on dramatic voyages across the world; and through the tragic devastation wrought by the Blitz on Plymouth. Full access and facilities for people with disabilities. Its a great adventure for all the family come rain or shine. Open: daily at 9am. Closed Christmas Day. Cafe. Shop.

YELVERTON BUCKLAND ABBEY
N.T. 11 miles north of Plymouth and 6 miles south of Tavistock to the west of A386 at Yelverton. Buckland's peaceful atmosphere belies its fascinating past. Once inside, the story of this 13th century monastery, which later became home to Sir Francis Drake, and his descendants, unfolds through exhibitions on monastic life, the Battle of the Armada and Drake memorabilia including his famous drum. The Tudor Great Hall features beautiful plasterwork and the Kitchen has a range of cooking utensils, open hearth and 'hams' hanging form the ceiling. Wonderful grounds. Open: 30th Mar-10th Oct daily except Thrus 10.30-5.30pm. Nov, Mar, Sat and Sun 2pm-5pm. Dogs in car park only, on leads. Licensed restaurant. Light refreshments in tea room at peak times. Shop.

DORSET

BOURNEMOUTH THE BOURNEMOUTH BEARS.
Tel: 01202 293544.
Explore the cuddly world of the teddy bear. Old bears, new bears, famous bears and designer bears. A fluffy wonderland for the young, a nostalgic journey for the not so young. Open daily all year round 9.30-5.30pm.

DORCHESTER TUTANKHAMON - THE EXHIBITION
Tel: 01305 269571.
An unforgettable experience can be had by all at Tutankhamon's Tomb and Treasures exhibition. Walk into the past to recapture the mystery and magnificence of ancient Egypt. Open daily all year round 9.30-5.30pm.

WEYMOUTH SEALIFE PARK
Tel: 01305 788255. Location: short walk from Weymouth town centre on A353 towards Wareham. Don't miss the chance to voyage to the bottom of the sea, take a wildlife trek through a tropical rain forest and brave the jaws of a giant shark in Captain Kid's World......all on the same day! In Neno's Discovery you'll experience the spine-tingling sensation of peering through the windows of a sunken wreck whilst special outdoor rock-pools provide 'hands on' encounters with a host of sturdy rockpool creatures like hermit crabs and starfish. With regular talks and feeding displays adding to the entertainment, along with a challenging quiz trail to test the fishy knowledge of young and old alike, the day is sure to be a fun-filled memorable adventure for everyone. Open from 10am seven days a week.

ESSEX

COLCHESTER ZOO
Tel: 01206 330253.
Award winning Colchester Zoo, set in 40 acres of beautiful grounds is home to 150 species of animals from around the world including Snow Leopards, Siberian Tigers, Orangutans, Elephants and breeding Chimpanzees. Children will enjoy the chance to stroke the animals in the centre's Children's Paddock and can also play among a menagerie of rescued animals and birds, open: daily from 9.30.

STANSTEAD HOUSE ON THE HILL TOY MUSEUM.
Tel: 01279 813237.
This interesting place is one of the largest toy museums in the world covering 7,000 square feet and housing a vast collection of toys, games and books from the late Victorian era, right up to the 1970s. The Museum offers a nostalgic trip back to childhood with a wealth of displays, some of them animated, there is a puppet theatre, moving Meccano fairground, military displays, space toys, books, comics, games and much, much more. Open: daily 13th Mar-13th Nov 10-4pm.

SOUTHEND ON SEA THE LYNN TAIT GALLERY
Tel: 01702 471737.
This wonderful gallery can be found in the heart of the historic old town of Leigh. In this lovely atmosphere of times gone by you can discover unusual gifts, local paintings and early local photographs from the turn of the century, all displayed on delightful arefacts from yester-year, including a magnificently restored Southend Pier Train. Open from 11am till dusk.

GLOUCESTERSHIRE

BERKELEY   BERKELEY CASTLE
off A38 Tel: 01453 810332
Perfectly preserved 800 year old castle. Keep, dungeons, staterooms, Great Hall kitchen, tapestries, furniture, silver. Ornamental gardens and Butterfly house. Open Apr-Sept Tues-Sun. October Sundays only.

BOURTON ON THE WATER   COTSWOLD MOTOR MUSEUM
Tel: 01451 21255.
30 motor vehicles and the largest collection of vintage advertising signs in Britain. Also Village Life exhibition. Open daily Feb-Nov.

BIRDLAND
Rissington Road. Tel: 01451 20689
Bird garden on the banks of the River Windrush. Penguins, waterfowl, tropical and sub tropical birds, many at liberty. Open daily all year.

BOURTON-ON-THE-WATER THE MODEL VILLAGE

Situated behind the Old New Inn, this is an incredible piece of work which delights and intrigues people of all ages from childhood upwards. The idea of building came from the late Mr C.A.Morris, landlord of the inn who in 1935 decided to turn his vegetable garden into something more decorative. It was not his intention to build a miniature model village but gradually the idea evolved and the model village was born. Every building and every feature of the landscape was built carefully to a scale of one ninth of the original and everything was erected exactly in position with the sole exception of the Church of St Lawrence, which stands at the far end of the model from the inn. One of the most fascinating aspects of the village is the miniature River Windrush, which is an artifical stream about three feet wide flowing from the working model of the mill through the whole length of the village. It is spanned by five little stone bridges, all of which are precise replicas of the famous bridges of Bourton. Now that the Model Village has been standing for some years the Cotswold stone of which all the buildings are constructed has begun to mellow. Each year it looks more and more like the original. OPEN; Summer 9-6pm. Winter 10-dusk. Not Christmas Day. Pets on leads. No access for disabled.

FOLLY FARM WATERFOWL

Off A436 near Bourton-on-the-Water. Tel: 01451 20285.
Collection of rare poultry breeds and waterfowl including endangered species, in natural Cotswold farm surroundings. Open daily all year.

CHELTENHAM CHEDWORTH ROMAN VILLA

Yarnworth. Tel: 01242 890256 Location: 10 miles south east of Cheltenham.
One of the best exposed Romano-British villas in Britain. Open March-end October Tues-Sun and Bank Holiday Monday 10-5.30pm Closed Good Friday. 2nd November -4th December: Wed-Sun 11-4pm. National Trust.

CHELTENHAM ART GALLERY & MUSEUM

Clarence Street. Tel: 01242 237431.
Important arts and crafts collection, including furniture, pottery and silver inspired by William Morris. Also local history and archaeology, rare Oriental porcelain and Dutch and British paintings. Admission free. Open all year. Mon-Sat plus Sunday afternoons in summer.

CHIPPING CAMDEN   HIDCOTE MANOR GARDENS

Hidcote Bartrim Tel: 01386 438333
Location: 4 miles east of Chipping Camden off B4632,
Internationally renowned, this memorable garden is, in reality, a series of smaller gardens. Each has its own special atmosphere and leads on to the next surprise. Open: April to end of Oct daily except Tues and Fri. 11-7pm. Closed Good Friday. Shop. Restaurant. Plant Sales Centre. National Trust.

RIFTSGATE COURT GARDENS

Tel: 01386 438777.
A magnificently situated house with fine views and trees. The garden, created over three generations, has many unusual shrubs and a good collection of old fashioned and specie roses including RosaFilipes Kiftsgate, the largest rose in England. Open: Wed, Thurs and Sun 2-6pm. Also Bank Holiday Mondays and Saturdays in June and July 2-6pm. 1st April-30th Sept.

COTSWOLD WATER PARK
Tel: 01285 861459.
The park lies to the south of Cirencester and offers exciting and varied activities based on a network of lakes formed as a result of 60 years gravel extraction. In addition to the variety of water-based activities including angling, windsurfing, sailing, water, skiing and power boat racing, there are lakeside walks and picnic sites provided at two country Parks. The area is recognised as being nationally important for nature conservation. A number of public and private nature reserves provide an opportunity to study the enormous variety of its wetland flora and fauna. Open all the year. Facilities for the disabled.

BARNSLEY HOUSE GARDEN
The Close Tel: 01285 740281
Spring bulbs, autumn colours. Mixed borders, climbing and wall shrubs. Knot garden, herb garden, laburnum walk (early June). Decorative vegetable potage. 18th century summer houses. House (not open) 1697. Interesting plants for sale. Carpark. Pub lunches available in Barnsley at the village pub.

GLOUCESTER   GLOUCESTER CITY MUSEUM
Brunswick Road Tel: 01452 524131 Famous Iron Age mirror, Roman sculptures and mosaics. Also Georgian silver, barometers, furniture and exhibitions. Admission free. Open Mon-Sat & Bank Holiday Mondays all year.

HOUSE OF THE TAILOR OF GLOUCESTER
9 College Court. Tel: 01452 422856.
The building chosen by Beatrix Potter to illustrate her famous story. Now a gift shop and exhibition. Admission free. Open Mon-Sat all year.

NATURE IN ART
On A38 2 miles north of Gloucester. Tel: 01452 713422.
Unique collection of wildlife art from all parts of the world and all periods. Specially commended in National Heritage Museum of the year awards. Nature gardens and outdoor sculptures. Full programme of artists in residence. Open Tues-Sun and Bank Holidays all year.

REGIMENTS OF GLOUCESTERSHIRE MUSEUM
The Docks, Tel: 01452 522682
Museum of the Year Award for the Best Small Museum 1991. New displays tell the story of Gloucestershire's soldiers in peace and war. Gift shop. Open Tues-Sun & Bank Holidays all year.

GLOUCESTER ANTIQUES CENTRE
Severn Road, Gloucester Docks Tel: 01452 529716
Collections of all kinds of antiques taking up four floors of a magnificent restored warehouse. Admission free. Open daily all year.

NEWENT   THE NATIONAL BIRDS OF PREY CENTRE
Tel: 10531 820286.
A full day out for the family is offered plus the chance to experience Birds of Prey at close quarters. The Daily Flying Demonstrations are undoubtedly the highlight of the day but there is

so much more to see and do. Coffee-shop. Book and Gift Shop. Children's Play Area and Picnic sites. No pets. Free parking. Open: 7 days a week 10.30-5.30pm Closed December-January. Facilities for the disabled.

THREE CHOIRS VINEYARD

Welsh House Lane. Tel: 01531 890555
Production of English Wine reviving the ancient tradition of Gloucestershire wine making. Admission free (Charge for tours) Open daily all year.

NEWENT BUTTERFLY & NATURAL WORLD CENTRE

Birches Lane off B4215 Tel: 01531 821800
Tropical Butterfly house, Nature Exhibition, Menagerie and Water Life. Spiders, snakes, rabbits, guinea pigs, rare breed fowl, waterfowl, pheasants, peacocks, parakeets and other small birds. Open daily Easter-October.

LYDNEY   DEAN FOREST RAILWAY

Norchard Steam Centre B4234 Nr. Lydney. Tel: 01594 843423.
Full size railway engines, coaches and wagons. Admission free to site. Open daily all year. Admission charge for steam rides (certain days throughout the year).

PAINSWICK   PAINSWICK ROCOCO GARDEN

The Stables, Painswick House. Tel: 01452 813204
18th century, 6 acre Rococo garden with garden buildings. Vistas and woodland paths. Open Feb-mid Dec. Wed- Sun.

PRINKNASH ABBEY

Nr. Painswick. On A46. Tel: 01452 812455.
Benedictine Abbey with world famous pottery worked by local craftsmen. Adjoined by Bird Park. Open daily all year.

SLIMBRIDGE   THE WILDFOWL AND WETLANDS TRUST

Off A38 Tel: 01453 890065.
World's largest collection of wildfowl in 73 acres of grounds. Tropical house. Permanent exhibition. Open all year. Closed Dec 24th & 25th.

STANWAY   STANWAY HOUSE

Near Cheltenham. Tel: 01386 73469
The jewel of Cotswold manor houses is very much a home rather than a museum. The mellow Jacobean architecture, the typical squire's family portraits, the exquisite Gate House, the old Brewery and medieval Tithe Barn, the extensive pleasure grounds and formal landscape contribute to the timeless charm of what Arthur Negus considered one of the most beautiful and romantic manor houses in England. Open: June, July, August Tuesdays and Thursdays 2-5pm.

WESTBURY

Tel: 01452 760461 Location: 9 miles south west of Gloucester on A48.
Laid out between 1696 and 1705, this formal Dutch water garden is a rare survival of its type in England. Historical varieties of apple, pear, plum, along with many other species of plants

introduced to England before 1700, make this a fascinating study for any gardener. Open: April-end October: Wed to Sun and Bank Holiday Monday 11-6pm. Closed Good Friday. National Trust.

WINCHCOMBE   HAILES ABBEY

Tel: 01242 602398 Location: 10 miles north east of Cheltenham off B4632. Picturesque ruins of great Cistercian Abbey and centre of pilgrimage. English Heritage. Open: April 1st- end September daily 10-6pm. Oct-March Tues-Sun 10am-4pm. Closed 24-26 December and New Year Bank Holiday. Museum may be closed on certain days from October-end of March for staffing reasons. Ring first.

SUDELEY CASTLE AND GARDENS

Tel: 01242 602308.
Once the residence of Queen Katherine Parr, Sudeley is now the charming home of Lord and Lady Ashcombe. Sudeley houses many fine antiques, civil war relics and old-master paintings. The gardens with the Queen's garden as their centrepiece, are quite magnificent and are complemented by 'Sudeley Castle Roses' a specialist plant centre. Also available: craft workshops, adventure playground, castle shop, licensed restaurant. Calendar of special events throughout the year. OPEN: Apr 1st-31st October. Grounds 11am-5.30pm. Castle apartments 12 noon - 5pm. Sudeley Castle Roses; 10am-5.30pm. Free parking for cars and coaches.

GLOUCESTERSHIRE - WARWICKSHIRE RAILWAY

Toddington, at intersection of B4632/A438. Tel: 01242 621405.
Restored GWR Station. Mainline steam rides. 8 miles round trip. Large rail complex, rolling stock under restoration. Admission free to site. Open daily. Admission charge for steam rides (Easter-October Sat, Sun & Bank Holidays) Open all year.

HAMPSHIRE

ANDOVER   THE HAWK CONSERVANCY.

4 miles west of Andover just off the A303 Tel: 01264 772252.
This is the largest and most comprehensive collection of Birds of Prey in Southern Englsnd. You can see and photograph Birds of Prey from all over the world, these include Hawks, Falcons, Eagles, Owls, Vultures and Kites. The Flying Demonstrations could be the highlight of your visit. These take place at 12 noon, 2-3pm & 4pm. (Weather permitting, as flying is not possible on wet days). Open: 1st March to last Sunday in October. 10.30-5pm spring and autumn. 10.30-5pm summer. Refreshments available. Children are not permitted unless accompanied by an adult. No dogs or pets allowed.

BEULIEU   THE NATIONAL MOTOR MUSEUM.

Tel: 01590 612123.
One of the world's most famous attractions. Inclusive admission covers The National Motor Museum, a superb exhibition of over 250 historic vehicles dating from 1895 to the present day and including Donald Campbell's 'Bluebird'. 'Wheels' an amazing journey throughout the history of motoring. Palace House, the ancestral home of the Montagu family since 1538 and former Gatehouse to Beaulieu Abbey, founded in 1204 by Cistercian monks, it lies mainly in

ruins today. It is a fantastic and thrilling outing. Open: Every day except Christmas Day. Easter to September 10-6pm. October- Easter 10-5pm.

ROMSEY BROADLANDS
located on the A31 at Romsey. Tel: 01794 516878.

Famous as the home of Lord Mountbatten. Braodlands is an elegant Palladian mansion in a beautiful landscaped setting on the banks of the River Test. Visitors may view the house with its art treasures and mementoes of the famous, enjoy the superb views from the Riverside lawns or relive Lord Mountbatten's life and times in the Mountbatten Exhibition and spectacular Mountbatten A-V Presentation. Open: Easter to last Sunday in September, 12 noon-5.30pm. Closed Fridays except Good Friday and in August. Self service tearoom. Gift shop. Free parking.

SOUTHHAMPTON EXBURY GARDENS
(Beaulieu 3 miles). Tel: 01703 891203.

These 200 acres landscaped woodland gardens include an outstanding collection of Rhododendrons, Azaleas, Camellias and Magnolias. In addition to many other notable trees and shrubs they feature a Rock Garden, Heather Gardens, Daffoldil Meadow, Iris Garden, Ponds, cascades and unlimited walks. Lunches and cream teas. Free parking. Plant Centre. Gift shop. Open: March to October 10-5.30pm.

SOUTHAMPTON HALL OF AVIATION
Albert Road South. Tel: 01703 635830.

The official and the Supermarine Company. The museum dipicts the story of some 26 aircraft companies, the legendary Spitfire and the history of the biggest flying boat operation in the world. Fascinating. Open: 10-5pm Tues-Sat. 12 noon-5pm Sundays. Open 10-5pm Mondays during School Holidays.

WINCHESTER CITY MILL
foot of High Street beside City Bridge. Tel: 01962 870057.

Positioned over River Itchen the mill was rebuilt in 1744 using materials dating back to the 15th century. There is a delightful island garden and an impressive millrace. Open: 1st April to end Sept daily 11-4.45pm. Open Sat and Sun in October 12 noon-4pm. Shop open April-31 Dec daily 10-5pm.

HEREFORD AND WORCESTERSHIRE

DROITWICH HANBURY HALL
Tel: 01527 821214

Location: Off M5 Junction 5 to Droitwich, 4 miles east of Droitwich off B4090.

William and Mary style brick house, notable for the famous Thornhill staircase. Fine collection of porcelain. Re-creation of formal 18th century garden. Open: Easter to end October; Sat, Sun and Mon 2-6pm. Closed Good Friday. Aug: also open Tues and Wed 2-6pm. Shop, Tearoom, National Trust.

HEREFORD CITY MUSEUM & ART GALLERY

Broad Street.

Full of interest. Open: Tues, Wed, Fri 10am-6pm. Thurs & Sat 10-5pm 10-4pm in winter. Sunday May-September 10-4pm. Open Bank Holiday Mondays.

LEDBURY EASTNOR CASTLE

Tel: 01531 633160.

Splendid Georgian Castle in fairytale setting with Deer Park, lake and arboretum. Inside this family home tapestries, fine art, armour and furniture from the Italianate and Gothic in richly decorated interiors, many recently restored to critical acclaim. Home-made cream teas and ice cream. Open Sundays Easter to end September, Bank Holiday Mondays. Sunday to Friday during August 12 noon-5pm.

LEOMINSTER BERRINGTON HALL

Nr. Leominster. Tel: 01586 780246. Location: 3 miles north of Leominster. Signposted off A49. A classical elegant 18th century mansion by Henry Holland, set in a gracefully landscaped park by 'Capability' Brown. Park walk open July to end October only. Open Easter to end September; Wed-Sun (open Bank Holiday Mon. closed Good Friday) 1.30-5.30pm. October Wed-Sun 1.30-4.30. Grounds open from 12.30pm. Shop. Licensed restaurant. Dogs on leads in car park only. National Trust.

CROFT CASTLE

Tel: 01586 780246 Location : 5 miles north west of Leominster. Signposted off A49 and A4110. Just 5 miles from Berrington Hall, this Marcher Castle has been the home of the Croft family since Domesday (with a short break of 170 years). Ancient walls and castellated turrets house an interior shown as it was in the 18th century with fine ceilings and Gothic staircase. The surrounding parkland is open all year. Open: Easter Sat, Sun & Mon 2-6pm. Closed Good Friday. April and October Sat & Sun 2-5pm. May to end Sept: Wed-Sun and Bank Holiday Monday 2-6pm. National Trust.

BRINGSTY   LOWER BROCKHAMPTON

Tel: 01885 488099 Location: 2 miles east of Bromyard on A44.

A 14th century half timbered moated farmhouse with a very unusual gatehouse. Only the medieval hall and parlour are shown. Open: House; April-end September; Wed-Sun and Bank Holiday Monday. 10-5pm. Closed Good Friday. Oct: Wed-Sun 10am-4pm. Estate open all year.

ROSS-ON-WYE   THE BUTTON MUSEUM

Kyrle Street. Tel: 01989 566089

Unique award winnng Museum of Dress and Uniform Buttons, worn by ladies and gentlemen over the last two hundred years. Museum shop. Open 7 days a week 1st April-31st October 10-5pm.

SWAINSHILL   THE WEIR

Location: 5 miles west of Hereford on A438. Fine views of the River Wye and the Welsh Hills from a steep bankstudded with trees, shrubs and plants. Beautiful, particularly in springtime, with drifts of flowering bulbs. Open: Mid-February to end October; Wed to Sun (including Good Friday) and Bank Holiday Monday 11am-6pm. National Trust.

TENBURY WELLS -BURFORD HOUSE GARDENS Tel: 01584 810777 Fax: 01584 810673. Burford House is an early Georgian House built on the ancient site of Scrob's Castle, at the confluence of the River Teme and Ledwych Brook. It was acquired by the late John Treasure in 1954 as the ideal setting for his new garden. Since then and until his death in 1993 John Treasure transformed the grounds of this austere Georgian red brick house from a scattering of a few good trees and an elegant summerhouse into an eloquently defined twentieth century garden. Contrasting its spare symmetry on the north front with curving vistas and beds on its south side, he elegantly described the setting of the house in the fertile alluvial loam of the River Teme which weaves around the garden. As an architect by training he brought that all too rare combination of the positive discipline of design to a passion for plants and the result is a garden of quiet serenity and fascination.

John Treasure's high standards of discipline are revealed in the crisply edged and well groomed beds. This is a plantsman's garden, laid out to display myriads of forms and species in ordered frameworks. There are special combinations and ideas which gardeners of all kinds will be inspired to study and copy. Harmonising combinations of colour have been brilliantly achieved throughout the garden, and especial use made of clematis, a favourite of John Treasure. The garden now boasts over 150 varieties and is home to the National Collection.

There are so many kinds of plants to be seen especially those that grow on neutral to limey soils, and many marginal plants that grow along the stream gardens. Of the genera that are well represented there are, Hosta, Hydrangea, Philadelphus, grasses, hellebores, shrub roses, penstemons, birches, irises, astilbes, agapanthus, daylilies and hosts of bulbs and rarities, all grouped beautifully and new ideas and plants are finding homes here in this dynamic and graceful garden.

Many of the unusual plants in the garden can be found in Treasures Plant Centre adjacent, who specialise in clematis, herbaceous, shrubs, trees and climbers. There is a Gallery open in the House and a new Craft Shop in the grounds. The Burford Buttery serves hot and cold meals together with home-made cakes, tea and continental coffee throughout the day. Coach parties are welcome and The Buttery is happy to cater for special occasions. OPEN: Monday-Sunday 10am-6pm (Dusk if earlier).

WELLINGTON QUEENSWOOD GARDEN CENTRE

Wellington HR4 8BB Tel: 01432 830880. Fax: 01432 830833.

The Milne Family - Tony, Frank,Kathleen, Eric and Alexi own and operate this attractive garden centre which is far more than somewhere one comes just to buy plants. It is an outing that is thoroughly enjoyable and one from which you can gain gardening advice from an expert and helpful staff. The plants are second to none. The company offers all its customers a unique plant and gardening equipment ' finder service'. If they do not have a product in stock they will make every attempt to source it for their customers to collect or have sent to them by post. To help gardeners and those interested in horticulture a joint venture with Pershore College of Horticulture has been set up resulting in Pershore setting up a lecture hall at Queenswood and offering courses/qualifications to local people. All of this demonstrates how dedicated the Milne family and their staff are to the centre. A large pet shop on the site offering small domestic pets such as rabbits and guinea pigs and a huge selection of tropical and cold water fish attracts many people. Here too advice is top notch from PTIA trained staff. The Tea House is a favourite place for customers. Not only does it serve excellent tea but lunches and evening meals are available including cakes and specialities made on the premises. OPEN; Mon-Sat 1st April-30th June & 1st Dec-23rd Dec. 9am-8pm. 27th Dec-31st March & 1st July -30th Nov 9am-6pm. Sundays.

Teahouse & Outdoor Plant Area 9am-5pm. Main Building and Pet Shop 11am-5pm. Easy parking
- 500 spaces. Coaches welcome.

WORCESTER THE GREYFRIARS

Friar Street. Tel: 01905 23571
Still surviving in the heart of Worcester, this medieval timber-framed house has been carefully
restored. Delightful walled garden. Open: April-end October. Wed, Thurs and Bank Holiday
Monday 2-5.30pm. National Trust.

HERTFORDSHIRE

BROXBOURNE PARADISE WILDLIFE PARK

White Stubbs Lane, Broxbourne EN10 7QA   Tel: 01992 468001.
Paradise Wildlife Park is unique! As Britain's most interactive Wildlife Park it is an ideal place
to touch, feed and meet many animals - both domestic and exotic. You can learn a great deal
during the 'meet the animals' session where experienced keepers impart information about the
wonderful creatures and answer visitors questions. The 'Meet the Animals' experience includes:
foxes, birds of prey, reptiles, chinchilla, camels, llamas and zebras. There are many other daily
events including Dr Do and Dr Little amazing animal facts show, the Sweetie man, the feeding
of the lions and tigers and lion and tiger cub talks. The friendly family run Park is very compact
and is set in the wonderful backdrop of Broxbourne woods. Other attractions on the site comprise
a Woodland Railway, Crazy Golf, Children's rides and Tractor Trailer rides for which there is a
fee of 50p per ride. FREE facilities include 3 superb adventure playgrounds, Fantasy Land,
Adventureland and Fun Land plus a woodland walk. There is a wide range of catering from
Mannings Snack Cabin, The Pembridge Cafeteria to a Barbecue and Bar area and The Pembridge
Restaurant. There are also ample picnic areas spread across the park. Paradise Wildlife Park also
offers the public the chance to meet their lion or tiger cubs. This is literally the opportunity of a
lifetime and is available outside the normal opening hours of the park. The money raised goes to
Project Life Lion, a registered charity which help to save African lions in the Serengeti from
Canine Distemper. The sessions last up to 30 minutes and are for a group of up to 4 people.
Priced at forty pounds a session - numbers are strictly limited. For further details or to book ring
01992 470490. The Park is located 6 miles from Junction 25 off the M25. Brown and White
tourist signs direct you to the Park from the A10 at the Broxbourne/Turnford Junction. Admission
prices are as at January 1996 £4.50adults, £4.00 senior citizens and £3.50 children (3-15). Opening
times are 10am-6pm (Summer) and 10am-dusk (Winter). Paradise Wildlife opens every day of
the year. Information line 01992 468001. Paradise Wildlife Park is a truly wonderful place with
something for everyone - whatever your age!

HATFIELD   MILL GREEN MUSEUM

Tel: 01707 271362.
This local museum is housed in what was for centuries the home of the millers who worked in
the adjoining water mill. Mill Green Museum has two permanent galleries where local items
from Roman times to the present day are on show - everything from pottery and craft tools to
underwear and school certificates. Open throughout the year Tues-Fri 10-5pm and Sat,Sun and
Bank Holidays 2-5pm Admission free.

HATFIELD HOUSE

Tel: 01707 262823.

Location: 21 miles north of London on the Great North Road (A1), seven miles from M25.

This celebrated Jacobean house, which stands in its own great park, was built between 1607 and 1611 by Robert Cecil, the first Earlof Salisbury and Chief Minister to King James I. It has been the family home of the Cecils ever since. The State Rooms are rich in world famous paintings, fine furniture, rare tapestries and historic armour. The beautiful stained glass in the chapel is original. Within the delightful gardens stands the surviving wing of the Royal Palace of Hatfield (1497) where Elizabeth I spent much of her childhood. Open 25th Mar-9th October weekdays from 12 4pm, Sun 1.30-5pm.

HATFIELD GARDEN

Tel: 01707 262823

Connected to Hatfield House, the West Gardens date back to the late 15th century when the Palace of Hatfield was built. Keeping in line with the manner of the garden of the 17th century, the garden has been planted with a great variety of sweet smelling flowers, bulbs, trees and shrubs for every season of the year. Although the West Garden is planted with mainly herbaceous plants, roses, irises and peonies, with a considerable number of rare and unusual plants. The West Gardens are open daily except Good Friday 11-6pm.

THE OLD PALACE, HATFIELD PARK

Tel: 01707 262055 Location: 31 miles north of London AI (M) junction 4.

Take an exciting trip back to Elizabethan times by visiting The Old Palace for an authentic Banquet. Set in the Great Hall people enjoy a magnificent five course meal of royal proportions including red or white wine and mead. From the moment you take your seat you are under the spell of a troop of costumed minstrels and players. Singing songs from the period, performing some of the picturesque ceremonies and customs of the Elizabethan era, they move from table to table serenading you as you dine. The authentic setting, the cuisine, the atmosphere and spectacle combine to make this not just a feast of entertainment but an unforgettable experience too. The Banquets are held every Tues, Thurs, Fri and Sat evenings.

KNEBWORTH   KNEBWORTH HOUSE & GARDENS

Tel: 01438 812661 Location: entrance direct from Junction 7 of the AI (M) at Stevenage.

Hours of fun can be had by all the family at the historic home of the Lytton family since 1490. The house contains many beautiful rooms, and magnificent paintings, fine furniture and objects d'art. As well as a visit to the historic house children can enjoy hours of fun at the giant Adventure Playground which includes a fort, suspension slide, bouncy castle and miniature railway, or a trip around the 250 acres of Parkland to see the herds of Red and Sika deer. Open daily 26th March-17th April and 28thy May-4th September. 11-5.30pm.

ROYSTON   WILLERS MILL WILD ANIMAL SANCTUARY

Tel: 01763 262226

Moulded out of a wilderness of nettles, rubbish, and an old deserted cottage, between the railway line and the village cricket pitch of Shepreth, Terry and Gill Willers have created a wonderful setting for their animal sanctuary. Here between a duck pond and in a totally enclosed environment, young children are able to come into direct contact with a variety of animals, often for the first time, and are able to touch and handle all species, much to their obvious enjoyment. It is a place for unwanted or injured animals to live in safety and to be well cared for, just as homes exist for unwanted cats and dogs. The animals come from a variety of sources, such as road, gun and gassing casualties, unwanted pets, research centres, zoos, safari parks and meat markets. Some even arrive by themselves! The majority of the animals have the run of the sanctuary and can indeed leave at any time if they wish to. However, some have to be kept in enclosures for their own protection as their injuries prevent them from leading a normal life. The more exotic species require special diets and a heated environment to keep them healthy. Willers Wildlife Park receives no form of government grant or other help. Entrance fees are its sole source of revenue so please do go and visit. OPEN; Summer 10am-6pm every day. Winter: 1st Nov-28th Feb 10-5pm every day. Closed Christmas Day.

STEVENAGE   STEVENAGE MUSEUM
Tel: 01438 354292.
When you step inside you enter another world. Fascinating collections of everyday objects tell the story of Stevenage from pre-history to the present. There are hundreds of objects for you to see including a 1950s living room, a perfect 1930s dolls house, gas masks, old farm tools and a Roman silver coin hoard. Open Mon-Sat 10-5pm. Free admission.

WELWYN GARDEN CITY   PANSHANGER GOLF COMPLEX
Tel: 01707 333350.
Set in some of Hertfordshire's most delightful countryside this offers one of the most popular 'Pay as you Play' courses in the country. The Herts Golf Academy offers men, women and children of all ages the opportunity to learn to play golf or improve their skills. The golf course offers a scenic and challenging eighteen hole par 72 golf course, nine hole pitch and putt, putting green and cafe open from 9am providing excellent refreshments. Open daily.

WHITEWELL   WATERHALL FARM & CRAFT CENTRE
Tel: 01438 871256.
Open all year round this farm and craft centre offers adults and children the opportunity to take a step back to nature to see how many farm animals live today. A wide range of quality gifts and souvenirs is always available from the craft shop including antiques, bric-a-brac and pine furniture. A visit can also be made to the tea-room which serves a selection of light lunches, delicious cream teas and home-made cakes. Open Wed-Sun 10-5pm March-October and all Bank Holidays.

SCUNTHORPE   ELSHAM HALL COUNTRY PARK
Tel: 01652 688698.
Elsham Country Park was opened in 1970 by Captain and Mrs Elwes because they wanted visitors to enjoy the Park and appreciate wildlife, Rural Crafts and Arts. The award-winning facilities now include the Granary Restaurant and Tea-Rooms, the 'Haybarn Centre', the new Garden Centre; Monk's Wood Arboretun; Children's Animal Farm and Pets Corner. There are also many special events and Arts Exhibitions throughout the year. Why not take a look for yourself. Open Easter Sat- mid Sept 11-5pm and mid-Sept-Easter Sun 11-4pm. Closed Good Friday and Winter Bank Holidays.

LEICESTERSHIRE

CASTLE DONNINGTON   AEROPARK AND VISITOR CENTRE
Tel: 01332 810621

See the action from this 12 acre park next to the taxiway at the eastern end of the airport. Aircraft exhibitions in the Aeropark include a Lightning jet fighter, Vulcan bomber, Canberra bomber, Argosy freighter and Whirlwind helicopter. There is also a viewing mound, themed children's play area and picnic tables. Open Easter-October Mon-Fri 10-5pm Sat 11-4pm Sun 11-6pm.

COALVILLE   SNIBSTON DISCOVERY PARK
Tel: 01530 510851

Built on the 100 acre site of a former colliery, Snibston Discovery Park is Leicestershire's largest attraction where finding out is a great day out for everyone. The Exhibition Hall contains five galleries exploring the Industrial Heritage of Leicestershire including transport, engineering, extractive industries, textiles and fashion. Follow fashion through the ages, travel through time from 1600 until the present day or see what it was like for a miner in the mid 19th century. Open daily all year round from 10-6pm.

HINCKLEY   ASHBY CANAL
Tel: 01455 232789

The Ashby-de-la-Zouch Canal was a relative latecomer being completed in 1804 but had many of the attributes of the earliest navigations. It follows the contours of surrounding countryside and has no locks throughout its lengths. The Canal is home to a wonderful variety of creatures and plants, including ducks, fish, dragonflies, waterlilies, kingfisher and many more. Open daily it is a great escape from the hustle and bustle of everyday life.

THE GUILDHALL
Tel: 01533 532569

The Guildhall is within five minutes walk of the City Centre. From the Clock Tower, turn into East Gate, and turn left onto Silver St. The Guildhall is on Guildhall Lane, the continuation of Silver St. It is a unique Grade I listed building and has been the scene of many significant events in Leicester's history. The Building comprises the following rooms: THE GREAT HALL: The timber framed Great Hall is the original Guildhall of the Gild of Corpus Christi dating back to c1390 and evokes a wonderful sense of space and time. As well as direct promotions, the Hall, outside museum hours, is available for public hire. THE MAYOR'S PARLOUR; The ground floor of the West Wing c1490 contains the Mayor's Parlour, a smaller civic room, remodelled in 1563. The room is oak panelled with a beautifully carved and painted overmantle above the fireplace.
THE JURY ROOM; The west wing also contains The Jury Room, above the Mayor's Parlour and was originally the retiring room for the Jury after Quarter Sessions. It now houses the Library of the Leicestershire Archeological and Historical Society founded in 1855. The room is available as a study and meeting room and seats 30 people. THE LIBRARY; The upper floor of the East Wing houses the Town Library. The Library is the third oldest public library in the country and was established in 1632. THE POLICE STATION; Leicester's first police force was established in 1836 and is the third oldest in Great Britain. The Borough Police Force was based at the Guildhall, and originally had 3 cells. The Cells have 2 replica criminals based on real criminals

of the Victorian period. THE RECORDER'S BEDROOM; The office of Recorder was established in 1464 and the Recorder was required to visit the borough at least 4 times a year to preside over the Quarter Sessions. A bedroom was granted to the Recorder and it's fitting out is recorded in the Chamberlain's records for 1581-82. THE CONSTABLE'S HOUSE: The brick built house off the side of the courtyard was built in 1836 for Leicester's first Chief Constable and is now the administrative base of the Guildhall and will shortly be converted into a new exhibition hall. GUIDED TOURS; Available on request. PUBLIC HIRE; Available for both community and commercial hire. PERFORMANCES AND CONCERTS; Magical atmosphere with its audience capacity of 100 people. SPECIAL EVENTS;Throughout the year. OPEN; Mon-Sat: 10am-5.30pm Sundays:2-5.30pm. Admission Free.

THE CATHEDRAL
Tel: 01533 625294
The Church of St Martin's was one of six parish churches recorded in Leicester in 1086. Extended in the 14th and 15th centuries and restored in the 19th century it was hallowed as the Cathedral of Leicester in 1927. Visitors are invited to tour the building and see its impressive roof, stained glass windows and stone and wood carvings. Inside the chancel is a memorial to King Richard III. Outside the graveyard has been laid out as a garden containing many interesting slate headstones. Open every day.

CASTLE GARDENS & CASTLE MOTTE
This used to be a low-flying marshy area of reeds and willows. At the end of the 19th century the land was drained and used for allotments before being opened as public gardens in 1926. The Motte is a man-made mound built by Leicester's first Norman Lord in about 1070. It may originally have been several metres higher and would have had timber fortification on the top. The Motte is open to the public and in the gardens is the statue of Richard III which commemorates his links with Leicestershire. Garden open daily during daylight hours.

RIVERSIDE PARK
This eight mile stretch of footpaths along the banks of the River Soar and Grand Union Canal passes through Castle Park and allows an insight into Leicester's early industrial history. The dominant Pex Building was originally a worsted spinning factory providing yarn for the knitting trade. Goods were brought to and from the City by the major waterway network. Flood alleviation work to the river in the late 19th century formed the 'Mile straight' on which rowing regattas are held annually. The line of the Great Central Railway has now been developed as a pedestrian walk and cycleway.

FARMWORL
Stoughton Farm Park, Gartree Road, Leicester LE22FB. Tel:01162 710355
This is an exciting day out for every age group. You will find it 3 miles SE of Leicester City Centre and 6 miles off the M1/M69 Junction 21. Follow the southerly ring road. Signposted 'Farm Park' from A6 and A47. It is a real working Dairy Farm with acres of Parkland for pleasure and play. There are Shire horses and cart rides, rare farm animals, lakeside and woodland walks, a picnic area, Toy Tractor park and indoor sandpit. A special Children's Farmyard and Playground. You are invited to the Milking Parlour to watch the herd being milked and to try your hand at operating a milking machine. The Craft workshops are fascinating and quite frequently there are demonstrations. Add to this lots of lovable pets, an EdwardianAle House, Audio Visual Theatre and Exhibitions and

displays featuring the countryside at work and it becomes very clear why Farmworld is so popular. In keeping with Leicester's innovative and go ahead thinking, Farmworld also offers a unique Conference venue. It is housed in beautifully restored and converted 18th century farm buildings and equipped with a wide range of modern facilities to provide for every business requirement. For further details please ring 01162 710355 or Fax: 01162 713211 FARMWORLD IS OPEN; Daily 10am-5.30pm (Winter 5pm) except December 25th &26th and January 1st. Dogs cannot be admitted. (Except Guide dogs) Disabled access. Gift Shop. Wheatsheaf Cafe.

MARKET BOSWORTH TWYCROSS ZOO
Tel: 01827 880250
This is an ideal day out. There is a wide variety of animals including gorillas, chimps, orangutans, gibbons, elephants, lions and giraffes. There is also an adventure playground, pets corner and penguin pool. Open daily from 10-6pm all the year round.

OAKHAM   RUTLAND FARM PARK
Tel: 01572 756789
In 18 acres of beautiful parkland Rutland Park Farm has a wonderful selection of farm animals, goats, poultry and wildfowl for the whole family to see. Apart from visiting the animals and old farm vehicles why not stroll through the countryside and look at the fern, bamboo and wildflower meadow. Open 3rd April-18th Sept 10-5pm.

RUTLAND WATER ANGLIAN WATER BIRD WATCHING CENTRE AND RUTLAND WATER NATURE RESERVE.
Egleton, Oakham, Rutland, Leicestershire LE15 8BT Tel: 01572 770651
Rutland Water has become one of the most importnt wildfowl sanctuaries in Great Britain, regularly holding in excess of 10,000 waterfowl of up to 28 species. It is a Site of Special Scientific Interest and has received recognition of its international importance by the European Community and has been designated as a globally important wetland. It covers an area of 450 acres and the wide variety of habitats ensures that many species of birds are present throughout the year, but the reserve is best known for the thousands of wildfowl which flock to spend the winter on the lagoons and open water. Gadwall shoveler, teal, tufted duck, pochard and shelduck are present all year round; in winter they are joined by pintail, goldeneye, goosander, wigeon and other, rarer ducks, such as smew, red-breasted merganser and long-tailed duck. Rare grebes and divers are frequent visitors. In summer common terns and cormorants breed communally on the lagoons. During spring passage, little gulls, Arctic terns and black terns pass through, often in their hundreds, while rare Caspian and white-winged black terns have been recorded. Wader passage may bring up to 19 species in a single day. Birds of prey include breeding kestrel and sparrowhawk; osprey and harriers during migration; regular sightings of peregrine and merlin in winter; and spectaculr views of hobbies in summer as they feed on insects over the lagoons. Three lagoons and 9 miles of shore and open water are overlooked by a total of 17 hides. Other attractive wildlife habitats contain species rare elsewhere; wildflowers, butterflies and dragon flies. Old hay meadows, rough grassland, hedges, plantations and woodland invite wildlife and visitor alike. On both reserves, trails lead to the hides through all these habitats. Car parking is provided free to reserve visitors at Egleton and Lyndon. There are toilets in bothreserves. Disabled facilities at Egleton. Dogs not allowed at Egleton. At Lyndon they must be on a lead. Disabled visitors access is available at Egleton at the Anglian Birdwatching Centre and Shoveler hide and at Lyndon Centre using Teal and Swan hides.

LINCOLNSHIRE

GRANTHAM   BELVOIR CASTLE
Tel: 01476 870262 Location: Near Grantham signposted off A607.
Home of the Duke and Duchess of Rutland, Belvoir Castle is superbly situated overlooking the Vale of Belvoir. The house has magnificent staterooms, containing notable pictures, tapestries and fine furniture. The Queen's Royal Lancers Museum is also situated within the Castle. Open April 1st -29th Sept. Tue, Thurs, Sat, Sun & Bank Holidays 11-5pm.

LINCOLN LINCOLN CATHEDRAL
- is one of the largest in England and has many attractive features including the magnificent open nave, St Hugh's Choir, the Angel Choir and beautiful stained glass windows including the 14th century 'Bishop's Eye'. The Chapter House Cloisters, Wren Library and Treasury are other interesting features and all visitors are invited to seek out the Lincoln importance... Services are held daily and there are generally guided tours and tower tours.

LINCOLN CASTLE
- is on the site of the original Roman fortress and the present castle dates back to 1068. Interesting architectural features include the keep known as the Lucy Tower, Cobb Hall which was the site of the public gallows, and the Observastory tower which offers tremendous views of the cathedral and city as a whole. The Victorian prison includes a unique prison chapel with separate pews like upright coffins. This building also houses an original version of the famous Magna Carta from 1215, and an exhibition interpreting the history of this document and its importance to modern freedoms and democracy. Guided tours and wall walks are available.

MIDDLESEX

EPPING LEE VALLEY PARK.
Tel: 01992 700766. Location: along M25 from Potters Bar.
The Lee Valley is Britain's first regional park devoted entirely for the enjoyment of leisure and recreation and the conservation of countryside and natural environment. Only a walk or boat trip away is splendid countryside, a Wildlife Oasis and Sporting Paradise along with the fascinating history and secrets of the Lee Valley industrial heritage. Admission free. Open throughout the year.

NORFOLK

AYLSHAM BLICKLING HALL & GARDEN
One and a half miles west of Aylsham on the B1354, signposted off the A140 Cromer Road. Tel: 01263 733084.
One of the most spectacular Country Houses in East Anglia. 17th century red brick house, extensive colourful garden, surrounded by wonderful parkland and woodland. National Trust. Open: Easter to end October Tues/Wed/Fri/Sat/Sun & Bank Holiday Mondays 1-5pm. Closed Good Friday. Garden same as Hall and also open daily in July and August.

BURE VALLEY RAILWAY

Tel: 01263 733858.

Travel in style through 9 miles of beautiful Norfolk countryside as the Bure Valley Railway takes you from the historic market town of Aylsham to Wroxham. Regular services run most days from Easter to October. There is a unique Boat-train service that combines a trip on the train and a cruise on the Broads.

CROMER   CARTING ACTION SPORTS,

The Avenue, Northrepps, Nr Cromer. Off A 149 opposite Aldis Service Station.
Tel: 01931 111819.

If you are aged 12 and over and have ever wanted to be a Formula One or Rally Driver, Grass Carting can satisfy your ambitions. Its fast, fun and above all affordable. Whether you are a novice or an accomplished driver you are bound to gain both experience and pleasure from this sport. Wise to book in advance.

THE NORFOLK SHIRE HORSE CENTRE & COUNTRYSIDE COLLECTION

West Runton Stables, West Runton. Tel: 01263 837339.

See Heavy Horses bred, preserved and protected. Show Itinerary every day. Indoor Area for wet weather demonstrations. Museum of farm equipment and bygones. Picnic area, cafe. Open 10-5pm. Easter to end October. Closed Saturdays unless Bank Holiday weekends.

EARSHAM   THE OTTER TRUST

A unique wonderland of waterfowl, Otters, Night Herons and Muntjac Deer, on the banks of the River Waveney. The worlds largest collection of otters in natural enclosures where the British Otter is bred for re-introduction to the wild. Open daily 1st April-31st October 10 One mile south-east of Fakenham, clearly signposted off the A1067 Norwich road. Tel: 01328 851465. In two hundred acres of beautiful reserve, Pensthorpe brings visitors and wildlife close together. Outside the visitor centre explore waterside walks and nature trails.

There are excellent access facilities for the elderly and disabled, quiet picnic areas and plentiful seating. Courtyard Restaurant. Children's Adventure Playground, wildlife, brass rubbing centre and discovery areas. Open 7 days a week (except Christmas Day) from mid-March to beginning of January. Weekends only January, February to mid-March. Dogs not allowed (Guide dogs excepted).

THE THURSFORD COLLECTION

Thursford Green, Thursford. Tel: 01328 878477.

Wonderful, exciting collection and constant live musical shows. Christmas is especially magical. Open daily April-May-Sept-Oct 1pm-5pm. June-July-August 11am-5pm. Off the A148 Fakenham to Holt road.

THE LIVING JUNGLE

Central Sea Front, Marine Parade. Tel: 01493 842202.

The Genesis Experience takes you back to the beginning before mankind, to give you an insight into what heaven must be like. You will see a lush tropical jungle garden, butterflies, birds and fish. You will hear the sound of the garden's creatures and the gentle trickle of warm waters. Open daily March to end October 10am.

HEACHAM   NORFOLK LAVENDER

Caley Mill. Tel: 01485 70384.

England's working Lavender Farm and the home of the National Collection of Lavenders. Excellent cream teas and home-made cakes. Shops selling lavender products + plants and herbs, gifts. Free Admission and Car Parking. Open daily 10-5pm (Closed for 2 weeks at Christmas). On A149 3 miles south of Hunstanton. Guided tours from end of May to end of September.

KENNINGHALL.   THE PARTICULAR POTTERY

Church Street, Kenninghall Nr16 2EN

Tel: 01953 888476

Kenninghall is a delightful conservation village with a lovely old market place. The Pottery is in quaint Church Street. Built in 1807, it was formerly the Particular Baptist Chapel which accounts for the name of the Pottery. It is both the workshop and the home of potter, David Walters and his family. In addition it provides a superb gallery environment for the work of many of East Anglia's finest crafts people. In creating a home, some changes were inevitable but the result is exciting. David works exclusively in Porcelain, creating hand-thrown bowls of all sizes, as well as large platters, vases and urns. **OPEN;** Tuesday to Saturday 9AM-5PM. Also Bank Holiday Weekends. If the family are there on Sundays, they are usually open. Please ring first to be sure or take pot luck! Off street parking. Disabled access. Affordable workshop prices. Visa/Access/ American Express welcome. Children should be accompanied by an adult.

KING'S LYNN   THE OLD GAOL HOUSE

Saturday Market Place. Tel: 01553 763044.

Let your imagination run riot as your personal stereo guide takes you through King's Lynn 1930's Police Station and into the cells beyond. Open daily Easter and Spring Bank Holiday until the end of September 10-5pm. Closed Wednesdays and Thursdays October-Easter.

BIRCHAM WINDMILL

6 miles from Sandringham. Tel: 01485 23393

Bakery, Tea Rooms, Cycle Hire, Free Parking. Open daily Easter-30th September 10-6pm (Tea Rooms and Bakery closed Saturdays).

LANGHAM   LANGHAM HAND-MADE CRYSTAL

The Long Barn, North Street, Nr Holt Tel: 01328 830511.

Glassmaking Mon-Fri Nov-March. Sun-Friday April-October 10-5pm. Free parking. Live Glass Making Museum. Adventure Playground. Restaurant/Cafe.

LONG SUTTON   BUTTERFLY AND FALCONRY PARK- signposted off A17 Kings Lynn-

Seaford road. Tel: 01406 363833 Stroll through one of the largest tropical Butterfly Houses in Britain. A wealth of tropical, Mediterranean and temperate flowers and foliage set around ponds, streams and waterfalls adds to the enjoyment. A small insectarium contains scorpions, tarantulas and giant stick insects all safely housed behind glass. In the Falconry Centre watch the stunning flying displays. Tea Room and Tea Garden.Adventure playground. Animal Centre & Nature trail. Mouse house. Picnic area. Open mid-March-October 31st daily 10-6pm Sept & Oct 10-5pm.

NORWICH   THE MUSTARD SHOP

3 Bridewell Alley Tel: 01603 627889

Trace the history of Colman's Mustard over 150 years. Buy a sample of the extensive range of mustards or browse through the kitchen ware and other items in the shop. Open: Mon-Sat 9.30-5pm. Closed all day Sunday and Bank Holidays.

NORFOLK WILDLIFE CENTRE & COUNTRY PARK

Gt Witchingham. On A1067 Europe's mammals and waterfowl in 40 acres beautiful parkland. Rare and unusual trees and flowering shrubs. Command and Adventure Play area. Woodland Steam Railway. No dogs. Open daily April 1st-31st October.

CASTLE MUSEUM

- houses one of the country's finest regional collections of natural history, archaeology and art. Busy programme of temporary exhibitions and free talks, tours and activities for all the family. Open: Mon-Sat 10-5pm Sun 2-5pm.

NORWICH & BROADS CRUISES

Southern River Steamers from Elm Hill Quay and Foundry Bridge Quay. Tel: 01603 624051. Enjoy a cruise to Surlingham Broad through historic Norwich. Either cruise to Surlingham Broad via Brundall or take a trip under Norwich bridges, daily throughout the season. Ring for times.

SANDRINGHAM SANDRINGHAM HOUSE, GARDENS & MUSEUM

Tel: 01553 772675

The private country retreat of Her Majesty the Queen is at the heart of the beautiful estate which has been owned by four generations of Monarchs. All the main rooms used by the Royal Family are open to the public. The Museum contains fascinating displays of Royal memorabilia ranging from photographs to vintage Daimlers and an exhibition of the Sandringham Fire Brigade. Sandringham Country Park is open daily all year 10.30-5pm. House, Grounds and Museum open daily from Good Friday until the beginning of October with certain exceptions. Grounds 10.30-5pm House and Museum 11-4.45pm. Dogs except Guide Dogs not permitted in Grounds. Sandringham Visitor Centre open daily Easter to end of October.

WELLS-NEXT-THE-SEA NORTH NORFOLK RAILWAY

Tel: 01328 710227.

One of Britain's most majestic stately homes, situated in a deer park. This classic 18th century Palladian style mansion is a living treasure house of artistic and architectural history. Apart from a tour of this stunning house with its superb alabaster entrance hall, there are Bygones Museum, Pottery, 18th century Walled Garden. Deer Park & Lake and a sandy beach. Open daily (except Fridays and Saturdays) from the beginning of June to end of September 1.30-5pm, also Easter, May, Spring and Summer Bank Holiday Sundays and Mondays 11.30-5pm.

WELLS & WALSINGHAM LIGHT RAILWAY

Tel: 01328 856506.

Visit the longest 10 1/4 inch narrow gauge steam railway in the world. See the unique Garratt Locomotive 'Norfolk Hero' which was specially built for the four mile journey between the seaside town of Wells and the pilgrimage town of Walsingham. Open dailyfrom Easter - 30th September. Free parking. Follow the Brown Tourist signs on the A149 coast road.

WROXHAM   NORFOLK DRIED FLOWER CENTRE

Willow Farm, Cangate, Neatishead. Tel: 01603 783588

A dazzling display of dozens of varieties and colours. Flower arranging classes and demonstrations. Free admission and parking. Two miles east of Wroxham just off the A1151 and follow the Brown Tourist signs on the A149 coast road.

BROADS TOURS

The Bridge Tel: 01603 782207

Enjoy a relaxing trip on the Norfolk Broads on luxurious passenger boats. Ring for details.

NORTHAMPTON FLAMINGO GARDENS & ZOOLOGICAL PARK

Tel: 01234 711451

This has been built over the last three decades by its owner, Mr Christopher Marler, into one of the finest bird collections in the country. In lovely natural surroundings the gardens are situated in the peaceful stone village of Weston Underwood, one mile from the market town of Olney. The flowers and blossom in the spring and autumn make the gardens an attractive alternative to the avian beauty; but the breathtaking colour of the Flamingos must surely make a lasting impression on the visitor. Open: Good Friday & Bank Holiday Mondays, Sat,Sun,Wed & Thurs until end of June. Every day except Mondays in July & August. Opening hours 2-7pm.

ST GILES   CHILTERN OPEN AR MUSEUM

Tel: 01494 871117

Many wonderful aircraft to be seen which would otherwise have been destroyed. These have been re-erected in 45 acres of countryside. The buildings illustrate everyday life and work of planes in the Chiltern region. Open 2-6pm 1st April-31st October.

NORTHUMBERLAND

BAGPIPE MUSEUM

Tel: 01670 519466. Location: Morpeth Chantry.

This unusual museum specialises in the history and development of Northumbrian small pipes and their music from India to Inverness. Small admission charge. Open Mon-sat 9.30-5.30pm Mar-Dec, Mon-Sat 9.30-5.30pm Jan-Feb. Closed between Christmas and New Year.

KIELDER WATER CRUISES.

Tel: 01434 240398.

Enjoy a 10 mile cruise in comfort on Europe's largest man-made lake in a covered ferry with commentary, licensed bar and light refreshments on board. Take a round trip calling at places of interest or use the ferry as access to self-guided walks on the north side of the lake. Open throughout mid-Mar to 31st Oct, weather permitting.

CHANTRY SILVER.

Tel: 01670 511323. Location: Just off the A1 15 miles north of Newcastle.

Housed within the Chantry Court Yard one can purchase hand-made jewellery and silver from Chantry Silver. Also on view and for sale are original paintings, tapestries and glass engravings by many local artists. Admission free. Open Mon-Sat 9.30-5.30pm.

WALLINGTON HOUSE.

Tel: 01670 74283. Location: 12 miles west of Morpeth (B6343).

Built in 1688 and altered in the 1740s, the house features exceptional plasterwork; fine collections of porcelain and dolls houses and the Museum of Curiosities. The house is set in 100 acres of lakes, lawns and woodland with a beautiful Walled Garden. Admission to House, Walled Garden and Grounds £4.00. Open daily 1st Apr-31st Oct, except Tues 1-5.30pm. Last admission 5pm.

OXFORDSHIRE

BURFORD   COTSWOLD WILD LIFE PARK

Tel: 01993 823006

Situated in 180 acres of gardens and woodland around an old English manor house, a large and varied collection of animals from all over the world can be seen in spacious grassed enclosures. There is also a reptile house, aquarium, tropical house, exhibition of fruit bats, picnicking areas, narrow gauge railway (Apr-Oct), adventure playground, bar, restaurant, children's farmyard, insect house and gift shops. Special events during summer months. Open; Daily (except Christmas day) from 10-6pm or dusk (whichever is the earlier).

OXFORD   THE OXFORD STORY

6 Broad Street Tel: 01865 790055

Created by Oxford University and the people behind York's 'Jorvik' Viking Centre, this is an extraordinary exhibition about Oxford's 800 years past. Now recognised as the best short introduction to Oxford. The Oxford Story uses a ride through the streets from the past, from medieval Oxford to Inspector Morse, Magnus Magnusson or Timothy Mallett (for children) provide the commentary. Open: April-October 9.30-5pm. July-August 9.30-7pm. Nov-March 10-4pm. Closed Christmas Day.

WITNEY   COGGES MANOR FARM MUSEUM

Church Lane. Tel: 01993 772602

A working museum of Victorian rural Life on a 20 acre site, close to Witney town centre. The historic site includes the manor house with room displays, walled garden, orchard, riverside walks, farm buildings housing traditional breeds of animals, exhibitions in the barns, daily demonstrations of cooking on the kitchen range and special weekends and activities. Buttery serving light lunches and teas, gift shop and car park. Open: April-end October, Tues-Friday abd Bank Holiday Mondays 10.30-5.30pm. Saturday and Sunday 12 njoon- 5.30pm.

WOODSTOCK BLENHEIM PALACE

Tel: 01993 811091

Home of the 11th Duke of Marlborough, birthplace of Sir Winston Churchill. A visit to Blenheim is a wonderful way to spend a day. An inclusive ticket covers the Palace tour, and Gardens, Butterfly House, Motor Launch, Train, Adventure Play Area and Nature trail. Optional are the Marlborough Maze and Rowing Boat hire on Queen Pool. Car parking is free for Palace visitors. Shops, Cafeterias and Restaurant. Special events include the Blenheim Audi International Horse Trials. Mid- March- 31st October daily 10.30-5.30pm.

SUFFOLK

BURY ST EDMUNDS MANOR HOUSE MUSEUM
Honey Hill. Tel: 01284 757072.
A new museum of art and horology in refurbished Georgian Mansion. Colliection of clocks, watches, paintings, furniture, costumes and ceramics. 'Hands On' Gallery. Cafe & shop. Open all year Mon-Sat 10-5pm Sun 2-5pm. Closed Godd Friday, Christmas Day and Boxing Day.

ST EDMONDSBURY CATHEFRAL
Angel Hill 11th century Mother church of Suffolk with fine hammer beam roof and a display of 1,00 embroidered kneelers. Open Jun-Aug 8.30-8pm Sept-May 8.30-6pm. Exhibitions in the Cloisters.

CLARE PRIORY.
Ruins of 13th century Monastery and Monastic Church. Open: daily.

COTTON MECHANICAL MUSIC MUSEUM
- off B1113 south of Diss. Tel: 01449 613876.
Extensive collection, includes organs, street pianos, polyphones, gramophones, music boxes, musical dolls, fruit bowls and even a musical chair. Also the mighty Wurlitzer Theatre pipe organ in specially reconstructed cinema. Open: Jun-Sept 2.30-5.30pm.

IPSWICH TOLLY COBBOLD BREWERY & BREWERY TAP
Cliff Road. Tel: 01473 281508.
Taste the malt, smell the hops and enjoy a complimentary glass of beer at one of the country's oldest breweries. A must for those interested in beer, heritage and history. Artefacts from 1723. Guided tours. Open: Easter & May-Sept daily 12 noon. (Extra tours weekends). Oct-Apr: Fri, Sat, Sun 12 noon. Min age 14. Public bar/food.

LOWESTOFT SOMERLEYTON HALL.
Tel: 01502 730224.
Rebuilt in Anglo-Indian style in 1840s. Fine state rooms, period furnishings and paintings. Superb gardens with famous maze. Deer Park. Tea Room. Picnic area. Hall open: Easter-Sept, Thurs, Sun and Bank Holidays. Also July & August: Tues, Wed 2-5pm. Gardens and tea room open from 12.30pm. Miniature railway Sun, Thurs, Bank Holidays from 3pm Guided tours of house, gardens, Luncheons, suppers, by prior arrangement. Lord and Lady Somerleyton hope that you will enjoy your day here and also that you will pay a visit to Fritton Lake Countryworld, part of the Somerleyton Estate, which is only a 10 minute drive and is open from 10am every day during the season.

NEWMARKET NATIONAL HORSE RACING MUSEUM
High Street. Tel: 01638 667333.
Story of the development of horse racing over 300 years, house in Regency subscription rooms. Arts, bronzes, development of the rules, institutions and the great men of the sport. Also British Sporting Art Trust Vestey Gallery. April-end of November Tues-Sat 10-5pm Sun 2-5pm except July, Aug 12-5pm. Also Bank Holiday Mondays and July, August Mondays 10-5pm. Various guided tours of the gallops, training grounds. National Stud, Jockey club, musuem and historic town by prior arrangement.

SUDBURY GAINSBOROUGH'S HOUSE

Gainsborough Street. Tel: 01787 372958.

Birthplace of Thomas Gainsborough RA 1717-88. Georgian fronted town house, with attractive walled garden, displays more of the artist's work than any other British Gallery. 18th century furniture and memorabilia. Open: Easter-Oct Tues-Sat 10-5pm Sun & Bank Holiday Monday 2-5pm Nov-Easter Tues-Sat 10-4pm Sun 2-4pm. Closed between Christmas and New Year, Good Friday.

SHROPSHIRE

IRONBRIDGE JACKFIELD THE MUSEUM

Tel: 01952 433522

One of the several museum sites within the famous Ironbridge Gorge which no one should miss. . Within the Gorge you will find hours of pleasure and fascinating features to absorb. Jackfield the Museum was a world centre of the decorative tile industry. The museum houses an impressive collection of wall and floor tiles ranging from the Victorian era, through the art deco periods, to a range of attractive silk-screened designs from the 1950s. Open daily all year round.

IRONBRIDGE TOY MUSEUM

Tel: 01952 433926

Overflowing with toys, games and childhood memorabilia from magic lanterns to Bayko building sets, clockwork trains to Rupert Bear can all be seen at this wonderful museum. See how toys reflect our lifestyle from houses, cars, fashion and TV culture. Also visit the well-stocked shop selling high quality traditional toys, collectors' models, dolls and teddies, children's books and greeting cards. Open daily from 10am.

IRONBRIDGE

Tel: 01952 433522

This is one of Britain's 11 World Heritage Sites, where the modern world began over 250 years ago. This was the birthplace of the Industrial Revolution, and here were made the first iron railing the first iron wheels and even the first high pressure steam locomotive. Today the Ironbridge Gorge Museum shows 20th century visitors how and why these events took place and how people lived during those momentous years. Open daily through the year 10-5pm.

MUCH WENLOCK   MUCH WENLOCK MUSEUM

Tel: 01952 727773

Interesting local museum, housed in former market hall. It contains new displays on the geology and natural history of Wenlock Edge, local history, exhibits including the Wenlock Olympics and information about Wenlock Priory. Open Apr-Sept Mon-Sat.

WENLOCK PRIORY

Tel: 01952 727466

Much Wenlock is a picturesque market town lying between Wenlock Edge and the Ironbridge Gorge in some of the most attractive countryside in Shropshire. Set amongst smooth lawns and ornamental topiary, are the magnificent remains of Wenlock Priory. A prosperous and powerful monastery in its time and a place of pilgrimage, Wenlock is an inspiring place to visit. There is plenty to explore and the Priory church still dominates the scene. The Norman Chapter House has some superb decorative arcading and you can also see the remains of the Cloister, once the bustling hub of daily life. Open daily 1st April-31st October 10-6pm 1st November-31st March Sun & Wed 10-4pm

THE AEROSPACE MUSEUM
Tel: 01902 374112 Locaton: On A41 just one mile from junction 3 on the M54.
One of the largest aviation collections in the UK with over 70 aircraft on display, including many unique examples, together with missiles, engines, uniforms and aviation memorabilia. Open all year round.

WYRE FOREST
Tel: 01299 266302
This magnificent 6000 acre forest nature reserve is home to a variety of wildlife, including deer, butterflies and wild flowers. A visitor centre includes forest information, exhibitions and a shop and cafe. Explore the forest on a range of way-marked paths, including a special wheelchair route. Open daily all year round. Visitor Centre open 11-4pm.

CHURCH STRETTON   ACTON SCOTT WORKING FARM
Tel: 01694 781306.
A visit to Acton Scott will enable visitors to experience life on an upland farm at the turn of the century. The waggoner and his team of shire horses work the land with vintage farm machines. Daily demonstrations of rural crafts complete the picture of estate life 100 years ago. There are weekly visits from the wheelwright, farrier and blacksmith and children will love the cows, pigs, poultry and sheep in the farmyard and fields. Open 29th Mar-3oth Oct Tues-Sat 10-5pm Sun and Bank Holidays 10-6pm.

MARKET DRAYTON   HODNET HALL GARDENS
Tel: 01630 685202
Over 60 acres of brilliantly coloured flowers, magnificent forest trees, sweeping lawns and a chain of ornamental pools which run tranquilly along the cultivated garden valley to provide a natural habitat for waterfowl and other wildlife are just some of the many attractions on offer. No matter what the season, visitors will always find something fresh and interesting to ensure a full and enjoyable days outing. Open from 1st April-end September Mon-Sat 2-5pm. Sun & Bank Holidays 12-5.30pm.

SHREWSBURY ATTINGHAM PARK
Tel: 01743 709203.
Attingham Park is one of the finest houses in the country, set in its own grounds of 250 acres, and offers the whole family a wealth of things to see and do. Explore the landscaped park, take a gentle stroll by the river or through the woods, discover the estate history at the Bothy exhibition, enjoy the elegant house and its beautiful furnishings, learn about the Berwick family and end your visit with home-made refreshments in the tea-room or purchasing a gift or souvenir from the shop. The Park and House are open throughout the year from the end of March until the end of September. 1.30-5pm, last admission 4.30pm.

BUILDWAS ABBEY

Tel:01952 433274

Founded in the 12th century Buildwas Abbey was largely untouched by the great events of history though periodically attacked by raiders from across the Welsh border. Its simple, sturdy buildings give a powerful impression of both grandeur and the austerity of monastic life, with its fine vaulted roof and unusual medieval floor tiles, depicting birds and animals. Open 1st April-30th September 10-6pm daily.

WROXETER ROMAN CITY

Tel: 01743 761330

To visit Wroxeter today is to step back in time to the heyday of Roman Britain. The centrepiece is the remains of the extensive bath complex, one of the best preserved in England. The enormous hill which divided the baths from the exercise area still stands, and whilst walking around you can recreate the everyday activities of the thriving Roman City. Open; April 1st - 31st October 10-6pm.

TELFORD   BOSCOBEL HOUSE

Tel: 01902 850244.

A visit to Boscobel House will take you to the scene of one of the most romantic stories in English history. King Charles II sought refuge in an oak tree at Boscobel House when he was chased by Cromwell's soldiers after the Battle of Worcester in 1651. The Royal Oak can be seen to this day painted on signs outside countless pubs all over the country, and you can still see a direct descendant of the famous oak itself now nearly 300 years old, in fields surrounding the house. A visit to the house will show that it has retained its romantic character. There are panelled rooms and hiding places, including the 'sacred hole' in the attic where Charles is said to have stayed at night. Open daily from 1st April-31st October 10-6pm. 1st Nov- 31st Dec & 1st Feb - 31st March Wed 7 Sun 10-4pm.

WALES

BEDDGELERT   SYGUN COPPER MINE

Beddgelert, LL55 4NE Tel: 01766 890595

24 hour info/line: 01766 890564.

Sygun is one mile from the village of Beddgelert on the A498 road to Capel Curig. Sygun Copper Mine is one of the wonders of Wales - a remarkable and impressive example of how part of our precious industrial heritage can be reclaimed, restored and transformed into an outstanding family attraction. The mine provides an excellent and informative experience of the underground world of the Victorian miner. The mine, a unique modern day reminder of 19th century methods of ore extraction and processing, is situated in the glorious Gwynant Valley - the heart of the stunning Snowdonia National Park - and on probably the most popular tourist route in Wales. The incomparable scenery captured the imagination of movie-makers, who turned the mountainside surrounding Sygun into a Chinese village in 1958 for the filming of 'The Inn of the Sixth Happiness' which starred the late Ingrid Bergman. Sygun offers a rare opportunity for those with a sense of adventure and curiosity, from the young to the elderly, to discover for themselves the wonders it still shelters after being abandoned in 1903. Audiovisual tours allow you to explore the old workings on foot in complete safety. There are winding tunnels and large chambers, magnificent stalactite and stalagmite formations and copper ore veins which contain traces of gold, silver and other precious metals. It usually takes about 40 minutes to complete the quarter mile route which rises 140feet via stairways to emerge at the Victoria level for a breathtaking view of the Gwynant Valley and surrounding Snowdonia mountain range. A shorter, less demanding tour can be arranged. Refreshments and a wide range of souvenirs are available in the visitors centre.

OPEN; All year. Oct, Nov, Feb, March 10.30am-4pm. (11am Sunday) Dec, Jan 11-3.30pm. Main season: Easter or late March - Sept inc. 10am-5pm (11am Sun. & 4pm Sat.) Visa/ Access/ Switch. Flat soled shoes advisable. Dogs not permitted underground.

BLAENAU FFESTINIOG LLECHWEDD SLATE CAVERNS
Blaenau Ffestiniog,LL41 3NB Tel: 01766 830306 Fax:01766 831260.

This is a day out to remember. Winner of all Britain's top tourism awards, Llechwedd Slate Caverns have been visited by five million people, including Edward VIII when he was Prince of Wales, the Princess Margaret, the Duchess of Gloucester and the Crown Prince of Japan. The spectacular underground lake has been used for a Walt Disney film set. Other sites have endeavoured, unsuccessfully, to copy the magic of Llechwedd - where the tourist operation has the benefit of historic authenticity while also remaining part of the biggest working slate mine in Wales. Here you can take two quite different rides, one exploring the complexities of old slate mining skills, the other the triumph, humour, religious fervour, and the pathos of the Victorian miner. Visitors are at liberty to take either or both.

Add to that an exploration of the Victorian Village, and some refreshment at one of the wide selection of catering facilities, and there is no reluctance to spend at least a day at Llechwedd. A very interesting and informative little book about Llechwedd written by Ivor Wynne Jones, a Director, is well worth acquiring. Not only does it tell you about the mine but also about the history of slate, and relates Llechwedd Slate Caverns' unexpected contribution to the conservation of Wales' endangered wild life. Choughs' Cavern which visitors see while the Miners' Tramway, was named after the shy crow-like birds which nested there for many years, returning in 1969, disappearing in the 1970s but rediscovering the same unlikely spot in 1991, since when annual nesting has been re-established. On the surface hovering kestrels are a common sight and buzzards nest on the northern rock face. One of nature's most beautiful contributions is rhododendron ponticum which bursts into flower each spring.

An interesting highlight of a visit to Llechwedd is the facility for spending Victorian coins, at Victorian prices, in the village shops and the ever popular Miners Arms. This journey back in time begins at the Old Bank of Greenway & Greaves. This is a banking museum, preserving the appearance of a small country branch early in the last century. The Llechwedd 'bank' has a shop counter where five pre-decimal coins may be purchased. They show correct designs on the reverse, but with modern dating. All prices in the Victorian Village -Pentre Llechwedd - are shown in old and new currencies, enabling such experiences as buying a 'pennorth' of sweets or a 3d pint at the Miners' Arms. In 1972 when a half-mile level section of the Miners' Tramway was opened to the world revealing the vast workings, it was immediately given the top awards of both the British Tourist Authority and the Wales Tourist Board. Boarding a train in a corner of the original slate slabbing mill of 1852, visitors now ride into an 1846 tunnel, hauled by battery-electric locomotives.

Entering through the side of the mountain, this journey into the early Victorian past remains on the level, and traverses some spectacular caverns. Passengers alight at various points to learn something of the strange skills needed to extract slate. There is a sound and light tableaux deep underground and guides describe the other chambers. OPEN: Daily 10am including Sundays. (Closed on Christmas Day, Boxing Day and New Year's Day) Last tours into mines: 5.15pm March to September 4.15pm October to February. Access, Visa, Switch. Special terms for parties of 20 or more. Free car parking, free surface exhibitions. Dogs not allowed on either ride. Separate cafe. Victorian Pub and Licensed restaurant.

CAERNARFON   CAERNARFON AIR WORLD

Museum and Pleasure Flights

Caernarfon Airport, Dinas Dinlle, Nr Caernarfon, Gwynedd LL545TP Tel: 01286 830800.

In the great hangar here you can see planes and helicopters in landscaped settings, aircraft engines, ejector seats and over two hundred model aircraft. If you enjoy the history and nostalgia associated with planes and flying, this is the place for you and it is 'Hands On'. You can sit in cockpits, take the controls in the Varsity Trainer and wander round full size planes. There are also exhibitions featuring Local Aviation History, the story of the Dambusters, Welsh Flying V.C's, the first RAF Mountain Rescue Service, fascinating wartime newspapers and historic First Day Covers.

There is a cinema where you can watch aviation shorts and full length films. The well stocked museum shop has been extended, and for small children there is a themed adventure playground, built around a Dragonfly helicopter. Pleasure Flights will provide you with a unique experience in North Wales. Take a bird's eye view of mountains, castles and coastline in a Cessna or the Vintage de Havilland Dragon Rapide. There are three standard flights, but you canalways plan your own. The first is a ten minute flight over the Menai Strait around the 13th century Caernarfon Castle and back over the 18th century Fort Belan. The second flight is a breathtaking 25 minute experience flying over the mountains of Snowdonia, over the summit of Snowdon, the highest peak in England and Wales, over Crib Coch and the Llanberis Pass, then back to the airport taking in Caernarfon Castle and Fort Belan. The third is another 25 minute flight that is offered if weather conditions do not favour a mountain trip. This one flies over the Menai Strait and the lovely island of Anglesey, taking in the foothills of Snowdonia and Caernarfon Castle on the return journey.

OPEN; MUSEUM Daily 1st March -31st October 9am-5.30pm. PLEASURE FLIGHTS Daily, weather permitting throughout the year. Check by phone prior to visit. RESTAURANT Open daily all year. Coffee Shop open from Easter to 31st October.

COLWYN BAY   EIRIAS PAR

Colwyn Leisure Centre, Colwyn Bay LL29 8HG Tel: 01492 533223

Here you will find something for all the family. With over half a million visitors annually to Eirias Park its popularity as a tourist and recreational attraction cannot be questioned. Set in 50 acres of beautiful parkland, the facilities on offer provide a unique recreational experience and offer an outstanding day out for all ages. Facilities available all year round include: Leisure Pool/Waterchute, Sports Halls, Squash Courts, Sauna/Solarium Suite, Function Room, Fitness Room, Lounge Bar/Cafe, Athletics Stadium, Indoor/Outdoor Tennis Courts and Synthetic Pitch. Facilities available throughout the summer season include: Crown Green Bowling Greens, Boating Lake with small and large pedaloes, Model Yacht Pond, Mini Golf Par Putting, Children' Play Area, Picnic Areas and Dinosaur World.

From a promotional point of view, the facilities within Eirias Park, serve as an ideal location for the hosting of a corporate day and last year such days were organised on behalf of the Inland Revenue for Wales and the Post Office, North West. Simply choose from the available facilities or allow the competent, friendly staff to arrange a programme of activities to suit your company's personal needs. To complement the days activities, the Catering Manageress will be delighted to arrange a buffet with a wide selection of menus to choose from.

From its commanding position overlooking the promenade and beach, the park is easily accessible by road via the A55 Expressway which links North Wales with the UK Motorway network and by rail with regular inter-city services from all parts of Britain. Easy access for the disabled. Free Car Parking.

CWMBRAN GREENMEADOW COMMUNITY FARM

Green Force Way, Cwmbran NP44 5AJ Tel: 01633 862202

In the early 1980's a group of local people formed an action committee in a bid to protect one of the last green spaces in Cwmbran from further development. The group came up with the exciting prospect of establishing a Community Farm. Today, the original, fully refurbished c17th farmstead with 150 acres of land throughout Cwmbran, offers a magnificent rural retreat in an urban setting. It is a place full of excitement where you will see traditional farm animals and Rare Breeds, a well-stocked aviary, an Exhibition Barn with ever changing exhibits.

On the woodland trails you will see a surprising variety of wildlife and the Pets Corner is a place in which children have a chance to make friends with the smaller animals. All visitors are encouraged to feed and handle selected farm animals. The Farm House Tea Room offers traditional home-made fare. The Sheep Dip Bar is open every evening and the 16th century Cordell's Restaurant is ideal for an intimate meal. It opens every evening 7-10pm and for Sunday lunch. Special events are organised throughout the year. OPEN; All year except Christmas Day Summer 10-6pm Winter 10-4.30pm. Disabled people welcome. Pets allowed. Licensed. Conference facilities.

DOLGELLAU GWYNBFYNYDD GOLD MINE

The Marian, Dolgellau, Gwynedd LL40 1UU Tel: 01341 423332 Fax: 01341 423737

To get to the mine take the courtesy bus from Welsh Gold in Dolgellau and enjoy the short guided journey through some of the most beautiful countryside in Wales. Here you will see the place where a huge bonanza of gold was found a century ago: worth £5 million if found today. As far as one can tell Gwynfynydd Gold mine is the only working gold mine open to the public. Gold ore is mined daily but actual gold is very rare ; the mine yields about 25g per month on the whole but most times it can be less. 8 full time miners work here with additional staff to guide people through the mine during the summer season.

Once you arrive at the mine you are presented with protective clothing which include a hard hat, waterproof jacket and boots. (It is advisable to take a sweater with you as it can be quite cold underground.) On the tour itself you can experience the roar and thunder of modern machinery, the blast of explosions, and take away your own free sample of a Welsh Goldmine ore. You will also see how they mined in the olden days, by candle light. After being underground for around one hour you will see the Gold Smelting room, where gold is melted down to a small gold bullion. At the end of your tour you may pan for gold, should you find any, which is normally found in small pieces of rocks, you may take it home!! The retail shop sells Welsh Gold Jewellery which is displayed amongst other crafts from Wales. It is advisable to book in advance for tours throughout the year.

The gold centre is open throughout the year 9.30am until 5.00pm, later on some occasions in the summer. It is open 7 days from Easter to September and closed on Sundays during the winter.

HOLYWELL   HOLYWELL LEISURE CENTRE

Fron Park, Holywell CH8 7UZ

An exciting Leisure Centre offering something for every age. The 6 lane swimming pool incorporates broad shallow steps for easy access. Contained within the pool hall is a small shallow water area where toddlers can play in safety and a splash pool which provides a safe landing area to the 42 metre corkscrew water slide. The swimmng pool is open from 10am each day but closes each weekday between 3.45pm and 5.15pm for junior swimming classes. Indeed there is a whole range of classes for swimmers of all ages and all stages.

The Silhouette Fitness Centre and the Silhouettes Health Suite are both excellent for anyone and supervised by an experienced and caring staff. Both open from 10am-10pm seven days a week. The Sports Hall has five a side football, basketball, volleyball and four badminton courts, bookable from 10am-10pm each day. The Dance Studio has a comprehensive range of dance classes and some popular aerobic and step aerobic sessions. This multi use area is excellent for small theatrical productions, drama workshops, film shows, seminars and training courses. The Hall is also used for Karate,Thai Boxing, Kung Fu, 50+ Exercise classes and children's birthday parties. Open from 10am-10pm seven days a week. The Snooker Room has 6 tables. For Bowling, two crown greens, one of which is floodlit are available for casual use from the beginning of April to the end of October. There is an Outdoor Area, two floodlit tennis courts, and a Synthetic Pitch for soccer. The Cafeteria is open from 9.30am-9.30pm each day and there is a comfortable lounge bar which opens from 7.30pm each evening. For further details please ring 01352 712027.

LLANDRINDOD WELLS THE RADNORSHIRE MUSEUM

Temple Street, Llandrindod Wells, LD1 5LD Tel: 01597 824 513

Situated in the centre of Llandrindod Wells, the museum houses exhibits relating to the history of the old mid-Wales county of Radnorshire. Displays illustrate the largely rural farming lifestyle of the area as well as the development of Llandrindod Wells as a country Spa Resort during the Victorian and Edwardian Era. The museum also displays material relating to Fine Art, costume and the Prehistoric, Roman and Medieval history of the area: including the Roman Fort of Castell Collen. New for 1995 was the Red Kite Centre: set on the museums first floor, this exhibition highlights the lifestyle and successful fight back from the edge of extinction of Britons most beautiful bird of prey. The exhibition also includes a thirty minute video on the Red Kite and computer information station on the birds of Europe.

OPEN; 10-12.30 and 2-4.30. Closed Wednesday (all year) and Saturday afternoon and Sunday (winter only).

TEIFI VALLEY RAILWAY

Henllan Station, Henllan, Nr Newcastle Emlyn SA44 5TD Tel/Fax: 01559 371077

The only Famous Little Trains of Wales in West Wales gives hours of pleasure to people of all ages. A 40 minute train ride experience for which you pay once and ride all day (if seats available). Facilities include Woodland Theatre (Phone for details), Woodland Trails, Cafe. Shop, Pictorial Museum, Crazy Golf/Quoits/Skittles, Childrens'Play Areas, Picnic and Barbeque Areas. W.C's, large Car Park, Coaches Welcome. Usual Coach Driver Facilities.

OPEN; Easter-Oct inc 10.30am-6pm. Closed: Saturdays. Apr 13/20/27 May 4/11/18 Oct 5/12/ 19. TRAINS: Apr. May. June Oct. 10.30,11.30, 12.30, 2pm, 3pm, 4pm. July, Aug-Sept Last train 5pm + Bank Holidays. SPECIAL EVENTS: April 6th, Aug 17th, 25th and 26th, Oct 26th, December - SANTA SPECIALS Entrance/Parking 50p (Adults) £3.50 (Children) £1.50(OAP) £3 Dogs 50p. Opending hours: daily Easter -26th October.

LLANGOLLEN   MODEL RAILWAY WORLD & DR WHO EXHIBITION
Lower Dee Mill Llangollen LL20 8SE Tel: 01978 860584.

These two exciting attractions opened in the summer of 1995 and rapidly drew attention from visitors to the area as well as curious locals! The Model Railway World Museum is based around the original Hornby Dublo Factory from Binns Road, Liverpool. You will see 24 large superb layouts with 1000s of models on display. You can try shunting in the hands-on section and watch and talk to experts about building these models. Fascinating and educational. Dapol Ltd design and manufacture precision model railways and a widerange of toys including Dr Who models. The move to Lower Mill not only enabled Dapol to improve its manufacturing but also to realise the life-long dream of its Managing Director, David Boyle - to establish a National Model Railway Museum. Over the years David has amassed a huge collection of model railway artefacts and memorabilia including the original design drawings, art work, photographs, lathes, jigs, etc from Hornby, Dublo, Mainline,Wrenn. Airfix. All these are displayed together with the working layouts resulting in a unique exhibition relating to the history of model railways from the very beginning to the present day.

The DR WHO exhibition adds yet another fascinating dimension at Lower Dee Mill. It was opened by former Dr Who actor, Colin Baker on the 17th June 1995 and has been mounted in association with the BBC who have provided the original costumes, Daleks, Cybermen monsters, visual effects (many of which are priceless). In consultation with BBC Dr Who producer, John Nathan-Turner the exhibition, covering three huge rooms, has been designed more as an experience than an exhibition with a full size working TARDIS and original sound effects give a fascinating insight into how the longest running science fiction series in the world was made for television. Please ring 01978 860584 for opening times.

LLANGOLLEN   LLANGOLLEN HORSE DRAWN BOAT TRIPS
Llangollen Wharf, Llangollen

Tel: 01978 860702 for general enquiries. 0169 175322 for Group bookings, Day Boats and Holiday Hire.

To take a trip on one of these boats eases you back to the days of leisure as you glide noiselessly through the spectacular scenery of the Vale of Llangollen. You may find yourself being pulled along by one of five horses who are all friendly and have names. Spot is the old boy who only works occasionally and then there is Fred, Sam, Stan and Arthur. They seem to enjoy their work as they go slowly along the towpath. In this timeless setting, the horse-drawn canal trips are as relaxing today as they were when the first pleasure boats slipped away from the Wharf in 1884. On the Wharf, you will find the Canal Exhibition Centre, telling the Canal Story with words, pictures and models. It is good to wander among the gaily painted canal ware in the gift shop and delightful to take tea on the terrace overlooking the town. Llangollen Wharf is a fascinating place for a day out. The popular cruise on the luxury narrowbat Thomas Telfrod includes a crossing of the Pontcysllte Aqueduct.

OPEN; Daily for 45 minute horse-drawn boat trips and exhibition visits from Easter to September with limited opening in October.

LLANGOLLEN   LLANGOLLEN RAILWAY
Abbey road, Llangollen LL208SN Tel:01978 860979

Llangollen is at the junction of the A5 and A539. The railway station is by the bridge over the River Dee. The nearest car parks are in Market Street in the town and at Lower Dee Mill on the A539 approaching from Ruabon. The nearst British Rail station is 5 miles away at Ruabon. Bryn

Melyn buses operate hourly to Llangollen from Wrexham and Ruabon, two hourly on Sundays. The Llangollen Railway Society rescued this delightful line and have spent years bringing the track, the station and the trains back to their original beauty and splendour. The Railway you see at Llangollen today is a direct result of the dreams and aspirations of the former Flint and Deeside Railway. The work has been done mainly by volunteer enthusiasts who removed masses of undergrowth and rubble from the trackbed and vandalised buildings without water or supplies to be restored. The journey in the restored carriages through the countryside with the River Dee appearing constantly, is both beautiful, exciting and relaxing. Thrilling for youngsters and an outstanding experience for steam railway enthusiasts. There are opportunities for people to spend two hours on the footplate on 14 miles of firing and driving. Full hot meals for the trainee and light refreshments for up to six guests. Try the Llangollen Steam Driving Course - something you will never forget or regret. There are special dining opportunities and Sunday Lunches aboard the Berwyn Belle. Friends of Thomas Events, Santa Specials and much more. Ring for further information 01978 860979.

COWBRIDGE   TASKFORCE PAINTBALL GAMES
(147 Ynysddu, Pontyclun CF7 9UB office) Tel:01443 227715 Fax:01443 225803

Situated just off the A48 west of Cowbridge, part of a large three and a half thousand acre estate at Penllyn. With easy access from the M4, just 10 minutes away, it can be reached with ease from most of the south west's major towns via the motorway network. Task Force is set in 30 acres of woodland within a deep undulating valley. It has been a venue for Paintball games since 1989 and during this period has had many special features added to it to create an exciting and varied site to play. Amongst its many varied features and scenarios are numerous bunkers, dugouts, a helicopter, bridges and a HUGE 'woodland village'. Your day will begin with a comprehensive briefing, followed by the issuing of all the equipment you will need for the day. Then once you are all kitted up and have had a practice on the firing range, you are ready for battle to commence. During the day you will play approximately 12 games. You do not need a special amount of players to book. There is an excellent Junior Paintball Game exclusively for 11-16 year olds. Open; Saturday and Sunday or during the week if you have a group of 15 or more people. Credit Cards: Visa/Delta/Access/Master .

LLANDYSUL   TY HEN FARM
Llwyndafydd, Nr New Quay, Llandysul SA44 6BZ West Wales.
Tel: 01545 560346

Approached by a bumpy lane and set on a sheep farm in peaceful countryside close to the Cardigan coast, near Cwmtudu, this attractive Guest House which also offers delightful, converted self-catering cottages is wonderful for people who want to relax, be well cared for and within easy reach of a whole host of exciting places. The main house has well appointed en suite bedrooms, the self-catering cottages and apartments are around the farmyard and so too is The Pits Centre which houses the restaurant and leisure facilities which comprise an indoor heated pool, well equipped gymnasium, sunbed, sauna, changing rooms, toilets, bowls/skittle alley, coin operated washing machine and drier. Good food is part of the reason this excellent place was awarded 3 Crowns and the farm-house award.

OPEN; Mid-Feb - Mid-Nov. Residential & Table Licence. Pets by prior arrangement. Disabled Access. Visa/Mastercard. Children welcome

MACHYNLLETH   KING ARTHUR'S LABYRINTH

Corris, Machynlleth, SY20 9RF Tel: 01654 761584 Fax: 01654 761575

King Arthur's Labyrinth is a fairly recent visitor attraction which has delighted people since it opened in 1994. An underground boat takes visitors deep into the spectacular caverns under the Braichgoch mountain at Corris. As visitors walk through the caverns, Welsh tales of King Arthur are told with tableaux and stunning sound and light effects. The journey ends with a return trip along the beautiful subterranean river into the grounds of the Corris Craft Centre.

This exciting centre is the starting point for King Arthur's Labyrinth and home to six craft workshops at which visitors are invited to see at first hand the skills of the craft workers and, if they wish, to buy from the displays of woodcraft, toy making, jewellery, leather work and hand-made candles, while the Labyrinth shop provides a range of souvenirs, books and gifts on the Celtic Arthurian theme. The Crwbyr Restaurant provides full meals, teas and refreshments throughout the day.

There is also a picnic area in the gardens and an extensive children's play area. Visitors to the Labryinth are advised to wear warm clothing as the underground caverns are cool. The 45 minute tour of the caverns involves a walk of about half a mile along level gravel paths unsuitable only for the very frail. However the variety of craft shops, gardens and refreshments within the Corris Craft Centre and the stunning scenery of the Corris valley provide ample enjoyment for everyone. Group bookings are welcome.

OPEN; 10-5pm daily from April to October.

MACHYNLLETH   MEIRION MILL

Dinas Mawddwy, Nr Machynlleth SY20 9LS Tel: 01650 531311

In a wonderful setting in the mountains of the Snowdonia National Park, shopping becomes a sheer delight when you see what wonderful goods, clothing, crafts and gifts are on offer.There is a tremendous range of wool products all under one roof: traditionally woven tweeds and rugs, skirt lengths, wool jackets, knitwear from black sheep, warm jumpers, subtle blended colours in ties and hats, sheepskin slippers, hats and gloves and of course, sheepskin rugs. The shelves are full of locally produced honey and jams, slate gifts, Celtic jewellery, lovespoons, jumping sheep and small items for children to collect. They also stock Portmeirion Pottery. Meirion Mill has everything going for it; parking couldn't be simpler nor the access easier.

The Old Station Coffee Shop has a restaurant licence and serves delicious home-cooked fare. There is a level entrance to the shop and all areas are accessible by wheelchair. You will find Meirion Mill situated on the Powys/Gwynedd border at the southern end of the National Park. The Mill site was originally the terminus for the old Mawddwy railway which ran for six miles down the valley to join the main railway at Cemmaes Road. The double arched Pack Horse Bridge spans the RiverDyfi next to the entrance gate. Heavily laden donkeys were led across this narrow bridge transporting bolts of flannel to be sold over the border. OPEN: Daily early March to late November. Mon-Sat 10am-5pm. Sun: 10.30am-5pm. Times do vary in the early and late season. Current times can be obtained by phoning 01650 531311. Normally closed during winter months. Amex/Visa/Access/Mastercard/Delta/Switch. Childrens Play Area. Picnic area. Dogs not allowed in play area, shop or coffee shop.

CENARTH   THE NATIONAL CORACLE CENTRE

Cenarth Falls, Newcastle Emlyn

NEWCASTLE
EMLYN SA389JL Tel: 01239 710980

Rescued from decay by Mr and Mrs Martin Fowler in 1983, Cenarth Mill was re-roofed in 1991 and the National Coracle Centre stands in the grounds of the 17th century flour mill where the mill pig stys and workshops once were. The mill is included in your visit here. An organised tour of the Centre takes you back to one of the earliest forms of transport, and presents a unique display of Coracles from many parts of the world. As well as nine varieties of Welsh Coracle and those from other British rivers, you can see examples from Iraq, Vietnam, India and North America. The workshop is an important part of the Centre and the ancient craft of Coracle making is displayed here. Coracles can be seen on the river during the summer holidays, and trips in one can sometimes be arranged. Viewing areas and pathways allow easy access for disabled people and provide wonderful views of the falls, salmon leap and 200 year old bridge. **OPEN;** Easter-October Sunday to Friday 10.30am-5.30pm and other times by appointment. Gift Shop. Tea rooms.

PORT DINORWIC
Y FELINHELI   THE GREENWOOD CENTRE
Tel: 01248 671493 Fax: 01248 670069

Indoors and outdoors the Award Winning Greenwood Centre is all about discovering the fascinating World of Trees. It is an enjoyable and educational experience for all ages. You can find out how trees work, how they clean the air, visit the Rainforest and hear its sounds, see a banana plant and find stick insects. Try out your sense of smell at the scent boxes and see if you can identify the fragrances. Find out about the history of forestry in Wales. Explore the rhododendron maze, tree nursery, root circle. See the wildlife pond and make friends with the rabbits in pets corner, and in the main holiday season, watch forest craft demonstrations and try out a Welsh Longbow from May to September.Enjoy a picnic outdoors or sample some of the tasty snacks and light lunches in the Tea Room. OPEN; Daily 10am-5.30pm March to October inclusive. Winter visits by arrangement. Dogs on leads welcome. Free car & coach park. Disabled and baby changing facilities.

PORTMEIRIO
Gwynedd LL48 6ET Tel: 01766 770228

One single word, Portmeirion, conjures up a magical place, somewhere that everyone should visit at least once in a lifetime. It is the realisation of a dream by its creator Sir Clough Williams-Ellis who had long nurtured the idea of one day building his own ideal village on some romantic coast. Eventually he was offered the Aber la peninsula, only five miles from his ancestral home-a perfect place to prove that the development of a naturally beautiful site need not necessarily lead to its defilement. Work began when he ws 42 in 1925 and when Sir Clough died in 1978 at the age of 95 he was content in the knowledge that his dream had become a reality. For people like myself the sheer beauty, colour and charm of Portmeirion is enough to make me want to just stand and stare. There are different vistas at every turn and each one you think cannot be more beautiful than the last, but it always is. Portmeirion is a world apart and you may come here as a day visitor - not the best way because you cannot see and absorb all it has to offer. Portmeirion has six different shops including the Seconds Warehouse, which is the only place in Wales selling second quality Portmeirion Pottery, designed by Susan Williams-Ellis. The Ship Shop sells best quality Portmeirion Pottery plus a wide range of design led gifts for all ages. There is also a Papur a Phensal for cards, the Golden Dragon bookshop, and Pot Jam selling Portmeirion preserves and confectionery. The Six of One shop specialises in The Prisoner TV series. The village has a licensed self-service restaurant with a pleasant terrace for meals outside. There is an ice-cream parlour and several ice-cream kiosks. The Hotel restaurant on the quayside welcomes non-residents and provides reasonably priced two and three course lunches.

RHAYADER WELSH ROYAL CRYSTA

5 Brynberth, Rhayader LD6 5EN Tel: 01597 811005

Winner of Wales Tourism Awards 1995 'Highly Commended' Welsh Royal Crystal is the Principality's own complete manufacturer of hand-crafted lead crystal products in tableware,stemware, presentation trophies and gift items. All production processes are undertaken on the one manufacturing site situated in Rhayader in the heartlands of Wales. Welsh Royal Crystal melts glass containing a lead content in excess of 30% (known as Full Lead Crystal) which is considered to be the best quality glass from which fine quality crystal glass products are made - weight and feel, definition of cutting and polishing brilliance are very much enhanced. Welsh Royal Crystal's range of products is traditional and the decoration combines classic florals (intaglio) with straight diamond cuts. A unique range of Celtic themes reflecting the design images of the Welsh Celtic heritage has been successfully introduced. The design and supply of presentation trophies and gifts is an expanding area of the Company's business. Welsh Royal Crystal can number within its customer portfolio important corporate customers in Wales and is pleased to be associated with the Cardiff Singer of the World Competition sponsored by British Petroleum, the Young Welsh Singer Competition sponsored by the Midland Bank and more recently, the Welsh Women of the Year sponsored by the Western Mail and HTV. In addition to supplying our fine Welsh crystal to over 100 retail accounts in Wales, sales are increasing across the borders of the Principality into England, Scotland, Saudi Arabia, North America, Australia and Canada. Time spent in theWelsh Royal Crystal Visitor Centre provides an opportunity to see the WELSH MASTERS OF FIRE AND GLASS handcraft full lead crystal products to the finest quality. A visit to the Welsh Crystal Shop presents an enviable opportunity to purchase quality crystal manufactured in Wales, whether it be a valuable centre piece or small gift item.

OPEN; All year round 9am-12.30pm and 1.30-4.30pm. Glass blowing demonstrations may not be available on some weekdays, Saturdays and Sundays.

MUMBLES   THE LOVESPOON GALLERY

492 Mumbles Road, Mumbles, Swansea SA348X Tel: 01792 360132.

You will find this unique gallery located on the right opposite the 1st Car Park just before the mini-roundabout in Mumbles. Do not miss the opportunity of visiting The Lovespoon Gallery. It is the world's first gallery devoted entirely to Welsh Lovespoons. Until you have seen the astonishing range you will have no idea that there are literally hundreds of designs made by some of the very best carvers in Wales. The Lovespoon has a well earned reputation for having only genuine carved Lovespoons and is known world wide. A Lovespoon makes a wonderful gift for special occasions like weddings, anniversaries christenings, birthdays and any important event. For 400 years this has been a Welsh tradition which is another good reason for buying one. When you examine the spoons you will see what wonderful artistry is employed when they are carved. They are certainly collectors' items.

OPEN: 10am-6pm Sunday opening in August. Children welcome. Credit cards: Visa.Mastercard. Suitable for the disabled, just one small step. Assistance given. Amex and Diners.

SCOTLAND

ABERDEEN
STORYBOOK GLEN, Maryculter. Tel: 01224 732941.
Children will be in their element in this 28 acre children's fantasy land. There are nursery rhyme and fairytale characters everywhere. Adults will also enjoy the chance to become children again. A delightful area surrounded by trees, flowers and waterfalls. Open 1st Mar-31st Oct, daily 10-6pm. Nov-end Feb, Sat and Sun only 11-4pm.

BALLETER
DEE VALLEY CONFECTIONERS, Station Square. Tel: 013397 55499.
Delicious traditional hand-made sweets. Free viewing area. Open: Sweet Factory, all year Mon-Thurs 9-5.30pm. Shop open daily 9am-9pm.

BANCHORY
CRATHES CASTLE. Scottish National Trust. Tel: 01330 844525.
Beautiful Castle and Gardens with a Castle Visitor Centre, adventure playground, restaurant and shop. You may also like to purchase some plants from the plant sales, to transform your garden. Open: all year round daily 9.30-sunset.

DUFFTOWN
THE GLENFIDDICH DISTILLERY.
A good point at which to start of the Malt Whiskey Trail which stretches for 70 miles and takes in seven distilleries and the Speyside Cooperage at Craigellachie. All the distilleries have gift shops, audio-visual, exhibitions and picnic areas, some have tea rooms. A wonderful experience to view whiskey in the making. Make sure there is someone to do just the driving.

GALSTON
LOUDOUN CASTLE PARK. Tel: 01563 822296.
This wonderful visitor attraction is set in the most magnificent parkland and woods. The imposing castle ruin is surrounded by farm livestock, aviary, playgrounds, adventure playground, and picnic area. There is also a Coach House restaurant and gift shop for those important souvenirs. It holds Britain's largest carousel. Open: from Easter daily 10.00-dusk.

GRETNA GREEN
THE FINE ARTS GALLERY, Headless Cross. Tel: 01461 338066.
Beautiful ceramics figurines all hand painted. Daily painting demonstrations throughout the summer. Open: daily.

HUNTLY
LEITH HALL, Kennethmont. Scottish National Trust. Tel: 01466 831216.
A 17th century mansion house. Inside it contains a military collection belonging to the Leith family. Wonderful gardens, picnic area tea room and disabled toilet. Open: House: 14th Apr-1st Oct daily 1.30pm-5.30pm (last admission 4.45pm). Garden and grounds: all year daily 9.30-sunset.

IRVINE

SCOTTISH MARITIME MUSEUM. Tel: 01294 275059.

Here you can see quite a unique collection of machinery, craft and buildings all from the 19th century. For visitors there is 'hands on' where you are encouraged to climb aboard the different vessels including the world's oldest clipper ship the 'Carrick'. In the main hall is an exhibition. Open: 1st Apr-31st Oct 10-5pm.

KILLIN

THE BREADALBANE FOLKLORE CENTRE. TEL: 01567 820254.

In the heart of Scottish mountain territory is the beautiful village of Killin, where legend has told of giants, saints, sinners, soothsayers spirits and warrior clans populated the area. A Celtic monk, Saint Fillan an early Christian missionary and Irish prince, settled here by the roaring waters of the Falls of Dochart, where he performed his wonders. Robert the Bruce gave credit to the Saint for the victory at Bannockburn, and stones which he blessed are said to heal different parts of the body. All this can be seen in the Centre, along with videos and artefacts from the past and wonderful stories from Gaelic folk tradition. A restored water wheel, Tourist Information Centre and a souvenir shop. Open: Mar-Jun and Sept-Oct daily 10-5pm. Jul-Aug daily 9-6pm. Nov-Dec and Feb weekends only 10-4pm. Closed January.

KILMARNOCK

DEAN CASTLE AND COUNTRY PARK. TEL: 01563 522702/534580.

The Castle is set in some 200 acres and is surrounded by woodland with rivers, nature trail, children's corner, picnic areas adventure playground, a riding centre and tea room. The Castle has the most fascinating array of medieval arms, armour, tapestries, musical instruments from an early European era, and a display of manuscripts belonging to Robert Burns. Open: all year round. Daily 12 noon-5pm.

MAYBOLE

CULZEAN CASTLE AND COUNTRY PARK. National Trust of Scotland. Tel: 01655 760274/760269.

The Castle was designed by Robert Adam in 1777, and is magnificently furnished. A special presentation explains General Eisenhower's part in European History. Not so long ago the Country Park was named as the 'most beautiful country park in Britain'. It has a deer park, swan pond, walled garden, aviary, and a ranger service with guided walks. Restaurant and tea room. Open: all year.

MOFFAT

THE MOFFAT POTTERY, Gerry Lyons, 20 High Street. Tel: 01683 220793.

See the 'Singing Potter' at his wheel and listen to the fine selection of songs from the operas. Once of the Scottish Opera Company, he now spends his time crafting beautiful item from clay. Take your time and peruse the individual designs in the studio. Open: Mon-Sat 9.00-5pm.

MOTHERWELL

BARON'S HAUGH NATURE RESERVE. RSPB. Adele Street. Tel: 0131 5573136.

The marsh meadowland has been flooded to give ideal conditions and habitat for the many species of birds. Here you can quietly watch the different wildlife from special hides which look out over the lake. A visit here will be an enchanting experience whether you are an expert bird watcher or just a beginner. The disabled have not been forgotten and certain parts of the reserve are accessible for wheelchair users. Also available are expert staff to offer help and information. A super day out.

ORKNEY

The are 18 inhabited islands, and on all of them history abounds. There are many Stone Age tombs where the communities buried their dead. There are underground earth houses where Iron Age families lived. The Farm and Folk Museum, here you can see the evolution of farm buildings with traditional breeds of sheep and poultry. The Wireless Museum has exhibits of early crystal sets to the present day radio, and much more. In 1850 a Stone Age Mainland village was discovered having been buried by sand for over 4000 years, a wonderful piece of history.

SKARES

DOON VALLEY RARE BREEDS CENTRE. Tel: 01290 421553.
With over 60 different breeds of waterfowl, poultry and animals to see, this is a wonderful experience and very educational too. Tea room and car park. Open: 1st mar-31 Nov. Daily 10-6pm. Dec-Feb by appointment only.

Congleton	466	Ditchling	352
Coniston	468	Doccombe	272
Cookham	373	Docklands	380
Copinsay	504	Doncaster	489
Corfe	322	Dorchester	319 & 371
Cotswolds	369	Dornie	506
Coventry	436	Dovedale	436
Covent Gardens	379	Dover	398
Cowdrey	348	Drewsteignton	271
Cranborne	324	Drumnadrochit	505
Cranborne Chase	322	Dulverton	263
Crawley	351	Dunbar	501
Crewkerne	264	Dundee	506
Crick	450	Dunsford	272
Cricklade	332	Dunstable	374
Cromer	403	Dunster	264
Cuckfield	351	Durham	490
Culborn	263	Durlston	322
		Duxford	402

D

Danebury	338	**E**	
Darlington	490	Eardisland	434
Dartmeet	273	Eastbourne	354
Dartmoor	267	East Bergholt	400 & 406
Dartmouth	290	East Grinstead	350
Daventry	445	East Head	347
Dawlish	270	East Hendred	371
Deal	398	East Knoyle	325
Dedham	400	East Linton	506
Derby	450	East Looe	283
Devizes	329	East Manley	274

Godney	263	Hawkhurst	357
Goodison	466	Haworth	483
Goring	371	Haywards Heath	351
Gorran Churchtown	281	Helensburgh	501
Gosport	344	Helston	279
Goudhurst	358	Henley-on-Thames	371
Grafton Underwood	445	Hereford	433
Granchester	401	Hernhill	397
Grasmere	468	Hickstead	352
Great Charfield	334	Highclare	338
Great Hampden	374	High Wycombe	374
Great Tew	371	Hindhead	378
Great Torrington	274	Hinton Ampner	336
Greenwich	379	Hixton	402
Gretna Green	508	Hodnet	443
Guildford	377	Hogs Back	377
		Holcombe Rogus	274
		Holdenby	444
H		Holne	273
Hackington	397	Holsworthy	274
Hadleigh	400	Holyhead	420
Hambledon	344	Hook Norton	372
Handcross	351	Horncastle	451
Hanley	437	Horning	404
Harbledown	397	Horsham	351
Hardham	349	Hove	352
Harrogate	484	Hoveton	405
Hartland	276	Huddersfield	483
Harwich	400	Humberside	489
Hastings	355	Huntingdon	402
Hatherleigh	274	Hythe	398
Hawkeridge	334		

Lerwick	504	Lyme Regis	315
Lesnewth	277	Lymington	341
Letchworth	375	Lyndhurst	342
Lewes	354	Lyne Down	433
Leyburn	488	Lynmouth	275
Lilleshall	438	Lynton	275
Lindfield	352		
Lindisfarne	489	**M**	
Littlehampton	350	Machynlleth	421
Little Stretton	440	Maidenhead	373
Littleton	336	Malmesbury	332
Liverpool	466	Manaccan	279
Llandeilo	423	Manaton	272
Llandudno	420	Manchester	467
Llandudno Junction	420	Marazion	279
Llangollen	423	Margate	398
Llanrhaedr-ym-Mochnant	442	Market Bosworth	446
London Colney	376	Market Deeping	451
Longnor	437	Market Drayton	443
Longton	437	Market Harborough	446
Lostwithiel	282	Market Rasen	451
Louth	451	Marlborough	330
Lower Beeding	351	Marlow	374
Lubenham	447	Marsden	490
Ludgershall	330	Marshfield	258
Ludlow	440	Mary Tavy	271
Lulworth Cove	322	Matlock	450
Lundy Island	275	Melbourn	402
Lutterworth	446	Melcombe Bingham	322
Lybster	505	Mells	260
Lydford	271	Melton Mowbray	447

Otley	486	Port Isaac	277
Ottery St Mary	268	Portesham	317
Oundle	445	Porthcurno	278
Overwallop	339	Porthmadog	422
Oxford	371	Portland	318
		Portmeirion	422
P		Portpatrick	502
Padstow	277	Portsmouth	344
Paignton	269	Postbridge	272
Parracombe	275	Poundsgate	273
Paul	278	Powerstock	317
Pembridge	434	Preston	467
Penally	277	Princetown	272
Penrith	469	Puddletown	322
Pentargen	277	Pulborough	349
Penzance	279	Purbeck	322
Perranorworthal	280	Purse Caundle	321
Perranporth	278	Puttey	433
Pershore	434	Pycombe	532
Perth	506		
Petersfield	337	**R**	
Petworth	348	Radstock	258
Pewsey	329	Redruth	280
Pickering	487	Ramsgate	398
Piddlehinton	322	Ringwood	340
Piddletrenthide	322	Ripon	484
Pilsdon Pen	316	Robin Hood's Bay	483
Plymouth	266	Rochester	399
Polperro	283	Rock	277
Poole	315	Rockingham	445
Porchester	344	Rode	261

Romney Marsh	398	Selkirk	507
Romsey	342	Selsey	347
Ross-on-Wye	433	Sennen	278
Royal Forest of Dean	370	Shaftsbury	321
Royal Lemington Spa	435	Shaldon	270
Royal Tunbridge Wells	398	Sheepwash	274
Runnymede	377	Sheffield	483
Rutland	447	Sherborne	320
Rydal	468	Sheringham	404
Rye	356	Shetland	502
Rye Foreign	356	Shifnal	438
		Shilston	271
S		Shipston-on-Stour	435
Salcombe	270	Shrewsbury	441
Sale	404	Shugborough	437
Salisbury	327	Sidmouth	268
Salisbury Plain	326	Silsoe	375
Sandringham	404	Sissinghurst	357 & 398
Sandwich	398	Sixpenny Handley	324
Saunton	275	Skye	502
Sawrey	468	Sleaford	451
Saxmundham	406	Slimbridge	370
Saxtead	406	Slindon	349
Sayers Common	352	Slough	373
Scapa Flow	504	Snape	406
Scarborough	483	South Kensington	378
Scilly Isles	279	South Molton	275
Seaton	268	South Shields	490
Seatown	316	South Thoresby	451
Selborne	337	Southbourne	322
Selby	484	Southampton	342

Southsea	344	Stoke Gregory		260
Southwell	449	Stoke Poges		374
Southwold	406	Stoke-in-Teignhead		270
Speyside	502	Stoke-on-Trent		438
Spitalfield	379	Stonehaven		501
St Abbs	504	Stonehenge		328
St Albans	376	Stopham		349
St Austell	281	Stourhead	261 &	325
St Germans	282	Stourpaine		321
St Ives	278	Stow-cum-Quy		401
St Just	278	Strand		380
St Just-in-Roseland	280	Stratford-Upon-Avon		435
St Kevern	279	Stratton		276
St Leonards	355	Strood		399
St Levan	278	Studland		322
St Margaret's Bay	398	Swaffham		404
St Mawes	280	Swallowcliffe		324
St Winnow	282	Swanage		322
Staithes	483	Swansea		419
Staffa	506	Swaston		402
Stafford	436	Swindon		331
Stamford	450	Symonds Yat		433
Stanton	371			
Steep	337	**T**		
Stenness	504	Tangmere		347
Stirling	506	Taplow		373
Stockridge	339	Tarbolton		507
Stocksfield	490	Taunton		264
Stogumber	265	Tavistock		271
Stoke	437	Teffont Evias		325
Stoke Bruerne	444	Teffont Magna		325

Westhay	262	Windsor	372
West Cliff	398	Wing	447
West Dean	347	Winsford	264
West Firle	353	Wingham	398
West Grinstead	350	Winterbourne	260
West Kennet	331	Witney	372
West Looe	283	Woburn	375
West Stoke	346	Wolverhampton	436
West Wittering	347	Wolverton	374
Westminster	380	Woodbridge	406
Weston-Super-Mare	259	Woodhall Spa	451
Weston-under-Lizard	438	Wootton	444
Weymouth	318	Woolacombe	275
Wheelock	466	Worcester	434
Whipsnade Heath	375	Wroxham	405
Whitby	483	Wylam	490
Whitchurch	338 & 443	Wylye	326
Whitchurch Canonicorum	316		
Whiteley	377	**Y**	
Whitstable	398	Yelverton	267
Whittington	442	Yeovil	261 & 264
Widecombe-in-the-Moor	273	York	484
Willoughbridge	438		
Wilmcote	435	**Z**	
Wilmington	353	Zennor	278
Wilton	326		
Wimbledon	378		
Wimborne Minster	322		
Wimborne St Giles	322		
Winchelsea	356		
Winchester	355		

ALLERGY

The Institute of Allergy Therapists, maintains a Register of Practitioners specialising in Allergy Diagnosis and Treatment. For Information and local lists of therapists, please write , telephone or fax 01974 241376. Institute of Allergy Therapists, Llangwyryfon, Aberystwyth, Dyfed SY23 4EY.

ALEXANDER TECHNIQUE

THE PROFESSIONAL ASSOCIATION OF ALEXANDER TEACHERS: practices throughout Britain, private lessons, introductory courses etc. Four year examined training course in Birmingham. Contact the secretary on (0120) 426 2108.

AROMATHERAPY

Aromatherapy Trade Council. The ATC enforces a code of practise to raise standards of safety and Quality in Aromatherapy Products. Send sae for list of members:
The ATC, PO Box 52, Market Harborough, Leicester LE16 8ZX.

International Society of Professional Aromatherapists, ISPA House, 82 Ashby Road, Hinckley, Leicestershire LE10 1SN. Tel: (01455) 637987. The largest Aromatherapy association, with professional and student membership, and accredited schools of high standard throughout the UK. S.A.E. for information. Local lists and hotline service F.O.C. Journals and national register at cost.

The Register of Qualified Aromatherapists, PO Box 6941, London N8 9HF.   (0181) 341 2958.

The Aromatherapy Organisations Council, is the UK governing body for aromatherapy, representing 13 professional associations and 85 training establishments. Professionally qualified romatherapists in complementary medicine should have trained to AOC standards implemented in 1994.
For General Information Booklet, send A5 SAE to: The Secretary, 3 Latymer Close, Braybrooke, Market Harborough, Leicester LE16 8LN.

ARTHRITIS RELIEF

The Arthritic Association, (Registered Charity No. 292569) First Floor Suite, 2 Hyde Gardens, Eastbourne, BN21 4P (0171) 491 0233. Provides Dietary Guidance with homoeopathic and herbal treatment to help relieve those suffering from arthritis and rheumatism

BACH FLOWER REMEDIES

The Dr. Edward Bach Foundation, Mount Vernon, Sotwell, Wallingford, Oxon, OX10 0PZ. Tel:(01491) 834678. Professional register of fully qualified therapists trained at the Bach Centre. Details of local practitioners on request.

CHIROPRACTIC

The British Chiropractic Association, 29 Whitley Street, Reading RG2 0E9. Tel: (01734) 757557. It represents the majority of chiropractors in Britain. Members registered with the BCA have completed a minimum of four years' full-time training. They have graduated with the following qualifications: DC.B App Sc (Chiro), Bsc Chiropractic. British Association for Applied Chiropractic, The Old Post Office, Stratton, Audley, Near Bicester, Oxon OX6 9BA. Tel: (01869) 277111.

Mc Timoney Chiropractic Association, 21 High Street, Eynaham, Oxon, OX8 1HE, Tel: 01865 880974. Please send large S.A.E. for information pack.

The Scottish Chiropractic Association, 30 Raeburn Place, Edinburgh, EH12 5NX. The SCA represents the majority of chiropractors in Scotland. Members registered with the SCA complete a minimum of four years' full time training and graduate with DC, BAppSC(Chiro) or BSc(Chiro)_

COLONIC HYDROTHERAPY

Colonic International Association (HH), 16 Englands Lane, London NW3 4TG.

GENERAL

HEALTH PRACTITIONERS ASSOCIATION, 3 Stoneleigh Drive,
Carterton, Oxford, OX18 1EE. Tel:(01933) 845805/ (01993)842422. Fax: 0181 313 1009. A multi-disiplinary organisation founded in 1935 to represent professional interests and to set standards of training and education for the benefit of patient and practitioner.

HEALING

World Federation of Healing, The membership Secretary, Mrs Doris Jones, (HH) 10 Gallards Close, London Road, Southborough, Tunbridge Wells, Kent TN4 0NB. Tel: (01892) 514342. This is the federation for all therapists in the field of healing.

The British Alliance of Healing Associations, Member of the Confederation of Healing Organisations. For membership or Healer in your area contact: Mr Wallace on (01502) 742224 or (01372) 733241..

International Self-Realization Healing Association (ISRHA), 1 Hamlyn Road, Glastonbury, Somerset BA6 8HS, UK. Healer and Progressive Counsellor referral service in the UK and abroad. Also membership details and information on professional training courses. Please send an sae for further information or Tel: (01458) 831353 or Fax: (01458) 835148.

HERBALISTS

The General Council and Register of Consultant Herbalists Diploma courses leading to professional registration in Herbal Medecine-Homoeopathy. Initial home study followed by Intensive clinical training. 'Pay as you learn' scheme available. Modular study designed to suit a wide variety of student proficiencies. For a prospectus please send 6 1st class stamps to: The Registrar, GCRCH, PO Box 10388, London N16 9BQ. Telephone 0171 503 7980.

HOLISTIC MASSAGE

The Massage Training Institute, 24 Highbury Grove, London N5 2DQ. High quality professional training in Holistic Massage. National Register of M.T.I. Practitioners (ethical and insured).

HOMOEOPATHY

The Homoeopathic Society, Hahnemann House, 2 Powis Place, London, WC1n 3HT. Tel: 0171 837 9469. Send for a free copy of the leading magazine "Health and Homoeopathy", an information pack on how to obtain treatment on the NHS and a list of Homoeopathic doctors. Please quote ref HH95/96.

The Society of Homoeopaths. RSHom or FSHom; 500 practitioners; member of CCAM. For register and information leaflet *Homoeopathy Simply Explained*, send large sae to 2 Artizan Road, Northampton, NN14HU (Tel: 01604 21400).

The United Kingdom Homoeopathic Medical Association, Administration Office, 6 Livingstone Road, Gravesend, Kent DA12 5DZ. Tel & Fax 01474 560 336. "Qualified Homoeopaths (MHMA) bound by a code of ethics, covered by professional indemnity insurance. Register on request."

HYPNOTHERAPY

Association of Professional Therapists (APT) 57 The Spinney, Sidcup, Kent, DA14 5NE. Tel: 0181 308 0249. Nationwide register of hypnotherapists with high standards of training and ethics.

British Council of Hypnotist Examiner. Established 1982. Certified Caring Practitioners. Please ring 01723 585960 or Fax 01723 585959 for practitioners in your area.

Central Register of Advanced Hypnotherapists, 28 Finsbury Park Road, London, N4 2JX.(0171) 359 6991. Membership by full practical and theoretical training, postgraduate clinical supervision and continuing professional education programs. Send an sae for explanatory leaflets and details of your local therapist(s).

For Qualified Hypnotherapists contact British Council of Hypnotist Examiners. Telephone 01723 585960. BCHE - Lambourn Court, look under stress Management heading for details.

The National Association of Counsellors, Hypnotherapists and Psychotherapists. For information and local list of therapists, please write (SAE), Telephone or Fax: 01974 241 376. NACHP, Flynnonwen, Llangwyryfon, Aberystwyth, Dyfed, SY23 4EY.

The Academy of Curitive Hypnotherapists Limited. For a list of Practitioners in your area or details of therapist training (student to advanced diploma - recognised qualifications) and weekend workshops, please contact administrative office: 75 Spring Bank, Stalybridge, SK15 2EQ. Telephone and Fax: 0161 303 371.

IRIDOLOGY

Guild of Naturopathic Iridologists, 94 Grovener Road, London SW1V 3LF Tel. (0171) 834 3579. Affiliated to Holistic Health College & ICM Qualified & experienced Irodologists & Naturopathic Practitioners. Code of ethics. Professional Insurance. SAE for register, £1.50 in stamps for courses.

KINESIOLOGY

The Kinesiology Federation PO Box 7891, London Sw19 1ZB - Tel/Fax 0181 545 0255. Kinesiology promotes optimum physical, emotional and spiritual health, restoring balance to the subtle energy channels and stimulating the body's natural healing process.

Association of Systematic Kinesiology 39 Browns Road, Surbiton, Surrey KTS 8ST. Applied Kinesiology uses gentle muscle testing to discover sub-clinical functional imbalances, massage, diet, lifestyle changes to correct them, relieving pain, stress, enhancing health and well being.

NUMEROLOGY

Association Internationale de Numerologistes 5 Ayot House, Ayot St. Lawrence, Welwyn, Herts AL6 9BP. To receive a list of qualified members and information on courses please send a stamped address envelope to the above address.

NUTRITIONAL THERAPY

Society for the Promotion of Nutritional Therapy (SPNT), PO Box 47, Heathfield, East Sussex TN21 8ZX. Tel: 01435 867007. Represents the majority of nutritional therapists in the UK. Send sae + £1 for information and a list of your nearest qualified registered practitioners. SPNT also has lay and student members. Services for members include journal and Independent advice on training.

The Institute for Optimum Nutrition, educational trust, Blades Court, Deodar Road, London SW15 2NU Tel:(0181) 877 9993. ION an independent charity, exists to help you achieve optimum health. ION offer short courses, homestudy courses, books, a magazine, consultations - and a Nutrition Consultants Diploma Course.

Nutrition Consultants Association.
Professionally qualified, Indemnified and bound by stringent Codes of Ethics and practice. Director of practitioners (£2.00) NCA (HH), 34 Wadham Road, London SW15 2LR.

OSTEOPATHY
Natural Therapeutic Osteopathic Society and Register - 14 Marford Road, Wheathampstead, Herts, AL4 8AS. Tel: (01582) 833950. Send a large sae for a register of members who use letter DO and MNTOS.

PALMISTRY COUNSELLORS
Association of Palmistry Counsellors, Private/Postal readings, Party Bookings, Tuition, Talks. SAE to Green-Havens, 71 Broad Street, Chesham, Bucks, HP2 3EA   Ph: 01494 792381

POLARITY TRAINING
The Federation of Polarity Training is an organisation providing Information on polarity training in the UK and a register of qualified practitioners. Send s.a.e. to 7 Nunney Close, Cheltenham, Glos. GL51 0TU.

RADIONICS
The Radionic Association - Est 1943. Reg. member CHO & BCMA. Incorporates The School of Radionics for training in Holistic Distant Healing. Send large s.a.e. + £1 for practitioners list to the secretary, Baerlein House, Goose Green, Deddington, Oxon. OX15 0SZ. Tel/Fax 01869 338852.

REBIRTHING
British Rebirth Society, 5 Manor Road, Catcott, Bridgwater, Somerset TA7 9HT. Tel: (01278) 722536. Send an sae for register of qualified practitioners and training courses.

REFLEXOLOGY
Association of Reflexologists, 27 Old Gloucester Street, London WC1 3XX. Tel: 0990 673320. Reflexology, for reliable information about: Registered Professional Practitioners; Accredited Training Courses; Membership - including quarterly journals, seminars and support groups; speakers and presenters. Please send a 9" x 7" stamped addressed envelope to the above address.

The Scottish Institute of Reflexology
Looking for a qualified Reflexologist, look no further. The Scottish Institute of Reflexology. For details of membership list contact the Secretary on (01292) 442923

International Institute of Reflexology
For a fully trained, insured, professional practitioner in reflexology in your area, with the use of the letters I.I.R.Dip or M.I.I.R regd., please contact LLR (UK) Tel:(01732) 350629.

The British Reflexology Association
Monks Orchard, Whitbourne, Worcester, WR6 5RB. Tel/Fax. 01886 821207. Register of members(£1.50). Details of training courses, books, charts (s.a.e. required). Reflexologists' Society. Founded in 1984 c/o Coed Ely Sub P.O. Elwyn Street, Tonyrefail, Mid Glamorgan CF39 8BL. Tel: 01 443 675557. A register of qualified and experienced Reflexology Practitioners is maintained. All practitioners operate under a Code of Practise with insurance. Please send SAE for Professional Practitioners or a list of affiliated schools who meet our high standards .

SHIATSU
The Shiatsu Society, 5 Foxcote, Wokingham, Berkshire RG11 3PG. Tel: (01734) 730836. Fax: (01734) 732752. The umbrella organisation for all Shiatsu in the UK, Providing a Quarterly newsletter and overseeing the Professional Register of Shiatsu Therapists. Registered practitioners use initials MRSS and have trained at an approved school.

The European Shiatsu Network, Highbanks, Lockeridge, Marlborough, Wiltshire, SN8 4EQ. Tel: (01672) 861362.
Co-ordinates Comprehensive training courses throughout Europe leading to professional Shiatsu qualifications.

STRESS MANAGEMENT
Lambourn Court Stress Management Consultants. Stress, Emotional and Personal Development problems? we can help you develop effective personal programmes, to improve your life and remove those unwanted barriers. A register of Nationally licensed consultants can be obtained from Lambourn Court, PO Box 328, Huddersfield, HD4 5YP or phone 01484 461 462.

SUGARING
The Association of Professional Sugaring, Queen Anne House, Charlotte Street, Bath, Avon BA1 2NE Tel: 0181 224 9063. Send SAE for list of Practitioners.

YOGA THERAPY
Yoga Biomedical Trust. Yoga Therapy for low back pain, asthma, ME and other stress-related conditions; pregnancy & child birth. Yoga Therapy Centre, 60 Great Ormond Street, London WC1. Tel: 0171 833 7267.

The Kingsley Company

Freepost (PY2100)
The Hoe, Plymouth, Devon PL1 3BR
Tel: 01752 600929 Fax: 01752 600632

Dear Reader,

I hope you have enjoyed my choice of places of all kinds - I have certainly enjoyed researching them in order to write this book.

It would make the next edition much easier if you would help by suggesting places that could be included and your comments on any establishment or attraction you have visited, would be much appreciated.

    I enjoy corresponding with my readers and look forward to hearing from you.

Yours sincerely,

Joy David

Joy David
Editor

READERS COMMENTS

Please use this page to tell us about HOTELS, RESTAURANTS etc and PLACES OF INTEREST that have appealed to you especially. We will pass on your approval where it is merited and equally report back to the venue any complaints. We hope the latter will be few and far between.

We would also welcome your comments on the specialist chapters included in this publication and any suggestions you might have that you feel would improve future editions.

Please post to:
Kingsley Media, FREEPOST (PY2100)
The Hoe, PLYMOUTH, Devon, PL1 3BR

Name of Establishment:

Address:

Comments:

Your Name: (Block Caps Please)

Address:

HEALTHY OPTIONS

* Now an established publication in the Alternative Health Market.

* The 1998 edition will facilitate exposure to an ever increasing consumer interest in your trade.

* The 1998 edition will provide exposure for a full year.

* The 1998 edition will feature even more subjects, professionally written, to attract a vast increase in consumer use.

* The 1998 edition will facilitate exposure for a full year.

For details of the 1998 edition, simply telephone NICKY or SUE on

01752 600929 / Fax 01752 600632 *or*

Email:- kingsley@hotels.u-net.com
alternatively write to
Kingsley Media Ltd, Freepost PY2100,
The Hoe, Plymouth, PL1 3BR.

ACT NOW TO AVOID DISAPPOINTMENT
Copy Date 31/10/97

NOTES

NOTES

NOTES

NOTES

NOTES

NOTES

NOTES

NOTES